W9-BIB-944

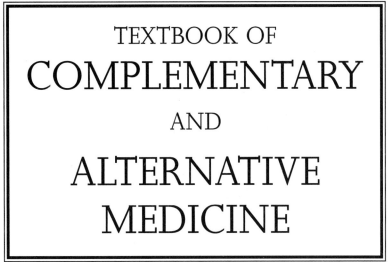

TEXTBOOK OF
COMPLEMENTARY
AND
ALTERNATIVE
MEDICINE

TEXTBOOK OF
COMPLEMENTARY
AND
ALTERNATIVE
MEDICINE

Edited by

Chun-Su Yuan, MD, PhD

Director
Tang Center for Herbal Medicine Research
University of Chicago Pritzker School of Medicine, Illinois

and

Eric J. Bieber, MD

Chairman
Department of Obstetrics and Gynecology
Geisinger Medical Center, Pennsylvania

The Parthenon Publishing Group
International Publishers in Medicine, Science & Technology

A CRC PRESS COMPANY
BOCA RATON   LONDON   NEW YORK   WASHINGTON, D.C.

Notice to readers: Our knowledge of medicine is constantly changing as a result of new developments. The editors, authors and publishers have taken every care to provide updated information compatible with standards at the time of publication, but cannot be responsible for any omissions or inadvertant errors, nor can they warrant that the work is accurate in every respect. The readers are advised to consult with their health-care professionals before the use of any complementary and alternative therapies.

Library of Congress Cataloging-in-Publication Data

Data available on request

Published in the USA by
The Parthenon Publishing Group
345 Park Avenue South, 10th Floor
New York, NY 10010, USA

Published in the UK and Europe by
The Parthenon Publishing Group
23–25 Blades Court, Deodar Road
London SW15 2NU, UK

Copyright © 2003
The Parthenon Publishing Group

British Library Cataloguing in Publication Data

Data available on request

No part of this book may be reproduced in any form without permission from the publisher, except for the quotation of brief passages for the purposes of review.

Typeset by Variorum Publishing, Lancaster and Rugby, UK
Printed and bound by Butler & Tanner Ltd., Frome and London, UK

ISBN 1-84214-134-1

Contents

List of contributors

Michael K. Ang-Lee, MD
Department of Anesthesia and Critical Care
University of Chicago
5841 S. Maryland Avenue, MC 4028
Chicago, IL 60637

Anoja S. Attele, DDS
Tang Center for Herbal Medicine Research
University of Chicago
5841 S. Maryland Avenue, MC 4028
Chicago, IL 60637

Han H. Aung, MD
Tang Center for Herbal Medicine Research
University of Chicago
5841 S. Maryland Avenue, MC 4028
Chicago, IL 60637

Toni Bark, MD
Department of Integrative Medicine
Good Shepherd Hospital
450 West Highway 22
Barrington, IL 60010
or
650 Vernon Ave, Glencoe, IL 60022

Patrick J. Barrett
Pritzker School of Medicine
University of Chicago
924 E. 57th Street
Chicago, IL 60637

Brent A. Bauer, MD, FACP
Complementary and Alternative Medicine
Mayo Clinic
200 First Street SW
Rochester, MN 55905

Eric J. Bieber, MD
Department of Obstetrics and Gynecology
Women's Service Line and Residency Program
Geisinger Health Systems
100 N. Academy Avenue
Danville, PA 17822

Mai T. Dang
Ben May Institute for Cancer Research
Department of Biochemistry and Molecular Biology
University of Chicago
5841 S. Maryland Avenue, MC 6027
Chicago, IL 60637

Lucy Dey, MD
Department of Anesthesia and Critical Care
University of Chicago
5841 S. Maryland Avenue, MC 4028
Chicago, IL 60637

David Dwyer
Department of Integrative Medicine
Good Shepherd Hospital
450 West Highway 22
Barrington, IL 60010

Jennifer S. Gell
Reproductive Endocrinology
Geisinger Wyoming Valley
Department of Obstetrics and Gynecology
Geisinger Health Systems
100 N. Academy Avenue
Danville, PA 17822

Jennifer L. Gnerlich
Pritzker School of Medicine
University of Chicago
924 E. 57th Street
Chicago, IL 60637

Richard A. Hiipakka, PhD
Ben May Institute for Cancer Research
Department of Biochemistry and Molecular Biology
University of Chicago
5841 S. Maryland Avenue, MC 6027
Chicago, IL 60637

Nancy A. Lass, MD, FAAP, FCP
Department of Medicine and Committee on Clinical
    Pharmacology
University of Chicago
5841 S. Maryland Avenue, MC 2115
Chicago, IL 60637

Shutsung Liao, PhD
Ben May Institute for Cancer Research
Department of Biochemistry and Molecular Biology
University of Chicago
5841 S. Maryland Avenue, MC 6027
Chicago, IL 60637

Spring A. Maleckar
Department of Anesthesia and Critical Care
and
Tang Center for Herbal Medicine Research
University of Chicago
5841 S. Maryland Avenue, MC 4028
Chicago, IL 60637

Sangeeta Mehendale, MD, PhD
Department of Anesthesia and Critical Care
and
Tang Center for Herbal Medicine Research
University of Chicago
5841 S. Maryland Avenue, MC 4028
Chicago, IL 60637

Jonathan Moss, MD, PhD
Department of Anesthesia and Critical Care
and
Institutional Review Board
University of Chicago
5841 S. Maryland Avenue, MC 4028
Chicago, IL 60637

Sarah Pessin, PhD
Department of Philosophy
California State University, Fresno
2380 E. Keats Avenue, M/S MB105
Fresno, CA 93740

Hemlata Pokharna, PhD
Department of Medicine
University of Chicago
5841 S. Maryland Avenue, MC 9025
Chicago, IL 60637

Victoria Rand, MD
Department of Medicine
University of California at San Francisco
650 29th Street
San Francisco, CA 94131

Michael F. Roizen, MD
Departments of Medicine and Anesthesia
SUNY Upstate Medical University
750 East Adams Avenue
Syracuse, NY 13210

Wallace Sampson, MD
Stanford University School of Medicine
and
The Scientific Review of Alternative Medicine
841 Santa Rita Avenue
Los Altos, CA 94022

David Schiedermayer, MD
Department of Medicine and Bioethics
Medical College of Wisconsin
Froedtert East Office Bldg., Suite 4200
9200 West Wisconsin Avenue
Milwaukee, WI 53226

Zuo-Hui Shao, MD
Section of Emergency Medicine
Department of Medicine
University of Chicago
5841 S. Maryland Avenue, MC 5068
Chicago, IL 60637

Matthew J. Sorrentino, MD, FACC
Section of Cardiology
Department of Medicine
Pritzker School of Medicine
University of Chicago
5841 S. Maryland Avenue, MC 6080
Chicago, IL 60637

Philippe O. Szapary, MD
Cardiovascular Risk Intervention Program
Division of General Internal Medicine
University of Pennsylvania School of Medicine
1222 Blockley Hall, 423 Guardian Drive
Philadelphia, PA 19104

Terry L. Vanden Hoek, MD
Section of Emergency Medicine
Department of Medicine
University of Chicago
5841 S. Maryland Avenue, MC 5068
Chicago, IL 60637

Jing-Tian Xie, MD
Tang Center for Herbal Medicine Research
University of Chicago
5841 S. Maryland Avenue, MC 4028
Chicago, IL 60637

Bob Xu, CMD, MS
Center for Holistic and Herbal Therapy
1109 Huntleigh Drive
Naperville, IL 60540

Wen Xuan, MD
Chicago First Chinese Acupuncture and Medical
  Center
Chinatown Square
2159-B S. China Place, 2nd Floor
Chicago, IL 60616

Yong Gao Wang MD, Dipl & L Ac
Department of Physiology
Loyola University of Chicago Maywood, Illinois
and
Chicago Acupuncture and Herbs Center
30 N. Michigan Avenue
Suite 523
Chicago, IL 60602

Ji An Wu, PhD
Department of Pharmaceuticals and New Technology
Pharmaceutical Products Division
Abbot Laboratories
100 Abbott Park Road
Abbott Park, IL 60064

Chun-Su Yuan, MD, PhD
Tang Center for Herbal Medicine Research
Department of Anesthesia and Critical Care
and
Committee on Clinical Pharmacology
Pritzker School of Medicine
University of Chicago
5841 S. Maryland Avenue, MC 4028
Chicago, IL 60637

Jennifer M. Zumsteg
Pritzker School of Medicine
University of Chicago
924 E. 57th Street
Chicago, IL 60637

Preface

Complementary and alternative medicine (CAM) can be defined as those health-care practices that are not currently considered an integral part of conventional therapies. People who use CAM therapies are usually seeking ways to relieve side-effects of conventional treatments and to improve their health and well-being. Although CAM therapies need to be proved safe and effective, the popularity of CAM has risen sharply over the past decade. This consumer/patient-driven movement affects all specialties of conventional medicine, influencing the decision-making and practice of allopathic physicians. However, medical professionals often do not have adequate CAM knowledge, and therefore are unable to provide informed responses to CAM questions from their patients. It is important for today's medical professionals to be familiar with the potential benefits and adverse effects of different CAM therapies; thus, patients will benefit from their doctors' awareness of CAM therapies.

This book originated from a CAM course offered to medical students at the Pritzker School of Medicine of the University of Chicago, and Chicago Annual CAM Meetings, organized by faculty members at the University of Chicago for the continuing medical education of practicing physicians. This book is designed for practicing physicians, medical students, other health-care professionals and interested individuals in general.

It is our intention to provide the most contemporary, evidence-based CAM information in this book, and the chapters are thoroughly referenced. Since CAM covers a broad range of healing therapies, approaches and systems, it is virtually impossible for any single book to cover all aspects of CAM. Section I of this book discusses some of the most commonly used CAM therapies such as herbal medicines, which may affect physicians' daily practice most. CAM therapies for common medical conditions are discussed in Section II of the book. For those CAM therapies and disorders that cannot be discussed at length, concise information is provided with a further reading list.

The work of this book was supported in part by the Tang Family Foundation, and NIH/NCCAM grants AT00381 and AT00563.

C.-S. Yuan
E. J. Bieber

Acknowledgements

The assembled text that you hold was born out of our personal hope that you the reader will gain from the experience of the many contributors. We have attempted to cover broad areas, often topics that you may or may not be familiar with, in a manner that will allow you to have a sense of the current state of the art. The broadly defined field of complementary and alternative medicine (CAM) continues to expand at an incredibly rapid pace. Given that most of us were not adequately trained in any of these areas, we conceived of this text as a primer for those looking to advance their knowledge and a reference text for those who have managed to stay current.

There are many contributors who have spent countless hours in an effort to provide you with current information. Without their input and energies this final product would not have existed. Many of these individuals are academicians who like you were not formally trained in most CAM concepts. We sincerely appreciate their time spent and their wisdom shared in bringing this project to fruition.

Many other individuals are also responsible for this text. We would like to thank David Bloomer, President of Parthenon Publishing, for his vision in seeing the value in this project and his continuing desire to disseminate medical knowledge in an effort to improve patient care and clinicians' armamentarium of knowledge and skills. Additionally, Pam Lancaster has spent countless hours with the editors in finalizing and bringing to closure the final text. Also, we would like to thank Gerald Myers for the cover design and Kate Lancaster for the original drawings.

Finally, we would like to thank our families for allowing us to take time away from our precious minutes with them. To my wife Xiaoyu, daughter Amanda, and to my parents, for your inspiration and guidance (CSY). To my wife, Edie and my children Brandon and Andrew, your untiring love has given me the support and enthusiasm to chase my dreams. To my parents George and Audrey and sister Kris, your constant encouragement to pursue knowledge in a tireless fashion and an unrelenting belief in me as a human being laid the foundation for all that I have and will accomplish (EJB).

C.-S. Yuan
E. J. Bieber

INTRODUCTION

Complementary and alternative medicine: prevalence and impact on conventional medicine

C.-S. Yuan, E. J. Bieber and M. K. Ang-Lee

Complementary and alternative medicine (CAM) means many things to many people. For practicing physicians who have in large part been trained in a Western culture, the concepts of CAM have been minimized. Unfortunately, most of us have been inadequately trained in these options and thus tend to minimize or neglect them in patient care. This text was devised not to advocate or minimize any of the plethora of options discussed but rather to open the dialogue to a more rational discussion of benefits and risks, pros and cons. Many studies are currently underway and our hope is that some of our readers will also begin (or continue) the process of performing well done prospective trials to add to the literature. Undoubtedly, many of the tenets we hold as indisputable today will be dispelled tomorrow. Unfortunately, lack of information should not cause us to also accept blindly that which should be further evaluated prior to widespread acceptance. We expect some readers to be uncomfortable with academicians and primary providers writing about the area of CAM. However, given the growing interest in complementary and alternative medicine it has become important to have reference texts that are timely and summarize in a non-polarizing manner what is and what is not presently known.

A therapy is called complementary when it is used in addition to conventional treatment, and a therapy is called alternative when it is used to replace conventional treatment. By conservative estimates, Americans spend approximately $27 billion per year on complementary and alternative therapies. More Americans visit CAM practitioners than primary care physicians[1]. The use of CAM is even more widely accepted in Europe, where, for example, herbal medicines are more frequently prescribed than conventional pharmaceuticals for certain conditions. The growing interest in CAM, however, has not been limited to patients. One study showed that over half of US physicians have tried some form of CAM[2].

Researchers, clinicians and the US government are aware of the potential benefits of CAM and the need for more research. A major step in meeting this need was the establishment of the National Center for Complementary and Alternative Medicine (NCCAM) at the National Institutes of Health in 1998. Moreover, many major universities now have entire centers devoted to CAM research, and CAM courses have been included in medical schools' curricula. As a result of the increased resources devoted to CAM research, four times as many alternative medicine-related studies were published in 2001 than a decade before in 1991.

The practices encompassed by CAM are broad and heterogeneous. The NCCAM has grouped complementary and alternative medicine practices into five major domains:

(1) Alternative medical systems;

(2) Mind–body interventions;

(3) Biologically based treatments;

(4) Manipulative and body-based methods;

(5) Energy therapies.

What specifically constitutes an 'alternative' practice is also constantly evolving as CAM therapies are integrated into conventional medicine. For example, diet, exercise and behavioral medicine, practices that were once considered unconventional, are now considered beneficial medical therapies by most physicians.

There are many reasons why patients with access to conventional medicine use CAM. It has been suggested that the use of alternative therapies represents dissatisfaction with conventional medicine and that patients who are turning to CAM are turning away from conventional medicine. The truth is that most patients who use CAM are complementing rather than replacing conventional therapies. Hence, practitioners of conventional medicine should not feel threatened by the growing interest in CAM. Another myth that should be dispelled is that of the ignorant or gullible CAM user. In fact, CAM users tend to be better educated and more financially well off than their counterparts who use conventional medicine. CAM users generally see CAM as better able to fulfill their desire for more 'holistic' medical care. Most importantly, CAM users believe in the effectiveness and safety of complementary and alternative therapies.

While CAM promises to provide patients with more health-care options, it is not without risks. Complementary and alternative therapies and their practitioners may not be subject to the same regulations as their conventional counterparts. Safety issues relating to alternative therapies such as herbal medications, acupuncture and spine manipulation are well documented. Safety issues include not only direct harm but also interactions with conventional therapies and delay in receiving appropriate medical therapy in some instances. In addition, physicians who recommend complementary and alternative therapies or refer their patients to CAM practitioners may, in rare instances, be held liable in the event of patient injury[3]. On the other hand, physicians could also be liable for failure to disclose the availability and benefits of CAM[4].

Potential interactions between herbal medications and prescription drugs may also affect patients. Herbal medications were classified as dietary supplements in the Dietary Supplement Health and Education Act of 1994[5]. This exempts them from the proof of safety and efficacy required of prescription drugs regulated by the Food and Drug Administration. However, like prescription medications, many also consist of pharmacologically active constituents. As we know, natural products are the most consistently successful source of new drug leads, with almost 50% of today's best-selling drugs being derived from natural products. Therefore, it is obvious that components from herbs can act directly on different organ systems and/or interact with medications prescribed by physicians[6]. To complicate matters, studies indicate that patients often do not inform their doctors of herb medications they are using[7,8].

In summary, today's physicians are practicing in a contemporary environment of widespread CAM use. It is important for medical professionals to know basic aspects of CAM therapies, and to be familiar with the medical literature on CAM treatment. Thus, physicians will be able to differentiate between CAM therapies that are potentially effective and those that may be unsafe.

References

1. Eisenberg DM, Davis RB, Ettner SL, *et al.* Trends in alternative medicine use in the United States, 1990–1997: results of a follow-up national survey. *J Am Med Assoc* 1998;280:1569–75

2. Burg MA, Kosch SG, Neims AH, Stoller EP. Personal use of alternative medicine therapies by health science center faculty. *J Am Med Assoc* 1998;280:1563

3. Studdert DM, Eisenberg DM, Miller FH, Curto DA, Kaptchuk TJ, Brennan TA. Medical malpractice implications of alternative medicine. *J Am Med Assoc* 1998;280:1610–15

4. Ernst E, Cohen MH. Informed consent in complementary and alternative medicine. *Arch Intern Med* 2001;161:2288–92

5. 103rd Congress. Dietary Supplement Health and Education Act of 1994. Public Law 103-417. 108 Stat. 4325. 1994

6. Ang-Lee MK, Moss J, Yuan CS. Herbal medicines and perioperative care. *J Am Med Assoc* 2001;286:208–16.

7. Eisenberg DM, Kessler RC, Foster C, Norlock FE, Calkins DR, Delbanco TL. Unconventional medicine in the United States. *N Engl J Med* 1993;328:246–52

8. Kristoffersen SS, Atkin PA, Shenfield GM. Uptake of alternative medicine. *Lancet* 1996;347:972–3

SECTION I

Commonly used CAM therapies

Most commonly used herbal medicines in the USA

1

M. K. Ang-Lee

ALOE

Common names: aloe, Barbados aloe, Cape aloe, Curaçao aloe, Zanzibar aloe, kumari (Sanskrit name), lu hui (Chinese name).

Background

Aloe, a member of the lily (Liliaceae) family (Figure 1), has been used medicinally for thousands of years. Of the several hundred species, *Aloe vera* is the most extensively used topically. Other species such as *Aloe barbadensis* (Curaçao aloe) and *Aloe capensis* (Cape aloe) are more frequently used internally.

Uses

Aloe gel, a clear jelly-like substance obtained from the inner parenchymal tissue of the leaf, is used for topical wound healing. It has been investigated for use in wounds caused by incisions[1], burns[2], radiation[3], dermabrasion[4], frostbite[5], pressure[6] and psoriasis[7]. The healing effect of aloe has been shown in animal models[8]. In humans, however, clinical trials have reported inconsistent results. An aloe extract in hydrophilic cream improved healing of psoriatic skin lesions[7]. Aloe gel accelerated wound healing in patients who underwent full-face dermabrasion[4]. In patients with aphthous stomatitis, aloe did not deter the development of oral mucosal ulcers[9], but acemannan, an isolated aloe gel polysaccharide, accelerated healing of ulcers and reduced pain[10]. *Aloe vera* gel did not prevent skin injury from radiation therapy[3]. In patients

with wounds healing by secondary intention, aloe may have been detrimental to wound healing[1]. These inconsistent results may be explained by differences in preparations, treatment regimens, patient populations and study methodologies.

In addition to topical administration, aloe is also taken orally. The latex of the plant, a yellow juice extracted from the superficial pericyclic cells, contains anthraquinones. Anthraquinones, particularly aloe-emodin, induce the active secretion of water and electrolytes into the lumen of the bowel. Laxative effects follow approximately 9 h after ingestion. Oral aloe has been advocated to heal gastrointestinal ulcers[11], treat AIDS[12], lower blood sugar in patients with diabetes[13], treat and prevent cancer[14] and lower blood lipid levels[15]. Although preliminary data suggest that aloe is potentially effective in some of these conditions, more evidence is necessary before clinicians should recommend oral aloe.

Phytochemistry and pharmacology

Aloe extract contains many compounds, not all of which have been characterized. Identified compounds include polysaccharides, lectins, anthranoids, salicylates, cholesterol, triglycerides, magnesium lactate and carboxypeptidase. Of these compounds, the polysaccharides and lectins are the most important. Acemannan, a proprietary aloe polysaccharide, has been used in several clinical trials.

Many mechanisms have been proposed to explain the wound-healing effects of aloe. The simplest of these is that aloe acts as a moisturizing agent. However, many aloe constituents are pharmacologically

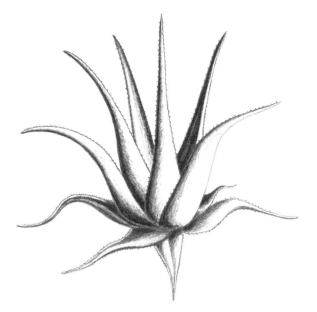

Figure 1 *Aloe vera*

active, and some have anti-inflammatory effects[16]. For example, magnesium lactate inhibits the production of histamine by blocking the enzyme histidine decarboxylase. Aloe also contains natural salicylates, and other substances may inhibit the production of inflammatory mediators such as bradykinin and thromboxane. Furthermore, aloe may have antibacterial[2] and antiviral activity[17]. The gel polysaccharides, particularly acemannan, have immunostimulatory effects *in vitro*[18]. Some constituents of aloe may have antimutagenic effects[19]. Aloe may alter vascular tone, improving blood supply to wounded tissue.

Safety

The topical use of aloe is generally safe, although cases of allergic dermatitis and minor burning sensations have been reported[20–22]. The internal use of aloe is contraindicated in cases of intestinal obstruction, inflammatory bowel disease, appendicitis and abdominal pain of unknown origin[23]. Long-term internal use can lead to electrolyte loss and dehydration and increase the risk (relative risk of 3.0) of colorectal cancer[24].

Internal use during pregnancy or by nursing mothers is not recommended.

Preparations and dosage

Aloe is an ingredient in a wide variety of cosmetic and health-care products. The benefits of commercially available products are unknown, because many only contain minimal amounts of aloe[25]. However, some aloe gel products are available that contain more than 95% pure aloe gel. For topical use, recommendations are to apply liberally as needed. When used internally, the typical dosage is 20–30 mg of anthraquinones/day[26].

ECHINACEA

Common names: purple coneflower, red sunflower, black sampson.

Background

There are nine species of *Echinacea*, a member of the daisy family (Figure 2). Three species, *Echinacea angustifolia*, *Echinacea purpurea* and *Echinacea pallida*, are used for medicinal purposes. The most commonly studied is *Echinacea purpurea*, used for the prophylaxis and treatment of viral, bacterial and fungal infections, particularly those of upper respiratory origin. Compelling evidence supporting its use in upper respiratory infections is lacking, however[27]. Echinacea is also used as an immunostimulant after chemo- and radiation therapy, an adjunct in cancer treatment and a topical promoter of wound healing.

Phytochemistry and pharmacology

Echinacea contains alkylamides, alkaloids, caffeic acid esters, polysaccharides, flavonoids, polyacetylenes and essential oils. Pharmacological activity cannot be attributed to a single compound, although the lipophilic fraction, which contains the alkylamides (primarily the increased production of immunoglobulins (Ig)G and M in rats[30].

Safety

Echinacea appears to have a low potential for toxicity and mutagenicity[31], and in a preliminary investigation it was not harmful during pregnanacy[32]. It has been associated with allergic reactions, including one reported case of anaphylaxis. Therefore, echinacea should be used with caution in patients with asthma, atopy or allergic rhinitis[33]. Its immunomodulatory effects may diminish the effectiveness of immunosuppression in patients such as organ transplant recipients. Moreover, immunosuppression is possible if echinacea is taken long-term (> 8 weeks)[34].

Although the pyrrolizidine alkaloids in echinacea lack the 1,2-unsaturated necrine ring system associated with hepatotoxicity in other pyrrolizidine alkaloid-containing plants such as comfrey, concerns of potential hepatotoxicity have also been raised[35].

The pharmacokinetics of echinacea have not been studied.

Preparations and dosage

Several preparations are available. The fresh ariel parts of the plant can be pressed to yield a juice that is stabilized with alcohol. The usual dosage is 6–9 ml of expressed plant juice or its equivalent as an extract per day. Preparations can also be made from plant root, and the usual dosage is 0.9 g of cut root several times daily.

EPHEDRA

Commmon names: ma huang, epitonin.

Background

Ephedra is an herbal medication obtained from the woody stems of *Ephedra sinica* (Figure 3), a shrub

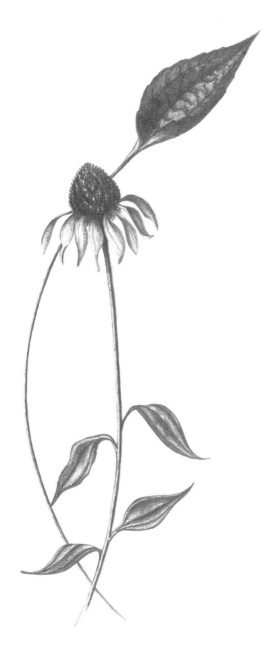

Figure 2 *Echinacea purpurea*

dodeca-2,4,8,10-tetraenoic acid isobutylamides), polyacetylenes and essential oil, appears to be more active than the hydrophilic fraction.

Echinacea has a number of immunomodulatory effects. *In vitro*, it activated immune cells, increased cytokine production and inhibited hyaluronidase[28]. *In vivo*, it activated natural killer cells in humans[29] and

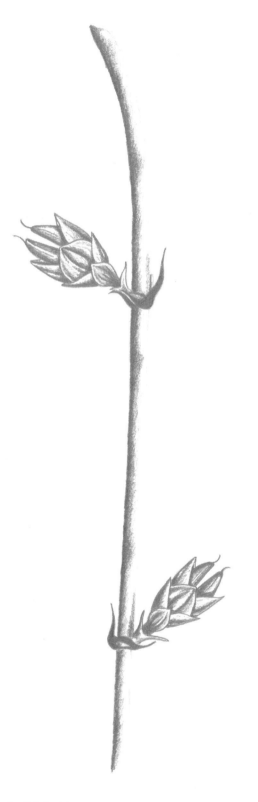

Figure 3   *Ephedra sinica*

native to the semiarid and desert areas of Asia, Europe and Africa. *Ephedra sinica* is the most commonly used species for medicinal purposes, but other species have also been described. This herbal medication has a long history in traditional Chinese medicine, in which it is known as ma huang.

Uses

Ephedra was traditionally given to induce perspiration and to treat respiratory conditions including asthma, bronchitis, allergic rhinitis and upper respiratory tract infections. Today, it is still used to treat respiratory disorders. The German Commission E has approved ephedra for diseases of the respiratory tract with mild bronchospasm in adults and children over the age of 6[31]. The World Health Organization has determined its effectiveness in treating nasal congestion and asthma[36]. The known pharmacological effects of ephedrine, the major active alkaloid in ephedra, suggest that ephedra is an effective bronchodilator.

Recently, ephedra has gained popularity as an aid to weight loss. In 1998, 2% of obese Americans and 1% of the general population took over-the-counter weight-loss products containing ephedra[37]. These figures are likely to increase in the future, particularly in light of a Food and Drug Administration (FDA) proposal in 2001 to withdraw approval of phenylpropanolamine, another popular over-the-counter drug for weight loss. Ephedrine is often combined with caffeine to promote weight loss by increasing thermogenesis and reducing appetite[38,39]. In a randomized controlled trial, an ephedra/caffeine preparation produced significant weight loss in obese subjects[40]. However, in that study, 23% of the actively treated subjects withdrew because of side-effects.

Ephedra has also gained popularity as an ergogenic (physical performance enhancing) aid. Individual ephedrine alkaloids did not affect physical performance[41], but the combination of ephedrine and caffeine improved physical performance as determined by exercise time to exhaustion[42]. This combination of ephedrine and caffeine may be unsafe, because it also causes greater tachycardia than either placebo or ephedrine alone. Moreover, ephedrine is a banned substance in amateur sporting events and is likely to disqualify athletes in drug-tested events[41].

'Herbal ecstasy' preparations that are advertised as safe alternatives to illegal street drugs contain ephedra[43]. The labels of such preparations claim or imply that they produce euphoria and increase awareness, energy and sexual sensation.

Phytochemistry and pharmacology

Unlike those in many herbs, the pharmacologically active constituents in ephedra are well characterized. They consist of ephedrine and ephedrine-related alkaloids, primarily pseudoephedrine, norephedrine, methylephedrine and norpseudoephedrine. Commercial preparations may be standardized to ephedra alkaloid content, but content can vary considerably among manufacturers[44].

Ephedrine, the primary alkaloid in ephedra, is a non-catecholamine sympathomimetic agent that exhibits α_1, β_1 and β_2 activity by acting directly at adrenergic receptors and by indirectly releasing endogenous norepinephrine (noradrenaline). Ephedrine has caused dose-dependent increases in blood pressure and heart rate[45]. However, ephedra inconsistently increased heart rate and blood pressure in healthy, normotensive volunteers after a single dose[46].

The pharmacokinetics of ephedrine have been studied in humans. It has an elimination half-life of 4.85–6.47 h and is excreted unchanged in urine[47]. The pharmacokinetics of ephedrine do not depend on whether it is taken alone or in unprocessed ephedra[46].

Safety

The use of ephedra has raised serious safety concerns. Its sympathomimetic effects have been associated with adverse events in the central nervous and cardiovascular systems including hypertension, arrhythmias, stroke, seizures and death[48]. Most of these adverse events have occurred in healthy young or middle-aged adults who used ephedra for weight loss

and for increasing energy[49]. In at least one case, ephedra has also been associated with eosinophilic myocarditis[50]. As a result, ephedra should be avoided by those with hypertension, cardiovascular disease, cerebrovascular disease, seizure disorders, thyrotoxicosis or pheochromocytoma. It should not be taken with caffeine or other stimulants. It should also be avoided by pregnant or nursing women and by those taking monoamine oxidase (MAO) inhibitors and cardiac glycosides.

The long-term abuse of dietary supplements containing ephedrine has been reported to cause radiolucent kidney stones that, by some estimates, account for 0.064% of all cases of nephrolithiasis[51].

In 1997, the FDA[49] proposed:

(1) To restrict the amount of ephedrine alkaloids in dietary supplements to 8 mg or less;

(2) To limit intake of ephedra alkaloids to 8 mg in a 6-h period and 24 mg in a day;

(3) To require a warning against use for more than 7 days;

(4) To require the label statement 'Taking more than the recommended serving may result in heart attack, stroke, seizure, or death';

(5) To prohibit the combination of ephedrine alkaloids with other stimulants.

These proposals were subsequently withdrawn, owing to criticisms by the General Accounting Office that the scientific evidence supporting them was weak[52]. In spite of the criticism, some states have individually adopted regulations similar to those proposed by the FDA.

Preparations and dosage

Ephedra should be used with caution, especially when it is in combination with caffeine. It should not be taken for prolonged periods. Daily doses of ephedra alkaloids should be limited to 24 mg/day.

GARLIC

Common names: stink weed, ajo, da suan (Chinese name), rashona (Sanskrit name), clove garlic.

Background

Garlic is the common name for *Allium sativum*, a member of the lily family (Figure 4). It is predominantly consumed for its aromatic qualities in food but has a history of medicinal use dating back to Egyptian times.

Uses

Garlic has been studied for its potential to modify the risk of atherosclerosis by reducing blood pressure, thrombus formation, and serum lipid and cholesterol levels. It may even promote the regression of atherosclerotic plaque[53]. Garlic has also been promoted for treatment and prevention of cancer and infectious diseases.

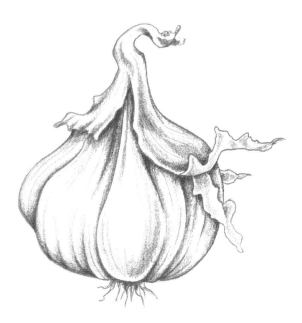

Figure 4   Garlic (*Allium sativum*)

Evidence of the therapeutic efficacy of garlic in lowering serum cholesterol is compelling, although the effect appears to be modest[54]. A meta-analysis determined that the consumption of one-half to one clove of garlic per day decreased total serum cholesterol levels by an average of 9%[55]. In a German multi-center randomized controlled trial, standardized garlic powder tablets reduced serum cholesterol levels by 12% and triglyceride levels by 17% in patients with hyperlipidemia[56]. However, not all studies have found that garlic reduced serum cholesterol[57–59]. It did not have a significant effect on children with familial hyperlipidemia[60]. Differences may be explained by variations in treatment regimens, patient populations, study methodology and publication bias.

Little is known about the mechanism of the cholesterol-lowering effect of garlic. In isolated rat hepatocytes, garlic inhibited acetate uptake and interfered with cholesterol biosynthesis[61]. This mechanism has yet to be demonstrated in humans[58]. Garlic may also decrease the susceptibility of lipoproteins to oxidation[62]. The cholesterol-lowering effect of garlic may be mediated by a reduction in food intake[63].

Although garlic lowers blood pressure in animals, there is insufficient evidence to support the antihypertensive effect of garlic[64,65]. Garlic may be useful in cases of mild hypertension but should not replace lifestyle modification and drug therapy. In nulliparous parturients, garlic therapy during the third trimester reduced the incidence of hypertension but not the incidence of pre-eclampsia[66].

Phytochemistry and pharmacology

Garlic contains organosulfur compounds, adenosine, trace minerals and amino acids. The pharmacological effects are attributed to the sulfur-containing compounds, particularly allicin and its transformation products. When garlic is cut or crushed, alliin, the first compound found in nature to display optical isomerism at a sulfur as well as a carbon atom, is exposed to the enzyme alliinase and converted to allicin.

Garlic's constituents and their transformation products inhibit platelet aggregation dose-dependently.

This activity is predominantly attributed to allicin[67], ajoene (4,5,9-trithiadodeca-1,6,11-triene-9-oxide)[64] and methyl allyl trisulfide[68,69]. The inhibition of platelet aggregation by ajoene appears to be irreversible[70] and may potentiate the effect of other compounds such as prostacyclin, forskolin, indomethacin and dipyridamole[71]. The mechanism behind these effects is unclear, although some investigators have implicated the cyclo-oxygenase pathway[64]. Others have found a direct interaction with the platelet fibrinogen receptor[72]. Still other possibilities surround the exogenous adenosine in garlic[73] and inhibition of endogenous adenosine deamination and cyclic AMP phosphodiesterase[64]. The extent of garlic's antiplatelet activity *in vivo* is uncertain. In volunteers, inhibition of platelet aggregation to 5-hydroxytryptamine was transient but potent[61]. Another study showed no such activity[74]. Garlic may also act as an anticoagulant by promoting fibrinolysis, which has been demonstrated in volunteers[75].

Little is known about the mechanism by which garlic may lower blood pressure. This effect may be mediated by nitric oxide[76,77] or by an as yet unknown mechanism[78]. Allicin decreased pulmonary vascular resistance in isolated rat lungs independently of nitric oxide, ATP-sensitive potassium channels, activation of cyclo-oxygenase and changes in bronchomotor tone.

The pharmacokinetics of garlic's constituents are poorly understood. Allicin is not found in the blood after garlic consumption[79]. It is unstable and converts readily into mono-, di-, tri- and polysulfides, sulfur oxide and other compounds such as ajoene[80]. These organosulfur compounds readily react with cysteine in the intestinal tract or circulation[81]. The sulfur-containing compounds found in the body after consumption of garlic are not known. Pharmacokinetic studies in animals have provided little insight[82,83].

Safety

The anticoagulant effect of garlic has raised concerns about bleeding in garlic users. One elderly patient developed a spontaneous epidural hematoma that was attributed to frequent garlic ingestion[84]. Although unreliable, bleeding times were significantly elevated when the patient was hospitalized and returned to normal 3 days after the discontinuation of garlic.

Preparations and dosage

The usual dosage is 4 g (approximately two cloves) of fresh bulb or its equivalent as an extract or tincture per day[85]. Much larger doses (up to 28 cloves/day) have been advocated, and the development of concentrated garlic preparations has made these doses achievable[86]. Commercial garlic preparations may be standardized to a fixed alliin and allicin content.

GINKGO

Common names: maidenhair, yin-hsing (Chinese name), silver apricot, duck foot tree, fossil tree.

Background

Ginkgo is derived from the leaf of *Ginkgo biloba* (Figure 5), also known as the maidenhair or fossil tree. It is the oldest living species of tree in existence today; fossils of the Ginkgo tree date as far back as 200 million years. An individual tree can live as long as 1000 years. In traditional Chinese medicine, *Ginkgo biloba* was used to make medicinal teas.

Uses

Ginkgo is primarily used to treat cognitive impairment, particularly Alzheimer's disease. A multicenter, randomized, placebo-controlled, double-blind trial showed that ginkgo extract (EGb 761) stabilized or improved cognitive function in patients with Alzheimer's disease and multi-infarct dementia[87]. In a meta-analysis of studies investigating the use of gingko for dementia or cognitive impairment, researchers concluded that ginkgo had a small but significant effect on objective measures of cognitive function in patients with Alzheimer's disease[88]. Whether ginkgo can improve cognitive function in healthy people is

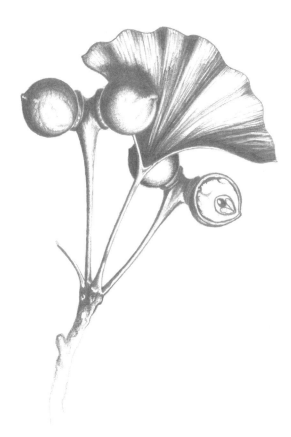

Figure 5   *Ginkgo biloba*

under active investigation; although results are mixed, preliminary evidence is generally promising[89–92].

The use of ginkgo has also been advocated for the treatment of peripheral vascular disease[93], age-related macular degeneration[94], vertigo[95], tinnitus[96], sexual dysfunction[97] and altitude sickness[98].

Phytochemistry and pharmacology

Ginkgo contains a number of active compounds. Those believed to be responsible for its pharmacological effects are the terpenoids and flavonoids. The terpenoids include the sesquiterpene bilobalide and ginkgolides A, B, C and J. The flavonoids are ginkgo-flavone glycosides that include kaempferol, quercetin and isorhamnetin derivatives.

Ginkgo appears to alter vasoregulation[99], to act as an antioxidant[100], to modulate neurotransmitter and receptor activity[101,102] and to inhibit platelet-activating

factor (PAF)[103]. The antioxidant and free radical scavenging effects have been attributed to the flavonoids, because they inhibit the expression of inducible nitric oxide synthase[104,105]. Ginkgolide B was a potent inhibitor of PAF in laboratory animals and humans[106]. PAF is an ether-linked phospholipid that mediates a diverse number of processes including stimulation of the inflammatory response, induction of platelet aggregation and modulation of neuronal function[107]. Inhibition of PAF protects against hypoxia-induced neuronal injury[108,109]. Ginkgo may also have a non-PAF-mediated inhibitory effect on platelet aggregation in stressed laboratory animals, a finding that, if confirmed in humans, may be significant[110]. Ginkgo inhibited MAO in laboratory animals[111,112], but not in humans[113].

Bilobalide and ginkgolides A and B are highly bioavailable when administered orally. Glucuronidation appears to be part of the metabolism of the flavonoids[114]. Elimination half-lives of ginkgolides A and B and bilobalide after oral administration are 4.5, 10.6 and 3.2 h, respectively[115].

Safety

Although serious adverse effects have not been reported in clinical trials in relatively small numbers of patients, the anticoagulant effects of ginkgo have been associated with bleeding complications. There are four reported cases of spontaneous intracranial bleeding[116–119], one case of spontaneous hyphema[120] and one case of post-operative bleeding[121] associated with ginkgo use.

Hypersensitivity to ginkgo preparations is possible. Use during pregnancy or by nursing mothers is not recommended.

Preparations and dosage

Ginkgo is usually prepared as a dried leaf extract. The two ginkgo extracts used in clinical trials, EGb 761 and LI 1370, undergo extensive processing and are standardized to ginkgo-flavone glycoside and terpenoid content. The recommended dosage of ginkgo extract is 120–240 mg/day in two or three divided doses.

GINSENG

Common names: Panax, redberry, tartar root, five fingers, American ginseng, Chinese ginseng, Korean ginseng, Asian ginseng.

Background

Ginseng is an herbal medication derived from the root of the *Panax* genus of plants (Figure 6). It has been used for several thousands of years in Asia and its purported medicinal properties have reached mythic proportions. The use of ginseng in America dates

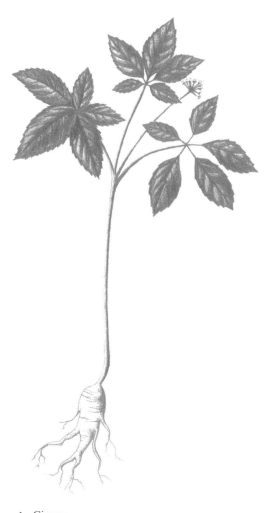

Figure 6   Ginseng

back to the 18th century. Daniel Boone traded ginseng, and in his diary, George Washington mentioned gathering the herb.

Among the species used for pharmacological effects, Asian ginseng (*Panax ginseng*), American ginseng (*Panax quinquefolius*) and Japanese ginseng (*Panax japonicus*) are commonly described. Other 'varieties' such as Siberian ginseng (*Eleintherococcus senticosus*) and Brazilian ginseng (*Pfaffia paniculata*) are unique plants with different pharmacological effects that may nevertheless be included in commercially available ginseng preparations.

Uses

Brekham, an early pioneer in the study of ginseng, labeled it an 'adaptogen' because it appeared to protect the body against stress and restore homeostasis[122]. Ginseng has been advocated for virtually every purpose including general health[123], fatigue[124], immune function[125], cancer[126], cardiovascular disease[127], diabetes mellitus[128], cognitive function[129], viral infections[130], sexual function[131] and athletic performance[132,133]. Although ginseng has therapeutic potential and measurable pharmacological activity, compelling evidence is lacking to support its use for any specific indication[134]. The German Commission E has approved ginseng as therapy for fatigue and decreased concentration and work capacity[135].

Phytochemistry and pharmacology

Constituents found in most ginseng species include ginsenosides, polysaccharides, peptides, polyacetylenic alcohols and fatty acids. Most pharmacological actions are attributed to the ginsenosides that belong to a group of compounds known as steroidal saponins, steroid molecules with attached sugar residues. More than 20 ginsenosides have been isolated.

The pharmacological profile of ginseng is broad and incompletely understood because of the many heterogeneous and sometimes opposing effects of different ginsenosides[136]. The underlying mechanism of action of the ginsenosides appears to be similar to that for steroid hormones. Actions on virtually every organ system have been described.

One of the most promising therapeutic uses of ginseng surrounds the regulation of carbohydrate metabolism and blood glucose. In patients with type 2 diabetes mellitus, ginseng lowered postprandial blood glucose compared to placebo when taken 40 min before or at the same time as a glucose challenge[128]. In healthy subjects without diabetes mellitus, ginseng lowered postprandial blood glucose compared to placebo only if taken 40 min before glucose challenge.

Data from animal studies suggest that ginseng may have beneficial effects in the central nervous system. Ginsenosides prevented scopolamine-induced memory deficits in laboratory animals by increasing central cholinergic activity[137,138]. The compounds may also protect neurons from ischemic damage[139] and facilitate learning and memory by enhancing nerve growth[140]. The effect of ginseng on pain pathways needs further investigation. Ginsenosides had non-opioid-mediated analgesic properties in laboratory animals[141,142], but attenuated the analgesic effects of opiates[143,144]. Ginsenosides appear to modulate neurotransmission through γ-aminobutyric acid (GABA)[145,146] and by inhibiting neurotransmitter reuptake[147].

The results of investigations of the cardiovascular effects of ginseng are often contradictory, depending on the compounds tested and the organ system in which they are tested[148]. Stimulation of endogenous nitric oxide release has been implicated in the cardiovascular and antioxidant effects of ginsenosides. In humans, normal doses of ginseng did not appear to affect blood pressure and heart rate, although extremely high doses were associated with hypertension[149]. Ginseng may protect against myocardial reperfusion injury. In a preliminary study, cardioplegia solution containing ginseng extract improved post-bypass myocardial function in patients having mitral valve surgery[150].

Ginsenosides have anticarcinogenic and immunomodulatory effects. Several individual ginsenosides suppressed tumor cell growth, induced cell differentiation, regulated programmed cell death and inhibited metastasis[136]. Results of a cohort study showed that ginseng consumers had a lower risk for several different types of cancer compared to those who did not consume ginseng, suggesting that ginseng may have non-organ-specific anticarcinogenic effects[151]. Ginsenosides also enhanced humoral and cell-mediated immune responses in laboratory animals[152–154] and potentiated the response to vaccination in humans[155].

The pharmacokinetics of ginsenosides Rg1, Re and Rb2 have been investigated in rabbits[156]. The elimination half-lives of these three ginsenosides ranged from 0.8 h for ginsenoside Re to 7.4 h for ginsenoside Rb2. The degree of protein binding may explain the wide variation in half-lives between different ginsenosides.

Safety

Early descriptions of a 'ginseng abuse syndrome'[149] characterized by hypertension and central nervous system excitation have since been challenged, although a number of case reports have cautioned against the indiscriminate use of ginseng. The estrogen-like effects of ginseng have been associated with postmenopausal vaginal bleeding and mastalgia[157–160]. An interaction between ginseng and the MAO inhibitor phenelzine resulted in headache, tremors and mania[161]. There is a case report of angiogram-confirmed, self-limited cerebral arteritis associated with ginseng overdose[162]. Ginseng was also associated with a significant decrease in warfarin anticoagulation in one case[163]. It is not known whether ginseng can cause the same side-effects as those described from long-term steroid use.

Another potential safety issue surrounding the use of ginseng concerns its effects on coagulation pathways. Ginsenosides inhibit platelet aggregation *in vitro*[164,165] and prolong both thrombin time and activated partial thromboplastin time in rats[166]. These findings await confirmation in humans.

Use during pregnancy or by nursing mothers is not recommended.

Preparations and dosage

Ginseng root is either dried to yield 'white ginseng' or steamed and then dried to yield 'red ginseng'.

Commercial ginseng extract preparations standardized to ginsenoside content are available. The recommended daily dose is 100–200 mg of ginseng extract once daily. Dosages of ginseng extract up to 600 mg three times daily have been advocated[167].

KAVA

Common names: intoxicating pepper, kawa, kava kava, ava pepper.

Background

Kava is an herbal medication derived from the dried root of the pepper plant *Piper methysticum* (Figure 7). Kava has a long history of use as a ceremonial intoxicant in the South Pacific islands. It was relatively unknown to the rest of the world until missionaries introduced it into Australian aboriginal society in the 1980s[168,169]. The missionaries intended kava to substitute for alcohol which was abused by the aboriginal population. Unfortunately, kava misuse became an additional public health problem, and it was eventually outlawed in many aboriginal communities. Australian physicians provided many of the earliest descriptions of the medical effects of kava[170,171].

Uses

Kava has gained popularity as an over-the-counter anxiolytic and sedative. It is purported to be a safe alternative to benzodiazepines. Kava and alcohol do not appear to have synergistic effects on cognitive and psychomotor impairment[172]. Several randomized controlled trials have compared kava to placebo for the treatment of anxiety (diagnosed by DSM-III-R criteria)[173], situational anxiety[174] and anxiety associated with menopause[175]. A meta-analysis of clinical trials suggested that kava has therapeutic potential in the treatment of the symptoms of anxiety[176]. Kava has been advocated for the treatment of insomnia, but its effect on sleep in humans has not been well characterized.

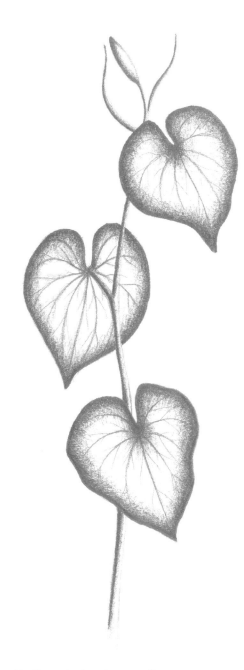

Figure 7 *Piper methysticum*, the source of kava

Phytochemistry and pharmacology

Kava contains many pharmacologically active constituents that act synergistically to produce effects greater than those achieved with any single compound[177–179]. The kavalactones, also known as kavapyrones or α-pyrones, are responsible for most of the pharmacological effects[180–183]. The six major kavalactones that have been identified are kawain, dihydrokawain, methysticin, dihydromethysticin, yangomin and desmethoxyyangonin.

Kava produces dose-dependent effects on the central nervous system. The antiepileptic and neuroprotective properties of kavalactones have been demonstrated in animal models[181,182,184]. Kavalactones produced centrally mediated skeletal muscle relaxation *in vivo* and smooth muscle relaxation *in vitro*[182]. Unlike other central nervous system depressants, kava does not depress cognitive function or electroencephalographic event-related potentials[176,185,186]. However, the ability of kavalactones to increase barbiturate sleep time significantly has been demonstrated in animals[178–187]. Kavalactones also have significant local anesthetic properties. Kawain is equipotent to cocaine in producing topical anesthesia[182].

The mechanism of action of kava has not been fully elucidated, but multiple effector sites are involved. The anxiolytic and sedative effects of kava suggest that it potentiates GABA inhibitory neurotransmission. The first investigation addressing this effect found no evidence of binding in the mouse brain frontal cortex or cerebellum[188]. A later investigation showed that kavalactones mediate their effect through $GABA_A$ in the limbic structures of the brain[177]. In that study, the kavalactones and pentobarbital also produced a synergistic effect on [³H]muscimol binding to GABA. Kavalactones inhibit voltage-dependent sodium and calcium channels *in vitro*, possibly explaining the antiepileptic and local anesthetic effects[189–192]. Kava may exert its effects through neurotransmitters such as dopamine and serotonin, but evidence of this is less compelling[193,194].

Peak plasma levels occur 1.8 h after an oral dose, and the elimination half-life of kavalactones is 9 h[195]. In rats, unchanged kavalactones and their metabolites undergo renal and fecal elimination[179].

Safety

In Germany, kava has been linked to 24 cases of liver toxicity culminating in one death and three liver transplants. At this writing, the regulatory status of kava in Germany remains uncertain. Kava may potentiate the sedative effects of prescription medications[196]. With frequent use, kava produces 'kava dermopathy', characterized by reversible scaly cutaneous eruptions[197]. Kava may have abuse potential, but whether long-term use results in addiction, tolerance and acute withdrawal after abstinence has not been satisfactorily investigated.

Use during pregnancy or by nursing mothers is not recommended.

Preparations and dosage

The recommended dose is 150–300 mg of kava extract divided into two doses or 50–240 mg of kavalactones per day[198].

MILK THISTLE

Common names: Marian thistle, St Mary's thistle, wild artichoke.

Background

Milk thistle is the common name for *Silybum marianum* (Figure 8), a member of the daisy family native to the Mediterranean. The therapeutic uses of milk thistle have been recognized for at least 2000 years. It was first used for liver and gallbladder disorders just as it is today. Silymarin, the biologically active flavonoid complex, is extracted from the seed of the plant.

Uses

Milk thistle has been advocated for the prophylaxis and treatment of liver disorders including cirrhosis and alcoholic, viral and toxic hepatitis. Although inconclusive, available evidence suggests that milk thistle is potentially useful in some clinical situations. In a randomized controlled trial, it was reported that silymarin significantly improved survival in patients with cirrhosis (4-year survival of 58% in the treatment group and 39% in the placebo group)[199]. The subgroup analysis in this study indicted that silymarin was effective in patients with alcoholic cirrhosis and in patients whose liver disease was initially rated as Child's Class A. Several clinical trials have demonstrated that silymarin significantly lowers serum liver enzyme and bilirubin levels in patients with cirrhosis and hepatitis[200–202]. In other controlled trials, however, silymarin did not improve survival or retard progression of disease in patients with alcoholic cirrhosis[203–205]. Milk thistle is effective in decreasing mortality caused by the ingestion of *Amanita phalloides*, the highly hepatotoxic deathcap mushroom[206].

Phytochemistry and pharmacology

The active compounds in milk thistle are the flavono-lignane isomers, silybin, silidianin and silichristine. Of these, silybin is the most prevalent and biologically active. Multiple mechanisms explain the hepatoprotective effects of milk thistle. Silymarin acts as an antioxidant, scavenging free radicals and inhibiting free radical production and lipid peroxidation[207–209]. Silymarin may protect against hepatotoxins by altering cell membrane permeability and receptor antagonism[210]. Data from *in vitro* studies suggest that silymarin may facilitate hepatocyte regeneration by effecting DNA expression[211].

Only 20–50% of silymarin is absorbed from the gastrointestinal tract. Peak plasma concentrations occur 2–4 h after an oral dose, and the elimination half-life is approximately 6 h[212].

Safety

Milk thistle is generally safe. The most frequently reported adverse effects are nausea and vomiting, urticaria, pruritis and dyspepsia. Allergic reactions may stem from the development of IgE and IgG antibodies[213]. No drug interactions with milk thistle have been reported.

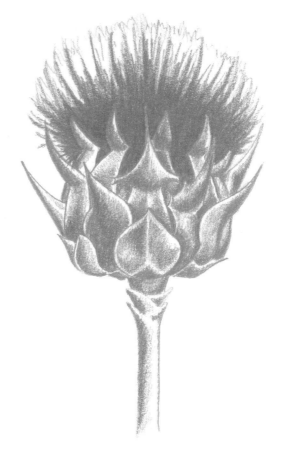

Figure 8 *Silybum marianum*, the milk thistle

Use during pregnancy or by nursing mothers is not recommended.

Preparations and dosage

Commerical extracts of milk thistle are typically standardized to a silymarin content of 70–80%. Tea preparations are not recommended because silymarin is poorly water soluble. The recommended dosage is 100–200 mg of silymarin twice daily.

SAW PALMETTO

Common names: dwarf palmetto, pan palm, sabal.

Background

Saw palmetto is the common name for *Serenoa repens* (Figure 9), a dwarf palm tree native to Florida and other parts of the southeastern USA. The urological effects of the saw palmetto berry were recognized by native Americans who used it as a source of food. Saw palmetto preparations today consist of refined extracts of the dried ripe berry.

Uses

Saw palmetto extract is used to treat symptoms associated with benign prostatic hypertrophy (BPH), a condition found in approximately 40% of men in their fifties and 90% of men in their eighties[214]. It is often used as first-line treatment for BPH in

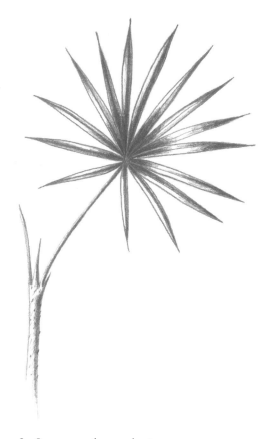

Figure 9 *Serenoa repens*, the saw palmetto

Europe[215], and in Germany herbal medications account for more than 90% of all drugs prescribed for the treatment of BPH.

In a meta-analysis of 18 randomized controlled trials that compared saw palmetto extract to placebo or standard medical therapies, saw palmetto extract improved urinary symptoms and flow measures significantly compared to placebo[216]. These improvements were comparable to those achieved with finasteride. Saw palmetto extract is less expensive and associated with a significantly lower incidence of impotence compared to finasteride[216]. Others have reached similar conclusions but caution that most trials were significantly limited by methodological flaws, small patient numbers and brief treatment intervals[217].

It is not known whether saw palmetto extract can prevent long-term complications of BPH such as acute urinary retention or the need for surgery. Saw palmetto extract does not affect levels of serum prostate-specific antigen[218].

Saw palmetto has been used to treat various other urological conditions and respiratory conditions such as chronic bronchitis laryngitis and nasal inflammation.

Phytochemistry and pharmacology

The major constituents of saw palmetto are fatty acids and their glycerides (triacylglycerides and mono-acylglycerides), carbohydrates, steroids, flavonoids, resin, pigment, tannin and volatile oil[219]. The pharmacological activity of saw palmetto has not been attributed to a single compound.

The mechanism of action of saw palmetto is not known, but multiple mechanisms have been proposed. Data from *in vitro* studies support the widely held belief that saw palmetto extract, like finasteride, inhibits 5α-reductase[217,220]. However, results of *in vivo* studies of inhibition of 5α-reductase by saw palmetto have been inconsistent[217]. Other hypotheses are that saw palmetto exerts its effects by inhibition of dihydrotestosterone binding to the androgen receptors in the prostate[221], inhibition of estrogen receptors[222], blocking of prolactin receptor signal transduction[223], interference with fibroblast proliferation[224], induction of apoptosis[225], inhibition of α_1 adrenergic receptors[226] and attenuation of the inflammatory response[227,228].

The pharmacokinetics of the constituents of saw palmetto have not been studied.

Safety

Adverse effects attributed to saw palmetto are mild and usually gastrointestinal in nature[221]. The long-term safety of saw palmetto extract has not been studied. However, it has a long history of safe use in Europe. Saw palmetto should be discontinued before undergoing surgery, because it may be associated with excessive intraoperative bleeding[229].

Use during pregnancy or by nursing mothers is not recommended.

Preparations and dosage

Liposterolic extracts are used in virtually all investigational studies. Commercial preparations may be standardized to fatty acid and sterol content. The recommended daily dose is 1–2 g saw palmetto berry or 320 mg of lipid soluble extract[219].

ST JOHN'S WORT

Common names: amber, goatweed, klamath weed, hardhay.

Background

St John's wort is the common name for *Hypericum perforatum* (Figure 10), a flowering plant that can be found in Europe, Asia, Africa, Australia and the Americas. It is so named because its yellow flower was traditionally gathered for the feast of St John the Baptist. The herbal medication comes from the aerial parts of the plant harvested shortly before or during flowering.

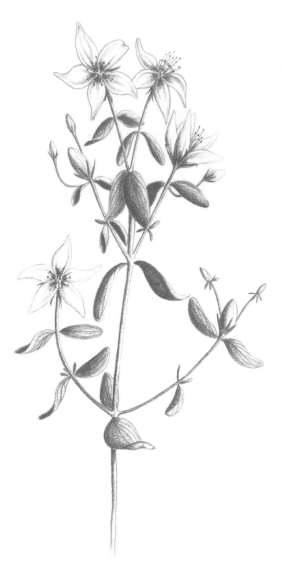

Figure 10 *Hypericum perforatum*, St John's wort

Uses

St John's wort has been used since the Middle Ages for neuralgia, depression and various 'nervous' conditions. Today, St John's wort is primarily used as an antidepressant. It has the largest market share of antidepressants in Europe with $6 billion in sales in 1988. The popularity of St John's wort is reflected in the large number of clinical trials, meta-analyses and reviews of its effectiveness as an antidepressant, which have concluded that it is more effective than placebo in the treatment of mild to moderate depression and has a low incidence of side effects[230–238]. In the treatment of major depression, however, St John's wort is not effective[239]. Moreover, it is unclear whether St John's wort is as effective as conventional antidepressants. Some reviews concluded that St John's wort and the older tricyclic antidepressants were equally effective[230–232]. Others concluded that St John's wort was less effective than tricyclic antidepressants[235]. Still others believe that there is insufficient evidence to compare St John's wort to conventional antidepressants and have called for more studies comparing St John's wort to the newer serotonin reuptake inhibiting antidepressants[236]. The methodology of many studies has been criticized with the implication that firm conclusions about the efficacy of St John's wort are premature[231,239–243].

Phytochemistry and pharmacology

The constituents of St John's wort are the naphthodianthrones (hypericin and pseuodohypericin), acylphloroglucinols (hyperforin and adhyperforin), flavonol glycosides, biflavones, proanthocyanidins and phenylpropanes (chlorogenic acid and caffeic acid). Among these constituents, hypericin and hyperfornin have received the most scientific interest. Hypericin was originally considered the active component in St John's wort, and commercial preparations are standardized to hypericin content. Recent evidence suggests that hyperforin and its analogs play a larger role in the pharmacological effects[244,245]. Because hyperforin is an unstable compound and is susceptible to oxidative degradation, its concentration in St John's wort may vary considerably[246].

St John's wort inhibits reuptake of serotonin, norepinephrine and dopamine[244,247,248]. This property appears to be different from that found in conventional antidepressants. St John's wort also had antinociceptive effects in mice similar to those seen with tricyclic antidepressants[249].

Initially, MAO inhibition was considered a possible mechanism of action. Later studies have shown, however, that the inhibition of MAO by St John's wort is clinically non-significant[244,250,251]. Adverse events that would be expected with MAO inhibition have not been reported with St John's wort.

The pharmacokinetics of hypericum extract have been studied. After oral administration in human volunteers, the median half-life for absorption was 0.6 h, the median half-life for distribution was 6.0 h and the median half-life for elimination was 43.1 h[252]. In another study, peak plasma levels of hypericum extract were obtained 3–3.5 h after oral dosing, and the elimination half-life was 9 h. Plasma concentration time curves fit a two-compartment model[253]. Hypericin and pseudohypericin are most likely to be conjugated and excreted in the bile[252].

Safety

When St John's wort is taken by healthy patients, it is generally well tolerated. Adverse effects include photosensitivity, rash, nausea, fatigue and restlessness[235,254,255]. Serotonin syndrome was reported in patients taking St John's wort alone[254,256] or in combination with conventional antidepressants[257]. In patients who may have subclinical or undiagnosed bipolar disorder, induction of mania was also reported[258–260].

Patients taking prescription medications should be cautious taking St John's wort, since significant herb–drug interactions can occur. It induces cytochrome P450 enzymes and increases the metabolism of protease inhibitors, oral contraceptives, cyclosporin, warfarin, digoxin and many other concomitantly administered drugs. The metabolic activity of the cytochrome P450 3A4 isoenzyme is most affected, and its metabolic activity is approximately doubled[261,262]. This isoform is the most abundant hepatic enzyme, responsible for the oxidative metabolism of over 50% of all conventional medications subject to cytochrome P450 oxidative metabolism. Interactions with substrates of the 3A4 isoform including indinavir[263], ethinylestradiol[264] and cyclosporin have been documented. In one series of 45 organ transplant patients, St John's wort was associated with an average decrease of 49% in blood cyclosporin levels[265]. Another group reported two cases of acute heart transplant rejection associated with this particular pharmacokinetic interaction[266]. In addition to the 3A4 isoform, the cytochrome P450 2C9 isoform may also be induced. The anticoagulant effect of warfarin, a substrate of the 2C9 isoform, was reduced in seven reported cases.

St John's wort also affects digoxin pharmacokinetics, possibly by altering a P-glycoprotein transporter[267]. In volunteers, co-administration of St John's wort led to a 26% reduction in the C_{max} and a 33% reduction of the C_{trough} of digoxin.

Use during pregnancy or by nursing mothers is not recommended.

Preparations and dosage

St John's wort extracts are commercially available, and many are standardized to hypericin content. The recommended daily dose of St John's wort is 2–4 g of St John's wort or 0.2–1 mg of hypericin[268].

VALERIAN

Common names: all-heal, garden heliotrope, vandal root, capon's tail, amantilla, setwall.

Background

Valerian is the common name given to the herbal medication derived from the root of the *Valeriana* genus of plants, pink-flowered perennials (Figure 11) native to the temperate areas of the Americas, Europe and Asia. The different species of valerian used in various parts of the world – *Valerian officinalis* in northern Europe, *Valerian angstifolia* in China and Japan, *Valerian wallichii* in India – are all used for essentially the same purpose. *Valerian officinalis* is the species most commonly available and studied.

Uses

Valerian is used as a sedative to treat insomnia and anxiety. Virtually all herbal sleep-aid preparations

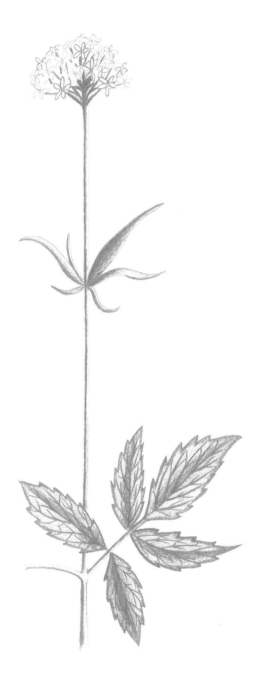

Figure 11 *Valeriana officinalis*, the source of valerian

contain valerian. During World War I, 'shell-shocked' soldiers were treated with valerian. Valerian also promotes smooth muscle relaxation and may be used to treat gastrointestinal hyperactivity.

Phytochemistry and pharmacology

Valerian contains multiple chemical constituents that act synergistically. These include volatile oils (sesquiterpenes and monoterpenes), valepotriates, alkaloids and lignans. The sesquiterpenes are considered the primary source of the pharmacological effects[269]. At least 17 sesquiterpenes have been characterized. Some commercial preparations are standardized to the content of valerenic acid, a sesquiterpene that is not known to exist elsewhere in nature. The valepotriates have also been characterized and consist of a furanopyranoid monoterpene skeleton found in glycosylated forms known as iridoids. At least 37 valepotriates have been isolated. They act as prodrugs that are metabolized into compounds more active than the parent compound. The pharmacological action of the other constituents of valerian is unclear. Seven alkaloids have been isolated but not well studied. GABA and various amino acids have been isolated from the aqueous portion of valerian, but their bioavailability remains in question[269].

Valerian produced dose-dependent sedation and hypnosis in preclinical studies[270,271]. The sesquiterpenes and, to a lesser extent, the valepotriates, increased barbiturate sleep time in animals. Valerian extract 11.2 g/kg was equivalent to diazepam 3 mg/kg in doubling hexobarbital sleep time in mice[272]. Valerian had weak anticonvulsant properties in mice[271]. In isolated guinea-pig ileum, relaxation of smooth muscle by valerian was peripherally mediated[273].

In humans, valerian produced dose-dependent electroencephalogram changes consistent with sedation[274]. The pharmacodynamic studies of valerian in humans have focused on the sleep setting. Modest improvements in subjective ratings of sleep were reported, but objective measurements were inconsistent[275–278]. Subjective and objective measurements of sleep improved after multiple but not single-dose treatment[279].

The biological activity of valerian is consistent with the modulation of GABA inhibitory neurotransmission. Constituents of valerian extract have effects at the $GABA_A$ receptor[280]. Valerian extract influenced presynaptic components of GABA-ergic neurons, although the mechanism of action was unclear. It also influenced GABA synaptosomal release[281,282], inhibited GABA reuptake[280] and inhibited GABA breakdown[283].

The pharmacokinetics of the active constituents of valerian have not been studied. The subjective effects of valerian are short-lived with no demonstrable psychomotor effects the morning after treatment[284]. Multiple doses per day are needed for treatment of anxiety, and the peak effect occurs 1–2 h after oral administration.

Safety

Short-term use of valerian is safe[285]. Because of its GABA receptor activity, the long-term use of valerian may be associated with a benzodiazepine-like withdrawal syndrome. In fact, valerian attenuated benzodiazepine withdrawal in rats[286]. In one patient, the long-term use of valerian was associated with a life-threatening benzodiazepine-like withdrawal syndrome after surgery[283].

Use during pregnancy or by nursing mothers is not recommended.

Preparations and dosage

Commercial valerian preparations consist of the dried extract of the root and may be standardized to a minimum level of valerenic acid or other selected constituents. As a sleep aid, the recommended dosage of valerian extract is 400–900 mg taken 30 min before bedtime. For anxiety, the recommended dosage of valerian extract is 220 mg of extract three times daily. The daily dosage of valerian extract should not exceed 1800 mg, and it is not meant for long-term use[285].

References

1. Schmidt JM, Greenspoon JS. *Aloe vera* dermal wound gel is associated with a delay in wound healing. *Obstet Gynecol* 1991;78:115–17

2. Rodriguez-Bigas M, Cruz NI, Suarez A. Comparative evaluation of aloe vera in the management of burn wounds in guinea pigs. *Plast Reconstr Surg* 1988;81:386–9

3. Williams MS, Burk M, Loprinzi CL, *et al.* Phase III double-blind evaluation of an aloe vera gel as a prophylactic agent for radiation-induced skin toxicity. *Int J Radiat Oncol Biol Phys* 1996;36:345–9

4. Fulton JE Jr. The stimulation of postdermabrasion wound healing with stabilized aloe vera gel–polyethylene oxide dressing. *J Dermatol Surg Oncol* 1990;16:460–7

5. McCauley RL, Heggers JP, Robson MC. Frostbite: methods to minimize tissue loss. *Postgrad Med* 1990;88:73–7

6. Thomas DR, Goode PS, LaMaster K, Tennyson T. Acemannan hydrogel dressing versus saline dressing for pressure ulcers. A randomized, controlled trial. *Adv Wound Care* 1998;11:273–6

7. Syed TA, Ahmad SA, Holt AH, *et al.* Management of psoriasis with *Aloe vera* extract in a hydrophilic cream: a placebo-controlled, double-blind study. *Trop Med Int Health* 1996;1:505–9

8. Reynolds T, Dweck AC. *Aloe vera* leaf gel: a review update. *J Ethnopharmacol* 1999;68:3–37

9. Garnick JJ, Singh B, Winkley G. Effectiveness of a medicament containing silicon dioxide, aloe, and allantoin on aphthous stomatitis. *Oral Surg Oral Med Oral Pathol Oral Radiol Endod* 1998;86:550–6

10. Plemons JN, Rees TD, Binnie WH, Wright JM, Guo I, Hall JE. Evaluation of acemannan in the treatment of recurrent aphthous stomatitis. *Wounds* 1994;6:40–5

11. Blitz J, Smith JW, Gerard JR. *Aloe vera* gel in peptic ulcer therapy: preliminary report. *J Am Osteopath Assoc* 1963;62:731–5

12. Montaner JS, Gill J, Singer J, *et al.* Double-blind placebo-controlled pilot trial of acemannan in advanced human immunodeficiency virus disease. *J Acquir Immune Defic Syndr Hum Retrovirol* 1996;12:153–7

13. Ghannam N, Kingston M, Al Meshaal IA, Tariq M, Parman NS, Woodhouse N. The antidiabetic activity of aloes: preliminary clinical and experimental observations. *Horm Res* 1986;24:288–94

14. Sakai R. Epidemiologic survey on lung cancer with respect to cigarette smoking and plant diet. *Jpn J Cancer Res* 1989;80:513–20

15. Vogler BK, Ernst E. *Aloe vera*: a systematic review of its clinical effectiveness. *Br J Gen Pract* 1999;49:823–8

16. Vazquez B, Avila G, Segura D, Escalante B. Anti-inflammatory activity of extracts from *Aloe vera* gel. *J Ethnopharmacol* 1996;55:69–75

17. Andersen DO, Weber ND, Wood SG, Hughes BG, Murray BK, North JA. *In vitro* virucidal activity of selected anthraquinones and anthraquinone derivatives. *Antiviral Res* 1991;16:185–96

18. Stuart RW, Lefkowitz DL, Lincoln JA, Howard K, Gelderman MP, Lefkowitz SS. Upregulation of phagocytosis and candidicidal activity of macrophages exposed to the immunostimulant acemannan. *Int J Immunopharmacol* 1997;19:75–82

19. Lee KH, Kim JH, Lim DS, Kim CH. Anti-leukaemic and anti-mutagenic effects of di(2-ethylhexyl)phthalate isolated from *Aloe vera* Linne. *J Pharm Pharmacol* 2000;52:593–8

20. Morrow DM, Rapaport MS, Strick RA. Hypersensitivity to aloe. *Arch Dermatol* 1980;116:1064–5

21. Shoji A. Contact dermatitis to *Aloe arborescens*. *Contact Dermatitis* 1982;8:164–7

22. Hunter D, Frumkin A. Adverse reactions to vitamin E and *Aloe vera* preparations after dermabrasion and chemical peel. *Cutis* 1991;47:193–6

23. Anon. Aloe. In Gruenwald J, Brendler T, Jaenicke C, eds. *PDR for Herbal Medicines*, 2nd edn. Montvale, NJ: Medical Economics Company, 2000:16–20

24. Siegers CP, von Hertzberg-Lottin E, Otte M, Schneider B. Anthranoid laxative abuse – a risk for colorectal cancer? *Gut* 1993;34:1099–101

25. Pribitkin ED, Boger G. Herbal therapy: what every facial plastic surgeon must know. *Arch Facial Plast Surg* 2001;3:127–32

26. Anon. Aloe. In Blumenthal M, Busse WR, Goldberg A, *et al.*, eds. *The Complete German Commission E Monographs: Therapeutic Guide to Herbal Medicines*, 1st edn. Boston, MA: Integrative Medical Communications, 1998

27. Melchart D, Linde K, Fischer P, Kaesmayr J. Echinacea for preventing and treating the common cold. *Cochrane Database Syst Rev* 2000;2:CD000530

28. Pepping J. Echinacea. *Am J Health-Syst Pharm* 1999;56:121–2

29. See DM, Broumand N, Sahl L, Tilles JG. *In vitro* effects of echinacea and ginseng on natural killer and antibody-dependent cell cytotoxicity in healthy subjects and chronic fatigue syndrome or acquired immunodeficiency syndrome patients. *Immunopharmacology* 1997;35:229–35

30. Rehman J, Dillow JM, Carter SM, Chou J, Le B, Maisel AS. Increased production of antigen-specific immunoglobulins G and M following *in vivo* treatment with the medicinal plants *Echinacea angustifolia* and *Hydrastis canadensis*. *Immunol Lett* 1999;68:391–5

31. Mengs U, Clare CB, Poiley JA. Toxicity of *Echinacea purpurea*. Acute, subacute and genotoxicity studies. *Arzneimittelforschung* 1991;41:1076–81

32. Gallo M, Sarkar M, Au W, *et al.* Pregnancy outcome following gestational exposure to echinacea: a prospective controlled study. *Arch Intern Med* 2000;160:3141–3

33. Mullins RJ. Echinacea-assoicated anaphylaxis. *Med J Aust* 1998;168:170–1

34. Boullata JI, Nace AM. Safety issues with herbal medicine. *Pharmacotherapy* 2000;20:257–69

35. Miller LG. Herbal medicinals: selected clinical considerations focusing on known or potential drug–herb interactions. *Arch Intern Med* 1998;158:2200–11

36. World Health Organization. *Herba Ephedra. WHO Monographs on Selected Medicinal Plants*, vol. 1. Geneva: World Health Organization, 1999:145–53

37. Blanck HM, Khan LK, Serdula MK. Use of nonprescription weight loss products: results from a multistate survey. *J Am Med Assoc* 2001;286:930–5

38. Astrup A, Breum L, Toubro S, Hein P, Quaade F. The effect and safety of an ephedrine/caffeine compound compared to ephedrine, caffeine, and placebo in obese subjects on an energy restricted diet: a double blind trial. *Int J Obes* 1992;16:269–77

39. Astrup A, Toubro S, Cannon S, Hein P, Madsen J. Thermogenic synergism between ephedrine and caffeine in healthy volunteers: a double-blind, placebo-controlled study. *Metabolism* 1991;40:323–9

40. Boozer CN, Nasser JA, Heymsfield SB, Wang V, Chen G, Solomon JL. An herbal supplement containing ma huang-guarana for weight loss: a randomized, double-blind trial. *Int J Obes* 2001;25:316–24

41. Bucci LR. Selected herbals and human exercise performance. *Am J Clin Nutr* 2000;72:624s–36s

42. Bell DG, Jacobs I, Zamecnik J. Effects of caffeine, ephedrine and their combination on time to exhaustion during high-intensity exercise. *Eur J Appl Physiol* 1998;77:427–33

43. Nightingale SL. From the Food and Drug Administration. *J Am Med Assoc* 1996;275:1534

44. Gurley BJ, Gardner SF, Hubbard MA. Content versus label claims in ephedra-containing dietary supplements. *Am J Health Syst Pharm* 2000;57:963–9

45. Hoffman BB, Lefkowitz RJ. Catecholamines, sympathomimetic drugs, and adrenergic receptor antagonists. In Hardman JG, Gilaman AG, Limbird LE, eds. *Goodman and Gilman's The Pharmacological Basis of Therapeutics*, 9th edn. New York, NY: McGraw-Hill, 1996:199–248

46. White LM, Gardner SF, Gurley BJ, Marx MA, Wang PL, Estes M. Pharmacokinetics and cardiovascular effects of ma-huang (*Ephedra sinica*) in normotensive adults. *J Clin Pharmacol* 1997;37:116–22

47. Gurley BJ, Gardner SF, White LM, Wang PL. Ephedrine pharmacokinetics after the ingestion of nutritional supplements containing *Ephedra sinica* (ma huang). *Ther Drug Monit* 1998;20:439–45

48. Haller CA, Benowitz NL. Adverse cardiovascular and central nervous system events associated with dietary supplements containing ephedra alkaloids. *N Engl J Med* 2000;343:1833–8

49. Nightingale SL. From the Food and Drug Administration. *J Am Med Assoc* 1997;278:15

50. Zaacks SM, Klein L, Tan CD, Rodriguez ER, Leikin JB. Hypersensitivity myocarditis associated with ephedra use. *J Toxicol Clin Toxicol* 1999;37:485–9

51. Powell T, Hsu FF, Turk J, Hruska K. Ma-huang strikes again: ephedrine nephrolithiasis. *Am J Kidney Dis* 1998;32:153–9

52. Anon. FDA backs away from elements of plan to regulate ephedrine supplements. *Am J Health-Syst Pharm* 2000;57:922

53. Koscielny J, Klussendorf D, Latza R, *et al*. The antiatherosclerotic effect of *Allium sativum*. *Atherosclerosis* 1999;144:237–49

54. Stevinson C, Pittler MH, Ernst E. Garlic for treating hypercholesterolemia: a meta-analysis of randomized clinical trials. *Ann Intern Med* 2000;133:420–9

55. Warshafsky S, Kamer RS, Sivak SL. Effect of garlic on total serum cholesterol. A meta-analysis. *Ann Intern Med* 1993;119:599–605

56. Mader FH. Treatment of hyperlipidaemia with garlic-powder tablets. Evidence from the German Association of General Practitioners' multicentric placebo-controlled double-blind study. *Arzneimittelforschung* 1990;40:1111–16

57. Gardner CD, Chatterjee LM, Carlson JJ. The effect of a garlic preparation on plasma lipid levels in moderately hypercholesterolemic adults. *Atherosclerosis* 2001;154:213–20

58. Berthold HK, Sudhop T, von Bergmann K. Effect of a garlic oil preparation on serum lipoproteins and cholesterol metabolism: a randomized controlled trial. *J Am Med Assoc* 1998;279:1900–2

59. Isaacsohn JL, Moser M, Stein EA, *et al*. Garlic powder and plasma lipids and lipoproteins: a multicenter, randomized, placebo-controlled trial. *Arch Intern Med* 1998;158:1189–94

60. McCrindle BW, Helden E, Conner WT. Garlic extract therapy in children with hypercholesterolemia. *Arch Pediatr Adolesc Med* 1998;152:1089–94

61. Gebhardt R. Multiple inhibitory effects of garlic extracts on cholesterol biosynthesis in hepatocytes. *Lipids* 1993;28:613–19

62. Steiner M, Lin RS. Changes in platelet function and susceptibility of lipoproteins to oxidation associated with administration of aged garlic extract. *J Cardiovasc Pharmacol* 1998;31:904–8

63. Kannar D, Wattanapenpaiboon N, Savige GS, Wahlqvist ML. Hypocholesterolemic effect of an enteric-coated garlic supplement. *J Am Coll Nutr* 2001;20:225–31

64. Ali M, Al-Qattan KK, Al-Enezi F, Khanafer RM, Mustafa T. Effect of allicin from garlic powder on serum lipids and blood pressure in rats fed with a high cholesterol diet. *Prostaglandins Leukot Essent Fatty Acids* 2000;62:253–9

65. Silagy CA, Neil HA. A meta-analysis of the effect of garlic on blood pressure. *J Hypertens* 1994;12:463–8

66. Ziaei S, Hantoshzadeh S, Rezasoltani P, Lamyian M. The effect of garlic tablet on plasma lipids and platelet aggregation in nulliparous pregnants at high risk of preeclampsia. *Eur J Obstet Gynecol Reprod Biol* 2001;99:201–6

67. Mohammad SF, Woodward SC. Characterization of a potent inhibitor of platelet aggregation and release reaction isolated from *Allium sativum* (garlic). *Thromb Res* 1986;44:793–806

68. Ariga T, Oshiba S, Tamada T. Platelet aggregation inhibitor in garlic [letter]. *Lancet* 1981;1:150–1

69. Boullin DJ. Garlic as a platelet inhibitor [letter]. *Lancet* 1981;1:776–7

70. Srivastava KC. Evidence for the mechanism by which garlic inhibits platelet aggregation. *Prostaglandins Leukot Med* 1986;22:313–21

71. Apitz-Castro R, Escalante J, Vargas R, Jain MK. Ajoene, the antiplatelet principle of garlic, synergistically potentiates the antiaggregatory action of prostacyclin, forskolin, indomethacin and dipyridamole on human platelets. *Thromb Res* 1986;42:303–11

72. Apitz-Castro R, Ledezma E, Escalante J, Jain MK. The molecular basis of the antiplatelet action of ajoene: direct interaction with the fibrinogen receptor. *Biochem Biophys Res Commun* 1986;141:145–50

73. Makheja AN, Bailey JM. Antiplatelet constituents of garlic and onion. *Agents Actions* 1990;29:360–3

74. Harenberg J, Giese C, Zimmerman R. Effect of dried garlic on blood coagulation, fibrinolysis, platelet aggregation and serum cholesterol levels in patients with hyperlipoproteinemia. *Atherosclerosis* 1988;74:247–9

75. Chutani SK, Bordia A. The effect of fried versus raw garlic on fibrinolytic activity in man. *Atherosclerosis* 1981;38:417–21

76. Kim-Park S, Ku DD. Garlic elicits a nitric oxide-dependent relaxation and inhibits hypoxic pulmonary vasoconstriction in rats. *Clin Exp Pharmacol Physiol* 2000;27:780–6

77. Das I, Khan NS, Sooranna SR. Potent activation of nitric oxide synthase by garlic: a basis for its therapeutic applications. *Curr Med Res Opin* 1995;13:257–63

78. Kaye AD, De Witt BJ, Anwar M, *et al*. Analysis of responses of garlic derivatives in the pulmonary valscular bed of the rat. *J Appl Physiol* 2000;89:353–8

79. Lawson LD, Ransom DK, Hughes BG. Inhibition of whole blood platelet-aggregation by compounds in garlic clove extracts and commercial garlic products. *Thromb Res* 1992;65:141–56

80. Dorant E, van den Brandt PA, Goldbohm RA, Hermus RJJ, Sturmans F. Garlic and its significance for the prevention of cancer in humans: a critical view. *Br J Cancer* 1993;67:424–9

81. Lawson LD, Wang ZJ. Pre-hepatic fate of the organosulfur compounds derived from garlic (*Allium sativum*). *Planta Med* 1993;59:A688–9 (abstr)

82. Lachmann G, Lorenz D, Radeck W, Steiper M. [The pharmacokinetics of S35 labeled garlic constituents alliin, allicin, and vinyldithiine.] *Arzneimittelforschung* 1994;44:734–43

83. Egen-Schwind C, Eckard R, Jekat FW, Winterhoff H. Pharmacokinetics of vinyldithiins, transformation products of allicin. *Planta Med* 1992;58:8–13

84. Rose KD, Croissant PD, Parliament CF, Levin MB. Spontaneous spinal epidural hematoma with associated platelet dysfunction from excessive garlic ingestion: a case report. *Neurosurgery* 1990:26:880–2

85. Anon. Garlic. In Blumenthal M, Goldberg A, Brinckmann J, eds. *Herbal Medicine – Expanded Commission E Monographs*, 1st edn. Newton, MA: Integrative Medical Communications, 2000:139–48

86. Agarwal KC. Therapeutic actions of garlic constituents. *Med Res Rev* 1996;16:111–24

87. Le Bars PL, Katz MM, Berman N, Itil TM, Freedman AM, Schatzberg AF. A placebo-controlled, double-blind, randomized trial of an extract of *Ginkgo biloba* for dementia. North American EGb Study Group. *J Am Med Assoc* 1997;278:1327–32

88. Oken BS, Storzbach DM, Kaye JA. The efficacy of *Ginkgo biloba* on cognitive function in Alzheimer disease. *Arch Neurol* 1998;55: 1409–15

89. Moulton PL, Boyko LN, Fitzpatrick JL, Petros TV. The effect of *Ginkgo biloba* on memory in healthy male volunteers. *Physiol Behav* 2001;73:659–65

90. Stough C, Clarke J, Lloyd J, Nathan PJ. Neuropsychological changes after 30-day *Ginkgo biloba* administration in healthy participants. *Int J Neuropsychopharmacol* 2001;4:131–4

91. Kennedy DO, Scholey AB, Wesnes KA. The dose-dependent cognitive effects of acute administration of *Ginkgo biloba* to healthy young volunteers. *Psychopharmacology (Berl)* 2000;151:416–23

92. Rigney U, Kimber S, Hindmarch I. The effects of acute doses of standardized *Ginkgo biloba* extract on memory and psychomotor performance in volunteers. *Phytother Res* 1999;13:408–15

93. Ernst E. [*Ginkgo biloba* in treatment of intermittent claudication. A systemic research based on controlled studies in the literature.] *Fortschr Med* 1996;114:85–7

94. Evans JR. *Ginkgo biloba* extract for age-related macular degeneration. *Cochrane Database Syst Rev* 2000:CD001775

95. Cesarani A, Meloni F, Alpini D, Barozzi S, Verderio L, Boscani PF. *Ginkgo biloba* (EGb 761) in the treatment of equilibrium disorders. *Adv Ther* 1998;15:291–304

96. Ernst E, Stevinson C. *Ginkgo biloba* for tinnitus: a review. *Clin Otolaryngol* 1999;24:164–7

97. Cohen AJ, Bartlik B. *Ginkgo biloba* for antidepressant-induced sexual dysfunction. *J Sex Marital Ther* 1998;24:139–43

98. Roncin JP, Schwartz F, D'Arbigny P. EGb 761 in control of acute mountain sickness and vascular reactivity to cold exposure. *Aviat Space Environ Med* 1996;67:445–52

99. Jung F, Mrowietz C, Kiesewetter H, Wenzel E. Effect of *Ginkgo biloba* on fluidity of blood and peripheral microcirculation in volunteers. *Arzneimittelforschung* 1990;40:589–93

100. Maitra I, Marcocci L, Droy-Lefaix MT, Packer L. Peroxyl radical scavenging activity of *Ginkgo biloba* extract EGb 761. *Biochem Pharmacol* 1995;49:1649–55

101. Hoyer S, Lannert H, Noldner M, Chatterjee SS. Damaged neuronal energy metabolism and behavior are improved by *Ginkgo biloba* extract (EGb 761). *J Neural Transm Gen Sect* 1999;106:1171–88

102. Huguet F, Tarrade T. Alpha 2-adrenoceptor changes during cerebral ageing. The effect of *Ginkgo biloba* extract. *J Pharm Pharmacol* 1992;44:24–7

103. Chung KF, Dent G, McCusker M, *et al.* Effect of a ginkgolide mixture (BN 52063) in antagonising skin and platelet responses to platelet activating factor in man. *Lancet* 1987;1:248–51

104. Oyama Y, Fuchs PA, Katayama N, Noda K. Myricetin and quercetin, the flavonoid constituents on *Ginkgo biloba* extract, greatly reduced oxidative metabolism in both resting and Ca(2+) loaded brain neurons. *Brain Res* 1994;635:125–9

105. Cheung F, Siow YL, Chen WZ, O K. Inhibitory effect of *Ginkgo biloba* on the expression of inducible nitric oxide synthase in endothelial cells. *Biochem Pharmacol* 1999;58:1665–73

106. Lamant V, Mauco G, Braquet P, Chap H, Douste-Blazy L. Inhibition of the metabolism of platelet activating factor (PAF-acether) by three specific antagonists from *Ginkgo biloba*. *Biochem Pharmacol* 1987;36:2749–52

107. Kornecki E, Ehrlich YH. Neuroregulatory and neuropathological actions of the ether–phospholipid platelet-activating factor. *Science* 1988;240:1792–4

108. Akisu M, Kultursay N, Coker I, Huseyinov A. Platelet-activating factor is an important mediator in hypoxic ischemic brain injury in the newborn rat. Flunarizine and *Ginkgo biloba* extract reduce PAF concentration in the brain. *Biol Neonate* 1998;74:439–44

109. Birkle DL, Kurian P, Braquet P, Bazan NG. Platelet-activating factor antagonist BN 52021 decreases accumulation of free polyunsaturated fatty acid in mouse brain during ischemia and electroconvulsive shock. *J Neurochem* 1988;51:1900–5

110. Umegaki K, Shinozuka K, Watarai K, *et al. Ginkgo biloba* extract attenuates the development of hypertension in deoxycorticosterone acetate-salt hypertensive rats. *Clin Exp Pharmacol Physiol* 2000;27:277–82

111. Sloley BD, Urichuk LJ, Morley P, *et al.* Identification of kaempferol as a monoamine oxidase inhibitor and potential neuroprotectant in extracts of *Ginkgo biloba* leaves. *J Pharm Pharmacol* 2000;52:451–9

112. Pardon MC, Joubert C, Perez-Diaz F, Christen Y, Launay JM, Cohen-Salmon C. *In vivo* regulation of cerebral monoamine oxidase activity in senescent controls and chronically stressed mice by long-term treatment with *Ginkgo biloba* extract (EGb 761). *Mech Ageing Dev* 2000;113:157–68

113. Fowler JS, Wang GJ, Volkow ND, *et al.* Evidence that *Ginkgo biloba* extract does not inhibit MAO A and MAO B in living human brain. *Life Sci* 2000;66:PL141–6

114. Watson DG, Oliveira EJ. Solid-phase extraction and gas chromatography–mass spectrometry determination of kaempferol and quercetin in human urine after consumption of *Ginkgo biloba* tablets. *J Chromatogr B Biomed Sci Appl* 1999;723:203–10

115. Anon. Ginkgo. In Mills S, Bone K, eds. *Principles and Practice of Phytotherapy*. New York, NY: Churchill Livingstone, 2000:404–17

116. Rowin J, Lewis SL. Spontaneous bilateral subdural hematomas associated with chronic *Ginkgo biloba* ingestion. *Neurology* 1996;46:1775–6

117. Vale S. Subarachnoid haemorrhage associated with *Ginkgo biloba*. *Lancet* 1998;352:36

118. Gilbert GJ. *Ginkgo biloba* [letter]. *Neurology* 1997;48:1137

119. Matthews MK Jr. Association of *Ginkgo biloba* with intracerebral hemorrhage [letter]. *Neurology* 1998;50:1933–4

120. Rosenblatt M, Mindel J. Spontaneous hyphema associated with ingestion of *Ginkgo biloba* extract [letter]. *N Engl J Med* 1997;336:1108

121. Fessenden JM, Wittenborn W, Clarke L. *Gingko biloba*: a case report of herbal medicine and bleeding postoperatively from a laparoscopic cholecystectomy. *Am Surg* 2001;67:33–5

122. Brekham II, Dardymov IV. New substances of plant origin which increase nonspecific resistance. *Annu Rev Pharmacol* 1969;9:419–30

123. Chong SK, Oberholzer VG. Ginseng – is there a use in clinical medicine? *Postgrad Med J* 1988;64:841–6

124. Wang BX, Cui JC, Liu AJ, Wu SK. Studies on the anti-fatigue effect of the saponins of stems and leaves of *Panax ginseng* (SSLG). *J Tradit Chin Med* 1983;3:89–4

125. Yang G, Yu Y. Immunopotentiating effect of traditional Chinese drugs – ginsenoside and glycyrrhiza polysaccharide. *Proc Chin Acad Med Sci Peking Union Med Coll* 1990;5:188–93

126. Shin HR, Kim JY, Yun TK, Morgan G, Vainio H. The cancer-preventive potential of *Panax ginseng*: a review of human and experimental evidence. *Cancer Causes Control* 2000;11:565–76

127. Chen X. Cardiovascular protection by ginsenosides and their nitric oxide releasing action. *Clin Exp Pharmacol Physiol* 1996;23:728–32

128. Vuksan V, Sievenpiper JL, Koo VY, *et al*. American ginseng (*Panax quinquefolius* L) reduces postprandial glycemia in nondiabetic subjects and subject with type 2 diabetes mellitus. *Arch Intern Med* 2000;160:1009–13

129. Lieberman HR. The effects of ginseng, ephedrine, and caffeine on cognitive performance, mood and energy. *Nutr Rev* 2001;59:91–102

130. Cho YK, Sung H, Lee HJ, Joo CH, Cho GJ. Long-term intake of Korean red ginseng in HIV-1-infected patients: development of resistance mutation to zidovudine is delayed. *Int Immunopharmacol* 2001;1:1295–305

131. Choi YD, Rha KH, Choi HK. *In vitro* and *in vivo* experimental effect of Korean red ginseng on erection. *J Urol* 1999;162:1508–11

132. Bahrke MS, Morgan WP. Evaluation of the ergogenic properties of ginseng. *Sports Med* 1994;18:229–48

133. Bahrke MS, Morgan WP. Evaluation of the ergogenic properties of ginseng: an update. *Sports Med* 2000;29:113–33

134. Vogler BK, Pittler MH, Ernst E. The efficacy of ginseng. A systematic review of randomised clinical trials. *Eur J Clin Pharmacol* 1999;55:567–75

135. Anon. Ginseng. In Blumenthal M, Busse WR, Goldberg A, *et al*., eds. *The Complete German Commission E Monographs: Therapeutic Guide to Herbal Medicines*, 1st edn. Boston, MA: Integrative Medical Communications, 1998

136. Attele AS, Wu JA, Yuan CS. Ginseng pharmacology: multiple constituents and multiple actions. *Biochem Pharmacol* 1999;58:1685–93

137. Benishin CG, Lee R, Wang LCH, Liu HJ. Effects of ginsenoside Rb1 on central cholinergic metabolism. *Pharmacology* 1991;42:223–9

138. Yamaguchi Y, Haruta K, Kobayashi H. Effects on ginsenosides on impaired performance induced in the rat by scopolamine in a radial-arm maze. *Psychoneuroendocrinology* 1995;20:645–53

139. Lim JH, Wen TC, Matsuda S, *et al*. Protection of ischemic hippocampal neurons by ginsenoside Rb1, a main ingredient of ginseng root. *Neurosci Res Suppl* 1997;28:191–200

140. Takemoto Y, Ueyama T, Saito H, *et al*. Potentiation of nerve growth factor-mediated nerve fiber production in organ cultures of chicken embryonic ganglia by ginseng saponins: structure–activity relationship. *Chem Pharm Bull (Tokyo)* 1984;32:3128–33

141. Mogil JS, Shin YH, McCleskey EW, Kim SC, Nah SY. Ginsenoside Rf, a trace component of ginseng root, produces antinociception in mice. *Brain Res* 1998;792:218–28

142. Nah JJ, Hahn JH, Chung S, Choi S, Kim YI, Nah SY. Effect of ginsenosides, active components of ginseng, on capsaicin-induced pain-related behavior. *Neuropharmacology* 2000;39:2180–4

143. Suh HW, Song DK, Huh SO, Kim YH. Modulatory role of ginsenosides injected intrathecally or intracerebroventricularly in the production of antinociception induced by kappa-opioid receptor agonist administered intracerebroventricularly in the mouse. *Planta Med* 2000;66:412–17

144. Huong NT, Matsumoto K, Yamasaki K, Duc NM, Nham NT, Watanabe H. Majonoside-R2, a major constituent of Vietnamese ginseng, attenuates opioid-induced antinociception. *Pharmacol Biochem Behav* 1997;57:285–91

145. Kimura T, Saunders PA, Kim HS, Rheu HM, Oh KW, Ho IK. Interactions of ginsenosides with ligand-bindings of GABA(A) and GABA(B) receptors. *Gen Pharmacol* 1994;25:193–9

146. Yuan CS, Attele AS, Wu JA, Liu D. Modulation of American ginseng on brainstem GABAergic effects rats. *J Ethnopharmacol* 1998;62:215–22

147. Tsang D, Yeung HW, Tso WW, Peck H. Ginseng saponins: influence of neurotransmitter uptake in rat brain synaptosomes. *Planta Med* 1985;3:221–4

148. Gillis CN. Panax ginseng pharmacology: a nitric oxide link. *Biochem Pharmacol* 1997;54:1–8

149. Siegel RK. Ginseng abuse syndrome. Problems with the panacea. *J Am Med Assoc* 1979;241:1614–15

150. Zhan Y, Xu XH, Jiang YP. [Protective effects of ginsenoside on myocardial ischemic and reperfusion injuries.] *Chung Hau I Hsueh Tsa Chih* 1994;74:626–8

151. Yun TK. Experimental and epidemiological evidence of the cancer-preventive effects of *Panax ginseng* C.A. Meyer. *Nutr Rev* 1996;54:S71–81

152. Yun YS, Moon HS, Oh YR, Jo SK, Kim YJ, Yun TK. Effect of red ginseng on natural killer cell activity in mice with lung adenoma induced by urethan and benzo(a)pyrene. *Cancer Detect Prev Suppl* 1987;1:301–9

153. Kim JY, Germolec DR, Luster MI. *Panax ginseng* as a potential immunomodulator: studies in mice. *Immunopharmacol Immunotoxicol* 1990;12:257–76

154. Kenarova B, Neychev H, Hadjiivanova C, Petkov VD. Immunomodulating activity of ginsenoside Rg1 from *Panax ginseng*. *Jpn J Pharmacol* 1990;54:447–54

155. Scaglione F, Cattaneo G, Alessandria M, Cogo R. Efficacy and safety of the standardised Ginseng extract G115 for potentiating vaccination against the influenza syndrome and protection against the common cold. *Drugs Exp Clin Res* 1996;22:65–72

156. Chen SE, Sawchuk RJ, Staba EJ. American ginseng. III. Pharmacokinetics of ginsenosides in the rabbit. *Eur J Drug Metab Pharmacokinet* 1980;5:161–8

157. Hopkins MP, Androff L, Benninghoff AS. Ginseng face cream and unexplained vaginal bleeding. *Am J Obstet Gynecol* 1988;159:1121–2

158. Palop-Larrea V, Gonzalvez-Perales JL, Catalan-Oliver C, Belenguer-Varea A, Martinez-Mir I. Metrorrhagia and ginseng [letter]. *Ann Pharmacother* 2000;34:1347–8

159. Greenspan EM. Ginseng and vaginal bleeding [letter]. *J Am Med Assoc* 1983;249:2018

160. Punnonen R, Lukola A. Oestrogen-like effect of ginseng. *Br Med J* 1980;281:1110

161. Jones BD, Runikis AM. Interaction of ginseng with phenelzine [letter]. *J Clin Psychopharmacol* 1987;7:201–2

162. Ryu SJ, Chien YY. Ginseng-associated cerebral arteritis. *Neurology* 1995;45:829–30

163. Janetzky K, Morreale AP. Probable interaction between warfarin and ginseng. *Am J Health-Sys Pharm* 1997;54:692–3

164. Kimura Y, Okuda H, Arichi S. Effects of various ginseng saponins on 5-hydroxytryptamine release and aggregation in human platelets. *J Pharm Pharmacol* 1988;40:838–43

165. Kuo SC, Teng CM, Lee JC, Ko FN, Chen SC, Wu TS. Antiplatelet components in *Panax ginseng*. *Planta Med* 1990;56:164–7

166. Park HJ, Lee JH, Song YB, Park KH. Effects of dietary supplementation of lipophilic fraction from *Panax ginseng* on cGMP and cAMP in rat platelets and on blood coagulation. *Biol Pharm Bull* 1996;19:1434–9

167. Anon. Ginseng. In Gruenwald J, Brendler T, Jaenicke C, eds. *PDR for Herbal Medicines*, 2nd edn. Montvale, NJ: Medical Economics Company, 2000:346–51

168. Anon. Kava. *Lancet* 1988;2:258–9

169. Cawte J. Parameters of kava used as a challenge to alcohol. *Aust N Z J Psychiatry* 1986;20:70–6

170. Cawte J. Macabre effects of a 'cult' for kava [editorial]. *Med J Aust* 1988;148:545–6

171. Mathews JD, Riley MD, Fejo L, *et al.* Effects of the heavy usage of kava on physical health: summary of a pilot survey in an aboriginal community. *Med J Aust* 1988;148:548–55

172. Herberg KW. [Effect of Kava-Special Extract WS 1490 combined with ethyl alcohol on safety-relevant performance parameters]. *Blutalkohol* 1993;30:96–105

173. Volz HP, Kieser M. Kava-kava extract WS 1490 versus placebo in anxiety disorders – a randomized placebo-controlled 25-week outpatient trial. *Pharmacopsychiatry* 1997;30:1–5

174. Neuhaus W, Ghaemi Y, Schmidt T, Lehmann E. [Treatment of perioperative anxiety in suspected breast carcinoma with a phytogenic tranquilizer]. *Zentralbl Gynakol* 2000;122:561–5

175. De Leo V, La Marca A, Lanzetta D, *et al.* [Assessment of the association of kava-kava extract and hormone replacement therapy in the treatment of postmenopause anxiety.] *Minerva Ginecol* 2000;52:263–7

176. Pittler MH, Ernst E. Efficacy of kava extract for treating anxiety: systematic review and meta-analysis. *J Clin Psychopharmacol* 2000;20:84–9

177. Jussofie A, Schmiz A, Hiemke C. Kavapyrone enriched extract from *Piper methysticum* as modulator of the GABA binding site in different regions of rat brain. *Psychopharmacology (Berl)* 1994;116:469–74

178. Keledjian J, Duffield PH, Jamieson DD, Lidgard RO, Duffield AM. Uptake into mouse brain of four compounds present in the psychoactive beverage kava. *J Pharm Sci* 1988;77:1003–6

179. Rasmussen AK, Scheline RR, Solheim E, Hansel R. Metabolism of some kava pyrones in the rat. *Xenobiotica* 1979;9:1–16

180. Cheng D, Lidgard RO, Duffield PH, Duffield AM, Brophy JJ. Identification by methane chemical ionization has chromatography/mass spectrometry of the products obtained by steam distillation and aqueous extraction of commercial *Piper methysticum*. *Biomed Environ Mass Spectrom* 1988;17:371–6

181. Klohs MW. Chemistry of kava. *Psychopharmacol Bull* 1967;4:10

182. Meyer HJ. Pharmacology of kava – 1. *Psychopharmacol Bull* 1967;4:10–11

183. Buckley JP, Furgiuele AR, O'Hara MJ. Pharmacology of kava – 2. *Psychopharmacol Bull* 1967;4:11–12

184. Backhauss C, Krieglstein J. Extract of kava (*Piper methysticum*) and its methysticin constituents protect brain tissue against ischemic damage in rodents. *Eur J Pharmacol* 1992;215:265–9

185. Heinze HJ, Munthe TF, Steitz J, Matzke M. Pharmacopsychological effects of oxazepam and kava-extract in a visual search paradigm assessed with event-related potentials. *Pharmacopsychiatry* 1994;27:224–30

186. Munte TF, Heinze HJ, Matzke M, Steitz J. Effects of oxazepam and an extract of kava roots (*Piper methysticum*) on event-related potentials in a word recognition task. *Neuropsychobiology* 1993;27:46–53

187. Jamieson DD, Duffield PH, Cheng D, Duffield AM. Comparison of the central nervous system activity of the aqueous and lipid extract of kava (*Piper methysticum*). *Arch Int Pharmacodyn Ther* 1989;301:66–80

188. Davies LP, Drew CA, Duffield P, Johnston GAR, Jamieson DD. Kava pyrones and resin: studies on GABA(A), GABA(B), and benzodiazepine binding sites in rodent brain. *Pharmacol Toxicol* 1992;71:120–6

189. Friese J, Gleitz J. Kavain, dihydrokavain and dihydromethysticin non-competitively inhibit the specific binding of [^{3}H]-batrachotoxinin-A 20-α-benzoate to receptor site 2 of voltage-gated Na$^+$ channels. *Planta Med* 1998;64:458–9

190. Magura EI, Kopanitsa MV, Gleitz J, Peters T, Krishtal OA. Kava extract ingredients, (+)-methystin and (±)-kavain inhibit voltage-operated Na(+)-channels in rat CA1 hippocampal neurons. *Neuroscience* 1997;81:345–51

191. Gleitz J, Friese J, Beile A, Ameri A, Peters T. Anticonvulsive action of (±)-kavain estimated from its properties on stimulated synaptosomes and Na$^+$ channel receptor sites. *Eur J Pharmacol* 1996;315:89–97

192. Gleitz J, Beile A, Peters T. (±)-Kavain inhibits veratridine-activated voltage-dependent Na(+) channels in synaptosomes prepared from rat cerebral cortex. *Neuropharmacology* 1995;34:1133–8

193. Baum SS, Hill R, Rommelspacher H. Effect of kava extract and individual kavapyrones on neurotransmitter levels in the nucleus accumbens of rats. *Prog Neuropsychopharmacol Biol Psychiatry* 1998;22:1105–20

194. Schelosky L, Raffauf C, Jendroska K, Poewe W. Kava and dopamine antagonism [letter]. *J Neurol Neurosurg Psychiatry* 1995;58:639–40

195. Pepping J. Kava: *Piper methysticum*. *Am J Health-Syst Pharm* 1999;56:957–8,960

196. Almeida JC, Grimsley EW. Coma from the health food store: interaction between kava and alprazolam. *Ann Intern Med* 1996;125:940–1

197. Norton SA, Ruze P. Kava dermopathy. *J Am Acad Dermatol* 1994;31:89–97

198. Anon. Kava kava. In Gruenwald J, Brendler T, Jaenicke C, eds. *PDR for Herbal Medicines*, 2nd edn. Montvale, NJ: Medical Economics Company, 2000:443–6

199. Ferenci P, Dragosics B, Dittrich H, *et al.* Randomized controlled trial of silymarin treatment in patients with cirrhosis of the liver. *J Hepatol* 1989;9:105–13

200. Lang I, Nekam K, Deak G, *et al.* Immunomodulatory and hepatoprotective effects of *in vivo* treatment with free radical scavengers. *Ital J Gastroenterol* 1990;22:283–7

201. Salmi HA, Sarna S. Effect of silymarin on chemical, functional, and morphological alterations of the liver. A double-blind controlled study. *Scand J Gastroenterol* 1982;17:517–21

202. Magliulo E, Gagliardi B, Fiori GP. [Results of a double blind study on the effect of silymarin in the treatment of acute viral hepatitis, carried out at two medical centres (author's transl)]. *Med Klin* 1978;73:1060–5

203. Pares A, Planas R, Torres M, *et al.* Effects of silymarin in alcoholic patients with cirrhosis of the liver: results of a controlled, double-blind, randomized and multicenter trial. *J Hepatol* 1998;28:615–21

204. Bunout D, Hirsch S, Petermann M, *et al.* [Controlled study of the effect of silymarin on alcoholic liver disease.] *Rev Med Chil* 1992;120:1370–5

205. Trinchet JC, Coste T, Levy VG, *et al.* [Treatment of alcoholic hepatitis with silymarin. A double-blind comparative study in 116 patients.] *Gastroenterol Clin Biol* 1989;13:120–4

206. Saller R, Meier R, Brignoli R. The use of silymarin in the treatment of liver diseases. *Drugs* 2001;61:2035–63

207. Dehmlow C, Murawski N, de Groot H. Scavenging of reactive oxygen species and inhibition of arachidonic acid metabolism by silibinin in human cells. *Life Sci* 1996;58:1591–600

208. Bindoli A, Cavallini L, Siliprandi N. Inhibitory action of silymarin of lipid peroxide formation in rat liver mitochondria and microsomes. *Biochem Pharmacol* 1977;26:2405–9

209. Feher J, Lang I, Nekam K, Csomos G, Muzes G, Deak G. Effect of silibinin on the activity and expression of superoxide dismutase in lymphocytes from patients with chronic alcoholic liver disease. *Free Radic Res Commun* 1987;3:373–7

210. Tuchweber B, Sieck R, Trost W. Prevention of silybin of phalloidin-induced acute hepatoxicity. *Toxicol Appl Pharmacol* 1979;51:265–75

211. Magliulo E, Carosi PG, Minoli L. Gorini S. Studies on the regenerative capacity of the liver in rats subjected to partial hepatectomy and treated with silymarin. *Arzneimittelforschung* 1973;23:161–7

212. Pepping J. Milk thistle: *Silybum marianum. Am J Health-Syst Pharm* 1999;56:1195–7

213. Walti M, Neftel KA, Cohen M, Winkler P, de Weck AL. [Radioimmunologic detection of IgE and IgG antibodies against drugs. Conclusions after experience with over 1200 patients.] *Schweiz Med Wochenschr* 1986;116:303–5

214. Berry SL, Coffey DS, Walsh PC, Ewing LL. The development of human benign prostatic hyperplasia with age. *J Urol* 1984;132:474–9

215. Buck AC. Phytotherapy for the prostate. *Br J Urol* 1996;78:325–36

216. Wilt T, Ishani A, Stark G, *et al. Serenoa repens* for benign prostatic hyperplasia. *Cochrane Database Syst Rev* 2000;(2)CD001423

217. Gerber GS. Saw palmetto for the treatment of men with lower urinary tract symptoms. *J Urol* 2000;163:1408–12

218. Gerber GS, Zagaja GP, Bales GT, Chodak GW, Contreras BA. Saw palmetto (*Serenoa repens*) in men with lower urinary tract symptoms: effects on urodynamic parameters and voiding symptoms. *Urology* 1998;51:1003–7

219. Anon. Saw palmetto berry. In Blumenthal M, Goldberg A, Brinckmann J, eds. *Herbal Medicine – Expanded Commission E Monographs*, 1st edn. Newton, MA: Integrative Medical Communications, 2000:335–40

220. Ichle C, Delos S, Guirou O, Tate R, Raynaud JP, Martin PM. Human prostatic steroid 5 alpha-reductase isoforms – a comparative study of selective inhibitors. *J Steroid Biochem Mol Biol* 1995;54:273–9

221. Plosker GL, Brogden RN. *Serenoa repens* (Permixon). A review of its pharmacology and therapeutic efficacy in benign prostatic hyperplasia. *Drugs Aging* 1996;9:379–95

222. Di Silverio F, D'Eramo G, Lubrano C, *et al.* Evidence that *Serenoa repens* extract displays an antiestrogenic activity in prostatic tissue of benign prostatic hypertrophy patients. *Eur Urol* 1992;21:309–14

223. Vacher P, Prevarskaya N, Skyrma R, *et al.* The lipidosterolic extract from *Serenoa repens* interferes with prolactin receptor signal transduction. *J Biomed Sci* 1995;2:357–65

224. Paubert-Braquet M, Cousse H, Raynaud JP, *et al.* Effect of the lipidosterolic extract of *Serenoa repens* (Permixon) and its major components on basic fibroblast growth factor-induced proliferation of cultures of human prostate biopsies. *Eur Urol* 1998;33:340–7

225. Vacherot F, Azzouz M, Gil-Diez-de-Medina S, *et al.* Induction of apoptosis and inhibition of cell proliferation by the lipodo-sterolic extract of *Serenoa repens* (LSESr, Permixon) in benign prostatic hyperplasia. *Prostate* 2000;45:259–66

226. Goepel M, Hecker U, Krege S, Rubben H, Michel MC. Saw palmetto extracts potently and noncompetitively inhibit human alpha-1-adrenoceptors *in vitro*. *Prostate* 1999;38:208–15

227. Brue W, Hagenlocer M, Redl K, Tittel G, Stadler F, Wagner H. [Anti-inflammatory activity of sabal fruit extracts prepared with supercritical carbon dioxide. *In vitro* antagonists of cyclooxygenase and 5-lipooxygenase metabolism.] *Arzneimittelforschung* 1992;42:547–51

228. Paubert-Braquet M, Mencia Huerta JM, Cousse H, Braquet P. Effect of the lipidic lipidosterolic extract of *Serenoa repens* (Permixon) on the ionophore A23187-stimulated production of leukotriene B4 (LTB4) from human polymorphonuclear neutrophils. *Prostaglandins Leukot Essent Fatty Acids* 1997;57:299–304

229. Cheema P, El-Mefty O, Jazieh AR. Intraoperative haemorrhage associated with the use of extract of saw palmetto herb: a case report and review of literature. *J Intern Med* 2001;250:167–9

230. Whiskey E, Werneke U, Taylor D. A systematic review and meta-analysis of *Hypericum perforatum* in depression: a comprehensive clinical review. *Int Clin Psychopharmacol* 2001;16:239–52

231. Kim HL, Streltzer J, Goebert D. St. John's wort for depression: a meta-analysis of well-defined clinical trials. *J Nerv Ment Dis* 1999;187:532–8

232. Linde K, Ramirez G, Mulrow CD, Pauls A, Weidenhammer W, Melchart D. St John's wort for depression – an overview and meta-analysis of randomised clinical trials. *Br Med J* 1996;313:253–8

233. Williams JW Jr, Mulrow CD, Chiquette E, Noel PH, Aguilar C, Cornell J. A systematic review of newer pharmacotherapies for depression in adults: evidence report summary. *Ann Intern Med* 2000;132:743–56

234. Hippius H. St. John's Wort (*Hypericum perforatum*) – a herbal antidepressant. *Curr Med Res Opin* 1998;14:171–84

235. Gaster B, Holroyd J. St John's wort for depression: a systematic review. *Arch Intern Med* 2000;160:152–6

236. Stevinson C, Ernst E. Hypericum for depression. An update of the clinical evidence. *Eur Neuropsychopharmacol* 1999;9:501–5

237. Josey ES, Tackett RL. St. John's wort: a new alternative for depression? *Int J Clin Pharmacol Ther* 1999;37:111–19

238. Kelly BD. St. John's wort for depression: what's the evidence? *Hosp Med* 2001;62:274–6

239. Shelton RC, Keller MB, Gelenberg A, *et al.* Effectiveness of St John's wort in major depression: a randomized controlled trial. *J Am Med Assoc* 2001;285:1978–86

240. Vitiello B. *Hypericum perforatum* extracts as potential antidepressants. *J Pharm Pharmacol* 1999;51:513–17

241. Deltito J, Beyer D. The scientific, quasi-scientific and popular literature on the use of St. John's wort in the treatment of depression. *J Affect Disord* 1998;51:345–51

242. Nangia M, Syed W, Doraiswamy PM. Efficacy and safety of St. John's wort for the treatment of major depression. *Public Health Nutr* 2000;3:487–94

243. Field HL, Monti DA, Greeson JM, Kunkel EJ. St. John's wort. *Int J Psychiatry Med* 2000;30:203–19

244. Muller WE, Singer A, Wonnemann M, Hafner U, Rolli M, Schafer C. Hyperforin represents the neurotransmitter reuptake inhibiting constituent of hypericum extract. *Pharmacopsychiatry* 1998;31(Suppl 1):16–21

245. Cott JM. *In vitro* receptor binding and enzyme inhibition by *Hypericum perforatum* extract. *Pharmacopsychiatry* 1997;30(Suppl 2):108–12

246. Verotta L, Appendino G, Jakupovic J, Bombardelli E. Hyperforin analogues from St. John's wort (*Hypericum perforatum*). *J Nat Prod* 2000;63:412–15

247. Calapai G, Crupi A, Firenzuoli F, *et al. Pharmacopsychiatry* 2001;34:45–9

248. Franklin M, Chi J, McGavin C, *et al.* Neuroendocrine evidence for dopaminergic actions of hypericum extract (LI 160) in healthy volunteers. *Biol Psychiatry* 1999;46:581–4

249. Apaydin S, Zeybek U, Ince I, *et al. Hypercium triquetrifolium* Turra extract exhibits antinociceptive activity in the mouse. *J Ethnopharmacol* 1999;67:307–12

250. Bladt S, Wagner H. Inhibition of MAO by fractions and constituents of hypericum extract. *J Geriatr Psychiatry Neurol* 1994;7(Suppl 1):S57–9

251. Thiede HM, Walper A. Inhibition of MAO and COMT by hypericum extracts and hypericin. *J Geriatr Psychiatry Neurol* 1994;7(Suppl 1):S54–6

252. Kerb R, Brockmoller J, Staffeldt B, Ploch M, Roots I. Single-dose and steady-state pharmacokinetics of hypericin and pseudohypericin. *Antimicrob Agents Chemother* 1996;40:2087–93

253. Biber A, Fischer H, Romer A, Chatterjee SS. Oral bioavailability of hyperforin from hypericum extracts in rats and human volunteers. *Pharmacopsychiatry* 1998;31(Suppl 1):36–43

254. Beckman SE, Sommi RW, Switzer J. Consumer use of St. John's wort: a survey on effectiveness, safety, and tolerability. *Pharmacotherapy* 2000;20:568–74

255. Schulz V. Incidence and clinical relevance of the interaction and side effects of *Hypericum* preparations. *Phytomedicine* 2001;8:152–60

256. Brown TM. Acute St. John's wort toxicity [letter]. *Am J Emerg Med* 2000;18:231–2

257. Lantz MS, Buchalter E, Giambanco V. St. John's wort and antidepressant drug interactions in the elderly. *J Geriatr Psychiatry Neurol* 1999;12:7–10

258. Barbenel DM, Yusufi B, O'Shea D, Bench CJ. Mania in a patient receiving testosterone replacement postorchidectomy taking St. John's wort and sertraline. *J Psychopharmacol* 2000;14:84–6

259. Moses EL, Mallinger AG. St. John's wort: three cases of possible mania induction. *J Clin Psychopharmacol* 2000;20:115–17

260. Nierenberg AA, Burt T, Matthews J, Weiss AP. Mania associated with St. John's wort. *Biol Psychiatry* 1999;46:1707–8

261. Obach RS. Inhibition of human cytochrome P450 enzymes by constituents of St. John's wort, an herbal preparation used in the treatment of depression. *J Pharmacol Exp Ther* 2000;294:88–95

262. Ernst E. Second thoughts about safety of St. John's wort. *Lancet* 1999;354:2014–16

263. Piscitelli SC, Burstein AH, Chaitt D, Alfaro RM, Falloon J. Indinavir concentrations and St. John's wort. *Lancet* 2000;355:547–8

264. Yue QY. Bergquist C, Gerden B. Safety of St. John's wort [letter]. *Lancet* 2000;355:576–7

265. Breidenbach T, Hoffmann MW, Becker T, Schlitt H, Klempnauer J. Drug interaction of St. John's wort with cyclosporine [letter]. *Lancet* 2000;355:1912

266. Ruschitzka F, Meier PJ, Turina M, Luscher TF, Noll G. Acute heart transplant rejection due to Saint John's wort [letter]. *Lancet* 2000;355:548–9

267. Johne A, Brockmoller J, Bauer S, Maurer A, Langheinrich M, Roots I. Pharmacokinetic interaction of digoxin with an herbal extract from St. John's wort (*Hypericum perforatum*). *Clin Pharmacol Ther* 1999;66:338–45

268. Anon. St. John's wort. In Blumenthal M, Goldberg A, Brinckmann J, eds. *Herbal Medicine – Expanded Commission E Monographs*, 1st edn. Newton, MA: Integrative Medical Communications, 2000:359–66

269. Houghton PJ. The scientific basis for the reputed activity of valerian. *J Pharm Pharmacol* 1999;51:505–12

270. Hendriks H, Bos R, Allersma DP, Malingre TM, Koster AS. Pharmacological screening of valerenal and some other components of essential oil of *Valeriana officinalis. Planta Med* 1981;42:62–8

271. Leuschner J, Muller J, Rudmann M. Characterization of the central nervous depressant activity of a commercially available valerian root extract. *Arzneimittelforschung* 1993;43:638–41

272. Sakamoto T, Mitani Y, Nakajima K. Psychotropic effects of Japanese valerian root extract. *Chem Pharm Bull (Tokyo)* 1992;40:758–61

273. Hazelhoff B, Malingre TM, Meijer DKF. Antispasmodic effects of valeriana compounds: an *in-vivo* and *in-vitro* study on the guinea-pig ileum. *Arch Int Pharmacodyn Ther* 1982;257:274–87

274. Vonderheid-Guth B, Todorova A, Brattstrom A, Dimpfel W. Pharmacodynamic effects of valerian and hops extract combination (Ze 91019) on the quantitative-topographical EEG in healthy volunteers. *Eur J Med Res* 2000;5:139–44

275. Leathwood PD, Chauffard F. Aqueous extract of valerian reduces latency to fall asleep in man. *Planta Med* 1985;2:144–8

276. Balderer G, Borbely AA. Effect of valerian on human sleep. *Psychopharmacology (Berl)* 1985;87:406–9

277. Leathwood PD, Chauffard F. Quantifying the effects of mild sedatives. *J Psychiat Res* 1982/83;17:115–22

278. Leathwood PD, Chauffard F, Heck E, Munoz-Box R. Aqueous extract of valerian root (*Valeriana officinalis* L.) improves sleep quality in man. *Pharmacol Biochem Behav* 1982;17:65–71

279. Donath F, Quispe S, Diefenbach K, Maurer A, Fietze I, Roots I. Critical evaluation of the effect of valerian extract on sleep structure and sleep quality. *Pharmacopsychiatry* 2000;33:47–53

280. Ortiz JG, Nieves-Natal J, Chavez P. Effects of *Valeriana officinalis* extracts on [³H]flunitrazepam binding, synaptosomal [³H]GABA uptake, and hippocampal [³H]GABA release. *Neurochem Res* 1999;24:1373–8

281. Santos MS, Ferreira F, Cunha AP, Carvalho AP, Ribeiro CF, Macedo T. Synaptosomal GABA release as influenced by valerian root extract – involvement of the GABA carrier. *Arch Int Pharmacodyn Ther* 1994;327:220–31

282. Santos MS, Ferreira F, Cunha AP, Carvalho AP, Macedo T. An aqueous extract of valerian influences the transport of GABA in synaptosomes [letter]. *Planta Med* 1994;60:278–9

283. Garges HP, Varia I, Doraiswamy PM. Cardiac complications and delirium associated with valerian root withdrawal [letter]. *J Am Med Assoc* 1998;280:1566–7

284. Kuhlmann J, Berger W, Podzuweit H, Schmidt U. The influence of valerian treatment on 'reaction time, alertness and concentration' in volunteers. *Pharmacopsychiatry* 1999;32:235–41

285. Anon. Valerian. In Gruenwald J, Brendler T, Jaenicke C, eds. *PDR for Herbal Medicines*, 2nd edn. Montvale, NJ: Medical Economics Company, 2000:783–6

286. Andreatini R, Leite JR. Effect of valepotriates on the behavior of rats in the elevated plus-maze during diazepam withdrawal. *Eur J Pharmacol* 1994;260:233–5

Other commonly used herbs

2

L. Dey and C.-S. Yuan

The preceding chapter discussed 11 most commonly used herbal medications, which account for over 50% of all single herb preparations among the 1500–1800 herbs sold in the USA. Table 1 is a brief summary of an additional 26 commonly used herbs in the USA.

Table 1 An additional 26 herbs commonly used in the USA

Herb	Actions	Common uses	Daily dose	Adverse effects/warnings
Bilberry, *Vaccinium myrtillus*	antioxidant; collagen stabilizer; astringent	eye disorder; diarrhea; circulatory disorders	60–120 mg anthocyanosides; 25% extract 240–480 mg	not reported
Black cohosh, *Cimicifuga racemosa*	estrogen receptor blocker; leutinizing hormone suppressant	menopausal symptoms; menstrual disorders	standard dose 40 mg; one product contained 1 mg triterpine glycosides	GI upset; avoid during pregnancy and lactation
Cascara sagrada, *Rhamnus purshiana*	laxative	constipation	20–30 mg hydroxyanthracene (cascaroside A)	nausea; vomiting; abdominal cramps; urine discoloration; avoid during pregnancy and lactation
Cat's claw, *Uncaria tomentosa*	immune stimulant; anti-inflammatory	arthritis; cancer; HIV	20–60 mg standardized dry extract	autoimmune illness; multiple sclerosis; avoid during pregnancy and lactation
Cayenne, *Capsicum annum*	substance P blocker; decreases lipids; decreases platelet aggregation	arthritis; muscle pain; neuralgia; post-mastectomy pain; psoriasis	0.025–0.075% extract; topical use	eye irritation; burning sensation; gastritis; diarrhea
Chamomile, *Matricaria recutita, Matricaria chamomilla*	antispasmodic effect; sedative effect; anti-inflammatory	GI complaints; skin inflammations; insomnia; stress and anxiety	3–4 cups of tea as needed; 0.9–2 g capsules; topical use	avoid if allergy to a member of daisy family (Asteraceae) such as ragweed, asters, chrysanthemums
Chaste tree, *Vitex agnus castus*	prolactin inhibitor; dopamine agonist; progestrogenic	menstrual disorder; promotion of lactation; infertlity	30–40 mg extract; 1–5 ml diluted tincture; 1–4 ml diluted extract; 1000 mg tablets	generally not significant; avoid during pregnancy and lactation
Cranberry, *Vaccinium macrocarpon*	antibacterial action	urinary tract infections	360–960 ml liquid; 300–400 mg standardized extract	not reported
Devil's claw, *Harpagophytum procumbens*	anti-inflammatory; analgesic; antirheumatic	rheumatic and arthritic conditions	400–500 mg extract	mild GI disturbances

continued

Table 1 *continued*

Herb	*Actions*	*Common uses*	*Daily dose*	*Adverse effects/warnings*
Dong quai, *Angelica sinensis*	phytoestrogen, antimicrobial effects; smooth muscle relaxant; IgE inhibition	dysmenorrhea; menopause symptoms; allergies	1–2 g dried root, 9–15 ml tincture	photodermatitis; uterine stimulant; contraindicated in the first trimester of pregnancy
Evening primose, *Oenothera biennis*	source of GLA	inflammation; premenstrual syndrome; menopause; fibrocystic breast; eczema	1.5–8 g	headache; GI symptoms; interaction with phenothiazines
Feverfew, *Tanacetum parthenium*	decreases platelet aggregation; smooth muscle relaxant; decreases prostaglandin from platelets and white blood cells	migraine prophylaxis and treatment	50–100 mg; 125 mg dried leaves or 2 fresh leaves	oral ulcers; rash; rebound migraine; avoid during pregnancy and lactation; interactions with warfarin
Flax seed, *Linum usitatissimum*	laxative; anticholesterolemic; anti-inflammatory	eczema; skin inflammation; hypertension; diabetes	1–6 tablespoons/day (58% standardized α-linolenic acid)	nausea; vomiting; diarrhea; hypersensitivity; avoid during pregnancy and lactation
Ginger, *Zingiber officinale*	antiemetic; positive inotropic	dyspepsia; emesis; loss of appetite; motion sickness	0.75–4.0 g extract	heartburn; avoid during pregnancy and lactation
Goldenseal, *Hidrastis canadensis*	antimicrobial	cold; diarrhea	0.75–1.5 g	mouth irritation; avoid during pregnancy and in diabetic patients
Grape seed extract, *Vitis vinifera*	antioxdant; antimutagenic; anti-inflammatory	retinopathy; allergies; prevention of atherosclerosis; cancer	40–80 mg of extract	not reported
Green tea, *Camellia sinensis*	antioxidant, stimulation of CNS; antibacterial; antimutagenic; cholestrol-lowering effect; inhibition of cell proliferation	cancer prevention; tumor progression; cardiovascular diseases; AIDS	6–10 cups; 3 capsules of standardized extract	insomnia; avoid during pregnancy and lactation
Hawthorn, *Crataegus laevigata*	cardiac glycoside effect; coronary dilatation; decrease peripheral resistance; ACE inhibition; mild diuretic; collagen stabilizer	congestive heart failure; hypertension; angina	0.9–2.3 g standardized extract	hypotension; arrhythmia
Hop, *Humulus lupulus*	sedative; antimicrobial	insomnia; nervous tension	0.5–1.0 g extract	allergic dermatitis; respiratory allergy; anaphylaxis; avoid during pregnancy and lactation
Horse chestnut, *Aesculus hippo castanum*	reduces lysozomal activity; improve venous tone; inhibits capillary permeability; diuretic	chronic venous insufficiency; hematoma; varicose veins; hemorrhoids	100–150 mg extract; topical use	pruritus; nausea; stomach complaints; bleeding; nephropathy; allergic reactions; avoid during pregnancy and lactation

continued

Table 1 *continued*

Herb	Actions	Common uses	Daily dose	Adverse effects/warnings
Licorice root, *Glycyrrhiza glabra*	laxative; expectorant; antispasmodic; anti-inflammatory; antimicrobial; estrogenic; adrenocorticotropic	gastric ulcer; catarrhs; cancer prevention; inflammation; antioxidation	750–1500 mg	nausea; vomiting; hypertension; edema; headache; weakness; hypokalemia; anorexia; hypersensitivity; avoid during pregnancy and lactation
Milk thistle, *Silybum marianum*	protection of hepatocytes; radical scavenger	liver diseases such as hepatitis, alcoholic cirrhosis	600 mg extract (70% silymarin)	diarrhea; avoid during pregnancy and lactation
Pycnogenol, *Pinus maritima*	antioxidant and antitumor actions; inhibition of tumor necrosis factor-α; inhibition of smoking-induced platelet aggregation	cardiac and cerebral infarction; antitumor; inflammation	not specified	avoid during pregnancy, lactation and in children
Soy, *Glycine max*	phytoestrogen; anticancer; anticholesterol	postmenopausal symptoms; prevention of osteoporosis and cancer; hypercholesterolemia	25–60 g of soy protein or 60 mg of isoflavones	nausea; bloating; diarrhea; abdominal pain; hypersensitivity reaction
Willow, *Salix* spp.	antipyretic; analgesic	fever; pain; rheumatic disorders	120–140 mg salicin	avoid during pregnancy and lactation, patients with salicylate intolerance; interaction with anticoagulants
Yohimbe, *Pausinystalia yohimbe*	penile vasodilatation via peripheral α_2 adreno receptor antagonism	erectile dysfunction	16–18 mg of yohimbine hydrochloride	nausea and vomiting; anxiety; hypertension; tachycardia; bronchospasm; avoid during pregnancy and lactation, and in psychiatric patients

GI, gastrointestinal; IgE, immunoglobulin E; GLA, γ-linoleic acid; CNS, central nervous system; ACE, angiotensin converting enzyme

Bibliography

Ernst E. *The Desktop Guide to Complementary and Alternative Medicine: an Evidence-based Approach*. London, UK: Harcourt Publishers, 2001

Foster S, Tyler VE. *Tyler's Honest Herbal: A Sensible Guide to the Use of Herbs and Related Remedies*. Binghamton, NY: The Haworth Herbal Press, 1999

Mills S, Bone K. *Principles and Practice of Phytotherapy: Modern Herbal Medicine*. London, UK: Churchill Livingstone, 2000

Schulz V, Hansel R, Tyler VE. *Rational Phytotherapy: a Physician's Guide to Herbal Medicine*, 3rd edn. New York, NY: Springer-Verlag, 1998

Sierpina VS. *Integrative Health Care: Complementary and Alternative Therapies for the Whole Person*. Philadelphia, PA: FA Davis, 2001

Skidmore-Roth L. In Como D, ed. *Mosby's Handbook of Herbs and Natural Supplements*. St. Louis, MO: Mosby, Inc. A Harcourt Health Sciences Company, 2001

RealAge – how do vitamins affect healthy behavior?

3

M. F. Roizen

THE EFFECT OF VITAMINS ON AGING

I often say to a patient that taking the right vitamins and minerals and avoiding the wrong ones can make him or her 6 years younger. The most important ones to take are folate, vitamin B_6, vitamin B_{12}, vitamin D, calcium, selenium, lycopene, vitamin C and vitamin E. It is important to avoid excess vitamin A and iron, unless demonstrated need is evident.

If the patient has not heard me speak before or read my writings, he or she usually says, 'I take brand X multivitamin. Isn't that enough?' or 'My doctor told me that a good diet is enough, isn't that correct?'

The answer is that most of us do not get the right amount of some vitamins, carotenoids or minerals for optimal health. There is an amount of vitamins, micronutrients and minerals that prevents deficiency disease and a different amount for optimal health. Through a basic diet, most of us get the right amounts to prevent deficiency disease except for folate, vitamin D, calcium and perhaps two carotenoids, lycopene and lutein. The patient often asks me to give an example. I ask the patient how many glasses of milk he or she consumes a day. Few say they have four, yet milk is the main source of vitamin D in the northern USA.

Virtually no one in those climates in the northern USA gets the right amount of vitamin D from either milk or the sun's conversions of an inactive vitamin D to active vitamin D in the winter months, so they need to take a supplement. Less than 30% consume the right amounts of calcium even with great media attention. Obtaining the right amount of calcium and vitamin D (whether from the sun's conversion of inactive vitamin D to active vitamin D, a supplement in milk, or supplement pill) makes the average 55-year-old's RealAge about 2.4 years younger (man) and 2.8 years younger (woman). Let us start at the beginning, to try to understand why I developed RealAge[1,2] as a currency for health, and how it can help motivate healthier behavior.

THE GENESIS OF RealAge AS A MOTIVATIONAL CURRENCY FOR HEALTH

One day in my internal medicine practice I was seeing a patient with hypertension. I do a peculiar thing in my practice: I have patients bring in the pills they take, not just tell me their names. The patient's blood pressure was 140/90 mmHg and he was consistently taking only one of the two medicines prescribed. I concluded that he was not taking these drugs as prescribed, because both pill bottles had the same refill date, although one bottle was half empty, while the other was barely touched. When discussing this 140/90 reading with him, he said to me, 'What difference does it make that I'm only taking one of my pills correctly? My blood pressure is 140/90 and most docs wouldn't treat that, would they?' I replied that this may be so, but his blood pressure of 140/90 made him live as though he were 9 years older. He asked me what I meant. Because he was not taking his pills as prescribed, he had a blood pressure of 140/90 rather than 115/75. Furthermore, because his blood pressure was not as low as it could be, his arteries delivered fewer nutrients, so he had the vitality and energy of someone who was 56 rather than his age of 47.

He then asked a key question, 'How many other things in medicine can you do this for?' I asked him why he wanted to know.

He replied, '...because people have told me that I might die a year or two sooner if I don't take my blood pressure pills, but no one told me before that I live with the vitality of someone 9 years older. That is meaningful to me. What other things in health can you explain this way?' After questioning me about the methods (he was a physics major in college), he decided to take his blood pressure pills correctly. The episode with this man made me understand how important the way a physician presents consequence to a patient is to a patient's adherence to recommendations.

SCIENCE BEHIND RealAge

As recently as 20 years ago, doctors largely believed that as soon as they understood genetics they would solve many basic medical problems. The overwhelming belief was that youth, health and longevity were determined from birth; there was nothing that could be done about it. However, from diseases as diverse as diabetes, Alzheimer's disease, many cancers, aging of the arteries, which leads to stroke, heart disease, memory loss, impotence and even wrinkling of the skin, we know that genetic components are involved. We all have the genes we were born with, but how we age is at least 70% up to us, and our choices have more influence as we get older.

How these choices affect our genes is unclear. We do not know whether they foster attachment for viruses, prevent or cause chromosome breaks, or activate specific components. We do know that these choices greatly affect the quality and length of life. RealAge takes the knowledge of how our choice influences how well and how long we live. RealAge then transforms it into a metric that lets people understand easily and simply how their choices affect their quality and length of life.

If the health and longevity and ultimately youth of a population age cohort (a group of people all born in the same year) are charted, it will be found that, with few exceptions, people age at a similar rate until they reach their late twenties and mid-thirties. With the exceptions of those who have inherited rare genetic disorders or who have been in serious accidents, everyone is basically healthy and able. Men reach the peak of their performance curve in their late twenties and women in their mid-thirties. That is when their bodies have fully matured and are at their strongest and most mentally acute.

Somewhere between 28 and 36 years of age, most people reach a turning point – a transition from 'growing' into 'aging'. If the population is examined as a whole and any one biological function is tracked – whether it be kidney function or cognitive ability – performance declines as we age. In general, each biological function decreases 3–6% per 10-year period after age 35. A 3–6% decrease is a measure of the average for the population, but averages are relatively useless because the variation is so great, especially for older populations, and the average does not measure anything about the individual.

If one looks at twins who have changed environments, or brothers who have changed environments, they age at very different rates. The variations between their aging, their ability to function, and their quality and length of life covers the entire range of possibilities. For every 80-year-old who is debilitated from cardiovascular disease, there is another who is running road races or traveling the globe.

I then set about to gather a group of experts, epidemiologists and biostatisticians to analyze the data and literature, and determine whether we could construct Kaplan–Meier survivor curves which reflected the quality and length of life, and find differences that behaviors caused in those survival or quality of life choices. It was easy for some behaviors. For example, regarding smoking, there were 11 studies that showed that smoking a pack a day makes you an average of 8 years older, and that quitting prior to age 35 reverses seven out of eight years of the aging cigarettes cause. That is, quitting causes you to be 7 years younger than if you continued smoking.

Blood pressure is another important age variable. The data (and plenty of them) show that we can control high blood pressure to a large degree and the aging it causes. Plentiful also were the data on vitamins and supplements.

Thus, RealAge is an information system. Instead of providing new scientific data, it is a way of making already published results understandable and motivating. We used data from the most up-to-date studies published in peer-reviewed journals. We stipulated that there must be four articles on any one subject with a preponderance of effect for us to say that some behavior has a RealAge effect.

RealAge translates the currently excellent available research into information we can use to motivate patients and can integrate into our own lives. Although my colleagues and I rely on scientific information for our calculations, the predominant data we use are from clinical studies of two types: large-scale, risk factor epidemiology studies and smaller-scale, randomized controlled trials. The large-scale studies look at many people, sometimes more than 100 000 individuals, and in one instance (the MR. FIT study) as many as 350 000 people. The researchers who co-ordinate these studies track huge populations of people for a given period of time, looking at one behavior or testable factor, such as blood pressure or vitamin D usage, and then associate these behaviors with risk of developing certain diseases with that behavior factor. These studies use statistics for a large population to obtain more accurate reflection of variations within the study sample. The drawback is that these studies do not provide very detailed information, and they are not controlled studies. The researchers are not able to regulate who takes a specific drug or engages in a specific behavior, which is why scientists conduct smaller controlled studies.

In randomized controlled studies, a study population of a few hundred to 100 000 people is randomly allocated to treatment or to control. Each group is assigned a certain task. For example, a third of the group may be asked to take the vitamin folic acid at 800 µg a day; a third of the group asked to consume 400 µg of folate a day; and a third might be asked to take placebos. Each participant's progress is tracked for a period of time, and his/her health status is recorded. At the end of the study, researchers compare the groups and evaluate the effects of a particular behavior or condition on the overall health of the group.

We select only factors that have been shown to make a quantifiable difference in the profile of risk (in other words, quality and quantity of life, or aging) in at least four peer-reviewed studies. RealAge integrates and compares studies that pertain to a certain issue; calculates what each study tells us about aging; assesses covariance and interactions; and finally determines a RealAge number that tells, in one 'easy-to-understand' number, the impact of each behavior in a number of years.

If a 55-year-old woman takes the ideal amount of calcium and vitamin D, she is 2.8 years younger, provided that she is taking average amounts of everything else. Adopting multiple healthy behaviors means benefiting less from each behavior but benefiting more overall[1–3]. While the calculations are complicated, modern computer programs that take into account interactions and covariances and store large amounts of data can make calculations quick, as can be seen on our website www.RealAge.com (this is a free website, but I should disclose that I have an equity interest in the company that runs the website).

THE RealAge EFFECT OF VITAMINS

Calcium and vitamin D

The proper daily intake of calcium and vitamin D makes the average 55-year-old man 2.4 years younger and the average 55-year-old woman 2.8 years younger. Why? The substances decrease the major cause of bone weakening and hip fractures, decrease the risk of some cancers and improve quality of life by lessening the risk and progression of arthritis.

Bone weakening or osteoporosis affects more than 30 million North Americans. It is the major underlying cause of hip fractures and bone breaks in the elderly – with about 1.4 million bone fractures and 350 thousand hip fractures yearly. Although osteoporosis affects woman disproportionately, especially small-boned woman of Northern European or Asian descent, we are all at risk. Twenty-five million women suffer from this disease, but so do more than 5 million American men. As men live longer, they are at increased risk of osteoporosis. We often forget that our bones are living tissues that need proper care. All living tissues are dynamic, being torn down and rebuilt. Bones, similarly, are not static 'steel beams', but are dynamic tissues being molded continuously. Calcium and vitamin D appear necessary and beneficial for that remodeling to be done without leading to arthritis and osteoporosis. While sun exposure alone can provide adequate conversion of inactive vitamin D to active vitamin D in the body, ultraviolet radiation during winter is inefficient in most locations (northern United States) to minimize the risk of osteoporosis and fracture[4]. Among patients admitted into a Boston hospital, 57% were deficient in vitamin D[5]. Among female adolescents in Finland during winter months, 75% either were vitamin D deficient or had low vitamin D concentrations[6]. This requirement of vitamin D and calcium emphasizes the difference between doses that prevent deficiency disease (rickets) and those that foster optimal health (fewer fractures, less arthritis).

Deficiency disease vs. optimal intake

Preventing scurvy, rickets or other deficiency diseases with daily diet is different from optimizing health. The amount of vitamin C, vitamin D or calcium needed to prevent deficiency diseases is different from the amount necessary for optimal living. What we have learned is that greater amounts of vitamins and nutrients (vitamin C, vitamin D, folate, vitamin B_6, vitamin B_{12}, calcium, selenium, lycopene and lutein) than prevent deficiency disease are needed to help us obtain optimal health. While the amount of vitamin C to prevent scurvy may be 60 mg a day, or vitamin D 200 IU to prevent rickets, larger doses are necessary to obtain the youngest RealAge. Vitamin C, vitamin D and calcium decrease bone loss, fracture and arthritis, and increase bone mineral density. It appears that vitamin D, when combined with vitamin C and calcium, has benefits in preventing premenstrual syndrome and possibly some forms of cancer in younger women[7–13].

For the youngest RealAge, the appropriate amount of vitamin D is 400 IU (one does not reach toxic levels until 2000 IU). Appropriate calcium intake is 1200 mg a day for men and 1600 mg a day for women, with an additional 20 mg for each 8 oz (225 ml) of caffeinated

beverage, and an additional 200 mg for every hour of 'sweat-producing' exercise.

Folate and the B vitamins decrease arterial aging and perhaps immune aging as well

It always surprises me to see that people are amazed that something that decreases heart disease also decreases memory loss, stroke and impotence. Whether it is the arteries to the brain, or to the heart, gonads or skin, they are arteries and keeping the arteries younger is associated with less heart disease, less stroke, less memory loss, less risk of impotence and even less risk of aging of the skin. Folate and the B vitamins appear to do so because they antagonize homocysteine. They also may do something more important than that relating to the immune system by decreasing chromosome breaks and, consequently, the risk of colon, breast and perhaps prostate cancer.

Homocysteine, a by-product of various metabolic processes, is an amino acid that may build up in the blood. As one ages, the homocysteine levels increase. No one is exactly sure how homocysteine affects arteries, but it is well established that people with high levels of homocysteine have considerably more arterial disease (atherosclerosis). People who take high doses of vitamins B_6 and B_{12} and folate have a decreased risk of arterial aging conditions[14–18]. Studies find that those with a higher intake of folate have a reduced rate of coronary artery disease, as well as stroke, impotence and memory loss. The appropriate amount of folate and vitamin B_6 for optimal RealAge appears to be 800 μg a day and 6 mg a day, respectively. Vitamin B_{12} is more problematic, because the elderly have inadequate vitamin B_{12} levels because of low gastric acidity and low intrinsic factor production. Thus, an intake of B_{12} greater than 400 μg, perhaps as large as 800 μg a day, an amount greatly above the recommended daily allowance (RDA) or daily value of 2–6 μg a day, might be necessary. Whether crystalline vitamin B_{12}, the form used in most supplements, requires intrinsic factor and gastric acid for absorption is a matter of debate. Clearly, if one takes 800 μg a day, one's blood homocysteine level will be lower.

Higher levels of folate are also associated with a lower risk of colon cancer[19] and breast cancer[20,21], particularly among persons who have one or two alcoholic drinks a day. Folate has the effect of decreasing neurotube defects by more than 70%. The net effect of folate and B vitamins on the average 55-year-old man is a RealAge effect of more than 2 years younger.

Many of us are deficient in folate and vitamins B_{12} and B_6. Chicken, banana, tomatoes, sunflower seeds, turkey and ground beef all contain 0.4 mg or more of vitamin B_6 per serving. Salmon and tuna contain 3 µg or more B_{12} per serving. For someone on a vegetarian diet, it is virtually impossible to get adequate vitamin B_{12}. The 800 µg I believe one should have a day is impossible to obtain from food. One hundred micrograms or more of folate is found in a serving of black-eye peas, brussel sprouts, artichokes and asparagus. Apples, lima beans, soybeans and avocado all contain about 50–80 µg of folate per serving, and bananas have 45 µg. It does not appear that one can get too much folate, whereas high doses of vitamin B_{12} are associated with diarrhea and hives. More than 500 mg per day of vitamin B_6 (more than 80 times what we recommend) is associated with neurotoxicity and photosensitivity.

Vitamins C and E

The benefits of vitamins C and E have stimulated controversy, which I believe started because some studies have not tested vitamins C and E together. Based on studies of vitamin E, I believe that 800 IU of vitamin E and around 1000 mg of vitamin C are optimal doses. The 1000 mg of vitamin C should not be taken in one dose, as one cannot absorb more than 500 mg at once without causing some degree of toxicity to DNA, as demonstrated in *in vitro* studies. Vitamin E (800 IU) can be taken all at once. The toxic doses of vitamin B_{12}, vitamin C and vitamin E are between 15 and 20 times the doses recommended as the daily value or RDA.

The controversy over vitamins C and E relates to separate use in studies. One prospective study demonstrated a large reduction in the rate of progression of intimal–medial (arterial aging) thickness among men randomly assigned to receive the vitamins C and E together[22]. Other studies that examined vitamins C and E independently have been less convincing; some have not shown any benefit[23]. Other studies have shown impressive benefit. In the CHAOS Study[24] 800 IU/day of vitamin E reduced the 1-year rate of non-fatal myocardial infarctions by 80% amongst patients with known coronary heart disease. A recent trial in dialysis patients of 800 IU/day of vitamin E showed a reduced risk of cardiovascular events, including myocardial infarctions[25]. Vitamin C supplements have also been associated with a lower risk of coronary heart disease in one large cohort study[26]. Vitamin E also appears to decrease prostate cancer, especially among smokers[27]. To re-emphasize, vitamin C appears to need to be taken with vitamin E for these optimal aging effects to manifest, and may have other benefits as well[28]. While the evidence of vitamins C and E is not as clear as the evidence of calcium and vitamin D, or folate and the B vitamins, vitamins C and E make your RealAge more than 1.4 years younger at age 55 (Table 1).

No vitamins have stimulated as much controversy as vitamin A and β-carotene. Opposite to their benefits, too much vitamin A not only can cause birth defects, but is also associated with risk of liver disease. Too much iron is associated with accelerating hemochromotosis in 1 in 250 Americans. It also seems to be associated with increased iron in the myocardium, thus decreasing myocardial performance.

LYCOPENE, LUTEIN AND SELENIUM

Studies on the carotenoids lutein and lycopene and the mineral selenium show benefits of increasing amounts over the usual American diet. With selenium one has to be careful about not getting above 2000 µg/day (ten times what we recommend), as toxicity results. There is more than a 1.7 year younger benefit in men and a 1.2 year younger benefit in women from increasing the intake of tomato products that contain lycopene, the eye benefits of lutein and the anti-cancer benefits of selenium. The large RealAge effect of lycopene on arterial aging shown in only

Table 1 Vitamin intake and RealAge effect

Optimal daily amount of vitamins/minerals/carotenoids for youngest RealAge	RealAge effect compared to average intake	
	Men aged 55	*Woman aged 55*
Vitamin D and calcium (400 IU; 1200–1600 mg)	2.4 years younger	2.8 years younger
Folate, vitamins B_{12} and B_6 (800 μg, 800 μg and 6 mg, respectively)	2.6 years younger	2.2 years younger
Vitamins C and E (together) (1000 mg and 400 IU, respectively)	1.6 years younger	1.4 years younger
Lycopene, lutein and selenium (see text, see text and 200 μg, respectively)	1.7 years* younger	1.2 years* younger
Vitamin A and iron (less than 8000 IU and none (unless iron deficient), respectively)	more than 2 years older	more than 2 years older

* Perhaps much more – data do not include arterial age-reducing benefits

three studies to date should not be disregarded. If a fourth study on lycopene and lutein indicates a similar benefit, then lycopene alone may have more than a 4-year RealAge benefit. The optimal lycopene amount is obtained by enjoying 10 tablespoons of tomato sauce or tomato paste a week with a little fat (the fat helps to absorb lycopene and lutein)[29–35].

DO WE NEED A MULTIVITAMIN?

The ideal amounts of vitamins, especially vitamins B_6, B_{12}, C, E, D and folate, selenium, calcium, lycopene and lutein, appear to be greater than the RDA. Do we get these optimal amounts from usual North American diets?

Over 3.7 million people have completed the nutrition part of the RealAge program on the RealAge website. These people are probably more health conscious than average. Less than 1% of these individuals consume the right amount of the above vitamins, minerals and carotenoids from their diet. Therefore, I have come to the conclusion that we all need a multivitamin that contains these amounts (hopefully in divided doses, so that one does not get too much calcium or vitamin C at one time) in order to have the youngest RealAge. If one adds the numbers up individually, one becomes more than 9 years younger by obtaining the right amount. Adopting other beneficial habits can decrease this 9-year effect. However, there is still a substantial benefit and a RealAge effect of obtaining the right vitamins and avoiding the wrong ones.

ACKNOWLEDGEMENTS

RealAge and Age Reduction are service marks registered by one of Dr Roizen's patients. The patient has formed a corporation to provide software to allow patients and physicians to calculate their RealAge. Dr Roizen is a paid consultant of and holds an equity interest in that corporation.

References

1. Roizen MF. *RealAge: Are You As Young As You Can Be?* New York, NY: HarperCollins, 1999

2. Roizen MF, LaPuma J. *The RealAge Diet: Make Yourself Younger With What You Eat.* New York, NY: HarperCollins, 2001

3. Website www.realage.com (A free website where this is explained)

4. Holick MF. Vitamin D and bone health. *J Nutr* 1996;126S: 1159s–64s

5. Thomas MK, Lloyd-Jones DM, Thadhani RI, *et al.* Hypovitaminosis D in medical inpatients *N Engl J Med* 1998;338:777–83

6. Outila TA, Karkkainen MU, Lamberg-Allardt CJ. Vitamin D status effects serum parathyiod hormone concentration during winter in female adolescence: associations with forearm bone mineral density. *Am J Clin Nutr* 2001;74:206–10

7. Thys-Jacobs S. Calcium caronate and the premenstrual syndrome: effects on premenstrual and menstrual symptoms. *Am J Obstet Gynecol* 1998;179:444–8

8. Dawson-Hughes B, Harris SS, Krall EA, Dallal GE. Effects of calcium and vitamin D supplementation on bone density in men and women 65 years of age or older. *N Engl J Med* 1997;337:670–6

9. Dawson-Hughes B, Harris SS, Krall EA, Dallal GE. Effect of withdraw of calcium and vitamin D supplements on bone mass in elderly men and women. *Am J Clin Nutr* 2000;72:745–50

10. Watson KE, Abrolat ML, Malone LI, *et al.* Active serum vitamin D levels are inversely correlated with coronary calcification. *Circulation* 1997;96:1755–60

11. Gloth FM III, Gundbert CM, Hollis BW, *et al.* Vitamin D deficiency on homebound elderly persons. *J Am Med Assoc* 1995;274:1683–6

12. McAlindon TE, Jacques P, Zhang Y, *et al.* Do antioxidant micronutrients protect against the development and progression of knee osteoarthritis? *Arthritis Rheum* 1996;39:648–56

13. McAlindon TE, Felson DT, Zhang Y, *et al.* Relation of dietary intake and serum levels of vitamin D to progression of osteoarthritis of the knee among participants in the Framingham Study. *Ann Intern Med* 1996;125:353–9

14. Pancharumiti N, Lewis CA, Sauberlich HE, *et al.* Plasma homocysteine, folate and vitamin B_{12} concentration and risk for early onset coronary artery disease. *Am J Clin Nutr* 1994;59:940–8

15. Selhub J, Jacques PJ, Bostom AG, *et al.* Association between plasma homocysteine concentration and extracranial carotid artery stenosis. *N Engl J Med* 1995;332:286–91

16. Rimm EB, Willett WC, Hu FB, *et al.* Folate and vitamin B_6 from diet and supplements in relation to risk of coronary heart disease among women. *J Am Med Assoc* 1998;279:359–64

17. Welch GN, Loscalzo J. Homocysteine and atherothromboses. *N Engl J Med* 1998;338:1042–50

18. Morrison HI, Schaubel O, Desmeules M, Wigle DT. Serum folate and risk of coronary heart disease. *J Am Med Assoc* 1996;275:1893–6

19. Giovannucci E, Rimm EB Ascherio A, *et al.* Alcohol, low-methionine low-folate diets, and the risk of colon cancer in men. *J Natl Cancer Inst* 1995;87:265–73

20. Zhang S, Hunter DJ, Hankinson SE, *et al.* A prospective study of folate intake and the risk of breast cancer. *J Am Med Assoc* 1999;281:1632–7

21. Rohan TE, Jain MG, Howe GR, Miller AB. Dietary folate consumption and breast cancer risk. *J Natl Cancer Inst* 2000;92:266–9

22. Salonen JT, Nyyssonen K, Salonen R, *et al.* Antioxidant Supplemention in Atherosclerosis Prevention (ASAP) Study: a randomized trial of the effects of vitamin E & C on 3 year progression on carotid atherosclerosis. *Ann Intern Med* 2000; 248:377–86

23. Stampfer MJ, Hennekens CH, Manson JE, Colditz GA, Rosner B, Willet WC. Vitamin E consumption and risk of coronary heart disease in women. *N Engl J Med* 1993;328:1444–9

24. Stevens NG, Parsons A, Schofield PM, *et al.* Randomized control trial of vitamin E in patients with coronary disease: Cambridge Heart Antioxidant Study (CHAOS). *Lancet* 1996;347:781–6

25. Yusuf S, Dagenais G, Pogue J, Bosch J, Sleight P. Vitamin E supplementation and cardiovascular events in high-risk patients. The Hearts Outcomes Prevention Evaluation Study Investigators. *N Engl J Med* 2000;342:154–60

26. Enstrom JE, Kanim LE, Klein MA. Vitamin C intake and mortality among a sample of the United States population. *Epidemiology* 1992;3:194–202

27. ATBC Investigators. The effect of vitamin E and beta-carotene on the incidence of lung cancer and other cancers in male smokers. The Alpha Tocopherol, Beta Carotene Cancer Prevention Study Group. *N Engl J Med* 1994;330:1029–35

28. Plotnick GD, Corretti MC, Vogel RA. Effect of antioxidant vitamins on the transient impairment of endothelium-dependent brachial artery vasoactivity following a single high-fat meal. *J Am Med Assoc* 1997;278:1682–6

29. Gann PH, Ma J, Giovannucci E, *et al.* Lower prostate cancer risk in men with elevated plasma lycopene levels results of a prospective analysis. *Cancer Res* 1999;59:1225–30

30. Chan JM, Stampfer MJ, Ma J, Rimm EB, Willett WC, Giovannucci EL. Supplemental vitamin E intake and prostate cancer risk in a large cohort of men in the United States. *Cancer Epidemiol Biomakers Prev* 1999;8:893–9

31. Giovannucci E. Tomatoes, tomato based products, lycopene, and cancer. Review of the epidemiology literature. *J Natl Cancer Inst* 1999;91:317–31

32. Kohlmeier L, Kark JD, Gomez-Garcia E, *et al.* Lycopene and myocardial infarction risk in the Euramic Study. *Am J Epidemiol* 1997;146:618–26

33. Clavel-Chapelon F, Niravong M, Joseph RR. Diet and breast cancer: review of the epidemiologic literature. *Cancer Detect Prev* 1997;21:426–40

34. Dorgan JF, Sowell A, Swanson CA, *et al.* Relationships of serum carotenoids, retinol, alpha-tocopherol, and selenium with breast cancer risk: results from a prospective study in Columbia, Missouri (United States). *Cancer Causes Control* 1998;9:89–97

35. Toniolo P, Van Kappel AL, Akhmedkhanov A, *et al.* Serum carotenoids and breast cancer. *Am J Epidemiol* 2001;153:1142–7

Herbal antioxidants: cardiovascular potential and danger

4

T. L. Vanden Hoek and Z.-H. Shao

INTRODUCTION

One important reason why herbal medication use has increased dramatically in the USA is the promise of youth. Many herbs contain antioxidant compounds which have great potential to lower the oxidant stress associated with aging. For example, 'To promote cardiovascular health' is one of the benefits posted on the bottle of some grape seed extracts. However, while oxidants may be associated with a number of disease processes associated with aging, they are also potentially beneficial in low levels as signaling molecules. Such oxidants are means by which communication between and within cells of the body can occur quickly, and they may help the body adapt to stress.

This dual role of oxidants, both as culprits of disease and messengers for healthy adaptation, may explain why so many clinical trials of antioxidants have had equivocal results on long-term cardiovascular health. Oxidants may also be useful in fighting infection and in preventing cancer by initiating apoptosis. Thus, although a number of medicinal herbs have antioxidative properties, like other antioxidants the long-term effect on health is unclear. Their effects in certain settings when the body is placed under greater stress becomes even more uncertain. For example, up to 32% of patients in the preoperative setting have been reported to use herbal medications[1]. In addition to possible adverse effects and drug interactions, possibly due to a number of these herbal medications[2,3], one could ask whether a potent antioxidant could interfere with useful oxidant signaling which probably occurs when the body undergoes the major stress of surgery. A more complete understanding of oxidant physiology and pathophysiology will be necessary to fully appreciate the best role for medicinal herbs in preventing cardiovascular disease without harmful side-effects.

In addition to the possible benefits of preventing long-term oxidant stress, the antioxidants found in herbal medications may have great potential benefit for a second reason. Oxidants probably contribute to the tissue damage associated with certain medical emergencies in which blood flow is suddenly stopped to either particular organs or the entire body. These emergencies include stroke, myocardial infarction, shock and cardiac arrest. The use of medicinal herbs for treating such medical emergencies has been less studied, but their antioxidant properties may be extremely useful in these particular settings. Traditional antioxidants such as vitamin E may not act quickly enough to be effective, whereas some herbal compounds may act fast enough to prevent rapid oxidant damage. Few studies have explored the potential for such acute treatment.

The goal of this chapter is to highlight these potential antioxidant benefits of herbal medications, both chronic and acute, and the potential dangers of interfering with the beneficial consequences of oxidants.

CARDIOVASCULAR DISEASE AND OXIDANT STRESS

Cardiovascular disease remains the leading cause of death in the USA, with 300 000 of these per year occurring outside the hospital as sudden cardiac arrest. While improvements in mortality have occurred, the actual numbers of people dying from cardiovascular diseases, including heart disease and stroke, have risen 37% since 1950 because of aging and population growth, while improvements in age-adjusted mortality have slowed to negligible levels in the 1990s. In addition, congestive heart failure affects almost 5 million people in the USA, with 400 000 new cases diagnosed per year and the prevalence is projected to increase 2–3-fold by 2010. Increased oxidant stress, when levels of oxidants within cells overwhelm antioxidant defenses, undoubtedly plays an important role in cardiovascular disease. Although critical for much life on our planet, oxygen has an important side-effect: it generates free radicals by interacting with sunlight, ionizing radiation, environmental chemicals and our own intrinsic metabolic processes when we digest food (Figure 1).

These free radicals, highly reactive molecules with unpaired electrons usually containing oxygen or nitrogen, may lead to a number of degenerative diseases associated with aging and tissue oxidation. In particular, oxidative modification of low-density lipoproteins (LDLs) probably plays a major role in the progression of atherosclerosis, which in turn predisposes to diseases of heart attack and stroke – leading causes of death and disability, respectively, in the USA. What we eat can alter this outcome, in part by shielding us against this constant barrage of free radicals. High intake of fresh fruits and vegetables rich in antioxidant flavonoids or nuts (rich in the antioxidant vitamin E) decrease cardiovascular risks of heart attacks, stroke and death[4–9].

CHRONIC EFFECTS OF ANTIOXIDANTS ON CARDIOVASCULAR DISEASE

Traditional antioxidants

Before discussing studies of the antioxidant cardiovascular effects of herbal medicines, much can be learned from research exploring the utility of traditional antioxidants, since this work has progressed further to multiple clinical trials. The use of antioxidant supplements to prevent cardiovascular disease has been an attempt to reproduce some of the benefits of a healthy diet. One of the most studied antioxidants is vitamin E, an antioxidant which affects smooth muscle proliferation and platelet adhesion, and in a number of smaller cohort studies appears to result in decreased risk of coronary artery disease[10,11]. However, a number of randomized clinical trials showed no benefit of vitamin E supplementation on coronary artery disease

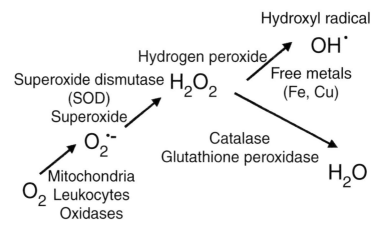

Figure 1 Simplified scheme of oxygen metabolism. Reactive oxygen species includes superoxide, hydrogen peroxide and hydroxyl radicals

risk[12–14], and while one study suggested that vitamin E may decrease the risk of non-fatal myocardial infarctions, it did not decrease cardiovascular mortality[15].

Another antioxidant commonly studied in human clinical trials is β-carotene. Carotenoids represent over 500 different colored plant pigments, with β-carotene the most abundant in nature. β-carotene, a highly effective free radical scavenger[16], has been associated with decreased LDL oxidation[17] and decreased risk of coronary artery disease[18]. However, prospective cohort studies have failed to show an association between carotenoid intake and coronary heart disease[19,20], and multiple primary prevention trials failed to show any reduction in coronary heart disease[21–24]. The potential dangers of antioxidants were highlighted in trials showing increased mortality among smokers taking β-carotene supplements[12,13].

In evaluating the potential benefits of herbal medications, the trials studying traditional antioxidants are very instructive. Although very promising as antioxidants in many models of free radical generation, antioxidants such as vitamin E and β-carotene have often failed to demonstrate a beneficial effect in human clinical trials. There may be many reasons for this failure, reasons which will need to be addressed in future evaluations of herbal medications.

First, currently, there is no single good assay that can quickly and reliably measure changes in oxidant stress in people. Thus, it is difficult to know if the dose of any antioxidant used is actually the most effective at reducing oxidants.

Second, there are many types of species of oxidants generated in different compartments of the cell (e.g. mitochondrial vs. cytosolic, lipid vs. water soluble phases) and body (e.g. organ-specific, liver vs. brain vs. heart). Since antioxidants have different mechanisms and sites of action, it is highly unlikely that any one antioxidant would be capable of attenuating oxidant stress in all cell compartments and organs of the body. Thus, a cocktail of antioxidants may be more beneficial than single agents. This is a potential advantage which herbal medicines possess. Many herbal formulations contain multiple phenolic compounds which may act in different ways to quench oxidant stress. They include flavonoids (over 5000 different compounds reported, including anthocyanidins,

catechins, flavanones, flavones, flavonols and isoflavones), tannins (ellagic acid, gallic acid), phenyl isopropenoids (e.g. caffeic acid, coumaric acids, ferulic acid), lignans, catechol, resveratrol (grape skins), rosmarinic acid (rosemary) and many others. (For a review of structures and antioxidant mechanisms see reference 25.)

Finally, the 'best' antioxidant(s) may not be the cocktail which quenches every trace of oxidants, including the beneficial effects of oxidants. Ideally, agents would augment oxidant defenses when needed but not decrease oxidant signaling, the use of oxidants to fight infections or the role of oxidants in apoptosis and prevention of cancer. Toward this end, more sophisticated assays to evaluate such effects will be useful in the future to predict which formulations will be most effective.

Herbal antioxidants

Far fewer and smaller studies have examined the potential protective effects of antioxidant herbal preparations. There are some examples of herbal therapies which have been tested in small clinical trials. While the greatest use of herbal medications occurs in the East, controlled trials there are lacking because in many instances the use of placebo is considered unethical[26]. Experience with some of these compounds is also greater in Europe than in the USA. In Germany, Commission E of the Ministry of Health is a committee of physicians, pharmacists, scientists and herbalists who evaluate the safety, quality and efficacy of herbs. A significant portion of these herbs are prescribed for cardiovascular conditions and are evaluated in ongoing reports published by the Commission, and circulated by the American Botanical Council, and the reference text *PDR for Herbal Medicines*. Below is a highlight of some herbal remedies with potential cardiovascular benefits due to antioxidant activity. Unfortunately, a complete summary of potential antioxidant and pro-oxidant effects of each compound is not possible given the page limitations of this chapter. The level of detail in each section depends in part on work done already in other chapters within this book, the amount of human experience with the herb as demonstrated by consumer interest and by clinical trials, and by work in our own laboratory with some of these compounds.

Danshen

Danshen (*Salvia miltiorrhiza*) has been used in traditional Chinese medicine for many years to promote blood flow and treat angina pectoris and acute myocardial infarction[27]. A constituent, terpene tanshinone, has been found to be a potent antioxidant against lipid peroxidation, including lipid peroxidation of LDLs[28] and myocardial mitochondrial membranes[29], without pro-oxidant effects[30]. Few placebo-controlled studies have been performed using danshen or its constituents. One double-blind study of 67 subjects reported symptomatic and electrocardiograph (ECG) improvement with tanshinone IIA. Adverse effects include acting as a vasoconstrictor of non-coronary arteries at higher doses[27], and a potentiation of warfarin when taken concurrently[31].

Garlic

Garlic (*Allium sativum*) is one of the over-the-counter preparations most widely used for medicinal reasons in the USA. The active substance in garlic is allicin, formed when alliin is broken down by alliinase as garlic is crushed[3]. Due to differences in bioavailability (in part due to preparation techniques and tablet composition) – with the additional difficulties of blinding studies and discontinuation by subjects due to odor – it has been difficult to perform randomized clinical trials to evaluate its possible effects on hyperlipidemia, hypertension, coagulation and atherosclerosis. These effects are reviewed elsewhere within this book and by others[3]. Of note, the anti-atherosclerotic activity of garlic may be independent of its lipid-lowering effects and more due to its inhibition of lipid peroxidation[32]. Garlic used in patients with peripheral vascular disease increased their pain-free walking distance[33], and has been reported to decrease atherosclerotic plaque detected in the femoral artery or carotid bifurcation[34].

Ginkgo

Ginkgo (*Ginkgo biloba*) is one of the best-selling herbal preparations in the USA, derived from the leaves of the maidenhair tree. It has had mixed results in the few clinical trials designed to test whether it can improve measures of cognition in patients with vascular dementia, and has been reported to treat claudication and antagonize platelet-activating factor. Constituents of ginkgo, including the terpenoid compounds bilobalide and ginkgolides A and B, have antioxidant properties and are reported to attenuate reperfusion injury following ischemia[35–37]. A small randomized, placebo-controlled trial of patients undergoing cardiopulmonary bypass or aortic valve replacement showed that high-dose pretreatment with *Ginkgo biloba* extract decreased indices of oxidant stress post-reperfusion (thiobarbituric acid-reactive species and electron spin resonance measures of the plasma ascorbate pool using dimethylsulfoxide/ascorbyl free radical levels)[38]. However, the clinical outcomes in this small study were not significant. However, this is one of the few herbal studies which used both placebo controls and indices of oxidant stress.

Other benefits and possible adverse effects are important as this herbal medicine is used extensively. Of note, particularly in preoperative patients, are possible effects on bleeding and potentiation of warfarin. These effects are discussed in more detail in other chapters.

American ginseng

American ginseng (*Panax quinquefolius*) is a perennial aromatic herb native to the northern region of the USA and Canada. It has a long, fleshy root, the shape of which somewhat resembles the human body. American ginseng extract is composed of a mixture of glycosides, essential oils and a variety of complex carbohydrates and phytosterols as well as amino acids and trace minerals[39]. The bioactive constituents of American ginseng are dammarane saponins, commonly referred to as ginsenosides which are present in root, leaf, stem and berries[40]. American ginseng extract contains more than 30 ginsenosides such as Rg$_1$, Re, Ro, Rb$_1$, Rc, Rb$_2$ and Rd[41,42]. Among them, Rb$_1$ is a major bioactive component[43]. Based on high performance liquid chromatography/mass spectrometry (HPLC/MS) detection, ginsenoside 24(R)-pseudoginsenoside F$_{11}$ is only present in American ginseng extract[44,45], while R$_f$ is only present in Asian ginseng (*Panax ginseng* C.A. Meyer)[40,46]. This is an important parameter used to differentiate American ginseng from Asian ginseng.

Ginseng is one of the most valuable natural tonics in the East and West. Asian ginseng has been used in the Oriental East for over 4000 years. Many studies have shown that Asian ginseng affects various biological processes and involves a wide range of pharmacological actions, including antiaging, antitumor and antistress effects[47]. Although many studies demonstrating beneficial effects of Asian ginseng can be found in the literature, relatively few studies have been performed with American ginseng. Until the last decade, researchers have found that American ginseng exerts beneficial effects on the cardiovascular system via its anti-ischemic, antiarrhythmic and antihypertensive actions, and these actions have been attributed to its antioxidant activity. Ginsenosides extracted from American ginseng increase plasma high-density lipoprotein (HDL) content and decrease the lipid peroxide levels in hyperlipidemic rats[48]. At a high concentration (mg/ml range), ginsenosides directly reduce LDL oxidation[49]. At a low concentration (μg/ml range), ginsenosides significantly lessen LDL oxidation and reduce CuSO$_4$-induced oxidative changes in the presence of vitamin C (0.1–1 μmol/l), and significantly decrease the impairment of endothelium function induced by oxidized LDL in rat aorta[50]. American ginseng extract also protected cultured rat cardiac myocytes from oxidative damage[51]. Similarly, ginsenoside Rb$_1$ protected hippocampal neurons against ischemic injury[39]. It has been reported that Rb$_1$, Rd, Ra$_1$ and Ro inhibit protein tyrosine kinase activity induced by hypoxia/reoxygenation in cultured human umbilical vein endothelial cells, suggesting ginsenosides may play a pivotal role in preventing hypoxia/reoxygenation injury[52]. In an *in vitro* study, American ginseng exhibited effective antioxidant activity in both lipid-soluble and water-soluble media

by its chelating and scavenging activities. It is known that Fe^{2+} and Cu^{2+} ions catalyze hydroxyl (OH$^.$) radical formation, and thereby accelerate lipid peroxidation. American ginseng extract has strong binding affinity to transition metal ions and inhibits the reduction of Fe^{3+} to Fe^{2+} and Cu^{3+} to Cu^{2+} to suppress the initiation of lipid peroxidation, and directly scavenges 1-diphenyl-2-picrylhydrazyl (DPPH) radicals and hydroperoxides (LOOH)[53].

Some work has been done in human trials to test whether the antioxidant effects of ginseng seen at the cellular level translate to the clinical setting. In a small randomized clinical trial of patients undergoing mitral valve replacement, the use of ginseng even more so than ginsenoside Rb in the cardioplegia improved post-bypass cardiac function (vs. control patients) as measured by transesophageal echocardiography[54]. However, no index of oxidant stress was used in this study.

Hawthorn

Hawthorn (*Crataegus* species) is the subject of one of the largest herbal clinical trials currently underway, approved by Commission E for use in treating New York Heart Association functional class II congestive heart failure. Hawthorn, a shrub native to both Europe and North America, contains a number of flavonoids and oligomeric procyanthin constituents within its leaves, flowers and berries which have been formulated into a standard extract WS 1442. In addition to acting as an inotrope, vasodilator and antihyperlipidemic agent, hawthorn also has potent antioxidant properties. It has been shown to decrease reperfusion injury in ischemic rat hearts[55]. Given its antioxidant properties, it may work in part via an attenuation of chronic reactive oxygen species released from nicotinamide adenine dinucleotide phosphate (NAD(P)H) oxidases and mitochondria – thought to be involved in the development and progression of heart failure[56]. Several clinical trials of hawthorn report improved symptoms and cardiac performance in patients with congestive heart failure[57,58]. These studies have culminated in the initiation of the Survival and Prognosis Investigation of

Crataegus Extract (SPICE) trial, an international (120 centers, seven countries) randomized placebo-controlled study of WS 1441 (450 mg/day for 24 months) in which it is hoped to enroll 2300 patients by this year with New York Heart Association (NYHA) functional class II and III[59]. Study endpoints include mortality, cardiac events and hospitalization.

Scutellaria baicalensis

Scutellaria baicalensis, known as 'Huang-Qin' in China and as 'Hwang-Gum' in Korea, is a widely used herbal medicine. The major constituents of *Scutellaria baicalensis* extract are flavonoids, a group of polyhydroxy phenols[60], such as baicalein, baicalin, wogonin and skullcapflavone I and II. These flavonoids have been shown to possess exceptional antioxidant activities[61–63]. Amongst the flavonoids, baicalein has attracted considerable attention, due to its phenolic hydrogens, and has been reported to exhibit anti-inflammatory, antihyperlipidemic and anti-arteriosclerotic effects.

Previous studies have shown that baicalein inhibits lipid peroxidation in rat liver homogenates[64], microsomes[65] and lecithin liposome membrane[66] and in brain cortex mitochondria[62]. It has been reported that baicalein prevents cell death induced by hydrogen peroxide in human neuroblastoma SH-SY5Y cells[63], dermal fibroblast[67] and protects against hippocampal neuronal death induced by 5 min of cerebral ischemia in gerbils[61].

In addition to preventing membrane and cell damage, *S. baicalensis* extract modulates nitric oxide (NO) production after concurrent treatment with interferon-γ (a NO inducer) in mouse peritoneal macrophages[68]. Baicalein has been shown to mediate the induction of quinone reductase and quinone reductase mRNA in the Hepa 1c1c7 marine hepatoma cell line[69]. A recent study has shown that *S. baicalensis* extract increases Bcl-2 protein, also known as anti-death factor, while it decreases Bax protein level (protein that induces apoptosis) in neuronal HT-22 cells during hydrogen peroxide exposure. Pretreatment with *S. baicalensis* extract increases cell viability and

reduces oxidant stress-induced protein carbonyl formation. Two-dimensional electrophoresis showed that *S. baicalensis* extract decreases oxidized protein by 15%. It appears that *S. baicalensis* extract confers an anti-apoptotic effect through the interaction of *Bcl-2* and *Bax* genes[70].

It has been demonstrated that *S. baicalensis* extract and baicalein directly scavenge superoxide, hydroxyl radicals, DPPH radical and alkyl radicals generated in chemical and enzyme systems[62,71]. Also, *S. baicalensis* extract inhibits xanthine oxidase, succinoxidase and NADH-oxidase to suppress free radical formation[72,73].

Oxidants such as reactive oxygen species (ROS) have been shown to participate in myocardial ischemia/reperfusion injury. Antioxidants are known to protect against the ROS-mediated tissue injury, e.g. in cardiac ischemia/reperfusion. Recently, our studies have demonstrated that *S. baicalensis* extract and baicalein confer cardioprotection in a perfused, cultured cardiomyocyte during brief hypoxia, simulated ischemia/reperfusion, and mitochondria electron transport chain complex III inhibition with antimycin A. The results have showed that *S. baicalensis* extract and baicalein attenuate oxidant generation during all conditions studied and significantly decrease cell death at reperfusion after ischemia. Very interestingly, we found that *S. baicalensis* extract and baicalein, given only during the reperfusion phase, attenuate a ROS burst at 5 min after 1 h simulated ischemia in a dose-dependent fashion (Figure 2a, b and c). Their protection may be related to the ability of the extracted chemicals to enter cells and orient in biomembranes. Baicalein, being free of sugar moieties, is more lipid soluble and may be able to penetrate the membrane with greater ease. An *in vitro* study revealed that *S. baicalensis* extract and baicalein possess potent ROS scavenging activity using electron paramagnetic resonance spectroscopy with spin trap 5-methoxy-carbonyl-5-methyl-1-pyrroline-*N*-oxide (MMPO) and biochemical cell free system (Figure 2d)[74,75]. These findings indicated that *S. baicalensis* extract and baicalein protect against oxidant-mediated cell injury in the ischemia/reperfusion model, presumably by virtue of its potent free radical scavenging ability and its ability to traverse cell membranes.

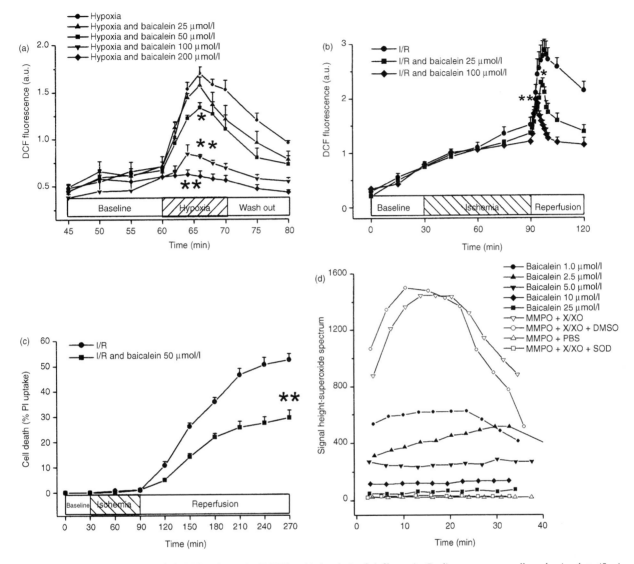

Figure 2 (a) Effect of baicalein on 2′,7′-dichlorofluorescin (DCFH) oxidation during brief hypoxia. Cardiomyocytes were allowed to incubate 45 min and perfuse 15 min with normoxia, and then exposed to 10 min of hypoxia ($pO_2 = 3$ torr) followed by a 10-min normoxia. Hypoxia increased in DCF fluorescence. By contrast, baicalein given during a 10-min period of hypoxia produced a concentration-dependent attenuation in DCF fluorescence. ⋆$p < 0.01$, ⋆⋆$p < 0.001$ compared to hypoxia. (b) Effect of baicalein on DCFH oxidation during ischemia/reperfusion (I/R). At 30 min of reperfusion following 1 h of ischemia, there was a rapid burst of DCF fluorescence. In cells treated with baicalein (25 μmol/l or 100 μmol/l), DCF fluorescence was attenuated. ⋆$p < 0.01$, ⋆⋆$p < 0.001$ compared to untreated cells. (c) Effect of baicalein on cell death during ischemia/reperfusion. When baicalein (50 μmol/l) was given only at reperfusion, PI uptake was significantly reduced at the end of 3 h of reperfusion. ⋆⋆$p < 0.001$ compared to untreated cells. (d) Effect of baicalein on the intensity of the electron paramagnetic resonance (EPR) spectrum of the 5-methoxycarbonyl-5-methyl-1-pyrroline-*N*-oxide (MMPO) spin trap adduct of superoxide. Superoxide anions (~ 10 μmol/l/min) generated by xanthine (X, 0.40 mmol/l) + xanthine oxidase (XO, 0.04 U/ml) were trapped by MMPO to yield a product with a characteristic EPR spectrum. The intensity of this spectrum was attenuated by baicalein in a dose-dependent manner. DMSO, dimethyl sulfoxide; PBS, phosphate buffered saline; SOD, superoxide dismutase

Possible pro-oxidant effects of herbal compounds

One important potential danger of herbal preparations is their ability to become pro-oxidants under certain conditions. For example, dietary polyphenols can be metabolized by peroxidases to form pro-oxidant phenoxyl radicals. Such radicals, particularly in the presence of Al, Zn, Ca, Mg and Cd can stimulate significant lipid peroxidation and have the potential to cause DNA damage[76,77]. Our own work has suggested that grape seed proanthocyanidin extract can at higher doses become a pro-oxidant, enough to cause cell death (Figure 3a and b). Since there are few dosing guidelines followed by consumers of these products, the notion that 'more is better' could potentially lead to higher oxidant stress in the long term. This also points out the value of measuring oxidant stress levels in antioxidant trials. For example, the trials showing increased mortality among smokers taking β-carotene supplements[12,13] may have resulted in part from increased oxidant stress rather than decreased. Without measures of oxidant stress, it is difficult to know what higher doses, or doses given in the context of other pro-oxidant agents, are doing to impact overall oxidant stress.

Why antioxidants may be detrimental: preconditioning

Preconditioning was described in 1986 as a paradoxical protective effect on the heart in which brief episodes of ischemia increase the heart's tolerance to a subsequent sustained perid of ischemia[78]. Originally, canine hearts were preconditioned with four 5 min occlusions of the coronary artery, each followed by 5 min of reperfusion[78]. When compared to controls, these hearts had 75% less infarcted myocardium after 40 min of occlusion. This early first window of preconditioning protection (within minutes to hours following the preconditioning stimulus) has been demonstrated in numerous *in vivo* models[79–85]. Since the work of Murry and colleagues, in which an antioxidant actually reversed the protective effects of preconditioning, it has become clear that oxidants may actually play an important role in the signaling induction of this protective adaptation[86]. Our own

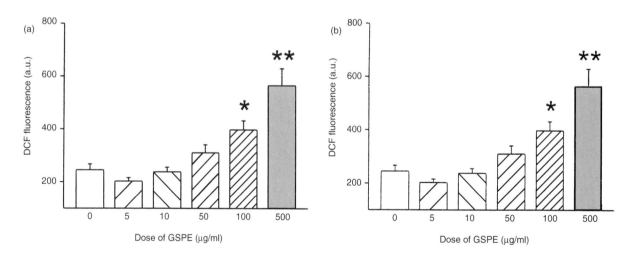

Figure 3 (a) Effect of increasing grape seed proanthocyanidin extract (GSPE) exposure on 2′7,′-dichlorofluorescin (DCFH) oxidation. Cardiomyocytes were exposed to GSPE (5, 10, 50, 100 and 500 μg/ml) for 8 h. DCF fluorescence was increased with increasing doses of GSPE at 100 and 500 μg/ml compared to non-GSPE-exposed cells (*n* = 10). ⋆*p* < 0.01; ⋆⋆*p* < 0.001. (b) Effect of increasing GSPE exposure on cell viability. Cardiomyocytes were exposed to GSPE (5, 10, 50, 100 and 500 μg/ml) for 8 h. Cell death was increased with increasing doses of GSPE at 100 and 500 μg/ml compared to non-GSPE-exposed cells (*n* = 10). ⋆*p* < 0.01; ⋆⋆*p* < 0.001

work shows that antioxidants attenuate oxidant signaling and abrogate preconditioning protection[87].

ACUTE EFFECTS OF HERBAL ANTIOXIDANTS ON CARDIOVASCULAR DISEASE

Herbal medications in treating acute cardiovascular disease

While much of the application of the antioxidant properties of herbal preparations has focused on chronic preventive effects, another important application is that of acute treatments particularly for ischemic emergencies. Such diseases include myocardial infarction, stroke, cardiac arrest and shock; and all involve ischemia and reperfusion – conditions which could quickly generate increased oxidant stress. The potential for impact by effective drugs which act quickly to attenuate oxidant stress is highlighted by cardiac arrest. Cardiac arrest affects 1000 women and men every day in the USA outside the hospital, occurring unexpectedly during their daily routines, with many under 50 years of age[88]. Survival is poor – usually less than 2–4%[89], most likely because irreversible injury to the brain and heart begins within minutes following global ischemia. This rapid rate of injury allows little time for all our modern efforts including mobile emergency medical services, cardiopulmonary resuscitation, trauma centers, and over 5000 emergency rooms to make a difference. The survival rate is particularly dismal after failed defibrillation and experts agree that a new approach is desperately needed[90].

Improving survival after cardiac arrest would have a significant impact on society and major causes of death, including treatment of other causes of arrest such as trauma and asphyxia, the leading causes of death in the young. In addition, any new therapy effective after such global ischemia would probably have a 'ripple' effect on the treatment of focal ischemic injuries to the heart and brain, i.e. myocardial infarction and stroke – leading causes of death and disability, respectively, in the USA[91]. The major barrier to treating all diseases of ischemia is time. During the global

ischemia of cardiac arrest, cells within key organs such as the heart and brain begin to die within 10 min under normothermic conditions. Antioxidant agents which rapidly gain intracellular access have the potential to improve survival from cardiac arrest if oxidants are found to play an important role in post-resuscitation injury. For every 100 cardiac arrest patients treated outside the hospital, approximately 30 regain a pulse; yet ultimately only five or less leave the hospital alive, most dying due to heart and brain dysfunction. Thus, improvement in post-resuscitation care would have the potential to improve survival from cardiac arrest as much as six-fold. Efforts to improve post-resuscitation care are justified since 75% of those discharged alive return to their communities with intact or only mildly impaired neurological function. A significant cause of the subsequent heart and brain dysfunction that kills these patients is probably due to oxidant injury and apoptosis. Recent evidence suggests that apoptosis occurs in the heart not during ischemia, but during the early events of reperfusion, i.e. in the post-resuscitation phase, suggesting an association with the reintroduction of oxygen and, thus, oxidant generation.

Antioxidants and acute treatment of reperfusion injury at the cellular level

Much work supports the concept of free radical-mediated reperfusion injury following myocardial ischemia[92–94]. Antioxidants decrease injury in many studies, and measures of free radical production have detected surges of reactive oxygen species, particularly the hydroxyl radical, during the first few seconds of reperfusion[95]. Controversy over the importance of reperfusion oxidants is due in part to the failure of antioxidant therapy to provide protection in a number of studies[96]. However, work by us and others suggests two possible explanations for this failure:

(1) Many antioxidants will not gain intracellular access fast enough to prevent reperfusion injury[96–98];

(2) Antioxidants could actually worsen ischemia/reperfusion injury in tissue by blocking oxidant

53

signaling which can induce adaptive protection in surrounding cells[86,98,99].

Other investigators have found significant protection in ischemia/reperfusion injury when oxidant stress is attenuated in ways which may not indiscriminately decrease signaling levels of oxidants. The work by Maulik, Yoshida and Das this past year in a perfused mouse heart model of ischemia/reperfusion injury and apoptosis showed significant protection in transgenic mouse hearts overexpressing glutathione peroxidase, and worsened injury in knockout mice without this antioxidant enzyme[100]. Studies such as these support the notion that reperfusion ROS play a critical role in whether cells live or die after ischemia.

Herbal medicines with potential for treating acute oxidant injury

Grape seed proanthocyanidins

Proanthocyanidins, oligomers or polymers of polyhydroxy flavan-3-ol units, are the major polyphenols in grape seeds and wine, particularly in red wine[101]. Over the past 10 years, increasing evidence has strongly suggested that moderate wine or alcohol consumption is associated with a reduced incidence of mortality and morbidity from coronary heart disease[102], possibly through the protective actions of polyphenolic compounds in grapes. The popular press carried stories on the beneficial constituents of red wine. People in Southern France consume more fatty foods in comparison to those in North America, and yet, they suffer less from heart diseases than people in North America or in the Northern regions of Europe. This incompatibility of a diet rich in fatty food with a decreased risk of heart diseases bears the name 'The France Paradox'[103].

Grape seed proanthocyanidins have gained considerable attention because of their wide range of biological and pharmacological properties, including the ability to scavenge free radicals[104,105]. Previous studies have demonstrated that grape seed proanthocyanidin extract (GSPE) inhibited TPA-induced lipid peroxidation and DNA fragmentation in mice brain homogenates and hepatic mitochondria. When compared with conventional antioxidants like vitamin C, E and β-carotene, GSPE proved to be a better antioxidant as evidenced by decreased ROS formation in the peritoneal macrophages of mice[106]. GSPE pretreatment also showed a cytoprotective effect against hydrogen peroxide-induced oxidant stress in cultured macro-

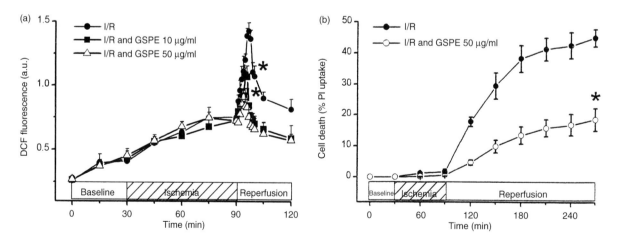

Figure 4 (a) Effects of grape seed proanthocyanidin extract (GSPE) on 2′,7′-dichlorofluorescin (DCFH) oxidation during ischemia and reperfusion (I/R). DCF fluorescence significantly increased during 30 min of reperfusion. When GSPEs were administered at the start of reperfusion, DCF fluorescence markedly decreased at reperfusion. $*p < 0.01$; $**p < 0.001$ compared to untreated ischemic cells. (b) Effects of GSPE on cell death during ischemia and reperfusion. A significant cell death occurred during 3 h of reperfusion. When GSPE was given during reperfusion phase, cell death was significantly reduced during 3 h of reperfusion. $**p < 0.001$ compared to ischemic untreated cells

phage J774A.1, neuroactive adrenal pheochromocytoma PC-12 cells[106] and in rat primary glial cultures, murine macrophage–derived RAW264.7 cells[107].

In recent years, GSPE was found to function as an antioxidant and confer the cardioprotection in oxidant-mediated injury. There is ample evidence indicating the beneficial effects of GSPE in promoting recovery of post-ischemic myocardium, possibly through its antioxidant effect. When hearts obtained from GSPE-fed rats were exposed to ischemia/reperfusion, post-ischemic ventricular function was significantly improved and the extent of myocardial infarction was significantly reduced. The cardioprotective effect of GSPE was explained by its ability to scavenge peroxyl radicals directly and inhibit xanthine oxidase during ischemia/reperfusion and ischemic arrest[108–110]. A similar study further supported the cardioprotective effect of GSPE[111]. In addition, GSPE significantly reduced severe arteriosclerosis in the rabbit aorta and inhibited oxidation of LDL[112], and increased total antioxidant plasma capacity to make the perfused heart less susceptible to ischemia/reperfusion damage in the young and aged rats[113]. A study has recently been reported showing that GSPE protected cardiomyocytes from apoptotic cell death by reducing the expression of proapoptotic genes, *JNK-1* and *c-Jun* during ischemia/reperfusion. The ischemia/reperfusion-mediated myocyte apoptosis is associated with enhanced expression of apoptotic factors, *JNK-1* and *c-Jun* and resulted in ROS generation. Treatment with GSPE reduced the expression of both *JNK-1* and *c-Jun* in the reperfused myocardium and ameliorated free radical formation by almost 50–75%, and simultaneously reduced the appearance of the apoptotic cardiomyocytes in ischemia/reperfusion heart. These data indicate that the cardioprotective effect of GSPE may be attributed to its ability to

block antideath signals by inhibiting pro-apoptotic factor and gene, *JNK-1* and *c-Jun*[110].

It has been reported that low-output NO can protect against ROS-mediated injury, whereas high-output NO may result in cytotoxicity. GSPE treatment alone can cause a low level of NO production in rat primary glial cells and murine macrophage-derived RAW264.7 cells, but did not show any cytotoxicity. However, GSPE can protect cells from lipopolysaccharide/interferon induced nitrosative stress by enhancing the endogenous glutathione (GSH) pool[107]. Recently, our own study has found that GSPE attenuates oxidant generation and confers cardioprotective effect against ischemia/reperfusion injury in cardiomyocytes (Figure 4a and b).

CONCLUSION

Given the importance of oxidants in both cardiovascular health and disease, it is likely that antioxidants will play important roles in both the chronic prevention and acute treatment of certain cardiovascular diseases. This chapter also highlighted recent thinking that some antioxidants at certain doses and under certain conditions can be harmful. Thus, it will be increasingly important to tailor our antioxidant therapies to attenuate harmful oxidants and not interfere with oxidants produced as part of healthy communication between cells and tissues. The promise of herbal medicines is great, as the numerous compounds they contain have the potential to treat quickly the oxidant stress of ischemic emergencies – an area not as extensively explored as chronic preventive therapy. In addition, they have been time-tested in some instances for centuries, and thus, may be safer as chronic therapies than even traditional antioxidants.

References

1. Kaye AD, Clarke RC, Sabar R, Vig S, Dhawan KP, Hofbauer R, *et al.* Herbal medicines: current trends in anesthesiology practice – a hospital survey. *J Clin Anesth* 2000;12:468–71

2. Ang-Lee MK, Moss J, Yuan CS. Herbal medicines and perioperative care. *J Am Med Assoc* 2001;286:208–16

3. Valli G, Giardina EG. Benefits, adverse effects and drug interactions of herbal therapies with cardiovascular effects. *J Am Coll Cardiol* 2002;39:1083–95

4. Hertog MG, Feskens EJ, Hollman PC, Katan MB, Kromhout D. Dietary antioxidant flavonoids and risk of coronary heart disease: the Zutphen Elderly Study. *Lancet* 1993;342:1007–11

5. Gillman MW, Cupples LA, Gagnon D, Posner BM, Ellison RC, Castelli WP, *et al.* Protective effect of fruits and vegetables on development of stroke in men. *J Am Med Assoc* 1995;273:1113–17

6. Key TJ, Thorogood M, Appleby PN, Burr ML. Dietary habits and mortality in 11 000 vegetarians and health conscious people: results of a 17 year follow up. *Br Med J* 1996;313:775–9

7. Hu FB, Stampfer MJ, Manson JE, Rimm EB, Colditz GA, Rosner BA, *et al.* Frequent nut consumption and risk of coronary heart disease in women: prospective cohort study. *Br Med J* 1998;317:1341–5

8. Strandhagen E, Hansson PO, Bosaeus I, Isaksson B, Eriksson H. High fruit intake may reduce mortality among middle-aged and elderly men. The Study of Men Born in 1913. *Eur J Clin Nutr* 2000;54:337–41

9. Bazzano LA, He J, Ogden LG, Loria C, Vupputuri S, Myers L, *et al.* Legume consumption and risk of coronary heart disease in US men and women: NHANES I Epidemiologic Follow-up Study. *Arch Intern Med* 2001;161:2573–8

10. Rimm EB, Stampfer MJ, Ascherio A, Giovannucci E, Colditz GA, Willett WC. Vitamin E consumption and the risk of coronary heart disease in men. *N Engl J Med* 1993;328:1450–6

11. Stampfer MJ, Hennekens CH, Manson JE, Colditz GA, Rosner B, Willett WC. Vitamin E consumption and the risk of coronary disease in women. *N Engl J Med* 1993;328:1444–9

12. Rapola JM, Virtamo J, Haukka JK, Heinonen OP, Albanes D, Taylor PR, *et al.* Effect of vitamin E and beta carotene on the incidence of angina pectoris. A randomized, double-blind, controlled trial. *J Am Med Assoc* 1996;275:693–8

13. Rapola JM, Virtamo J, Ripatti S, Huttunen JK, Albanes D, Taylor PR, *et al.* Randomised trial of alpha-tocopherol and beta-carotene supplements on incidence of major coronary events in men with previous myocardial infarction. *Lancet* 1997;349:1715–20

14. Yusuf S, Dagenais G, Pogue J, Bosch J, Sleight P. Vitamin E supplementation and cardiovascular events in high-risk patients. The Heart Outcomes Prevention Evaluation Study Investigators. *N Engl J Med* 2000;342:154–60

15. Stephens NG, Parsons A, Schofield PM, Kelly F, Cheeseman K, Mitchinson MJ. Randomised controlled trial of vitamin E in patients with coronary disease: Cambridge Heart Antioxidant Study (CHAOS). *Lancet* 1996;347:781–6

16. Vile GF, Winterbourn CC. Inhibition of adriamycin-promoted microsomal lipid peroxidation by beta-carotene, alpha-tocopherol and retinol at high and low oxygen partial pressures. *FEBS Lett* 1988;238:353–6

17. Jialal I, Norkus EP, Cristol L, Grundy SM. beta-Carotene inhibits the oxidative modification of low-density lipoprotein. *Biochim Biophys Acta* 1991;1086:134–8

18. Morris DL, Kritchevsky SB, Davis CE. Serum carotenoids and coronary heart disease. The Lipid Research Clinics Coronary Primary Prevention Trial and Follow-up Study. *J Am Med Assoc* 1994;272:1439–41

19. Kushi LH, Folsom AR, Prineas RJ, Mink PJ, Wu Y, Bostick RM. Dietary antioxidant vitamins and death from coronary heart disease in postmenopausal women. *N Engl J Med* 1996;334:1156–62

20. Evans RW, Shaten BJ, Day BW, Kuller LH. Prospective association between lipid soluble antioxidants and coronary heart disease in men. The Multiple Risk Factor Intervention Trial. *Am J Epidemiol* 1998;147:180–6

21. Blot WJ, Li JY, Taylor PR, Guo W, Dawsey S, Wang GQ, *et al.* Nutrition intervention trials in Linxian, China: supplementation with specific vitamin/mineral combinations, cancer incidence, and disease-specific mortality in the general population. *J Natl Cancer Inst* 1993;85:1483–92

22. Greenberg ER, Baron JA, Karagas MR, Stukel TA, Nierenberg DW, Stevens MM, *et al.* Mortality associated with low plasma concentration of beta carotene and the effect of oral supplementation. *J Am Med Assoc* 1996;275:699–703

23. Hennekens CH, Buring JE, Manson JE, Stampfer M, Rosner B, Cook NR, *et al.* Lack of effect of long-term supplementation with beta carotene on the incidence of malignant neoplasms and cardiovascular disease. *N Engl J Med* 1996;334:1145–9

24. Omenn GS, Goodman GE, Thornquist MD, Balmes J, Cullen MR, Glass A, *et al.* Effects of a combination of beta carotene and vitamin A on lung cancer and cardiovascular disease. *N Engl J Med* 1996;334:1150–5

25. Rice-Evans CA, Miller NJ, Paganga G. Structure-antioxidant activity relationships of flavonoids and phenolic acids. *Free Radic Biol Med* 1996;20:933–56

26. Hesketh T, Zhu WX. Health in China. Traditional Chinese medicine: one country, two systems. *Br Med J* 1997;315:115–17

27. Lei XL, Chiou GC. Cardiovascular pharmacology of *Panax notoginseng* (Burk) F.H. Chen and *Salvia miltiorrhiza*. *Am J Chin Med* 1986;14:145–52

28. Niu XL, Ichimori K, Yang X, Hirota Y, Hoshiai K, Li M, Nakazawa H. Tanshinone II-A inhibits low density lipoprotein oxidation *in vitro*. *Free Radic Res* 2000;33:305–12

29. Zhao BL, Jiang W, Zhao Y, Hou JW, Xin WJ. Scavenging effects of *Salvia miltiorrhiza* on free radicals and its protection for myocardial mitochondrial membranes from ischemia-reperfusion injury. *Biochem Mol Biol Int* 1996;38:1171–82

30. Ng TB, Liu F, Wang ZT. Antioxidative activity of natural products from plants. *Life Sci* 2000;66:709–23

31. Yu CM, Chan JC, Sanderson JE. Chinese herbs and warfarin potentiation by 'danshen'. *J Intern Med* 1997;241:337–9

32. Orekhov AN, Grunwald J. Effects of garlic on atherosclerosis. *Nutrition* 1997;13:656–63

33. Kiesewetter H, Jung F, Jung EM, Blume J, Mrowietz C, Birk A, *et al.* Effects of garlic coated tablets in peripheral arterial occlusive disease. *Clin Invest* 1993;71:383–6

34. Koscielny J, Klussendorf D, Latza R, Schmitt R, Radtke H, Siegel G, *et al.* The antiatherosclerotic effect of *Allium sativum*. *Atherosclerosis* 1999;144:237–49

35. Janssens D, Remacle J, Drieu K, Michiels C. Protection of mitochondrial respiration activity by bilobalide. *Biochem Pharmacol* 1999;58:109–19

36. Liebgott T, Miollan M, Berchadsky Y, Drieu K, Culcasi M, Pietri S. Complementary cardioprotective effects of flavonoid metabolites and terpenoid constituents of *Ginkgo biloba* extract (EGb 761) during ischemia and reperfusion. *Basic Res Cardiol* 2000;95:368–77

37. Zhou LJ, Zhu XZ. Reactive oxygen species-induced apoptosis in PC12 cells and protective effect of bilobalide. *J Pharmacol Exp Ther* 2000;293:982–8

38. Pietri S, Seguin JR, d'Arbigny P, Drieu K, Culcasi M. *Ginkgo biloba* extract (EGb 761) pretreatment limits free radical-induced oxida-

tive stress in patients undergoing coronary bypass surgery. *Cardiovasc Drugs Ther* 1997;11:121–31

39. Lim JH, Wen TC, Matsuda S, Tanaka J, Maeda N, Peng H, *et al.* Protection of ischemic hippocampal neurons by ginsenoside Rb1, a main ingredient of ginseng root. *Neurosci Res* 1997;28:191–200

40. Li T, Mazza, G, Cottrell, AC, Gao, L. Ginsenosides in root and leaves of American Ginseng. *J Agric Food Chem* 1996;44:717–20

41. Wang X, Sakuma T, Asafu-Adjaye E, Shiu GK. Determination of ginsenosides in plant extracts from *Panax ginseng* and *Panax quinquefolius* L. by LC/MS/MS. *Anal Chem* 1999;71:1579–84

42. Harkey MR, Henderson GL, Gershwin ME, Stern JS, Hackman RM. Variability in commercial ginseng products: an analysis of 25 preparations. *Am J Clin Nutr* 2001;73:1101–6

43. Li W, Gu C, Zhang H, Awang DV, Fitzloff JF, Fong HH, *et al.* Use of high-performance liquid chromatography-tandem mass spectrometry to distinguish *Panax ginseng* C. A. Meyer (Asian ginseng) and *Panax quinquefolius* L. (North American ginseng). *Anal Chem* 2000;72:5417–22

44. Chan TW, But PP, Cheng SW, Kwok IM, Lau FW, Xu HX. Differentiation and authentication of *Panax ginseng*, *Panax quinquefolius*, and ginseng products by using HPLC/MS. *Anal Chem* 2000;72:1281–7

45. Li W, Fitzloff JF. Determination of 24(R)-pseudoginsenoside F(11) in North American ginseng using high performance liquid chromatography with evaporative light scattering detection. *J Pharm Biomed Anal* 2001;25:257–65

46. Smith RG, Caswell D, Carriere A, Zielke B. Variation in the ginsenoside content of American Ginseng, *Panax quinquefolius* L., roots. *Can J Bot* 1996;74:1616–20

47. Attele AS, Wu JA, Yuan CS. Ginseng pharmacology: multiple constituents and multiple actions. *Biochem Pharmacol* 1999;58:1685–93

48. Li JP, Lu ZZ, Lu YF. Lipoprotein-cholesterol metabolism and anti-oxidative effects of *Panax quinquefolius* saponins on experimental hyperlipidemic rat. *Chung Kuo Yao Hsue Tsa Chi* 1993;28:355–7

49. Li J, Huang M, Teoh H, Man RY. *Panax quinquefolium* saponins protects low density lipoproteins from oxidation. *Life Sci* 1999;64:53–62

50. Li JP, Huang M, Teoh H, Man RY. Interactions between *Panax quinquefolium* saponins and vitamin C are observed *in vitro*. *Mol Cell Biochem* 2000;204:77–82

51. Yang SJ, Qu JB, Zhang GG, Zhang WJ. Protective effects of *Panax quinquefolius* saponins on oxidative damage of cultured rat cardiac cells. *Chung Kuo Yao Hsue Tsa Chi* 1992;17:555–7

52. Dou DQ, Zhang YW, Zhang L, Chen YJ, Yao XS. The inhibitory effects of ginsenosides on protein tyrosine kinase activated by hypoxia/reoxygenation in cultured human umbilical vein endothelial cells. *Planta Med* 2001;67:19–23

53. Kitts DD, Wijewickreme AN, Hu C. Antioxidant properties of a North American ginseng extract. *Molec Cell Biochem* 2000;203:1–1059

54. Zhan Y, Xu XH, Jiang YP. Protective effects of ginsenoside on myocardiac ischemic and reperfusion injuries. *Zhonghua Yi Xue Za Zhi* 1994;74:626–8, 648

55. Nasa Y, Hashizume H, Hoque AN, Abiko Y. Protective effect of crataegus extract on the cardiac mechanical dysfunction in isolated perfused working rat heart. *Arzneimittelforschung* 1993;43:945–9

56. Sorescu D, Griendling KK. Reactive oxygen species, mitochondria, and NAD(P)H oxidases in the development and progression of heart failure. *Congest Heart Fail* 2002;8:132–40

57. Leuchtgens H. Crataegus Special Extract WS 1442 in NYHA II heart failure. A placebo controlled randomized double-blind study. *Fortschr Med* 1993;111:352–4

58. Tauchert M, Gildor A, Lipinski J. High-dose Crataegus extract WS 1442 in the treatment of NYHA stage II heart failure. *Herz* 1999;24:465–74; discussion 475

59. Holubarsch CJ, Colucci WS, Meinertz T, Gaus W, Tendera M. Survival and prognosis: investigation of Crataegus extract WS 1442 in congestive heart failure (SPICE) – rationale, study design and study protocol. *Eur J Heart Fail* 2000;2:431–7

60. Kimura Y, Okuda H, Tani T, Arichi S. Studies on Scutellariae radix. VI. Effects of flavanone compounds on lipid peroxidation in rat liver. *Chem Pharm Bull* 1982;30:1792–5

61. Hamada H, Hiramatsu M, Edamatsu R, Mori A. Free radical scavenging action of baicalein. *Arch Biochem Biophys* 1993;306:261–6

62. Gao Z, Huang K, Yang X, Xu H. Free radical scavenging and antioxidant activities of flavonoids extracted from the radix of *Scutellaria baicalensis* Georgi. *Biochim Biophys Acta* 1999;1472:643–50

63. Gao Z, Huang K, Xu H. Protective effects of flavonoids in the roots of *Scutellaria baicalensis* Georgi against hydrogen peroxide-induced oxidative stress in HS-SY5Y cells. *Pharmacol Res* 2001;43:173–8

64. Kimuya Y, Kubo M, Tani T, Arichi S, Okuda H. Studies on Scutellariae radix. IV. Effects on lipid peroxidation in rat liver. *Chem Pharm Bull (Tokyo)* 1981;29:2610–17

65. Gao D, Sakurai K, Chen J, Ogiso T. Protection by baicalein against ascorbic acid-induced lipid peroxidation of rat liver microsomes. *Res Commun Molec Pathol Pharmacol* 1995;90:103–14

66. Gabrielska J, Oszmianski J, Zylka R, Komorowska M. Antioxidant activity of flavones from *Scutellaria baicalensis* in lecithin liposomes. *Z Naturforsch [C]* 1997;52:817–23

67. Gao D, Tawa R, Masaki H, Okano Y, Sakurai H. Protective effects of baicalein against cell damage by reactive oxygen species. *Chem Pharm Bull (Tokyo)* 1998;46:1383–7

68. Kim HM, Moon EJ, Li E, Kim KM, Nam SY, Chung CK. The nitric oxide-producing activities of *Scutellaria baicalensis*. *Toxicology* 1999;135:109–15

69. Park HJ, Lee YW, Park HH, Lee YS, Kwon IB, Yu JH. Induction of quinone reductase by a methanol extract of *Scutellaria baicalensis* and its flavonoids in murine Hepa 1c1c7 cells. *Eur J Cancer Prev* 1998;7:465–71

70. Choi J, Conrad CC, Malakowsky CA, Talent JM, Yuan CS, Gracy RW. Flavones from *Scutellaria baicalensis* Georgi attenuate apoptosis and protein oxidation in neuronal cell lines. *Biochim Biophys Acta* 2002;1571:201–10

71. Shieh DE, Liu LT, Lin CC. Antioxidant and free radical scavenging effects of baicalein, baicalin and wogonin. *Anticancer Res* 2000;20:2861–5

72. Hanasaki Y, Ogawa S, Fukui S. The correlation between active oxygens scavenging and antioxidative effects of flavonoids. *Free Radic Biol Med* 1994;16:845–50

73. Hodnick WF, Duval DL, Pardini RS. Inhibition of mitochondrial respiration and cyanide-stimulated generation of reactive oxygen species by selected flavonoids. *Biochem Pharm* 1994;47:573–80

74. Shao ZH, Li CQ, Vanden Hoek TL, Becker LB, Schumacker PT, Wu JA, *et al.* Extract from *Scutellaria baicalensis* Georgi attenuates oxidant stress in cardiomyocytes. *J Molec Cell Cardiol* 1999;31:1885–95

75. Shao ZH, Vanden Hoek TL, Qin Y, Becker LB, Schumacker PT, Li CQ, *et al.* Baicalein attenuates oxidant stress in cardiomyocytes. *Am J Physiol Heart Circ Physiol* 2002;282:H999–H1006

76. Galati G, Sabzevari O, Wilson JX, O'Brien PJ. Prooxidant activity and cellular effects of the phenoxyl radicals of dietary flavonoids and other polyphenolics. *Toxicology* 2002;177:91–104

77. Sakihama Y, Cohen MF, Grace SC, Yamasaki H. Plant phenolic antioxidant and prooxidant activities: phenolics-induced oxidative damage mediated by metals in plants. *Toxicology* 2002;177:67–80

78. Murry CE, Jennings RB, Reimer KA. Preconditioning with ischemia: a delay of lethal cell injury in ischemic myocardium. *Circulation* 1986;74:1124–36

79. Li GC, Vasquez BS, Gallagher KP, Lucchesi BR. Myocardial protection with preconditioning. *Circulation* 1990;82:609–19

80. Schott RJ, Rohmann S, Braun ER, Schaper W. Ischemic preconditioning reduces infarct size in swine myocardium. *Circ Res* 1990;66:1133–42

81. Cohen MV, Liu GS, Downey JM. Preconditioning causes improved wall motion as well as smaller infarcts after transient coronary occlusion in rabbits. *Circulation* 1991;84:341–9

82. Asimakis GK, Inners-McBride K, Medellin G, Conti VR. Ischemic preconditioning attenuates acidosis in isolated rat heart. *Am J Physiol* 1992;263:H887–94

83. Lawson CS, Downey JM. Preconditioning: state of the art myocardial protection. *Cardiovasc Res* 1993;27:542–50

84. Baxter GF, Yellon DM. Ischemic preconditioning of the myocardium: a new paradigm for clinical cardioprotection. *Br J Clin Pharmacol* 1994;38:381–7

85. Jenkins DP, Pugsley WB, Yellon DM. Ischaemic preconditioning in a model of global ischaemia: infarct size limitation, but no reduction of stunning. *J Molec Cell Cardiol* 1995;27:1623–32

86. Murry CE, Richard VJ, Jennings RB, Reimer KA. Preconditioning with ischemia: is the protective effect meditated by free radical induced myocardial stunning? *Circulation* 1988;78(Suppl II):77

87. Vanden Hoek TL, Becker LB, Shao Z, Li C, Schumacker PT. Reactive oxygen species released from mitochondria during brief hypoxia induce preconditioning in cardiomyocytes. *J Biol Chem* 1998;273:18092–8

88. Becker LB, Ostrander MP, Barrett J, Kondos GT. CPR Chicago: outcome of cardiopulmonary resuscitation in a large metropolitan area – where are the survivors? *Ann Emerg Med* 1991;20:355–61

89. Becker LB, Han BH, Meyer PM, Wright FA, Rhodes KV, Smith DW, *et al.* CPR Chicago: racial differences in the incidence of cardiac arrest and subsequent survival. *N Engl J Med* 1993;329:600–6

90. Weil MH, Becker LB, Budinger T, Kern K, Nichol G, Shechter I, *et al.* Workshop executive summary report: post-resuscitative and initial utility in life saving efforts (PULSE). *Circulation* 2001;103:1182–4

91. National Heart, Lung and Blood Institute. *Morbidity and Mortality: Chartbook on Cardiovascular, Lung, and Blood Diseases.* Bethesda, MD: US Department of Health and Human Services, Public Health Service. National Institute of Health, Bethesda, Maryland, 1992

92. Zak R, Rabinowitz M. Metabolism of the ischemic heart. *Med Clin N Am* 1973;57:93–103

93. Hearse DJ. Stunning: a radical re-review. *Cardiovasc Drug Ther* 1991;5:853–67

94. Das DK. Cellular biochemical and molecular aspects of reperfusion injury. *Ann NY Acad Sci* 1994;723:116–27

95. Zweier JL, Flaherty JT, Weisfeldt ML. Direct measurement of free radical generation following reperfusion of ischemic myocardium. *Proc Natl Acad Sci USA* 1987;84:1404–7

96. Opie LH. Reperfusion injury and its pharmacologic modification. *Circulation* 1989;80:1049–62

97. Vanden Hoek TL, Shao Z, Li C, Zak R, Schumacker PT, Becker LB. Reperfusion injury in cardiac myocytes after simulated ischemia. *Am J Phys* 1996;270:H1334–41

98. Vanden Hoek TL, Becker LB, Shao Z, Li C, Schumacker PT. Preconditioning in cardiomyocytes protects by attenuating oxidant stress at reperfusion. *Circ Res* 2000;86:534–40

99. Das DK, Engelman RM, Maulik N. Oxygen free radical signaling in ischemic preconditioning. *Ann NY Acad Sci* 1999;874:49–65

100. Maulik N, Yoshida T, Das DK. Regulation of cardiomyocyte apoptosis in ischemic reperfused mouse heart by glutathione peroxidase. *Mol Cell Biochem* 2000;196:13–21

101. Ricardo da Silva JM, Darmon M, Fernandez Y, Mitjavila S. Oxygen free radical scavenger capacity in aqueous models of different procyanidins from grape seeds. *J Agric Food Chem* 1991;39:549–52

102. Rimm EB, Giovannucci EL, Willett WC, Colditz GA, Ascherio A, Rosner B, *et al.* Prospective study of alcohol consumption and risk of coronary disease in men. *Lancet* 1991;338:464–8

103. Renaud S, de Lorgeril M. Wine, alcohol, platelets, and the French paradox for coronary heart disease. *Lancet* 1992;339:1523–6

104. Bagchi D, Bagchi M, Stohs SJ, Das DK, Ray SD, Kuszynski CA, *et al.* Free radicals and grape seed proanthocyanidin extract: importance in human health and disease prevention. *Toxicology* 2000;148:187–97

105. Bagchi M, Kuszynski CA, Balmoori J, Joshi SS, Stohs SJ, Bagchi D. Protective effects of antioxidants against smokeless tobacco-induced oxidative stress and modulation of *Bcl-2* and *p53* genes in human oral keratinocytes. *Free Radic Res* 2001;35:181–94

106. Bagchi D, Garg A, Krohn RL, Bagchi M, Bagchi DJ, Balmoori J, *et al.* Protective effects of grape seed proanthocyanidins and selected antioxidants against TPA-induced hepatic and brain lipid peroxidation and DNA fragmentation, and peritoneal macrophage activation in mice. *Gen Pharmacol* 1998;30:771–6

107. Roychowdhury S, Wolf G, Keilhoff G, Bagchi D, Horn T. Protection of primary glial cells by grape seed proanthocyanidin extract against nitrosative/oxidative stress. *Nitric Oxide* 2001;5:137–49

108. Facino RM, Carini M, Aldini G, Berti F, Rossoni G, Bombardelli E, *et al.* Procyanidins from vitis vinifera seeds protect rabbit heart from ischemia/reperfusion injury: antioxidant intervention and/or iron and copper sequestering activity. *Planta Med* 1996;62:495–502

109. Sato M, Maulik G, Ray PS, Bagchi D, Das DK. Cardioprotective effects of grape seed proanthocyanidin against ischemic reperfusion injury. *J Mol Cell Cardiol* 1999;31:1289–97

110. Sato M, Bagchi D, Tosaki A, Das DK. Grape seed proanthocyanidin reduces cardiomyocyte apoptosis by inhibiting ischemia/reperfusion-induced activation of JNK-1 and C-JUN. *Free Radic Biol Med* 2001;31:729–37

111. Pataki T, Bak I, Kovacs P, Bagchi D, Das DK, Tosaki A. Grape seed proanthocyanidins improved cardiac recovery during reperfusion after ischemia in isolated rat hearts. *Am J Clin Nutr* 2002;75:894–9

112. Yamakoshi J, Kataoka S, Koga T, Ariga T. Proanthocyanidin-rich extract from grape seeds attenuates the development of aortic atherosclerosis in cholesterol-fed rabbits. *Atherosclerosis* 1999;142:139–49

113. Facino RM, Carini M, Aldini G, Berti F, Rossoni G, Bombardelli E, *et al.* Diet enriched with procyanidins enhances antioxidant activity and reduces myocardial post-ischaemic damage in rats. *Life Sci* 1999;64:627–42

Evidence-based medicinal action of male hormones and green tea catechins

5

S. Liao, M. T. Dang and R. A. Hiipakka

INTRODUCTION

Male hormones (androgens) are probably the oldest (> 2000 years) drugs used in purified forms. As early as 200 BC, the Chinese were using highly purified androgenic preparations to treat individuals lacking 'maleness activity'. Joseph Needham, a distinguished biochemist in England, stated that this was the most important pre-biochemical discovery. Tea extracts are among the most widely used ancient (> 3000 years) medicinal agents in man's history (Figure 1). In oriental cultures, it has been widely believed for a long time that tea has medicinal efficacy for prevention and treatment of many diseases. Scientific and medical evaluation of tea, however, started only very recently. Our studies also indicate that specific green tea catechins can modulate androgen actions *in vivo*, and therefore might be medically important for treating male hormone-related abnormalities. Androgens and major green tea catechins also modulate the growth of androgen-dependent and -independent prostate cancers, as well as other hormone-related abnormalities.

BIOMEDICAL ACTIVITIES OF GREEN TEA CATECHINS

A comprehensive review of the biochemical and biological studies of the health benefits of green tea is now available[1]. Green tea catechins have been noted for their benefit in treating various cancers, cardiovascular diseases, hypertension, allergy, asthma, arthritis, diabetes, nervous system disorders including memory loss, tooth decay, osteoporosis, and bacterial and viral infectivity. Most of these studies, however, need more thorough re-evaluation.

Epidemiological studies of the health benefits of green tea have been equivocal. Such studies are often complicated by variations in diets, environmental conditions, socioeconomic factors and living habits, such as smoking and alcohol consumption. Since catechins are unstable to air oxidation, the qualities of green tea and its beverage are usually not assessed or standardized. Numerous studies of the molecular and cellular activities of purified catechins have been reported. These investigations include modulation of enzyme activities *in vitro* and antiproliferative effects of catechins on cells in culture. Findings from this research may provide potentially important leads to the understanding of the molecular or cellular bases of green tea benefits. However, many of these effects were observed with the concentrations of catechins that are difficult to attain through oral consumption of green tea beverage, and therefore it is difficult to determine whether these *in vitro* effects represent the *in vivo* action of green tea catechins.

CONTROL OF MALE HORMONE ACTION

In the early 1960s, it was found that androgens can rapidly enhance RNA synthesis in target organs, such as the ventral prostate of rats, suggesting that androgens act by modulating gene expression[2]. Subsequent

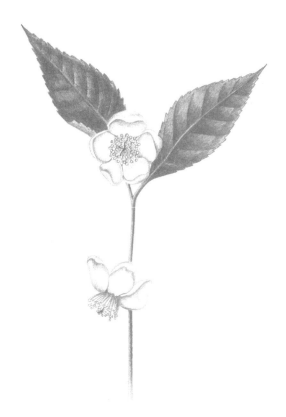

Figure 1   The tea plant

studies have shown that, in some androgen-sensitive organs, testosterone, the major androgen produced by the testis and circulating in blood, is converted by 5α-reductase to 5α-dihydrosterone (DHT), which binds to a specific nuclear androgen receptor (AR)[2,3]. The DHT–AR complex, in conjunction with other chromosomal proteins, then regulates the synthesis of specific RNA and modulates cellular activities and organ functions. Mutations in the genes for 5α-reductase or the AR and loss of their functions have been shown to be responsible for androgen-insensitivity syndromes[4–7].

The molecular steps required for androgen action provide two effective methods for the control of testosterone-regulated responses: first, the use of a 5α-reductase inhibitor to suppress DHT production; and second, the use of an antiandrogen to block the interaction of DHT with AR. Both methods are now being utilized as therapies for androgen-related disorders[3].

NATURAL 5α-REDUCTASE INHIBITORS FOR TREATMENT OF SKIN DISORDERS

A number of natural compounds that inhibit 5α-reductase have been found. The first one we reported was γ-linolenic acid[8], an essential fatty acid in many plant oils including evening primrose and borage oil that are being used as health food products. In cell-free assay systems, γ-linolenic acid is far more active than many dozens of other fatty acids tested and is active at concentrations lower than 5 μmol/l. Green tea catechin gallates, such as (−)-epigallocatechin-3-gallate (EGCG) and (−)-epicatechin-3-gallate (ECG) are also active at concentrations less than 5 μmol/l[9]. The gallate group is important for inhibitory activity. Non-gallated catechins, such as (−)-epicatechin (EC) and (−)-epigallocatechin (EGC), are not active. However, gallic acid and the methyl ester of gallic acid are not active.

The biological activity of γ-linolenic acid and EGCG has been tested *in vivo* using flank organs of male hamsters as animal models. When hamsters are castrated, flank organ growth is clearly suppressed. Topical application of testosterone on the flank organ stimulates the growth of the organ, but this growth is effectively suppressed by topical application of γ-linolenic acid[10] or EGCG[11]. Other natural compounds, including alizarin and curcumin, are also 5α-reductase inhibitors and inhibited flank organ growth. However, EC and EGC, which are not gallated and are not 5α-reductase inhibitors, also inhibited flank organ growth. These compounds may act by a mechanism other than inhibition of 5α-reductase. Since topical application of these inhibitors of flank organ growth does not appear to exhibit systemic effects and can inhibit sebum production from human forehead skin, they may be potentially useful for treatment of human skin problems including acne and baldness.

SUPPRESSION OF PROSTATE TUMORS BY ANDROGEN

Since prostate cancer is initially androgen-dependent, hormonal therapy pioneered by Charles Huggins more than 60 years ago using castration[12] or more recently antiandrogens, has been the front-line therapy for prostate cancer. More than 70% of patients benefit from this therapy. However, prostate cancer recurs in most of these patients in 1–3 years as tumors that do not need androgen for growth. For lack of effective therapy, patients die from this androgen-independent cancer.

During the past 10 years, we established that androgen-independent cancer cells can develop from clonal androgen-dependent cancer cells during long-term (1–3 years) culture in androgen-depleted media[13,14]. This transition to androgen independence is accompanied by dramatically increased AR expression without gene amplification or new mutation in the AR gene. Surprisingly, the growth of these cells is inhibited by physiological levels of androgens.

These androgen-independent prostate cancer cells grow as tumors in castrated athymic mice but not in normal athymic male mice. Administration of androgen to castrated mice prevents tumor growth and suppresses prostate tumors already present in these animals[15]. The 5α-reductase inhibitor, finasteride (Proscar®), or anti-androgens, such as Casodex®, block the repressive effect of testosterone on these xenografts and stimulate tumor growth, suggesting that the growth suppression requires conversion of testosterone to DHT and binding of DHT to AR. If testosterone has a role in suppressing prostate cancer growth in patients, the use of these drugs may enhance the growth of certain prostate cancers.

The DHT-dependent suppression of prostate cancer cell proliferation appears to be dependent on cell cycle arrest due to increased levels of Cdk2 inhibitors including p27[16].

SUPPRESSION OF PROSTATE AND BREAST TUMORS BY EGCG

Green tea consumption has been linked to a lower incidence of cancer of the stomach and certain organs, and numerous studies have shown tumor suppression by lengthy use of green tea beverage in animals[1]. However, many epidemiological studies have not provided strong evidence that green tea is clearly antitumorigenic in humans.

For better understanding of green tea's ability to control cancer growth, we injected purified catechins intraperitoneally into tumor-bearing mice. Human prostate cancer cell lines, PC-3 (AR-negative and androgen insensitive) and LNCaP 104-R (androgen repressive), inoculated subcutaneously into nude mice produced prostate tumors. Green tea EGCG, injected intraperioneally, significantly inhibited the growth and rapidly (within a week) reduced the size of human prostate tumors in athymic mice. Structurally related catechins, such as ECG that lack only one of the eight hydroxyl groups in EGCG, are totally inactive. EC and EGC are also not antitumorigenic[17].

Both androgen-dependent and androgen-independent prostate tumors respond to tumor suppression by EGCG, suggesting that EGCG action is not related to modulation of androgen activity. In addition, the growth of human breast tumors in nude mice produced by human breast cancer MCF-7 cells was also clearly inhibited during the first week of intraperitoneal injection of EGCG.

It is possible that the low clinical incidence of prostate and breast cancer in some Asian countries is related to high green tea consumption. The frequency of the latent, localized prostate cancer does not vary significantly among geographically different populations, but the clinical incidence of metastatic prostate cancer varies considerably between countries (low in Japan and high in the USA). If consumption of green tea beverage is related to this difference, EGCG may play an important role in preventing the progression or metastasis of prostate cancer cells.

MODULATION OF FOOD INTAKE AND OBESITY BY EGCG

In Asian countries, long-term use of green tea beverage is considered to be beneficial for keeping a healthy body weight. However, clear scientific evidence has not been available until recently. We have shown that EGCG, given to rats by intraperitoneal injection, could within 2–7 days reduce body weight by about 20–30%[17,18]. Other structurally related catechins, such as EC, EGC, or ECG, are not effective at the same dose. Body weight loss is reversible; when EGCG administration is stopped, animals regain body weight. Reduction of body weight appears to be due to EGCG-induced reduction in food intake. The loss of appetite might involve neuropeptide(s) other than leptin, since EGCG is effective in reducing body weight of both lean and obese (leptin receptor-negative) female and male rats.

Various hormones including cholecystokinin, glucagon-like peptide-1, glucagon, substance P, somatostatin and bombesin have been reported to inhibit food intake, and it has been reported that plasma cholecystokinin levels are elevated in rats given a diet supplemented with tea polyphenols. Further study is required to determine whether the expression of other hypothalamic or gastrointestinal neuropeptide genes that control appetite are altered by EGCG and are perhaps responsible for the effect of EGCG on food intake. Since EGCG can also selectively reduce body fat accumulation[11,18,19], EGCG may be useful for acute treatment of obesity.

MODULATION OF ENDOCRINE SYSTEMS BY EGCG

The effects of tea on endocrine systems have not been carefully evaluated until recently. We demonstrated that rats injected intraperitoneally with EGCG showed significant changes in various endocrine parameters[19]. Seven days after injection of EGCG, circulating levels of testosterone in male rats and 17β-estradiol in female rats were reduced by 40–70%. In these animals, the weight of androgen-sensitive organs, such as ventral prostate, seminal vesicles, coagulating and preputial glands, and the weight of estrogen-sensitive organs, such as the uterus and ovary, were reduced by about 50%. These changes in the weight of sexual organs are catechin-specific, with EGCG showing the largest effect. The effect of EGCG on the prostate or uterine weight loss is due to reduced sex hormone levels and not a direct effect of EGCG on the organs; the organ weight loss is completely reversed with externally supplied sex hormones. With male and female rats treated with EGCG for 7 days, the serum levels of luteinizing

hormone (LH) were significantly reduced by 40–50%, suggesting that low LH levels led to the reduced production of sex hormones.

In both male and female rats, 7 days of EGCG treatment also caused significant reduction in blood levels of leptin, insulin-like growth factor (IGF)-I and insulin. The effect of EGCG on these peptide hormones was not mimicked by structurally similar catechins, EC, EGC or ECG at an equivalent dose. In EGCG-treated male rats, the serum level of protein, fatty acids and glycerol were not altered, but significant reductions in serum glucose (−32%), lipids (−15%), triglycerides (−46%) and cholesterol (−20%) were observed. Based on proximate composition analysis, rats treated daily with EGCG for 7 days had no change in percentage of water and protein content, a moderate decrease in carbohydrate content, but a very large reduction in fat content, decreasing from 4.1% in controls to 1.4% in the EGCG-treated group. Within 7–8 days, EGCG treatment decreased subcutaneous fat by 40–70% and abdominal fat by 20–35% in male rats[19].

CONCLUDING REMARKS

The effects of EGCG on body weight loss, hormone level changes and food intake depend on the route of administration. The effects of EGCG observed when EGCG was administered by intraperitoneal injection were not present when the same amount of EGCG was given to rats orally. This may be due to inefficient absorption of EGCG or metabolism in the digestive tract, and suggests that the effects of intraperitoneal administration of EGCG are not caused by interaction of EGCG with food or by EGCG action inside the gastrointestinal tract.

Although oral administration of EGCG is less effective, long-term oral consumption of green tea or EGCG-containing extracts may mimic some of the acute EGCG effects caused by intraperitoneal administration of EGCG and may be beneficial to health. Based on oral and intraperitoneal effects of EGCG on serum hormones and nutrients, long-term consumption of green tea may influence the incidence and provide therapies for various diseases.

By lowering plasma levels of sex steroids and other endocrine factors, such as IGF-I, long-term use of EGCG or green tea may be effective in prevention and suppression of the growth of hormone-dependent and hormone-independent cancers of various organs.

Green tea beverage originated many thousands of years ago as a medicinal tonic. Although the historically long use of many folk remedies does not necessarily prove their medical usefulness, recent scientific evidence appears to support the possibility that green tea catechins are medically valuable. However, it is important to consider also the potential adverse effects that may accompany the use of green tea or catechins.

For example, alteration of endocrine systems may have serious consequence in pregnant woman and small children.

Androgen may be the first natural medicine used in purified form for therapy. It provides the best example that traditional Chinese medicines are not necessarily effective only in combination. Unfortunately, many Chinese medicine researchers and practitioners are not aware of this great discovery and still strongly support an antimolecular approach. It is time to correct this misconception. This is the era to promote science in herbal medicine. Both unorthodox and orthodox medicinal researchers and practitioners should work together for 'one medicine' that benefits all[20].

References

1. Liao S, Kao YH, Hiipakka RA. Green tea: biochemical and biological basis for health benefits. *Vitam and Horm* 2001;26:1–94
2. Liao S, Fang S. Receptor proteins for androgens and the mode of action of androgens on gene transcription in ventral prostate. *Vitam Horm* 1969;27:17–90
3. Hiipakka RA, Liao S. Molecular mechanism of androgen action. *Trends Endocrinol Metab* 1998;9:317–24
4. Imperato-McGinley J, Guerrero L, Gautier T, Peterson RE. Steroid 5α reductase deficiency in man. *Science* 1974;186:1213–15
5. Sai T, Seino S, Chang C, *et al.* An exonic point mutation of the androgen receptor gene in a family with complete androgen insensitivity. *Am J Hum Genet* 1990;46:1095–100
6. Wilson JD. Syndromes of androgen resistance. *Biol Reprod* 1992;46:168–73
7. Russell DW, Wilson JD. Steroid 5α-reductase: two genes/two enzymes. *Annu Rev Biochem* 1994;63:25–61
8. Liang T, Liao S. Inhibition of 5α-reductase by specific aliphatic unsaturated fatty acids. *Biochem J* 1992;285:557–62
9. Liao S, Hiipakka RA. Selective inhibition of steroid 5α-reductase isoenzymes by tea epicatechin-3-gallate and epigallocatechin-3-gallate. *Biochem Biophys Res Commun* 1995;214:833–8
10. Liang T, Liao S. Growth suppression of hamster flank organ organs by topical application of γ-linolenic and other fatty acid inhibitors of 5α-reductase. *J Invest Dermatol* 1997;109:152–7
11. Liao S, Lin J, Dang, MT, *et al.* Growth suppression of hamster organs by topical application of catechins, alizarin, curcumin, and myristoleic acid. *Arch Dermatol Res* 2001;293:200–5
12. Huggins C, Steven RE, Hodges CV. Studies on prostate cancer II. The effects of castration on advanced carcinoma of the prostate gland. *Arch Surg* 1941;43:209–23
13. Kokontis JM, Takakura K, Hay N, Liao S. Increased androgen receptor activity and altered *c-myc* expression in prostate cancer cells after long-term androgen deprivation. *Cancer Res* 1994;54: 1566–73
14. Kokontis JM, Liao S. Molecular action of androgen in the normal and neoplastic prostate. *Vitam Horm* 1999;55:219–307
15. Umekita Y, Hiipakka RA, Kokontis JM, Liao S. Human prostate tumor growth in athymic mice: inhibition by androgens and stimulation by finasteride. *Proc Natl Acad Sci USA* 1996;93:11802–7
16. Kokontis JM, Hay N, Liao S. Progression of LNCaP prostate tumor cells during androgen deprivation: hormone-independent growth, repression of proliferation by androgen, and role for p27[kip1] in androgen-induced cell cycle arrest. *Mol Endocrinol* 1998; 12:941–53
17. Liao S, Umekita Y, Guo J, Kokontis JM, Hiipakka RA. Growth inhibition and regression of human prostate and breast tumors in athymic mice by tea epigallocatechin gallate. *Cancer Lett* 1995;96: 239–43
18. Kao YH, Hiipakka RA, Liao S. Modulation of obesity by a green tea catechin. *Am J Clin Nutr* 2000;72:1232–3
19. Kao YH, Hiipakka RA, Liao S. Modulation of endocrine systems and food intake by green tea epigallocatechin gallate. *Endocrinology* 2000;141:980–7
20. Liao S. Putting science into herbal medicine. *Bio/Pharma Q* 2000;5: 2–3

Homeopathy

6

T. Bark and D. Dwyer

INTRODUCTION

Here is an ancient story about healing.

There was a doctor in China, one among a family of physicians, who was the medical advisor to a local leader. When asked by his patient which brother was most skilled in the medical arts, he replied as follows:

'My eldest brother sees the spirit of sickness and removes it before it takes shape, so his name does not get out of the house. My elder brother cures sickness when it is still extremely minute, so his name does not get out of the neighborhood. As for me, I puncture veins, prescribe potions, and massage skin, so my name gets out and is heard among the lords.'

The two older brothers obviously practiced homeopathy and, with few exceptions, the history of this fine and beautiful healing art is populated with 'eldest' or 'elder' brothers and sisters, who, because of their compassion and skill in healing without dramatics or fanfare, are not heard of outside the practice of homeopathy; their names do not get out of the 'neighborhood' or even the house. Hahnemann, Kent, Vithoulkas, Hering and countless others have quietly and successfully practiced the art and science of Homeopathy, curing countless thousands of patients, and teaching thousands of other successful practitioners. Outside the limelight of popular medicine, progress within homeopathy has been quiet, subtle, steady and powerful.

As quantum physics differs from classical physics, homeopathy differs from allopathic thought and practice. Homeopathy is, in fact, energy medicine. The operative theories in the field of homeopathy are based in quantum theory. In our practice, healing always begins at the electromagnetic or quantum mechanical level. As a result, our remedies are very effective, are much safer in both chronic or acute situations and have far fewer side-effects than those routinely used in mainstream medicine.

Long before my medical school experience, I (T. B.) had developed an interest in health and disease prevention through healthy eating and daily exercise. In the course of my training, I acquired a fascination with acupuncture and herbs. I assumed that I would study these disciplines after my medical school training. After medical school came residency training and then a job as the director of a pediatric emergency room. My naive dreams as they pertained to better nutrition, wise lifestyle choices and alternative treatments seemed to fall by the wayside then, but in the year I worked as a director of the pediatric emergency room, I took a course in medical hypnotherapy with Dr Erica Fromm. I became fascinated with the power hypnosis had in regards to healing and decided to revisit the study of acupuncture. I prepared to enroll at the Midwest School of Acupuncture and Oriental Medicine, but a slight, unexpected change in direction brought me suddenly into my present vocation. I attended the annual conference of the National Center for Homeopathy, which happened to be in Chicago that year.

The conference piqued my interest to such an extent that I enrolled in summer school at the Center and finally found my true passion in medicine. It has been a challenging and enlightening journey. I hope, after this most basic presentation, you will also find, and ultimately practice, this precise and elegant science.

HISTORICAL SUMMARY

The old old-timers

Hippocrates wrote, 'By similar things a disease is produced and through the application of the like, it is cured.' He also described the symptoms of disease as the expression of Nature's healing powers – the view of modern homeopathy. Aristotle may have touched upon the homeopathic principle when he wrote that 'often the simile acts upon the simile'. Another Greek physician, Galen, wrote of 'natural cure by the likes'.

The old timers

A year after the voyage of Columbus, the Swiss medical reformer Theophrastus Bombastus von Hohenheim was born. He adopted the name Paracelsus, for obvious reasons, and in his writings elucidated the principle that 'likes must be cured by likes. . .'. He also rejected the heroic principle of opposite-acting remedies. Later, in the 17th century, the physician George Stahl wrote, 'To treat with opposite acting remedies is the reverse of what it ought to be. I am convinced that disease will yield to, and be cured by, remedies that produce similar affections'. According to Trevor Cook, author of *Homeopathic Medicine Today*[1], Dr Stahl's statement was 'the first enunciation of the fundamental homeopathic principle'. Cook pointed out that the first clear, concise statement of this powerful principle was largely ignored by Stahl's contemporaries, who certainly considered themselves the 'scientific' thinkers of their day. The medical arts, as they were then and as they continued to be practiced, consisted of 'venesection or bloodletting, augmented by stomach-rending emetics, laxatives and massive doses of often poisonous medicines, many of which caused serious side effects'. Then, as now, too often the major side-effect of treatment was sudden death.

Fearless leader

Samuel Hahnemann brought the gift of homeopathy to the world of medicine and that world thanked him with a nice big kick in the face (Figure 1). His is the archetypical case of the tortured genius. While we do not have time in this small chapter for biographical niceties, we feel it is essential to cover the major events and turning points in Samuel Hahnemann's life and career.

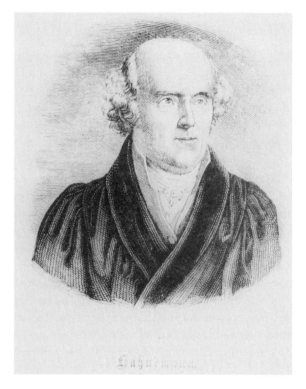

Figure 1 Samuel Hahnemann, 1755–1843. Courtesy of the National Library of Medicine

Samuel Hahnemann was born into the Lutheran faith on 10 April 1755 in Meissen, Germany. His upbringing was typical of the strict social and political traditions practiced at the time. His family was poor, and his schooling was interrupted sporadically when he had to help make ends meet. His situation was not unusual, and did not set Samuel apart from his contemporaries. There were, however, two qualities of character that did stand out: academic intensity and an inexorable restlessness, which would be his constant companions from grammar school days until his death at the age of 90. Hahnemann had an exceptional facility for languages, and was fluent in six at the age of 20. He worked as a translator and studied medicine, such as it was, moving often and changing schools, gaining experience in hospitals and other related situations where he could. A large measure of his dissatisfaction may have been from his experience with both the medical and the educational environment of his time. He felt strongly that the educational standards of his day were myopic and offered no respect for the inherent potential of the human mind. With regard to the state of medical science of his day, Hahnemann's early observations evolved into an individual revolutionary war he would carry on until his death.

In order to develop a true appreciation of Hahnemann and his struggle to bring this great gift to the world of medicine, it is important to understand the state of medical science at the time. Based on his own observations – and his powers of observation are very well documented – Hahnemann believed that more people were dying from their treatment than from their disease. While there is no uncontested body of hard, statistical data to prove this belief, the commonly accepted allopathic methods of treatment are a proven historic fact. The core concept in medicine in the 18th century was to *purge disease from the body*. Bloodletting was the industry standard. Medical education of the time recommended 'repeated and copious venesections until the patient faints' for nearly all types of conditions including whooping cough and pregnancy. 'Blood-sucking leeches, stomach rending emetics, and violent laxatives and enemas' were routine procedures deliberately and persistently prescribed to purge conditions and causes that were not understood in the least. These cures were then followed up with massive doses of murderous remedies that would finish the job, one way or the other.

Hahnemann, in an essay published in 1784[2], wrote his first public criticism of the medical profession. It was also the first elucidation of his developing holistic approach to health. In *Directions for Curing Old Diseases* he stressed the need for 'adequate sleep, regular exercise, and a sensible diet. Houses should be spaced apart, should be light and admit plenty of fresh air; sewage should be properly treated, and public hygiene is of great importance'. Soon thereafter, fortune smiled and Hahnemann became the Medical Officer of Health for Dresden. In the years to follow, he published two popular books and developed his unique and revolutionary view of medical practice.

Restlessness and trouble followed Hahnemann and his family at every turn, but in the midst of great misfortune, his brilliant insight prevailed. Hahnemann was translating a book, *A Treatise on Materia Medica* by William Cullen[3]. This book was an account of the drug Cortex Peruvianus, or Cinchona, which was used to treat malaria. During the translation work, Hahnemann was inspired to try an experiment. He took large doses of the drug for several days, observing and noting the symptoms. He discovered that Cinchona produced exactly the symptoms of malaria, and the first known experimental proof for the first principle of homeopathy – cure like with like – was completed. This great discovery, made in 1790, was recognized only by a note made by Hahnemann in the translation of the Cullen book. 'Cinchona bark, which is used as a remedy for intermittent fever acts because it can produce symptoms similar to those of intermittent fever in healthy people.' It would be some time before the full significance of his discovery was known, even to himself.

In his essay, *New Principles for Ascertaining the Curative Power of Drugs*[4], published in 1796, Hahnemann stated the first principle of homeopathy, as such, for the first time: *Simila similibus curentur*. For the next 13 years, he would write many essays relative to the thought and practice that would become the elements of modern homeopathy. The most important book in homeopathy is the *Organon of the Healing Art*, which was first published by Samuel Hahnemann in 1810[5].

The typhus test

Three years after the first cohesive description of homeopathy in the *Organon*, Napoleonic ambition gave homeopathy its first true test and its first great opportunity. In October 1813, the battle of Leipzig left approximately 80 000 soldiers dead and an equal number of wounded. After the battle there was a typhus outbreak. Hahnemann worked day and night, using homeopathic treatments alongside colleagues using conventional medicine. When the verified results were published, the rate of mortality for the conventionally treated typhus patients was over 50%; the rate for those treated homeopathically was less than 2%. This incident gave homeopathy its first real foothold in its battle with the mainstream medical community. 'It is the duty of physicians to distinguish subtle variations of every individual case – that is to specialize and individualize in each personal case, instead of treating the disease.' This is a quote from Hahnemann's *Materia Medica Pura*[6], written and published in six volumes between 1811 and 1821. He realized that the commonly held concept of 'disease' was little more than a convenient artificial construct, an idea. Further, he realized that the medical profession of the day, for their own convenience and to make a better living at their trade, found it to be of critical importance not only to continue to treat this intellectual invention with their own misguided conventional wisdom, but also to defend themselves against all homeopathic thinkers and their holistic notions about treating the patient instead of the disease concept. Hahnemann, therefore, wrote detailed accounts of each homeopathic medicine and its application in the treatment of the patient.

In 1812, Hahnemann published *Chronic Diseases: Their Peculiar Nature and Their Homeopathic Cure* in two volumes[7]. In the first volume he further articulated homeopathic thought and practice, including the essential holistic approach to the patient. In the second volume, he introduced the Vital Force, a central concept in homeopathic thought. Here he also introduced his Psora theory, which describes an inherited predisposition to certain imbalances.

The cholera test

An outbreak of cholera in 1831 brought on an epidemic all through Russia and Europe that would claim several hundred thousand lives before it was over. Hahnemann wrote an analysis of the problem along with the homeopathic cure, and published his work in four separate locations lest the establishment succeed in sabotaging his efforts as they had in the past. In one of those essays, the holistic revolutionary wrote, 'In order to render the spread of cholera impossible, the garments, linen, etc. of all strangers must be quarantined (whilst their bodies are cleansed with baths) and heated for two hours at a stove heat of 80 degrees centigrade – this represents the temperature at which all known infections and consequently the living miasms are annihilated…cholera infection is most probably caused by a swarm of infinitely small, invisible living organisms so murderously hostile to human life'.

As with the typhus epidemic, the homeopathic solution proved itself most effective. In several European cities where statistics were kept, the series of remedies suggested by Hahnemann failed only 4% of the time, while conventional treatments failed at least 50% of the time. Quietly, in his writing and private practice, Hahnemann continued his great work and his remarkable and restless personal life. In 1835, at the ripe old age of 80, Hahnemann married a 30-year-old patient, Melanie D'Hervilly. His quiet genius, combined with her talent for promotion, produced a booming practice within a few years, and continued as such until his death at the age of 90.

While the history and development of our subject, especially Hahnemann's life, is interesting, the most exciting and substantive developments are happening all over the world right now. The work that Hahnemann began with his essay *New Principles for Ascertaining the Curative Power of Drugs* in 1796[4] is just now gaining worldwide momentum. Hahnemann spent his entire life engineering the great revolution that is just now beginning.

It may be surprising to know that, owing to the early success in homeopathy, by the turn of the century there were 22 homeopathic medical schools in the USA. The North American Academy of Homeopathic Healing Arts in Allentown, Pennsylvania was the first of these. This first school was set up by Dr Constantine Hering, who, in 1844, also established the American Institute of Homeopathy. It is the oldest professional medical association in this country. While not the first to practice Homeopathy in the USA, Hering was certainly one of the most notable pioneers. It is said that Hering discovered, understood and made Homeopathy his life's work while researching a book he had been commissioned to write. Ironically, in that book, it was Hering's assignment to discredit the work of Samuel Hahnemann.

The popularity of the homeopathic arts made a quantum leap in the 1860s during the yellow fever epidemic. This led to the establishment of the many homeopathic medical schools and over 100 homeopathic hospitals in the USA by the early 1900s. The future of homeopathy seemed very bright indeed at that time, but dramatic changes both inside and outside the field nearly led to the complete elimination of the practice. Early in the 20th century three major trends very nearly eliminated homeopathy. In 1909, the first specific antibacterial drug, Salvarsan, began a 'drug revolution' that has continued unabated until the present.

The small doses prescribed by homeopaths were soon overlooked and then ignored by a public and medical community interested in more dramatic results from their drugs. At the same time, mainstream medicine began to abandon the use of the most invasive and disturbing practices and procedures that had been the benchmark for previous centuries, and a favorable public image began to grow. Inside homeopathy, a rift developed concerning the philosophy and practice of posology, which concerns itself with the strength of the remedy prescribed. Prescription of the lowest effective dose possible, in any given case, is a principle central to the beliefs of Hahnemann and his disciples, but homeopaths began to use higher doses and to develop theories closer to allopathic thinking at the time. This seriously weakened the core of the homeopathic community in the USA until the last homeopathic hospital closed in 1951. It is estimated that, by 1960, there were only 100 practicing homeopaths across the country.

Fortunately, this downward trend has also been dramatically reversed, and today, homeopathy enjoys robust life and growth in the USA and throughout the world. This may be due, in large measure, to the fact that people are becoming ever more aware that the 'miracle drug revolution' begun in 1909 may prove to be a mixed blessing for many sufferers. Many pharmaceuticals and modern treatment modalities have produced serious side-effects. Drug resistance is climbing and there is a resurgence of old diseases. Strong drugs are becoming less effective in curing disease and more effective in rendering a weakened natural defense mechanism entirely helpless. For these and many other reasons, homeopathy is becoming a primary resource for those seeking sensible, effective heath care. There are many schools, workshops, associations and other organizations growing around the principles and practice of homeopathy.

ESSENTIAL HOMEOPATHIC THOUGHT

The Law of Similars

The Law of Similars, one of the defining principles of the theory that 'like cures like', is not limited to homeopathy. Immunization and allergy treatment, while not necessarily homeopathic, work on the same principle.

In the context of homeopathy, this is how it works. The patient has a collection of symptoms, which can be related directly, indirectly, or even obliquely, to their imbalance (or 'disease' in the allopathic vernacular). There is a substance in nature that will produce that same set of symptoms in a healthy person. That substance, when taken homeopathically, will provide the natural defense mechanism with the energy necessary to eliminate the symptoms and their underlying cause.

Samuel Hahnemann provided the first empirical evidence in support of this principle with his Cinchona experiment. Until then, the idea that 'like cures like' was just an intellectual construct without any real-life investigation or experimental evidence. Since that time, homeopaths have developed vast resources on toxicology as it relates to *Similia similibus curentur*.

'When I am able to correctly match the symptoms of a patient with symptoms produced in a healthy person in a homeopathic proving, the results are tremendous. The patient begins to improve in all ways and feels his overall health and vitality return. The old symptoms do not come back; there are no side effects, and the patient does not have to stay on the medicine in order to continue feeling well'[8], so states the author of *Homeopathy*, David Sollars, whose experience described above mirrors precisely the experience of thousands of homeopathic practitioners.

The theory of structure – quantum mechanics to metaphysics

Just as the success of quantum electrodynamics allowed the physical sciences to move beyond the narrow limits imposed by the laws of classical mechanics and into the modern technological world we experience today, modern homeopathic thought moves beyond the narrow limits of mainstream medicine to understanding and treatment far more complex than was previously imagined.

The classical allopathic perspective that the human being is, in essence, a neurochemical and biomechanical entity, that a problem-solving or engineering approach is the logical and reasonable path to health and well-being, is reaching its limits. It misses completely the fact that each human being is also a vibrant and complex system of energy and information in motion; a system that is fully integrated with, and inseparable from, the systems of chemical and biological matter that have been observable thus far.

Allopathic treatment, like Newtonian physics, is extremely effective within its range. Homeopathy, like quantum physics, is a science of deeper understanding based on a significantly more accurate view of the human being known as 'the patient'. The physical, mental, emotional and spiritual aspects of each patient are considered in 'homeopathic physics'. As a result of this vision, homeopathic treatment is as subtle as it is powerful.

Homeopathic remedies, which are classified as drugs by the Food and Drug Administration (FDA), are created by sequentially diluting and succussing the original substance or 'mother tincture'. The more diluted and succussed, the higher the potency and the lower the toxicity.

Homeopathy is energy medicine. As such, homeopathy seeks a cure on the electromagnetic, or quantum mechanical plane. The homeopathic remedy begins its healing activity on this plane. Two modern theories consider the concepts of resonant frequency and bioinformation as possible explanations for the effectiveness of homeopathic treatments. The 'resonant frequency theory' suggests that an accurately prescribed remedy will provide a strengthening of the electromagnetic condition of the patient, returning them to good health. 'Bioinformational theory' suggests that specific instructions for healing are provided to diseased cells through energetic pathways. As a substance is diluted and succussed, its electromagnetic imprint is magnified. While the technological ability necessary to provide experimental support for these theories is in its infancy, we

believe that these ideas are not mutually exclusive, but are probably two aspects of a much more intricate system of energy and the process of healing.

Regardless of theory, the interactions and equivalence of energy and matter within the patient are of primary importance to the homeopathic practitioner. Not long ago, this idea would have been considered metaphysical. Now, these ideas, known as quantum electrodynamics, are a part of everyday life, and soon will be recognized as such by the entire medical community.

The life force

There is a life force in nature that may be generally defined as the animating force that directs all aspects of life in the organism. On the purely physical level, the life force may be thought of as the patient's electromagnetic profile or character. The terms 'life force' and 'vital force' will be used interchangeably here. George Vithoulkas, a respected modern-day teacher and clinician, believes that the vital force manifests itself in the form of an electromagnetic field that is unique to each individual, and characterizes the patterns of health and illness inherent in the individual.

'Some animating force or principle enters the organism at the time of conception, guides all of the functions of life and then leaves at the time of death. What does occur at the moment of death? The organism is structurally intact, cells are busily functioning, chemical reactions are still proceeding, yet a sudden change occurs and the body begins to decompose! Reflection on this fact renders the concept of "vital force" not only understandable, but appealing'[9].

Vithoulkas' beliefs are firmly grounded in two areas: first, his direct observational experience in practice; and second, his intuitive understanding of quantum electrodynamics. In this brief chapter, we focus only on the second.

'It is not as if the dynamic plane is a separate fourth level of the organism. It has exactly the same relationship to the physical body as the electromagnetic fields have to matter.'

Central to homeopathic thought and practice is the understanding that, only by treating the central imbalance as it manifests itself on the dynamic plane, will the symptoms and the disease be completely and permanently eliminated.

In his book, *The Spirit of Homeopathy*, Rajan Sankaran, another respected teacher of homeopathy, describes the importance of this essential concept. 'Vital to developing the homeopathic vision is the understanding of what is to be cured in disease. It is to be able to perceive, to feel and to know as the truth that disease is not something local but a disturbance of the whole being. It is to have the unshakable conviction that if we treat *the disturbance at the center*, the local problems will be lessened. . . . These points need to be stressed repeatedly, explained and exemplified so that they become a part of our thought process. This and only this conviction can make us staunch and successful homeopaths and remove from our minds the confusions that arise in practice'[10].

The disturbance at the center referred to by Sankaran is a disturbance in the wave pattern or resonance of the electromagnetic field which characterizes the vital force. Through a framework of classical physics, homeopathic practice recognizes the patterns of health and illness, as these patterns occur on the mental, emotional and physical planes. These structures are built upon the foundation of the vital force, which is governed by the laws of quantum electrodynamics. Vithoulkas suggests that the dynamic plane of each patient has a characteristic resonant wave pattern, and that the mission of homeopathy is first, to identify that resonance by analyzing the totality of symptoms; second, to identify a substance of similar wavelength that will reinforce the wave pattern of the patient's vital force; and third, to determine the method of application of that substance[9].

Treatment with the substance of the correct electromagnetic resonance will eliminate the 'disturbance at the center' referred to by Sankaran[10]. By strengthening the patient's life force in this way, a return to soundness and health on the mental, emotional and physical levels can be accomplished. The organism is then returned to equilibrium, and the vital force can return to the performance of its primary function, which, according to Samuel Hahnemann[5], is to fine-tune and maintain a dynamic equilibrium among and through all of the fields or dimensions (referred to as 'planes' or levels).

Defense mechanism

While it is not the primary function of the vital force, there is within the dynamic plane a set of functions whose specific focus is the response to threatening stimuli. The term 'defense mechanism' is simply a term of theoretical convenience used to describe any set of responses produced by the vital force when a morbid stimulus is introduced to the organism through any of the physical, emotional or mental sub-dimensions. It is believed that most threats are dealt with on the dynamic plane quickly, efficiently and unnoticeably. If the threatening stimulus is 'stronger' than the defense mechanism, that is, if the new stimulus has a quality which causes material interference with the resonant frequency of the vital force, the defense mechanism begins to produce what are commonly known as symptoms.

The theory of symptoms

As with the holistic view of the patient, the quantum mechanical foundations, the vital force and the Law of Similars, a solid conceptual grasp of the homeopathic view of signs and symptoms is critical to any substantive understanding of the field.

To cure the symptoms is not to cure the disease. While mainstream medicine has always characterized the disease–symptom pattern as a direct cause-and-effect relationship, equating the cure of the symptoms with the cure of the disease, homeopathy takes another, very different point of view, 'The totality of the symptoms must be the principal, indeed the only thing the physician has to make note of in every case of disease and to remove by means of his art, in order that the disease shall be cured and transformed into health'.

The homeopathist sees signs and symptoms as clear reflections of activities of the defense mechanism in its efforts to deal with a threatening stimulus. Symptoms are not qualities of the disease, but qualities of the cure. The signs and symptoms must be painstakingly observed and evaluated, because in the totality of symptoms (the disease picture) the homeopathist discovers a pathway, not obvious at the start, but already established by the defense mechanism, which will give the homeopathist an accurate direction to the cure. Any substantial oversight in concept or practice here will cause a pernicious failure of the entire process.

In homeopathy, the totality of symptoms is really a skillful and comprehensive evaluation of the patient themself. All the mental, emotional and physical qualities of the patient's life and lifestyle, at that moment and in the past, are taken into careful consideration by the homeopathist in developing the theory of symptoms. An integral part of this process is the identification of the modalities of the symptoms, that is, the conditions that directly or indirectly affect a symptom in a positive or negative way.

'The cure', in homeopathy, is not that which ameliorates the symptoms, but that which enhances the strength of the defense mechanism/vital force through its resonant frequency. So strengthened, the vital force returns the patient to health without suppression or destruction. Any attempt at 'curing' the symptoms through suppression is at best risky, at worst fatal. Suppression therapy not only hides the symptoms, it changes the electromagnetic character of the curative frequency, therefore making the direction of the cure ever more elusive, and often inaccessible.

Other fundamental homeopathic concepts

Here are summary descriptions of several concepts that are fully integrated into the homeopathic spirit. We will use the terms disease, imbalance and disturbance interchangeably.

Treat the patient

In homeopathy, the disease, as it is commonly known, has no independent existence. Symptoms are not functions of the imbalance. The totality of symptoms describe a condition of the patient, not a quality of the disease, and it is the patient that needs to be understood fully and with compassion, not the disease.

The totality of symptoms is the patient's best effort to resolve an imbalance, so the patient must be assisted in the effort to resolve every symptom, modality and interactive influence associated with the imbalance.

This best effort is not to be dissipated by replacement or suppression with strong drugs or heroic therapies. Only by increasing the patient's overall strength will the disease imbalance be brought into equilibrium.

The holistic view

Mind, body and spirit are one. Divisions are the artificial products of cognition and language. Communications of all kinds are, within the patient, constant, fluid and instantaneous. In language and theory, a part of the being or a system within the being can be identified, evaluated and treated in relative isolation. In real life, this never happens. The symptoms of the condition as identified in isolation will apparently be reduced, suppressed, or even eliminated by direct and limited intervention. The patient experiences relief, but the energy pattern that created the symptom has only been moved to another location or system within the being. When this happens, the energy imbalance that caused the patient's system to create the symptom in the first place can be driven deeper and become more intense, elusive and destructive as a result.

Homeopaths were among the first in the medical arts to recognize the need to understand the entire patient and the patient's lifestyle before prescribing remedies and treatment procedures. A patient's asthma will never be cured if the patient works with certain caustic chemicals that may appear to be harmless or owns a heating system that is a breeding ground for microbes. While this example is deliberately simple and obvious, far more subtle effects can create, enhance or stabilize an initial imbalance to the point where it becomes a chronic condition that could never be resolved through replacement or suppressive therapy. The holistic point of view is not a trend that started in the 1960s. It is just medical common sense that has been practiced with compassion in homeopathy from the outset.

The energetic planes

Homeopathy is energy medicine. Energy, to our limited abilities and experience, is largely a mysterious subject. What do we know about energy? We know that it seems to move things around, and we know that it roughly conforms to a set of laws we call quantum electrodynamics. We know that the phenomenon we like to call energy exists, and that energy seems to take on some kind of pattern. We know much of the mechanics of energy as it relates to technology, but not much of its nature that it is 'there'. (We know that it is not nowhere, but we cannot say where it is or is not.) Where is 'there'?

When we talk about energy in terms of a living being, our minds seem to need a 'there' in order to form even the most vague visual pattern of existence. In homeopathy, the patterns of organic energy we are concerned with live on, and in, a series of dimensions or planes. These are characterized, in order of relative importance, as the dynamic, mental, emotional and physical planes. We further imagine that the mental, emotional and physical dimensions are encapsulated within the sphere of the dynamic dimension that could be imagined to be, like the surface of the earth, finite but unbounded.

These are not discrete entities; there are no well-defined borders. Because of this, disease patterns and the being's response to those patterns (symptoms) often do not follow a traceable linear pattern through the patient. Physical and emotional events ebb and flow. The brain produces thoughts: in one moment rapid-fire and at random, scattered across the other planes; in the next moment, the thought process slows to a trudging deliberation, turns inward on itself and becomes serious for no apparent reason. Energy flows where it will, and symptoms that begin as a subtle emotion become a physical event and then a pathological process resonating across all of the energetic planes. Wavelengths vary. Amplitudes vary. Even time is relative here. Past and future events can have a great effect on the patient, the imbalance, the defense mechanism, the symptoms, the modalities and the doctor who watches and listens with competence and compassion.

There is within the practice a theory, which assigns conceptual values to the energetic planes, and this hierarchy is illustrated clearly in the section on difficult cases (p. 75). In a general way, this theory describes the tendencies or probable directions of energy movement through the being. For example, a symptom on the physical dimension, tendonitis, may have begun as a disturbance on the mental plane. Therefore, a prescription for anti-inflammatories to replace the action of the natural defense mechanism may well eliminate the obvious symptom, but the energy pattern that created the symptom may migrate to the mental or emotional plane and then return to the physical plane. A new set of consequences may then evolve, becoming more serious and complex as they again resonate through the various planes. This kind of activity, apparent only through observation of results, has led homeopathy to establish a conceptual hierarchy of symptoms, which, in everyday practice, is used to establish both the essence and the totality of the symptoms.

THE BASICS OF THE PRACTICE

The art of the science

The homeopathic interview, or case-taking, is an intensely subjective and personal experience that produces the objective information necessary for the homeopathic science to do its work. In the interview there is no room for an observer to evaluate the process and the patient from an intellectually convenient distance. Long before the theory of quantum mechanics, the homeopathic community understood that the observer is an integral part of the process and product of the scientific method. In fact, the practitioner is encouraged to enter the interview with heightened awareness in order to participate fully in the process and to bring the patient's latent thoughts and emotions into the bright light of awareness. Only by total immersion in this process by both doctor and patient will the totality of symptoms – quality, quantity, modalities, and contributing factors – be accurately elucidated.

Beginner's mind

'To the beginner there is a world of possibilities, to the expert there are but few', so says Suzuki Roshi in his classic, *Zen Mind, Beginners Mind* [11]. A mind that is free of predispositions and judgements, however well founded and well intentioned, is critical to the success of the homeopathic interview. This is true for both the doctor and the patient, but for the practitioner, the cultivation of 'pure awareness' as the Zen masters say, is a most important element of daily practice.

From Rajan Sankaran [10], 'What are the requirements of case-taking? The only requirements are an unprejudiced mind, an observing mind and a mind that draws a very accurate picture. We must not fit people into slots; instead we have to just let the picture come out, without imposing our own ideas on what we see'. The doctor must be disciplined to observe and act on what they see and hear from the patient before them – not what they think about other patients who may have looked and sounded a lot like this one.

As long as it takes...

The homeopathic case-taking, or interview, may take 2 h or more, depending on many factors. Because this doctor is treating this unique patient and this unique totality of symptoms, an extremely detailed picture of *these* particular symptoms and *this* particular patient's life must be carefully drawn. The doctor must act as the catalyst in order to bring out the patient's life and struggle as vividly and precisely as possible. This is not a simple task. There are no convenient checklists or standardized testing. 'Yes or no' answers (and questions) are strongly discouraged and there is absolutely no latitude for leading the patient to the desired answer. (Indeed, if the doctor has an answer in mind, they must rid themself of it!) As in quantum physics, in homeopathy there are no clear lines or sharp corners to guide either the doctor or the patient in the direction of the cure. Nevertheless, the practitioner must observe and identify *all* of the symptoms, modalities and contributing factors if the correct remedy is to be found. Case-taking has all the complexity and difficulty of any fine art or science. For the dedicated and disciplined doctor, the results of the practice, as in science or the fine arts, are at once simple and elegant.

Taking the case properly requires the simultaneous abilities of active listening and keen observation.

Subtle nuances can be very important, and the way in which a patient describes their situation can be as important as the content of their portrayal. A good example of this principle would be the case of a long-time patient (Ms R), whose initial visit to me (T.B.) was about 7 years ago. She came to me for Lyme disease and its associated symptoms, and was successfully treated with calcarea carbonica. I became her family physician and successfully treated all the members of her family for many minor conditions. Recently, Ms R came to see me for an acute sore throat. She could not swallow and had persistent, intense pain. She had tried typical remedies for acute pharyngitis and related symptoms. As she struggled to describe in detail the modalities that affected her sore throat symptoms, I noticed that manner and speech were devoid of her usually spirited good humor. In that context, she appeared to be on the borderline of depression, a mental plane condition disproportionate to the physical symptoms of pharyngitis. I treated her for the mental state by prescribing aurum metallicum. This remedy is often used for patients with suicidal depression. Within 30 min of taking the medication, Ms R phoned the office to report a complete recovery from the sore throat symptoms, and again within a few days to report complete recovery from the depths of a depressive state so subtle and powerful that she could not even recognize it, much less extricate herself from it. Her slightly altered speech and body language provided the nearly imperceptible clues to the correct remedy.

In addition to careful, open-minded observation as demonstrated in the example above, active, careful listening will lead the doctor to ask the right questions at the right time. In this way, the doctor will get answers that are critical to the totality of the symptoms, but answers which the patient, in less skillful hands, might otherwise be loathe to give. A good example of this is a patient who came to me for recurrent Achilles tendonitis and heel pain. At the outset, without any direction from me, she wanted to describe in detail how the pain affected her leg and foot, how it affected her tennis game and her life in general. It was obvious to me that the injury went deeper, beyond the physical dimension, and that I would need to get her talking about her emotional and mental states. This patient had a proclivity for defensiveness when prompted to look at her condition on these deeper energetic levels. With gently framed questions – not suggestive of any answer – I guided her to look at the qualities of her life on the mental and emotional dimensions. This quiet persuasion required a second and even a third interview. After the determined early resistance, the real problem began to unravel as the truth spilled out. She finally admitted to having a marriage that was virtually non-existent. Her husband was chronically depressed. Uninvolved to the point that he was practically absent from her life, his only remaining participation in the relationship was a relentless pattern of verbal abuse. I had sensed serious problems at home, but also sensed that, if suddenly confronted with their full image, she would cut and run away from any treatment of the problems. Once she was brought out, though, I was able to find the correct remedy for her, lycopodium. At this time, her domestic situation has been resolved much to her benefit via divorce, and the tendonitis has not returned.

There are differing styles in case-taking. While it is vital to let the patient speak about themselves without fear or inhibition, it is also imperative to learn specific details about the patient. There are times when only carefully pointed questions will provide the necessary information. Some homeopaths ask few questions and let the silence motivate the patient's talk. Others use questions to bring the patient's story out. Often, both methods are required to get the whole picture. I find that I can learn much about my patient by the way they carry themselves, their general body language, specific gestures, patterns of speech, vocabulary, style of dress, and other visual and aural clues. By simply paying attention and being aware of these individual elements, I get a sense of the patient's 'presence' or their aura.

For example, a patient came to me impeccably groomed and dressed in very conservative clothes. His speech was condescending and his aura was ominous, threatening. He surrounded himself with an attitude that suggested a propensity towards violence: carefully cultivated, understated and undeniable. My colleague-in-training excused herself from the initial interview, based solely on her instinctive feeling about this patient.

During the interview, I asked him whether he was aware of this sinister quality and he immediately became defensive. After feigned innocence, he told me, 'I am a professional killer, not the murderer you suspect', and as the interview progressed, he elaborated that he had been a professional killer in a past life but now was so spiritually advanced – far more than most – that he would hurt no one in this life. He had few friends and had no intimate acquaintances. His central complaint was recurrent prostatitis, which was unresponsive to antibiotics. I prescribed *Veratrum album* based on the totality of his symptoms. In a follow-up interview 6 weeks later, he was doing better physically and psychically, and continued to describe mental and emotional problems as effecting his daily life. I prescribed a higher dose of *Veratrum album*, and in several weeks his threatening manner had disappeared along with his physical and friendship problems. It was his intimidating manner that led to the direction of the cure.

Difficult cases

Every case has its own particular difficulties and challenges, and in the ideal world, case-taking would be such a fine art that no generalizing would be necessary. Indeed, many of the great practitioners exhort their students to leave any assumptions and preconceived notions about the patient and the case behind when entering the office for an initial interview. George Vithoulkas is one such great teacher, who warns his readers and potential homeopathic practitioners not to fall prey to the temptation of substituting generalizations. In *The Science of Homeopathy*[9], however, Vithoulkas offers some rough guidelines about problem patients. He mentions three general profiles of difficult cases: the timid patient, the intellectual patient and the doctor-hopper.

With the *timid patient*, a very misleading symptom picture could easily be the result of the patient's reticence. The timid patient may be inherently inarticulate or simply self-contained. Spanning that broad range is a basic fear, which can lead the patient to give incomplete or inaccurate descriptions of symptoms or modalities, or, worse, entirely to leave out symptoms that might begin to expose or give any kind of energy to that basic fear. This is especially true when the patient is called on to explain symptoms and modalites which may originate in the mental or emotional planes. Here the doctor must become an even more studious and methodical observer, while showing enough compassion to lead the patient to full and accurate descriptions of his condition.

Vithoulkas mentions hypochondriacs as problem patients for obvious reasons, and goes on to talk about the *intellectual* patient. Here, the patient's mind gets in the way of an accurate description of his symptoms, modalities and other significant influences on his condition. The intellectual or highly educated patient has already done research and often wants to direct the course of the initial interview. As with the timid patient, the collection of useful information becomes difficult or even impossible. This patient is too articulate about dangerously small amounts of knowledge, and can make it impossible to find *any* symptom, much less an accurate totality of symptoms.

Akin to the intellectual patient is the *doctor-hopping* patient, who knows too little and too much at the same time. This patient's experience with other doctors, usually of all types, will almost certainly color the symptom picture in a way that will make the essence or the totality of symptoms impossible to evaluate.

For the homeopath, the very extensive case-taking procedure is a science and an art. They must gather critical and specific information from patients who are unwilling or unable to describe their conditions and lifestyle accurately. They must be practiced in the arts of open-mindedness, pure awareness and silence. They must be entirely objective while completely immersed, along with the patient, in the case-taking process. They cannot simply dismiss or bypass the effects of physical symptoms on the mental or emotional lives of their patients. They cannot send off a difficult case with a 5-min examination. They must take in more information than is possible and do so with insight and compassion. They must be relentless in their search for the truth for each patient's totality of symptoms.

Basic elements of case analysis

Once the homeopath is reasonably certain that the entire case has been taken, that is, every one of the symptoms, signs, modalities, lifestyle variables and potential obstructions to the cure are noted and organized, then the case analysis can move into a working analysis of the symptoms, the essence of the totality of symptoms.

Symptoms analysis

In homeopathy symptoms are gathered, analyzed and utilized in a manner that is very different from its allopathic counterpart. For example, when a patient complains of a headache to their allopathic physician, a few simple questions are asked related to the location, intensity and duration of the headache pain. Obvious physical abnormalities are checked visually, and a pain medication is prescribed. If there is no further complaint, the problem is considered solved. If that same patient were to approach the homeopathic physician with the same complaint, a very different set of responses would evolve. The doctor would schedule a case-taking interview. They would learn from the patient everything it is possible to know about the headache. They might begin with the question, 'What was going on in your life just before the headache began?' and follow with 'What time of day does the headache first appear?' or 'Does the headache sometimes surface under similar emotional conditions?' The patient might then describe a situation or situations in her daily life which seem to precipitate the headache. These descriptions would naturally lead the homeopath to ask of themself, 'Why is this patient *susceptible* to these headaches?' or 'How is the patient susceptible to the conditions that seem to bring on these headaches?' The doctor will also look for repeating patterns of disease. So, after the homeopathic symptom analysis is complete, the remedy prescribed will be based on the comprehensive symptom picture, not simply the chief complaint of headache pain as reported by the patient.

The case of Miss M was brought to me by her mother for the child's terrible case of asthma as well as a multiple history of anaphylactic reactions to foods. The child had been put on steroids with the last anaphylactic reaction and had been kept on them, because of an exacerbation of her asthma. I took the case, and found there to be redness, swelling and inflammation as a recurrent theme. I then queried into her personality and found her to be constantly busy as well as productive. I prescribed apis, a remedy made from bee venom known for its proclivity for work, heat, swelling and redness. The child did exceptionally well. She was off her steroids by the first follow-up 6 weeks later. Her asthma was gone for the first time in years and she was not having any allergic reactions. I have followed her for over a year, and her asthma is still much improved, with her needing no medications most of the year. She had an outbreak of molluscum contagiosum along with a bout of asthma midwinter which required a different remedy for that picture, antimonium crudum. She has done well and has even been exposed to nuts without any allergic response.

Modalities

The case of Miss M also provides a good, simple example of a modality, that is, a situation that has a modulating effect on the symptom being analyzed. A modality is a condition that will either aggravate or ameliorate a symptom. A given set of symptoms may, by itself, point to several potential remedies. Here, identification of specific modalities becomes critical. In the case of Miss M above, the fact that she was constantly red and swollen was the modality that led to the successful remedy. Without that critical bit of information, the selection and treatment may well have taken much longer.

Modalities are grouped into several major categories: physical, temperature, time, diet and locality. Identification of these general modalities provides a direction for the investigation into specific modalities. For example, a patient may experience the worsening of a symptom at 11.00 each day, or may experience the amelioration of a symptom only on warm summer days. To the untrained observer, these situations may appear to be coincidences or just peculiarities,

but to the homeopath skilled in thorough case analysis, these modulating factors are critical elements in the development of the symptom picture.

Interactive influences

In addition to symptoms, signs and modalities, the vigilant doctor must identify and analyze as many interactive influences as possible. It is very important for the observer to know of any diseases the patient may have had in both the recent and the distant past. Even conditions that may have apparently been completely eradicated can have an effect, however obliquely, on the energy imbalance behind the current symptoms. In fact, a 'cured disease' may even be the underlying cause of the patient's situation. Depending on the treatments used, an obscured disease may be responsible for the new symptoms.

In addition to past or existing diseases, the doctor must be thoroughly appraised of the methods of treatment used for those diseases. Broadly speaking, most of the treatments commonly used are suppressive in nature. We have mentioned how a condition, apparently cured through suppressive treatment, will surface at a later time on the same or on another of the energetic planes. This situation, in turn, will create new or intensified symptoms. These may again be treated typically, and apparently eliminated, only to surface again in another form. It is conceivable that the early treatments are a cause for the present symptoms, signs and modalities.

Vaccinations can be another factor contributing to the patient's malaise. For example, a vaccination is often overlooked as a potential catalyst or cause of physical or emotional problems that surface after the vaccination.

In the complete analysis of the patient, there are many non-pathological situations which must be considered in the case analysis. There may be serious nutritional imbalances of which the patient is completely unaware. For example, a patient may have adopted a vegetarian or vegan diet for moral or conscientious reasons, but have a physical constitution that is slowly deprived or starved of essential nutrients as a result, or a patient may be on a trend diet to lose weight and mask substantial emotional problems in the effort.

Often, too, patients who have become interested in their various conditions and symptoms prior to their visit to their homeopath may be on a course of self-prescribed medications.

When these or other lifestyle imbalances are added to another non-obvious imbalance, over-exercise or over-achieving, for example, a complex synergetic effect can take place that could easily be missed in a brief examination. Therefore, thoroughness is the watchword in homeopathy. Establishment of nothing less than the totality of symptoms is the single purpose of homeopathic case-taking and analysis, and for the conscientious and compassionate practitioner, nothing less will do.

AFTERWORD

Practicing homeopathy for the past several years has been an extremely rewarding addition to my (T.B.) practice of medicine. Prior to homeopathy, I would manage people on medications. They would feel better and their symptoms would be controlled; however, they would rarely be cured of their diseases (an exception would be acute infections).

Now that I have been practicing homeopathy for a few years and have had a fair amount of training and experience, I have the pleasure of seeing many patients responding beautifully to homeopathy, cured of the disease as well as the symptoms, whether they be physical, emotional or spiritual in nature.

I recently saw a 5-year-old girl for her juvenile rheumatoid arthritis. She had been managed at one of Chicago's prestigious children's hospitals by the rheumatology department. She had been managed with steroids and high doses of ibuprofen. When I saw her, she already had chronically inflamed and deformed knees, the right one being much worse than the left. She was in chronic pain in spite of the medications. I took her case and found her to be a 'textbook' picture of the remedy Pulsatilla – timid and sweet with wandering arthritic pains and unprovoked fears of men. I prescribed the remedy with confidence.

Three weeks later I received a great compliment, which, ironically, would have been the greatest insult just a few years previously. The child's mother phoned my nurse to say that her daughter was thriving without any medication for the first time in years. The chronic pain had disappeared entirely, and, devoid of pain, her knees had become strong and beautiful again. She then proceeded to ask my nurse if I was a witch.

Did I sell her daughter's soul to the devil? She claimed to be a very religious Catholic and did not understand how I did what I did. My nurse assured her that there was science behind homeopathy and that I was a fully degreed physician. My nurse actually cried tears when relaying the story to me, not out of laughter, but out of happiness for the little girl who was helped so much by homeopathy and was now out of pain and playing like a normal 5-year-old.

ACKNOWLEDGEMENTS

I want to thank my co-author David Dwyer. He started out as my ghost writer-editor. However, his brilliance, writing and organization skills contributed so much that I realized it would be a shame to list him as anything less than a co-author. In the beginning, he did not know anything about homeopathy; in the end, he became an intelligent scholar of homeopathy's philosophy and wisdom. Thank you, David.

Thank you to my first teachers in homeopathy, Drs Messer and Herrick, and thank you to my one and only supervisor, without whom I might have drowned under the massive learning curve, Dr Mitchel Fleisher. Thank you to my partner in homeopathic studies, Susan Slessinger. Thank you to my parents who always encouraged me equally whether it was in allopathic medicine or homeopathy. And thanks to all my patients, for without them, homeopathy would just be a theory.

References

1. Cook T. *Homeopathic Medicine Today*. Keats, 1989
2. Hahnemann S. *Directions for Curing Old Diseases*. 1784
3. Cullen W. *A Treatise on Materia Medica*. London, 1773
4. Hahnemann S. *New Principles for Ascertaining the Curative Power of Drugs*. 1796
5. Hahnemann S. *Organon of the Healing Art*. 1810
6. Hahnemann S. *Materia Medica Pura*. 1811–1821
7. Hahnemann S. *Chronic Disease: Their Peculiar Nature and Their Homeopathic Cure*. 1812
8. Sollars D. *Homeopathy*. Alpha Books, 2001
9. Vithoulkas G. *The Science of Homeopathy*. Grove/Atlantic, 1980
10. Sankaran R. *The Spirit of Homeopathy*. Homeopathic Educational Services
11. Roshi S. *Zen Mind, Beginners Mind*

Further reading

Capra F. *The Tao of Physics*. Shambhala Publications, 2000

Gerber R. *Vibrational Medicine for the 21st Century*. HarperCollins, 2001

Grossinger R. *Homeopathy. An Introduction for Skeptics and Beginners*. Berkeley, CA: North Atlantic Books, 1993

Kaufman M. *Homeopathy in America*. Baltimore: Johns Hopkins Press, 1971

Ullman D. *The Consumer's Guide to Homeopathy*. Jeremy P. Tarcher, 1996

Meditation

7

H. Pokharna

INTRODUCTION

Meditation is a process of healing and restoration of wholeness of mind, body and spirit. The words 'meditation', 'medicine' and 'medication' all share the same Latin root *medico*, meaning 'to cure'. Meditation is probably derived from the same root as the Latin word *mederi* meaning 'to heal'. The word 'heal' comes from the Indo-European root 'to make whole'. Studies have shown how the state of mind affects physical health. For example, anything that promotes a sense of isolation may lead to disease. The premise of meditation practice is that every individual has vast inner resources which, through meditation practice, can be mobilized to assist him or her in their healing.

One of the ancient health systems called Ayurveda, which is actively practiced in India, is a major promoter of meditation. The purpose of Ayurveda is to maximize human potential, defying sickness and aging through specific healing techniques, including the prescription of vegetarian foods, herbs, exercises, massages and meditation. Modern science is now beginning to accept what the ancient mystics and yogis have experienced through the ages, concerning the latent healing and rejuvenating powers of man. Yoga, meditation and relaxation, when supplemented with natural foods and vegetarianism, have proven to increase the productivity of the mind and body, and create a state of well-being and inner peace.

Meditation has been practiced and perfected as a health-enhancing technique for several thousand years in the Jain, Hindu and Buddhist practices. Meditation practices have also been used within the Western traditions, which include Judeo-Christian religious groups, as well as the Native Americans. 'Traditional' meditation is based on theoretical and spiritual concepts rooted on ancient Eastern philosophies, while 'modern' forms of meditation are concerned with efforts to explain meditation in terms of 'Western physiology'. The meditation practices that are without cultural or religious aspects were developed primarily for research purposes. Meditation gained widespread attention in the West after Maharishi Mahesh Yogi introduced transcendental meditation to the USA in 1959. In 1972, Herbert Benson and Keith Wallace published an article in the *Scientific American*, 'The physiology of meditation', which gave scientific credibility to an ancient spiritual practice that changes the body's metabolism, reduces stress and all its parameters and even offers a way of treating addictions. This search for healing of a problem, rather than control of symptoms, is one of the greatest attractions of alternative medicine, and meditation is no exception to this effect[1–3].

The scientific study of meditation and its applications in health care has focused on three specific approaches: transcendental meditation; the elicitation of the 'relaxation response', a generic approach to meditation formulated by Benson[4–6]; and mindfulness meditation, specifically the mindfulness-based stress-reduction program developed by Kabat-Zinn[7–9].

This chapter is an overview of meditation as a complementary medical approach to the treatment and prevention of health-related problems and for the promotion of health. This is intended to assist health-care providers in giving advice to their patients about meditation. Unlike approaches in complementary medicine such as biofeedback and acupuncture, most meditation practices were developed within various religious and spiritual contexts. However, as a health-care intervention, meditation can be effectively employed regardless of a patient's cultural and religious background.

WHY MEDITATE?

The main objective of meditation is to bring steadiness to the mind, which usually remains disturbed as it is constantly stimulated by the sense organs, sense objects and countless desires. In order for the mind to be relieved from the disturbance and confusion, it needs to move slowly towards calmness, clarity and focus. To reach this, one might sit in a solitary place, try to close the doors of all the sense organs and allow mental distractions to end.

One can make use of the following three key functions of meditation:

(1) To curb the existing thoughts and prevent new thoughts from rising in the mind, in order to become thoughtless;

(2) To have only desired thoughts in the mind;

(3) To observe thoughts in the mind as a witness.

These three functions of meditation are equally important. They are rooted in the three different branches of yoga: *jnana* (knowledge), *karma* (action) and *bhakti* (devotion).

WHAT IS MEDITATION?

The word 'meditation' has an infinite variety of associations. In the English language meditate is used as a verb 'to meditate about, or to meditate upon' implying that meditation is a mental or cerebral activity. In that sense 'to meditate' would be to focus one's attention exclusively on something predetermined by the person meditating. In English such an activity is called concentration and in Sanskrit it is referred to as *dharna*, meaning to hold, or sustain attention. On the otherhand, meditation, referred to in Sanskrit as *dhyana*, is a state of being in which there is an effortless and choiceless awareness of what life is within and around. By this conception meditation is a state of being, not an activity. Meditation can be said to be a non-cerebral activity, an activity of the consciousness. It does not involve

that part of the brain that is inhibited by conditioning through education, culture, civilization and the socioeconomic contents of life. Meditation is the inner journey, the spiritual journey and the journey towards the absolute or the journey towards divine love[10,11]. Meditation is a total way of living, not a partial or fragmentary activity. Meditation is not only ideally suited for optimum physical and mental health, but it confers a sense of self-reliance, a sense of harmony with laws of the universe, and an unfolding of one's latent potentialities, as well as the unfolding of capacities for healing and regeneration.

Meditation includes different kinds of practice, means something different to different cultures and traditions and includes both concentration and meditation practices. Some of the different forms include:

* Breath meditation

* Mantra meditation

* Vipassana or insight meditation

* Mandala/visual meditation

* Movement meditation, including Tai Chi, Qigong and Hatha Yoga

* Classic Zen Buddhist meditation

* Classic yoga meditation

* Prayer

* Mindfulness meditation

* Medical meditation as used in stress-reduction clinics and for other medical problems (creativity meditation, or art as meditation (journaling, writing, drawing, sculpting, etc.))

* Guided imagery

* Sufi dance

* Centering prayer

There are three elements basic to most traditional forms of meditation. These elements are:

- a comfortable or poised posture;

- an object for attention-awareness to dwell upon; and

- a passive attitude.

There are different meditation traditions and most systems can be grouped into two basic approaches: concentrative meditation and mindfulness meditation. Concentrative meditation focuses attention on the breath, an image or a sound (mantra). These techniques use a focus of attention towards one point, so that thoughts are no longer scattered and undirected. These meditations use verbal tools, such as mantras, and visual tools, such as mandalas, prayer beads, rosaries or candles to help enhance concentration and focus thoughts. Mindfulness meditation involves opening of the attention and awareness to sensations, feelings, images, thoughts, sounds and smells without thinking about them.

In other words, practicing meditation is practicing the art of observation, not to interpret, not to analyze, not to compare, not to judge as good or bad but to be aware of the movement of the mind in the same way one is aware of the sunset. One can learn to observe the thoughts as they come by devoting some time to this, by sitting comfortably and quietly in an upright sitting position or lying prone. The core requirement is that the spine and the neck be straight, so that the rhythm of breathing and blood circulation are not disturbed.

WE RELAX TO MEDITATE AND DO NOT MEDITATE TO RELAX

Meditation is not relaxation alone. Relaxation is a necessary component of meditation and is a preparatory step towards meditation, as it becomes a gateway to deep sleep, rest and meditation. It helps to cultivate a restful, alert and focused mind, which then opens the flow of natural life force also referred to as

prana, which is the subtlest form of biological energy. This life force is recognized in many cultural traditions; the Chinese know it as *chi* and control its flow through acupuncture, meditation and specialized exercises, such as tai chi. In Japanese, this force is referred to *ki*. If you have seen the movie Star Wars, the *force* is the same thing. Depletion or absence of *prana* is directly linked to aging and death. *Prana* includes intelligence and consciousness, the two vital ingredients that animate physical matter. *Prana* flows from spirit, or pure awareness, to bring intelligence and consciousness to every aspect of life.

Relaxation is usually equated with sleep or apathy, while meditation seeks to combine inner peace and awareness. Meditation restores energy and allows it to be used more effectively by causing one to be more mindful of what one is directing it to, thus fostering productivity while reducing tension. Being relaxed is not about avoiding responsibilities; rather, it is about developing skills and abilities to deal with responsibilities free of fears and tensions. The essence of meditation is to transform relaxation from a mechanical health chore to a reminder of personal beliefs, values and commitments conducive to increased calm. In the broadest sense, the art of meditation is to help a person discover a source of inner calm and tranquility in the midst of life's activities. This quality of relaxation leads to transcendence.

MEDITATION IS A PROCESS OF HARNESSING THE HEALING POWER

Hippocrates said, 'The natural force within us is the greatest healer of disease'. Meditation is a way of harnessing this natural force to maintain health and wholeness. Ancient sages have said that the *atman* (soul) is the source of all wisdom and, from that source alone, streams of wisdom flow into the heart. This flow of wisdom can be achieved only to the extent that the mind remains peaceful and undisturbed. The mind is a powerful ally in healing the body, and meditation keeps the mind primed. Yogis have believed and proved that our well-being depends on the energy fields within us that are far more subtle than the purely physical one. Of prime importance are the chakras or the spinning centers of etheric energy, which distribute the force throughout our entire being. The etheric energy field consists of a network of energy lines called *nadis* and where the lines intersect, the spinning energy centers are called the *chakras*.

In the Indian tradition there are seven major chakras, situated at different points on the spine, each spinning at its own rate. The seven are, in ascending order:

(1) Muladhara (coccygeal)

(2) Svadhishthana (sacral)

(3) Manipura (solar plexus)

(4) Anahata (heart)

(5) Vishuddha (throat)

(6) Ajna (brow)

(7) Sahasrara (head)

As shown in Table 1, each of these chakras is associated with a particular physiological system. For example, the heart chakra is associated with the physical heart and the circulatory system. The chakras are known to contribute energy to specific parts of the body. Meditation practices are known to open each of the chakras and allow the flow of *prana* or the healing force to circulate in the body, thus acting as energy transformers to distribute the *prana* energy to the

major glands, nerves and organs of the body. The root or the base chakra is the storehouse for the *prana* energy, also called the *kundalini*. This *kundalini* energy has the potential to cultivate and align all of the major chakras with the higher centers, bringing illumination and spiritual enlightenment as the proper sequence of chakras unfold[10,12].

COMPONENTS OF MEDITATION

Physiotherapeutic breathing

The ancient yoga tradition dedicated to breathing exercises is called *pranayama*. According to the philosophy of yoga, breathing controls the flow of *prana*, the cosmic life force, into the body. The nose is believed to be the proper instrument for breathing rather than the mouth. Yogic breathing methods teach breathing through the nose, rather than the mouth, and abdominal breathing in a slow and rhythmic pattern, rather than chest breathing. The followers of yoga believe that this form of breathing will facilitate the flow of prana. If one pays close attention to one's breathing, one will notice that it varies according to one's mood. One breathes differently, for example, when one is happy as opposed to sad, bored as opposed to excited, or calm as opposed to angry. Proper breathing can help to control destructive emotions, including anger, hatred, jealousy, grief and frustration.

In general, all meditation practices have the following in common:

(1) Awareness of the nasal function and of nasal breathing; encouragement to breathe through the nose;

(2) Awareness of the rate and rhythm of one's breathing; encouragement to practice slowing the breathing process;

(3) Awareness of the difference between thoracic and abdominal breathing; encouragement to breathe by contracting the diaphragm, rather than by expanding the chest.

Table 1 Associations of the seven chakras

Chakra	Physiological system	Endocrine system
Coccygeal	reproductive	gonads
Sacral	genitourinary	Leydig cells
Solar plexus	digestive	adrenals
Heart	circulatory	thymus
Throat	respiratory	thyroid
Brow or third eye	autonomic nervous system	pituitary
Head	central nervous system	pineal

All yogic techniques have certain outcomes, which include a state of deep relaxation in a short time; slowing of the body's metabolism (physiological process of utilizing oxygen and nutrients) as the oxygen is consumed; and a decrease in carbon dioxide production, respiratory rate, heart rate and blood pressure. In addition, lactic acid, a substance produced by the metabolism of skeletal muscles and associated with anxiety and tension, is reduced. There is an increase in the intensity and frequency of alpha brain waves, which are present with deep relaxation, and a change in state of arousal and awareness[13].

Cognitive processes

Cognitive processes are ways to assimilate information. Cognitive structures are the beliefs, values and commitments that underlie thoughts, speech and actions. Three cognitive processes are integral to initiating the process of meditation. *Focusing* is the ability to identify, differentiate, maintain attention on, and return attention to simple stimuli for an extended period. *Passivity* is the ability to stop unnecessary goal-directed and analytic activity. *Receptivity* is the ability to tolerate and accept experiences that may be paradoxical, uncertain or unfamiliar[14].

MANIFESTATIONS OF MEDITATION

Understanding the mind–body connection

More than 2000 years ago, Galen observed that tumor growth was more pronounced in melancholic women than in sanguine women. Thus, the seed of the idea that mental processes and emotional status are linked with physical health and disease has long been planted. An important advancement in constructing a scientific framework for understanding the pathways came with the descriptions by Cannon (1914) and Selye (1934) of the body's responses to and defenses against a variety of stressful stimuli. Cannon coined the term 'fight or flight' response, which is associated with a series of physiological reactions triggered when faced with a threatening environmental situation,

which includes dilatation of pupils, increased blood pressure, increased respiratory rate and heightened motor excitability. This mimics the increased sympathetic nervous system activity.

The terms 'stress' and 'stress syndrome' were first adopted some 66 years ago by Hans Seyle who, in an article in the science journal *Nature*, described a series of pathophysiological changes that typically develop in the rat following exposure to noxious stimuli as diverse as physical (cold, surgery), chemical (morphine, adrenaline (epinephrine)) or emotional challenges[15].

The anterior pituitary gland and its control center in the brain, the hypothalamus, together constitute the classical neuroendocrine system, which plays an important role in controlling the release of stress hormones, especially the powerfully immunosuppressive glucocorticoids, which can then communicate with the cells of the immune system, whether they be moving within the circulation or static in the primary and secondary lymphoid tissues. The products of the immune system can 'talk' to the neuroendocrine tissues. The hypothalamus is also a critical modulator of the behavioral responses to stress and of the autonomic nervous system, which is activated by stress and innervates tissues of the immune system. Stress hormones have a crucial role in maintaining body homeostasis in the face of an ever-changing external and emotional environment. If present at raised levels for prolonged periods, these hormones become immunosuppressive, thus predisposing an individual to a variety of diseases, including infection, autoimmune disorders, inflammatory diseases and cancers[16].

Relaxation response

Individuals possess an opposite, alternative response: the relaxation response, which counteracts the effects of stress. The relaxation response is believed to be an integrated hypothalamic response that results in generalized decreased sympathetic nervous system activity and this response consists of changes opposite to those of the fight or flight reaction. Hess called this response the 'trophotropic response'. When he stimulated cats with electrical stimulation of the hypothalamic area, the response resulted in decreased blood pressure, decreased respiratory rate and pupil constriction[17]. The major physiological elements of the relaxation response were first defined in humans during the practice of transcendental meditation: decreased oxygen consumption, carbon dioxide elimination and changes in heart rate, respiratory rate, minute ventilation and arterial blood lactate. Systolic, diastolic and mean blood pressures remained unchanged compared to control levels. Rectal temperature also remained unchanged, whereas skin resistance markedly increased and skeletal muscle blood flow slightly increased. The electroencephalogram demonstrated an increase in the intensity of slow alpha waves and occasional theta wave activity. These changes are consistent with generalized decreased sympathetic nervous system activity and are distinctly different from physiological changes noted during quiet sitting or sleep. These changes occur simultaneously and are consistent with those noted by Hess.

Physiological manifestations

Marked metabolic and circulatory changes accompany transcendental meditation, especially in long-term practitioners. Virtually none of the effects could be reproduced by sleep and unstylized eyes-closed rest. Jevning and colleagues proposed that the metabolic changes are probably mediated by circulating plasma effectors, and comprise an 'integrated meditation response'[13]. There appears to be a patterned physiological response of an overall decreased muscle mass, red cell metabolism, as well as decreased thyroid and adrenocortical hormone secretion. Electrophysiologically, increased galvanic skin resistance is inversely related to stress. These manifestations include increased cardiac output, probable increased cerebral blood flow, increased plasma rennin and prolactin and decreased carbon dioxide generation by muscles. Briefly, these findings emphasize that meditation may result in beneficial changes in physiological parameters, such as levels of adrenal hormones, platelet aggregation, autonomic tone and balance, blood pressure, brain biochemistry and cerebral blood flow.

Evidence–based clinical usefulness

Reductions in arousal through meditation or relaxation can be manifested in at least three ways: behaviorally, physiologically and through self-report. Relaxation response-based studies at the Mind/Body Medical Institute suggest that relaxation-based techniques can reduce the nausea and fatigue associated with chemotherapy, decrease insomnia, ease hot flushes and increase fertility in women with fertility problems. Studies by Benson and co-workers have shown that meditation can lower blood pressure in hypertensive patients[18]. Meditation may also be an effective complementary treatment for coronary artery disease (CAD). CAD patients practicing transcendental meditation showed significant increase in exercise tolerance, maximal workload and delay in the onset of ST-segment depression compared to controls. Ornish's programs on reversal of heart diseases include meditation as the central component[19,20].

Meditation has been effective in the treatment of chronic pain[21]. Chronic pain patients have reduced their physician visits by 36%. Mindfulness meditation facilitated significant reduction in pain symptoms, psychological pain and pain-related drug use. The reduction in pain with meditation may be attributed to the hypo-arousal and cultivation of detached and decreased attention to the cognitive–emotional alarm reactions to painful sensations. The emotional and cognitive components of the pain experience are lowered in patients trained in meditation, resulting in less suffering and distress[9,21].

A variety of exercises were developed for these patients who suffer from chronic obstructive pulmonary disease (COPD), including emphysema and cystic fibrosis. These included practicing *pranayama* (a special breathing technique) and other yogic meditative techniques. These patients have demonstrated fewer asthma attacks, less shortness of breath and greater control over their breathing[22].

Psychological and cognitive manifestations

Meditation can help reduce symptoms of anxiety and anxiety-related disorders[23]. Practitioners of all forms of relaxation, whether it be autogenic training, breathing or Zen meditation, are essentially doing the same thing: honing and refining their ability to attend to a limited stimulus; ceasing unnecessary goal-oriented and analytic activity; and tolerating and accepting experiences that may be uncertain, unfamiliar or paradoxical.

Spiritual benefits of meditation

When individuals practice meditation for over 6–7 weeks, they observe a shift toward personal and spiritual growth. Many individuals who initially learn meditation for its self-regulatory aspects find that as their practice deepens, they are drawn more and more into the realm of the 'spiritual'. The daily development of spiritual integration involves such factors as competent self-care, stress management, clarification of spiritual beliefs and the discipline of spiritually enhancing practices. Being aware and respectful of one's body by providing healthy food, exercise and rest supports the work of the physician. Meditation practices also give one the power to change one's attitudes and beliefs, and therefore one's reactions, in addition to making physical improvements. Meditation practices influence physical, mental, social and spiritual well-being. Borysenko and Chopra, pioneers in the mind–body connection, have observed for many cancer and AIDS patients that most are interested in meditation as a way of becoming more attuned to the spiritual dimension of life. Borysenko reported that many die 'healed', in a state of compassionate self-awareness and self-acceptance[24,25].

MEDITATION: MYTHS AND MISCONCEPTIONS

There has been a false impression in Western society that meditation is connected to Eastern mysticism, that by practicing meditation one might be doing something against God, that meditation is somehow a sin. It is true that meditation is embraced, professed and perfected in the East, but it can be found in all world religions, and it was this spiritual

omnipresence that prompted Benson and Wallace to research it initially[3].

PRESCRIPTION, WARNINGS AND PRECAUTIONS

It is recommended that concentrative meditation exercises should be avoided by individuals whose reality-testing function is poor, who are strongly paranoid, or who are likely to develop delusions of grandeur from the altered states of consciousness that these practices tend to produce. People with overwhelming anxiety should probably avoid insight meditations. Long periods of meditative practice (as in contemplative meditation) may precipitate psychotic episodes in susceptible individuals. Meditation practices may need to be closely monitored in patients with mental disorders. As emphasized throughout in complementary medicine, a patient's health and well-being encompasses more that just his or her physical health. Consequently, in order to treat the physical maladies manifested by psychological stress, one must consider the impacts on the patients' mental, social and spiritual health. Therefore, meditation and relaxation exercises are a valuable adjunct to our current therapies, and they are also useful as a preventive measure, as these offer an appropriate solution that includes all aspects of health. These exercises are effective, are readily available and have no side-effects, yet their incorporation into medical practice is slow. Merely studying meditation, as with exercise, will not produce the outcomes described here; practice and experience are essential. Familiarity with the simplicity and practice of these exercises tends to clear up misunderstandings, thus demystifying them. Probably the safest course for those in the healing professions is to experiment with meditation practices for themselves, and then share with clients and friends those they thoroughly understand. With all the advantages of meditation, one of the challenges follows the saying 'time is money'; most people do not feel that they have time to meditate or relax. In this case the physicians could encourage the patients to consider the wisdom of the Earl of Derby: 'those who cannot find time for bodily exercise will sooner or later have to find time for illness'[26].

APPENDIX

Relaxation response

(1) Pick a focus word or short phrase that is firmly rooted in your belief system. The repeat word could be a word, sound, prayer, phrase or muscular activity. (You can use a religious or other word that means something to you or you can use a neutral word such as: one, ocean, love, peace, calm, relax.)

(2) Sit quietly in a comfortable position.

(3) Close your eyes.

(4) Relax your muscles.

(5) Breathe slowly and naturally, and as you do, repeat your focus word, phrase or prayer silently to yourself as you exhale.

(6) Assume a passive attitude. When other thoughts come to mind, simply say to yourself, gently return to the repetition.

(7) Continue for 10–20 minutes.

(8) Do not stand immediately. Continue sitting quietly for a minute or so, allowing other thoughts to return. Then, open your eyes and sit for another minute before rising.

(9) Practice this technique once or twice daily.

Source: Herbert Benson. *Timeless Healing*. New York, NY: Simon and Schuster, 1990

Mindfulness meditation

This stress-reducing technique calls for meditating on different parts of the body to relax the mind. It can be done every day. Set aside 30–45 minutes for this exercise.

(1) Lie down on your back, with your legs uncrossed and your arms along your sides, palms facing up. Close your eyes.

(2) Become aware of your breathing, feeling your breath flow in and out of your body, noticing sensations at your nostrils, your chest or abdomen.

(3) Now, start to focus on the toes of your left foot. Notice what you feel as you remain aware of your breathing. Continue for at least 1–2 minutes. If you get distracted, return here.

(4) As you exhale, shift your focus to the bottom of your left foot as you continue to be aware of your breathing. Stay here for 1–2 minutes.

(5) Now, move to the top of your left foot, and do the same as before. Eventually, move up your left ankle, lower leg, knee, thigh and hip. Then, go back to the toes of your right foot, and start moving up from there.

(6) Once you return to the hip, move up through hips, the genitals, the buttocks and the rectum. Proceed up to the lower back, the abdomen, the upper back, ribs, chest, shoulder blades and shoulders.

(7) From the shoulders, move out to the fingers and hands on both sides (you can do both hands at same time), and then move up to the wrists, forearms, elbows and upper arms, and return to the shoulders.

(8) From the shoulders, move up to the neck, and then proceed to the head. Start with your face, focusing on the jaw, and move to the lips, teeth, gums, roof of your mouth, tongue, back of the throat, cheeks, nose, ears, eyes, eyelids, territory around the eyes, eyebrows, forehead, temples, scalp and the rest of the cranium.

(9) Having reached the top of your head, imagine exhaling through it. Then, imagine inhaling through the bottom of your feet and again

exhaling through the top of your head. Do this for a few minutes.

(10) Let go of any focus on the body and be aware of breathing at no particular location.

(11) Let go of the focus on breathing, and pay attention to whatever enters your awareness at the moment, whether thoughts, sensations of any sort, feelings, sounds, or silence. Perceive what they are, and let go of them, remaining in the moment.

Source: Kabat-Zinn J. *Full Catastrophe Living*. New York, NY: Doubleday & Co, Inc; 1990

GLOSSARY

Mindfulness is a form of meditation originally developed in Buddhist traditions of Asia but practiced today by many, from meditations in monasteries to physicians in stress-reduction clinics. Mindfulness can be defined as awareness of each moment as it occurs.

    Yoga, from the Sanskrit root *yuj*, meaning 'to yoke or join together,' is a 5000-year-old method of mind–body health with a goal of enlightenment. It has many paths or methods:

- Karma yoga, which emphasizes action and service to others

- Bhakti yoga, which emphasizes love of God

- Jnana yoga, which emphasizes intellectual striving

- Hatha yoga, which emphasizes balance through physical and mental exercise

- Raja yoga, which emphasizes techniques for controlling mind and body, including exercises, breathing and relaxation techniques and meditation

- Yama (moral commandments)

- Niyama (self-purification)

- Asana (posture)

- Pranayama (rhythmic breath control)

- Pratyahara (sense withdrawal)

- Dharna (concentration)

- Dhyana (meditation)

- Samadhi (higher unitive consciousness)

    Yogi is someone who practices yoga.

    Chakras are psychological–physical–spiritual centers of energy that exist between the base of the spinal column and crown of the head, according to yogic thought. Chakras are often described as the centers where astral or subtle body and physical body converge, where mass is converted to energy and vice versa.

    Mantras, wards chanted during meditation, resonate within the body and the chakras. The chanted words evoke and release specific energies.

    Prana, chi, ki are all names for life force energy that animates the body and the universe, and which, when unblocked and properly directed, can help the body to heal itself.

References

1. West M. Meditation. *Br J Psychiatry* 1979;135:457
2. Shapiro DH Jr. Overview: clinical and physiological comparison of meditation with other self-control strategies. *Am J Psychiatry* 1978;139:267
3. Wallace K, Benson H. The physiology of meditation. *Sci Am* 1972;226;84–90
4. Smith JC. *Relaxation Dynamics; A Cognitive–Behavioral Approach to Relaxation*. Champaign, IL: Research Press, 1989

5. Benson H. *The Relaxation Response*. New York, NY: Morrow, 1975

6. Benson H, Beary JF, Carol MP. The relaxation response. *Psychiatry* 1974;37:37–46

7. Kabat-Zinn J, Massion AO, Hebert JR. Meditation. In Holland JC, ed. *Textbook of Psycho-oncology*. Oxford: Oxford University Press, 1998

8. Kabat-Zinn J. Mindfulness meditation: what it is, what it isn't, and its role in health care and medicine. In Haruki Y, Suzuki M, eds. *Comparative and Psychological Study on Meditation*. Delft: Eburon, 1996

9. Kabat-Zinn J, Lipworth L, Burney R. Four-year follow-up of a meditation-based program for self regulation of chronic pain: treatment outcomes and compliance. *Clin J Pain* 1987;2:159–73

10. Krpalvanand S. *Science of Meditation*. Bombay, India: New Karnodaya Press, 1977

11. Le Shan L. *How to Meditate*. New York, NY: Bantam Books, 1974

12. Richard G. *Vibrational Medicine*. Santa Fe, NM: Bear and Company Publications, 1996

13. Jevning R, Wallace R, Beidebach M. The physiology of meditation: a review. A wakeful hypometabolic integrated response. *Neurosci and Biochem Rev* 1992;16:415–24

14. Smith JC. *Cognitive Behavioral Relaxation Training*. New York, NY: Springer Publishing Company, 1990

15. Selye H. A syndrome produced by diverse nocuous agents. *Nature (London)* 1936;138:32

16. Buckingham J, Gillies G, Cowell A. *Stress, Stress Hormones and the Immune System*. Chichester, UK: John Wiley and Sons, 1997

17. Hess WR. *Functional Organization of the Diencephalons*. New York, NY: Grune and Stratton, 1957

18. Benson H, Rosner BA, Marzetta BR, Klemchuk HM. Decreased blood pressure in pharmacologically treated hypertensive patients who regularly elicited the relaxation response. *Lancet* 1974;1:289–91

19. Eisenberg DM, Delbanco TL, Berkey CS, *et al*. Cognitive behavioral techniques for hypertension: are they effective? *Ann Intern Med* 1993;118:964–72

20. Ornish D, Scherwitz LW, Billings JH, *et al*. Intensive lifestyle changes for reversal of coronary heart disease. *J Am Med Assoc* 1998;280:2001–7

21. Benson H. Chronic pain patients reduce their physician visits. *J Chronic Pain* 1991;2:305–10

22. Hass A, Pineda H, Hass F, Axen K. *Pulmonary Therapy and Rehabilitation: Principle and Practice*. Baltimore, MD: Williams and Wilkins, 1979

23. Eppley KR, Abrahams AI, Shear J. Differential effects of relaxation techniques on trait anxiety: a meta-analysis. *J Clin Psychol* 1989;45:957–74

24. Borysenko J. *Minding the Body, Mending the Mind*. New York, NY: Warner Books, 1987

25. Chopra D. *Ageless Body, Timeless Mind*. Crown Publishers, 1993

26. Buckley J, Holmes J, Mapp G. *Exercise on Prescription: Cardiovascular Activity for Health*. Boston, MA: Butterworth-Heinemann–Reed Educational and Professional Publishing, 1999

Biofeedback

8

J. M. Zumsteg

INTRODUCTION

Biofeedback is a safe complementary therapy with rapidly increasing efficacious applications. This approach of general relaxation with awareness and voluntary control of physiology is gaining acceptance in the medical field, with many physicians listing biofeedback in a treatment category of successful therapies along with support groups, aerobic exercise and a healthy diet[1]. The director of the National Center for Complementary and Alternative Medicine (NCCAM) describes biofeedback as one of the 'mind–body approaches that have a well-documented theoretical and evidence base'[2].

Applied psychophysiology and biofeedback are often grouped into the same procedural or therapeutic category. The range of approaches and protocols in biofeedback is immense. There is a continuing discussion concerning the preferred definition of biofeedback[3], illustrating the difficulty of categorizing this versatile practice. Definitions range in their emphasis, depending on whether the application is therapeutic, research based, procedural, teleological, or having another application. A comprehensive definition of the approach often used in medically related issues was presented by Schwartz and Schwartz[4]:

> As a process, applied biofeedback is a group of therapeutic procedures that uses electronic or electromechanical instruments to accurately measure, process, and feed back, to persons and their therapists information with educational and reinforcing properties about their neuromuscular and autonomic activity, both normal and abnormal, in the form of analogue or binary, auditory and/or visual feedback signals. Best achieved with a competent biofeedback professional, the objectives are to help persons develop greater awareness of, confidence in, and an increase in voluntary control over their physiological processes that are otherwise outside awareness and/or under less voluntary control, by first controlling the external signal, and then with internal psychophysiological cognitions, and/or by engaging in and applying behaviors to prevent symptom onset, stop it, or reduce it soon after onset.

Although lengthy, the above statement is informative of the philosophy and nature of treatment in biofeedback. Applied psychophysiology requires, as a minimum, a biofeedback trainer/practitioner/therapist and the person participating in training. Since the focus in biofeedback training is wellness and training often takes place outside a traditional medical setting, the patient is most often referred to as a client. It is notable that biofeedback is useful therapeutically only if the information is meaningful to the patient; this is important when selecting training modalities and highlights the importance of the role of a well-trained biofeedback practitioner. Also, a significant component of successful biofeedback training is the movement from observing and manipulating an outside feedback signal to an awareness and direct enhanced control of one's physiology. The eventual goal is awareness and control of physiology without the need for feedback, equipment, or therapist intervention. This independence is achieved through the development of personal strategies; practice of techniques during training sessions and at home; and a heightened personal awareness of one's healthy physiology as compared to one's body state during disease and stress.

Achieving results with applied psychophysiology requires an interested client and a proficient trainer.

Certification as a biofeedback practitioner is available and recommended. General training requirements for certification through the Biofeedback Certification Institute of America (BCIA) reinforces delivery of quality services and include: a bachelor's degree or higher in a health-related field; 50 h of classroom instruction in specific topics; 100 h of supervised work as a biofeedback trainer; a course in human anatomy or physiology; and written and practical examinations. Re-certification is required to maintain BCIA status. Health-care providers or consumers can locate certified practitioners in their area by utilizing the search area of the BCIA website.

Frequently conducted in one-to-one, personal, small office settings, biofeedback has recently entered the 'telehealth' sphere. Now, when properly equipped, biofeedback training has the potential to occur with the practitioner and client in different locations[5]. Many practitioners expect this approach to increase access to biofeedback services, reduce cost and increase efficiency[6]. New technology and an interest in cost-effective care have encouraged both telehealth applications and increased research regarding the minimum number of biofeedback sessions required to achieve and maintain desired results.

A basic understanding of biofeedback as a complementary approach in health care is important, so that practitioners may refer patients to effective modes of treatment, and so that they understand the medical implications, positive or negative, for those already participating in training. Many health-care providers are unfamiliar with the practices of biofeedback and the range of disorders routinely treated through this modality; the result can be unnecessary hesitancy to utilize biofeedback services and difficulty discussing alternative approaches with patients. Confusion surrounding the range of applications, safety and efficacy of biofeedback has become evident through a number of studies. One survey investigating nurses' attitudes towards complementary and alternative medicine found that, while biofeedback was thought by the majority to have strong evidence supporting its effectiveness, a majority was also unsure of the safety of biofeedback[7]. Another survey, conducted at Gundersen Lutheran Medical Center, reported that over half the medical staff had referred

patients for either biofeedback or chiropractic care at some time and that biofeedback is a complementary therapy providers would like to offer their patients in the future[8]. Increasingly convenient resources should make the continued integration of biofeedback into medicine an easier task. Biofeedback is currently used to treat many disorders and is growing in its medical, business, education and peak performance (sports/music) applications.

As with many areas of alternative medicine, a growing number of applications, continuing research and increasing utilization of biofeedback services raise the question of who will pay for these additional health-care costs. Insurance coverage for biofeedback is quite variable. Health insurance companies may make a blanket decision about coverage or they may approve biofeedback for applications where the provider deemed the benefits of a treatment undeniable. In 2000, the Centers for Medicare and Medicaid Services (CMS) made one such specific decision, approving reimbursement for biofeedback training to treat urinary incontinence[9]. As more patients utilize alternative therapies there will be an increased demand for third-party payers to define benefits specifically. The present chapter addresses the essentials of understanding of biofeedback, including the general technology and modalities used; current and emerging medical applications; indications and contra-indications for participating in training; and an examination of the efficacy and safety of numerous applications of biofeedback.

FORMS OF FEEDBACK

As suggested by the definition cited above, feedback can take a variety of forms. When a new therapeutic relationship is created or when a new task in biofeedback is to be explored, it is common to establish the individual's baseline physiology and symptom patterns. If a specific disorder is being treated, baseline assessment often begins with monitoring of specific physiological indicators in a journal for a few weeks, which will then be reviewed by the trainer. The first session will usually be an intake interview and a sitting for physiological baseline assessment, often lasting at least 50 min. During this time the client is monitored in a fashion as close to the training situation as possible. Feedback is absent during baseline sessions; the client's computer monitor is blank and the audio signal is turned off. The therapist will introduce a series of mildly stressful tasks and then allow time for physiological recovery. Although there are many tasks for the clients to perform, the general categories of interest are baselines for situations of resting tension, resting arousal, reactivity, recovery and relaxation. There are numerous approaches to baselines, but clients may be asked to sit quietly with their eyes open or closed; to think of a stressful situation in their life; or may be directed to relax with the therapist in or out of the room. A mental task may also be introduced to monitor the physiological reaction to this type of stress. Serial sevens is commonly used; the client is asked to subtract 7 from 100 and to continue subtracting 7 from the result. There may also be changes in the environment, such as having the lights turned on or dimmed down. The computer system records the corresponding physiological changes and the information will be utilized in creating a personalized training approach. Baselines are especially important if multiple biofeedback sessions will be conducted[4]. Some practitioners may choose to include a short (5–7 min) baseline reading at the beginning of each session. Baselines are often a dramatic indicator of progress and a thorough baseline reading is often conducted as the terminating session, as a summary of the work and as a discussion tool for the physiological changes that occurred.

Although the interaction between trainer and client is essential to productive biofeedback, the choice of equipment is important to the structure of training sessions. The first wave of biofeedback equipment consisted of a monitor for each physiological indicator measured and feedback was presented through a meter, usually reading out voltage. Although these stand-alone units are sometimes still used, biofeedback today is dominated by integrated computer feedback systems. A myriad of computer software programs are available and the computer-based design allows for multiple channels of input to be analyzed and fed back to the client. Combining indicators permits bilateral training and synchronous feedback for more

than one modality, which is useful in applications such as breath training, which pairs trapezius electromyography (EMG) with heart rate or training for symmetry in hand temperature. Computerized feedback programs typically offer visual and auditory (digital and analog) feedback, programmable by the trainer. Quantified goals are redefined during each session through the trainer's entries on the computer. At least two video monitors are present during training, one to display feedback to the client and one for the therapist to view and enter training parameters. The feedback provided to the client changes as they near the current goal. Instant feedback and reward are desired to drive learning; a pitch may become progressively lower when muscles relax (decrease in voltage) or an image might gradually fill in on the monitor as the goal is approached. Some programs also include mazes, games and animation, which can be especially useful for pediatric applications. Usually, when the client reaches a set goal, there is an immediate endpoint reward such as winning the game, seeing the complete image filled in, or the start of an animation. The trainer will then change the parameters to set another goal and the process begins again. The client–trainer interaction is important in setting realistic physiological goals and in producing an experience that is rewarding and challenging, but not overly frustrating, for the client. Positive psychological interactions during biofeedback training and the experience of success in the first session can be essential for the long-term results in biofeedback training[10].

MODALITIES

Although there are some physiological concerns described below to consider before initiating biofeedback, indication for treatment relies predominantly on connecting an interested patient with an appropriate practitioner to address the client's health concerns. A practitioner will usually conduct a thorough interview, take a medical and personal history and sometimes perform a physical examination before accepting a new client[11]. Since the backgrounds of practitioners varies so greatly, the client profile will differ from practice to practice, depending on the training and interests of the professional staff.

Numerous tools are used in biofeedback, with the majority originating through applications in other fields. Nearly all instrumentation applied in biofeedback reads an indirect measure of a physiological process. For example, skin temperature is applied as an indicator of vasoconstriction. Commonly used measures in biofeedback include EMG, heart rate, blood pressure, electroencephalography (EEG), breath rate, skin temperature and electrodermal activity. Often multiple modalities are utilized during each training session. In any setting where multiple biofeedback sessions will occur, physiological monitoring devices should be positioned on the client in the same place each time. Consistency creates more accurate monitoring of progress across sessions. Certain modalities have been shown to be more effective for certain types of people or therapies, each of which are described later in this chapter.

Electromyography

EMG uses the difference in potential between two electrodes as an indicator of muscle contraction. Voluntary muscles are the focus in biofeedback EMG, and surface electrodes are placed over the belly of the muscle of interest[11]. The potential difference is usually reported in microvolts. Needle electrodes, such as those used for nerve conduction studies, are not regularly used in biofeedback. EMG levels are informative in biofeedback, since the amount of voltage measured is proportional to the magnitude of the action potentials of the underlying motor units. Electromagnetic interference may occur, making it important for a practitioner to distinguish artifacts from physiological readings. EMG instrumentation is especially vulnerable to reporting 60-Hz interference (such as fluorescent lights) and electrocardiogram signals. However, proper skin preparation and adequate quality of electronic instrumentation significantly reduces such artifacts. With some applications of EMG it is useful to train bilaterally, so that muscle contraction is symmetrical[11]. Portable instrumentation for EMG has been developed, and is used in biofeedback

applications where it is beneficial to have the patient be mobile. This technique, sometimes labelled dynamic EMG, is especially useful in gait training, posture exercises and sports/music performance applications, since the training is not limited to a still, sitting position.

Heart rate and blood pressure

Many people are readily aware of a change in their heart rate. Some clients will find this awareness of cardiac signals as a more obvious signal of sympathetic activation than cold sweaty hands or tense muscles. In biofeedback training, the photoplethysmograph[4] is employed as an indicator of heart rate. As with all biofeedback equipment, it is important to be consistent from session to session with the placement of the sensors. Phototransmission of blood through the skin is typically measured on the fingers, for reasons of accessibility.

Depending on the goals of training, blood pressure measurements may also be of interest. There are several direct and indirect assessments of pressure, which are briefly described in the section regarding biofeedback for hypertension. Blood pressure feedback has many applications and for some patients may be the most meaningful indicator of autonomic activity, stress level and effective relaxation techniques.

Skin temperature

Skin temperature training is usually focused on peripheral blood flow. For example, when more blood is present in the fingers, they are warmer. Changes in the peripheral circulation are meaningful indicators during training of autonomic activity and the sensors are accordingly placed most often on the fingers or toes[4]. Lower-extremity temperature training is potentially useful in patients with chronic peripheral vascular disease, for example from complications of diabetes[4,12]. Proper technique requires the sensor to be placed on the same fingertip for each session, usually slightly to one side of the fleshy pad[11]. For some people skin temperature may be the best indicator of arousal level and the primary focus of training. In the USA most feedback for skin temperature is reported in degrees Fahrenheit[4]. Common training techniques include warming the extremities, both during relaxation and after stress and bilateral temperature training if one side is significantly cooler than the other. Adjunctive techniques are useful in temperature training; a client may be asked to imagine their hands over a warm fire or participate in a progressive relaxation exercise to observe body temperature changes during relaxation.

Electroencephalography

With a design similar to EMG, EEG biofeedback measures general neuronal activity of the cortex through electrodes placed on the scalp. These potentials are converted using software into dynamic graphs of the electrical activity of the brain. There are many patterns, or montages, of electrode placement. A typical pattern may include 8–20 surface electrodes plus neutral reference electrodes, sometime pre-positioned in a cap that is worn by the client[11]. Once the electrodes are placed, two types of reading are used. Monopolar recordings compare one active electrode to one neutral electrode. The neutral location for an electrode is kept consistent with each client and may be an earlobe or part of the scalp. Bipolar recordings compare two active electrodes that are within about 2 in (5 cm) of each other. The selection of recording type differs with trainer preference and the purpose of the session. EEG is also prone to electrical artifacts, and most software programs include filters to lock out signals from eye blinks, 60-Hz sources, EMG and EKG signals.

EEG readings are sometimes referred to as 'brain-waves'. Labels for electrical frequencies have been devised for ease of communication (Table 1). Deep sleep is accompanied by a frequency of 0.5–4 Hz, which is called delta; 4–7 Hz is the range for theta waves and is observed in a state just between wakefulness and sleep. A predominance of theta waves is frequently recorded during reported moments of insight. Alpha waves have a frequency range of 8–12 Hz, and are associated with resting and

Table 1 Categorization of 'brainwaves'

Category	Frequency (Hz)	Associated state	Associated lobe
Delta	0.5–4	deep sleep	frontal
Theta	4–7	between wakefulness and sleep, insight	temporal
Alpha	8–12	resting, meditation	occipital–parietal
Beta	12–30	alert; indicates dominant hemisphere	—

meditation. Beta waves have a frequency between 12 and 30 Hz, and are indicative of an alert person. A predominance of beta waves usually shows which hemisphere of the brain is most active during that recording[11], although general patterns can also illustrate hemisphere dominance. Values measured during EEG training include frequency, amplitude and the percentage of time that each category of waveform is present. Recent studies have confirmed that biofeedback training can teach a person to manipulate and recognize changes in the electrical activity of his or her brain[13]. In a currently experimental application of EEG, several patients with amyotrophic lateral sclerosis (ALS) have been trained to use EEG frequency shifts as part of a design allowing communication without any voluntary muscle involvement[14]. Trainers who intend to utilize EEG with a client will often first facilitate general stress management so the person is more familiar with his or her physiology[11]. Specific trainer certification in EEG training is available from the BCIA.

Breath rate

Breath training in biofeedback is common and useful alone or paired with additional modalities. The reinforcement of attention to breath in other popular activities, including yoga and visualization, creates a special niche for biofeedback to expand on other experiences. Approaches to breath training, measurements of breath rate and feedback of associated muscle activity are only briefly described here. Respiration rate may be observed by direct or indirect methods.

Although a diaphragm-like device can be placed around the torso for direct measurement of breathing movements, it is more common to analyze breath patterns using shoulder (trapezius) EMG readings as a guide[11]. This is more comfortable for the patient and allows for useful visual feedback patterns. However, if a continuous record of breath rate is desired, direct methods should be utilized.

Electrodermal activity, skin conductance activity and galvanic skin response

All three of the above terms indicate indirect measures of sweat gland activity. As more sweat is produced, the amount of ions available to conduct electricity across the skin increases, and these changes can be measured[4]. Galvanic skin response (GSR) is the most commonly used term for this modality in biofeedback; units of electrical conductance are reported in micromhos, a measure of conductance. This scale is utilized to present more useful feedback to the patient; one micromho of conductance (ohm spelled in reverse) is equivalent to $(1 \text{ micro-ohm})^{-1}$ of resistance[11]. Using the scale of conductance allows for a convenient feedback signal that decreases with relaxation and seems to be a more useful form of feedback. Most practitioners do not discuss the origin of the skin conductance scale with their clients and simply explain that sweat gland activity is an indicator of arousal level. A standard electrodermal biofeedback sensor consists of two surface electrodes placed on different fingers that allow for an electrical circuit across the skin. The more activity of the sweat glands, the more electrical current is allowed to pass across the skin to complete the circuit[4]. Many people have very reactive GSRs, which make it both a sensitive modality as well as one that may be dynamic and difficult to train[11]. GSR training is usually not attempted until the client is adept at skin temperature control[11]. GSR can be useful as a monitor of progress and an indicator of stress, especially in psychologically related applications: biofeedback-assisted psychotherapy, systematic desensitization and stress management. These applications are described individually later in the chapter.

CONTRAINDICATIONS

Although the number of contraindications is minimal, certain physiological consequences of biofeedback result in a few situations where biofeedback is not generally recommended[11]. Biofeedback is viewed as a generally safe therapy with potential benefit and few mechanisms of harm. There is variability in views of exclusion criteria, but general guidelines may be useful to assist physicians in determining who may be appropriately referred for biofeedback. Some patients will have medical conditions that require increased communication between the biofeedback practitioner and other health-care providers (Table 2).

Owing to the low baseline physiological arousal of people with endogenous depression, biofeedback relaxation training is contraindicated. Recommendations are for the depression to be addressed by an appropriate health-care provider and biofeedback pursued once the depression is reasonably managed[11]. People with epilepsy are cautioned about biofeedback training, owing to the possibility of seizure during EEG training. However, there are practitioners with special training in biofeedback applications for epilepsy and some progress has been made in creating biofeedback protocols to reduce seizure frequency[4,15]. Those with epilepsy seeking biofeedback training should be aware of the risks involved and train only under the supervision of a practitioner with special training in addressing seizures.

Table 2 Contraindications to biofeedback

Condition	General recommendation
Depression	no relaxation training; delay biofeedback until depression is addressed appropriately
Epilepsy	advise of seizure risk during electroencephalogram training; seek a practitioner specially trained for epilepsy applications
Chronic medical conditions, especially hypertension, thyroid conditions, diabetes	maintain communication between primary physician and biofeedback trainer; frequent re-evaluation of medication requirements
Psychological factors	delay biofeedback training until issues surrounding relationship changes, motivation, compliance and secondary gain are resolved

Of more general concern is the potential for chemotherapeutic reactions for those simultaneously taking medications and participating in biofeedback training. It is imperative for the patient's physician and biofeedback trainer to stay in communication, to minimize this risk[11]. Some trainers will request a letter of approval for training from the physician if a new client has a chronic medical problem. Of particular concern are medications for hyperthyroidism, hypothyroidism, diabetes and hypertension[4]. Biofeedback may produce physiological effects that decrease or increase the need for medications, and monitoring by a primary care physician is required.

The broadest exclusion for participation in biofeedback training is for psychological reasons. Training is dependent on the participation and compliance of the patient, and factors that limit or interfere with his or her personal stake in the training suggest that biofeedback is not the best approach for such a client. Such people will often resist suggestion, may not notice physiological changes, may be distracted, may want to talk instead of practicing the techniques and frequently drop out of training[11]. There are individuals in specific situations that are contraindicated. These include those who are unable to experience hope, often because of learned helplessness, and those who are beginning or ending an intimate relationship, who need to readjust before seeking biofeedback training. Additionally, those who may experience secondary gain related to an illness, including continued leave from work or a pending lawsuit, are poor candidates for training, since they have a vested interested in remaining ill or disabled. At the simplest level, people who are unmotivated, do not wish to co-operate, or are non-compliant should not be considered as biofeedback clients until these other issues are resolved. The contraindications to biofeedback are not well defined and there is often intense debate within the biofeedback community about which patients and which treatments should be excluded or included in general practice[16].

CONDITIONS TREATED

There are currently two broad categories of conditions treated using biofeedback: common and emerging applications (Table 3). Conditions commonly treated through biofeedback often have specific, widely accepted therapeutic protocols. In these cases, trials or case studies have been conducted and published to establish a standard practice of treatment, and efficacy has often been investigated. The second category of applications, termed 'non-traditional'[4] or emerging, covers what is new in biofeedback or an approach that only a small group of practitioners have applied. Periodically, biofeedback is used as an assessment or therapeutic tool in more complicated studies, sometimes resulting in a single trial application of the new treatment. In the interest of effectively advising patients, physicians should be oriented towards the conditions routinely treated successfully by biofeedback. For any training exceeding basic stress management, patients should

Table 3 Common and emerging applications of biofeedback

Common
Attention deficit hyperactivity disorder
General stress management
Headaches (tension, migraine, pediatric, pregnancy)
Hypertension
Raynaud's phenomenon
Temporomandibular joint disorders

Emerging
Addiction
Anxiety
Arrhythmias
Asthma
Business
Chronic fatigue syndrome
Chronic obstructive pulmonary disease
Chronic pain
Diabetes type 2
Education
Epilepsy
Fecal incontinence
Insomnia
Neuromuscular re-education/gait training
Obsessive–compulsive disorder
Premenstrual syndrome
Psychodermatology
Psychotherapy
Sports/music performance
Torticollis
Urinary incontinence

search for a well-trained practitioner with a solid amount of experience appropriate to the patient's condition.

COMMON APPLICATIONS

Headache

Headaches are a common health concern, and the prolonged use of analgesics has unclear consequences[4]. Problems with conventional pharmacological treatment include possible 'rebound headaches' and interactions with other essential medications. Biofeedback is considered one of the approaches to treatment and prevention of chronic tension headaches[17]. One study discussed by Schwartz and Schwartz[4] reported biofeedback as a cost-effective treatment for headache with biofeedback-trained patients using less medication and reporting lower rates of health-care utilization (fewer emergency room visits, doctor's office visits and phone calls to physicians). Patients reportedly maintained their improvement during the 5-year follow-up period. Cost effectiveness was also linked to a protocol for biofeedback treatment of headaches named PLOT (prudent limited office treatment)[4]. This approach emphasizes home practice of relaxation techniques to accompany 7.5 h of in-office training time, phone consultations between office visits, plus audiotapes and manuals for guidance. In general, effective treatment of headache using biofeedback requires compliance by the client. Homework between sessions often includes extensive symptom, diet and activity journal keeping, plus extra independent practice of the relaxation techniques taught in the office. However, it is currently unclear how much home practice is required, if any, for improvement of headache symptoms. Monitoring improvement of headaches is usually accomplished by documenting headache frequency, intensity and duration.

Although increased hormones in the first trimester of pregnancy may offer protection against migraine headaches for some women, headache is often a continuing problem. Biofeedback has been cited as one of several safe and effective preventive approaches for reducing headache occurrence during pregnancy[18].

Tension headaches

It is recommended that training addressing tension headaches begin with 1 week of symptom journal keeping to establish a baseline of headache frequency and characteristics[4]. Training utilizes EMG of the frontalis and trapezius muscles to reveal sources of tension and to heighten the client's awareness of where she or he holds tension. Other common sites of EMG monitoring include occipital muscles and neck muscles. Relaxing stress-sensitive muscles is utilized as a preventive tool for tension headaches. Bilateral EMG training is useful for some patients. Treatment varies in the number of sessions provided; however, follow-up 2 weeks after sessions are completed is recommended. Data regarding the benefit of biofeedback and relaxation training for tension headaches are currently inconclusive, since most studies use biofeedback in conjunction with other cognitive modalities[4].

Migraine headaches

Treatment of migraine headaches begins with a 2-week symptom baseline, ideally including documentation of triggers and aggravating factors. Sessions focus on the vascular changes associated with migraine and often use skin temperature training as the primary treatment modality. A client practices warming his or her hands and can then use the skin temperature training to develop techniques for preventing the onset of a migraine. This approach is especially useful if headache warning symptoms are present[11]. Training may also focus on stress reduction if stress is involved in perpetuating the headache cycle. If the headaches are associated with muscle tension, EMG is used with an approach similar to training for tension headaches. Some headache sufferers are shallow breathers and in these cases breath training may be beneficial[11]. Several studies discussed by Schwartz and Schwartz[4] have indicated that biofeedback for migraine was advantageous over both no treatment and cognitive therapy alone.

Pediatric headache

Headaches in children are an area of interest in biofeedback since they are common and respond to relaxation; children with headaches often continue to experience them as adults. Biofeedback-assisted relaxation for pediatric headache is thought to be an effective primary and adjunctive therapy, with some studies reporting 80–90% of children treated showing an improvement in headache symptoms. Similar to other pediatric conditions, treatment of childhood headache is often dependent on the home environment. Accordingly, recommendations are that as much training as possible be done in-office with a practitioner[4]. It has been suggested that symptoms related to pediatric migraine can be improved through relaxation and hand temperature training. One particular study demonstrated sustained improvement after four training sessions and home practice[19]. Another study using EMG-assisted relaxation showed reduced headache symptoms and continued improvement at the 3-year follow-up[20].

Hypertension

Biofeedback for managing hypertension appears to be more cost-effective than conventional treatment[4]. Additionally, treatment of essential hypertension is reported to be efficacious[11]. Biofeedback is not recommended for those with secondary causes of hypertension, and training should be used as an adjunctive procedure in patients with established hypertension. Biofeedback is appropriate as a stand-alone intervention for patients with borderline hypertension[4]. Biofeedback is reportedly efficacious for the general treatment of hypertension as well as neurocardiogenic syncope[21]. There are indicators of who is best suited for biofeedback intervention for hypertension[4]. Patients with an increased anxiety level, elevated heart rate, increased cortisol levels, increased plasma rennin activity or decreased hand

temperatures often do better with training to manage hypertension. Heart rate may be an especially useful training target; one exercise study in normal volunteers suggested that some control over heart rate is possible for some individuals, even with minimal biofeedback input and training[22,23]. Another study suggested that biofeedback training was effective at minimizing cardiovascular responses to some types of stress[24]. There are other indicators of who will benefit from biofeedback. These include: young patients, those experiencing severe medication side-effects, those with lifestyle changes for hypertension that are unsuccessful, those for whom the physician does not want to prescribe medication and those engaged in research[4]. Biofeedback is also indicated when the patient is interested and realistic; has a family history of hypertension and wants to act preventively; or has a stressful lifestyle and shows a slow increase in blood pressure over time.

Patient education is an important component of preparing a hypertensive patient for biofeedback training. Also, a series of 20–40 blood pressure values is an important part of baseline information. Treatment plans often include thermal training, where the client learns to warm their fingers or toes, reinforcing a goal of vasodilatation. One study reported decreased norepinephrine levels with successful thermal training[25]. However, temperature training has been criticized on the basis that skin vasculature contributes little to total peripheral resistance.

Additionally, several practices have developed protocols for managing hypertension that include direct blood pressure feedback and EMG relaxation training. In direct blood pressure feedback a cuff is inflated to a pressure approximately equal to the patient's systolic blood pressure. The therapist then works with the client to find methods of reducing brachial artery sounds through lowering of blood pressure. Training usually spans 3 months and clients are asked to participate in home practice multiple times each day. The goal of direct blood pressure training is for a client to learn the sensations associated with lowering their blood pressure and then be able to apply strategies to maintain a lower blood pressure in situations that previously aggravated the hypertension. EMG relaxation training for hypertension is based on the assumption that minimizing blood vessel constriction will return blood to the extremities, an approach similar to temperature training. A typical practice regimen may include 15–20-min relaxation sessions twice a day. It has been suggested that increasing the blood supply to the muscles through relaxation can decrease blood pressure by lowering total peripheral resistance[4]. Respiration training is often employed to reinforce the relaxation process. Practitioners may work with physicians to reduce hypertension medication if a patient can maintain a blood pressure of 140/90 mmHg or better. The consensus is that consistent follow-up after initial biofeedback sessions is required for maintenance of blood pressure improvements.

A 1988 study reported in the *British Medical Journal* stated that general practitioners can effectively use relaxation therapy, significantly to reduce systolic blood pressure in patients with mild hypertension[26]. This study design consisted of ten weekly 1-h sessions. Time for each session was divided equally between patient education and physiological training in relaxation, breath work and skin conductance. Clients were asked to participate in daily home practice. Another study reported a decrease in systolic blood pressure in an elderly population after biofeedback training[27]. Treatment of mild hypertension, and perhaps more severe hypertension, appears to be a cost-effective therapy with potential benefits in several specific populations.

Raynaud's phenomenon

Raynaud's disease has a history of being difficult to treat, and attempts to use medication are often ineffective. As a result of these traditional difficulties, and promising results with biofeedback, applied psychophysiology is now considered to be the treatment of choice[11]. When participating in biofeedback training, clients are asked to record the frequency, severity and duration of their episodes. These indicators are used for baselines, monitoring of progress and follow-up. If cold weather is an aggravating factor, precipitating episodes, biofeedback should be started, if possible, in the late summer or early fall[11].

One mechanism of the disease is thought to be specific vasoconstriction in the hands, so the general goal of the biofeedback approach is to reduce sympathetic outflow. Temperature training, with benefits that appear to persist for at least a year, is recommended instead of general relaxation training[4]. Raising hand temperature can be very difficult for some patients and the psychological aspects of making progress in training, especially during the first session, weigh heavily in the usefulness of the training[10]. EMG or EEG training for general relaxation is indicated when a client has difficulty mastering temperature training[11]. One study suggested that introduction of a cold stimulus was better tolerated when warm water immersion of the hands accompanied home practice[28].

Available data indicate that Whites and men have an easier time learning to warm their hands than African-Americans or women[4]. It is unclear whether these findings are useful in distinguishing those who would benefit from biofeedback treatment for Raynaud's phenomenon.

Attention deficit hyperactivity disorder

As the popular media have noted, many children are being diagnosed with attention deficit hyperactivity disorder (ADHD) and often treated pharmacologically. Unfortunately, up to 25% of these children do not improve with medication[4]. Several years ago biofeedback practitioners began developing a neurophysiological approach to treat ADHD in response to reports that these children often had abnormal EEGs. One such study, by Mann and colleagues[29], reported that, especially during reading and drawing, boys with ADHD showed increased theta and decreased beta waves when compared to the control group. In this relatively new and specialized area of biofeedback training, practitioners should have ADHD-specific training and use equipment and instrumentation approved for this specific use. In general, biofeedback in a psychosocial context for children is viewed as a nontraditional treatment that should not be automatically accepted or rejected without further investigation[30,31].

By 1995, neurofeedback using EEG had been used in 300 different organizations with more than 3000 children treated[4]. Good candidates for this type of training are individuals with a primary diagnosis of ADHD, who are between 7 and 45 years of age and possess at least a low-average intelligence. Target areas for treatment during training include attention, focus, concentration, task completion, organization, impulsiveness and mild hyperactivity. This type of neurofeedback is contraindicated for those with mental retardation, childhood psychosis, severe unipolar or bipolar depression, seizures, untreatable hyperkinesis, learning disabilities not caused by ADHD and children with families who are not willing to participate in the training process. Training sessions for hyperactivity often involve learning to increase the so-called sensorimotor rhythm-associated frequencies of 12–15 Hz[4]. EEG training to reduce the percentage of beta waves correlates with alleviation of ADHD symptoms[32]. Improvement of reading disorders or poor concentration uses EEG feedback to enhance beta waves, specifically in the dominant hemisphere. The next step in reading training may involve using audio feedback to practice maintenance of desired EEG levels while completing a reading task. A more general approach is to practice increasing beta waves without producing excess theta waves. Some practitioners may also use EMG training to address ADHD[11]. Long-term follow-up is recommended with booster sessions scheduled as necessary.

Improvement of ADHD is monitored through reported increases in appropriate behavior, learning success, grades, job performance, investment in true personal potential, increased IQ scores and parent–teacher rating scales. It is reported that, after neurofeedback, many children with ADHD are better at correcting their behavior when someone explains why it is inappropriate[4]. Therefore, it has been suggested that this type of biofeedback could possibly introduce insights and resulting behaviors that non-ADHD children already normally practice.

Temporomandibular joint disorders

Treatment of disorders of the temporomandibular joint (TMJ) with biofeedback has a consistent protocol and is only superficially addressed here. Bilateral

EMG training is used to increase client awareness of tension in face and neck muscles and to learn to promote relaxation in these areas[11]. This first level of training almost always involves the masseter muscles, but may also include temporalis and neck muscles. As training progresses, feedback on additional neck muscles may be added[4].

EMERGING APPLICATIONS

Premenstrual syndrome

Current treatment of premenstrual syndrome (PMS) by Western medicine usually involves pharmaceuticals such as antidepressants, diuretics and hormone replacement, and with all pharmaceuticals there is a potential for side-effects and drug interactions. Women in the USA and the UK often seek out complementary and alternative therapies for PMS[33]. A recent review article compiled randomized controlled trials of alternative treatments for PMS and included evaluation of two studies involving a highly specific type of biofeedback: vaginal temperature feedback. The two studies reported improvement of PMS symptoms after feedback training. However, the same author reported these identical studies and the study design led the reviewers to question the reliability of the results. For reasons including lack of evidence and poor study design, the reviewers did not recommend any of the complementary or alternative therapies discussed for PMS. However, it was acknowledged that relaxation training using biofeedback may have a general benefit, and although its use has not been proven to alleviate PMS, the low risk associated with biofeedback presents it as a potential therapy to explore[33].

Chronic obstructive pulmonary disease

Chronic obstructive pulmonary disease (COPD) is a relatively new application of biofeedback, and is only briefly discussed in this chapter. Retraining of breathing patterns through biofeedback is one of several therapies that have been successful in reducing symptoms of shortness of breath in patients with COPD[34].

Type 2 diabetes

The role of biofeedback in controlling diabetes is to promote stress management and, in turn, better management the disease itself. This is a non-traditional application of biofeedback and is best suited for those who believe that stress has an impact on their blood sugar level[4]. A patient with newly diagnosed diabetes may easily be overwhelmed with the number of doctor's appointments, medications and time required for proper management of sugar levels. Therefore, current recommendations are to wait at least 1 year after diagnosis to begin biofeedback training. Monitoring blood glucose levels is essential to disease management and should be recorded as a baseline, as well as followed during treatment and follow-up. Documenting sugar levels will help the patient avoid hypoglycemia during training sessions. As an extra precaution, it is recommended that relaxation sessions should be avoided when the patient is hypoglycemic, within 1 h of exercising, at peak insulin times and after 21.00 in the evening[4].

A typical relaxation training program for a client with diabetes consists of 12 1-h sessions. Approaches include general relaxation and some EMG or thermal feedback. These relaxation techniques are then frequently applied at home, where the patient may be asked to relax for 15–20 min twice daily. Some trainers may recommend many short (30–60 s) relaxation exercises; for ease these are often paired with waiting during blood glucose testing. Thermal training focusing on fingers and toes may promote the peripheral circulation; however, the data regarding this modality as prevention for peripheral blood flow problems resulting from diabetes are inconclusive. One case study showed promising improvement in lower extremity blood flow and mobility after temperature training with sensor placement on the great toe[12].

Training success in these clients is often measured by tracking blood glucose levels as an indicator of how well they are managing their diabetes. Progress measures include average blood glucose level, the percentage of measurements that are above 200 mg/dl, the percentage of fasting glucose measurements that are between 80 and 120 mg/dl and the number of hypoglycemic episodes. Currently there are no data regarding the long-term effects of biofeedback on the management of diabetes. However, many authors suggest follow-up sessions to renew stress-management skills. Most studies have supported the use of relaxation training for people with diabetes, although a few provide contradictory evidence[4]. Although there have been no adverse outcomes with biofeedback training for management of diabetes, this approach is best utilized with people who routinely document their blood sugar levels.

Neuromuscular re-education and gait training

Biofeedback techniques can be used efficiently to improve musculoskeletal functioning. Some applications include recovery from surgery, loss of function from a lower motor neuron lesion, stroke rehabilitation and retraining after amputation[4]. EMG training has also been used after computer keyboard work-related injuries to retrain muscles properly and prevent further injury[35]. Biofeedback during postoperative rehabilitation can make patients more comfortable. The most common modality in musculoskeletal applications is EMG. Training through EMG with either video feedback or observation in a mirror can be helpful for clients with muscle tics. Some patients with Tourette's spasms become more aware of how to relax these muscles and identify triggers[11]. In a similar manner, biofeedback can be used to facilitate recovery of symmetrical muscle contraction after injury causing Bell's palsy. Clients with cerebral palsy may also find biofeedback useful for retraining muscle groups to perform specified tasks[11]. Biofeedback has been suggested as one of many useful treatment modalities after traumatic brain injury to improve motor function[36] and reduce ataxic tremor[37]. There has been some success in treating hand dystonia through audio EMG feedback when the muscles involved in writing are overactive[38].

In the physical therapy setting EMG monitoring of major muscle groups can demonstrate to both client and therapist that motor units are firing in a weak muscle prior to the observation of macroscopic movement. Such feedback is useful for reinforcing the therapy and can indicate correct attempts to contract the target muscle. Training is most effective beginning with large muscle groups and progressing to smaller ones as strength improves; surface EMG electrodes should be placed as close to the belly of the muscle as possible[11]. Audio feedback for EMG has been useful in restoring a normal gait pattern in patients with hemiplegia[39]. For patients with incomplete spinal cord injury showing Trendelenburg gait, gait training with EMG biofeedback showed almost normal gait at 2 months, while the clinical therapy group improved by only 50%[40].

In stroke rehabilitation, EMG training often begins with dorsiflexsion of the impaired foot[11]. A meta-analysis of biofeedback with range of motion for a paretic limb after stroke did not show significant improvement. However, the difficulties of pooling data may have masked a clinically important effect[41]. Auditory feedback has been shown to reduce body sway in patients who have had a single stroke in the previous 12 months[42]. Active learning is required for this approach. Auditory feedback for sway was not effective for those with multiple strokes or with strokes that occurred more than a year before initiating biofeedback. Success with several patients indicates that auditory feedback might also be useful for retraining movements in the upper extremity after stroke[43].

Current biofeedback EMG surface electrodes detect electrical events lasting at least half a second, and therefore training should focus on isometric contractions[4]. Stemming from this limitation, surface EMG training has been criticized as being too general, and training programs using force and range of motion measurements are sometimes favored[4]. Additionally, the delay between muscle contraction and feedback display makes EMG training best suited for simple new tasks; training loses its power with complex or automatic activities. Biofeedback for neuromuscular re-education should always be considered an adjunctive procedure and be used in conjunction with a standard, prescribed, monitored exercise regime[4].

Epilepsy

EEG training to promote frequencies between 12 and 16 Hz may act to reduce seizure frequency[11]. Although data are limited at this time because of a small number of studies, general relaxation was found to have no effect on seizure frequency or quality of life, although several studies using neurofeedback have shown improvement[44].

Psychodermatology

Many dermatological conditions have a psychological component. Referral of these patients to professionals such as a psychologist, biofeedback trainer or social worker may be worthwhile for the patient[45]. Recommendations from controlled studies include referrals to 'a skin-emotion specialist', which may be useful for psoriasis, rosacea, herpes simplex, body dysmorphic disorder, acne, eczema, urticaria, neurotic excoriations, excoriated acne, trichotillomania, dysesthetic syndromes, delusion parsitosis and other skin conditions[45]. However, it is emphasized that a cure should not be expected, and such approaches are an adjunct to traditional dermatological treatment. Physical and psychological changes should be monitored as treatment progresses.

Chronic pain

A common complaint after injury and during chronic illness is pain. Relaxation training to assist in the management of chronic pain can be especially successful if the pain increases with tension or stress. Although the mechanism of action for the benefits of biofeedback is unclear, training is thought to act by reducing the autonomic reaction to pain and thus interrupting the chronic pain cycle. Autonomic modulation may be facilitated by muscle relaxation. Biofeedback sessions for chronic pain usually focus on EMG, skin temperature and EEG alpha training to facilitate the relaxation process[11]. The success and length of effect of biofeedback training for common pain varies greatly with the approach used and condition being treated;

further studies are needed to examine large patient groups for specific therapeutic effects for chronic pain conditions such as chronic low back pain and fibromyalgia[46]. Phantom limb pain is another area where biofeedback training is being applied.

Low back pain is a common complaint and many methods have been sought to improve comfort. EMG biofeedback training has been suggested for use with both acute and chronic back pain. However, studies give conflicting data regarding the relative effectiveness of this approach[47].

Pain due to chronic pelvic disorders and vulvodynia in women is difficult to treat. Patients often seek out specialists for treatment of chronic pain and associated symptoms, such as urinary incontinence. Biofeedback, especially muscle relaxation, is one potential approach to managing chronic pelvic pain[48].

The pain associated with fibromyalgia is frequently disabling, and the search for effective pain relief to increase mobility is ongoing. One study in the Netherlands compared high-impact exercise to low-impact exercise plus biofeedback, and found no significant improvement in either experimental group[49]. These approaches also showed no benefit over standard care for fibromyalgia.

Chronic fatigue syndrome

One suggested application of the expanding area of neurofeedback is for the treatment of the symptoms associated with and diagnosis of chronic fatigue syndrome. An EEG training model has been applied and one case study resulted in improvement in many psychological and functional categories after neurofeedback training[50].

Arrhythmias

Although it is a non-traditional application, management of arrhythmias through biofeedback has gained some support through the reported success of hypertension management. However, so-called 'feedback cardiography' should be facilitated only by a trainer with special training and experience. The treatment

approach is centered on general relaxation and stress management, and can be integrated into the general model of cardiac rehabilitation[11]. As with many relaxation approaches, the most common modalities used are EMG, EEG and skin temperature training.

Torticollis

Biofeedback shows some promise in successfully teaching clients to balance the spastic and flaccid muscles in the neck. This approach should be used in a physical therapy setting and usually consists of EMG training to strengthen one muscle group and relax the opposing muscles[11].

Psychotherapy

Biofeedback is a useful tool to combine with psychotherapy. This pairing is often termed biofeedback-assisted psychotherapy or psychotherapy-assisted biofeedback, depending on which process dominates the sessions. Biofeedback can facilitate relaxation during therapy sessions, and can be used to detect small physiological changes indicating topics that need to be addressed. EMG of the frontalis muscle indicates facial expression changes and GSR often detects small stress changes during discussions[11]. These combination sessions are usually run by one individual trained in both biofeedback and psychotherapy. Utilizing this approach obviously requires the full interest and trust of the client. The connection of chronic grief and physiological stress points to biofeedback as an appropriate approach for processing loss[51].

Addiction

Alcoholism is the most common type of addiction treated with biofeedback. However, biofeedback may be a useful component in other drug rehabilitation programs. The biofeedback approach may be particularly successful for those whose drug dependence has an element of learned helplessness. General relaxation training can renew a sense of control in the client and provide alternative ways of dealing with stress[11].

Anxiety

Biofeedback is a successful approach in managing many types of anxiety and related conditions. Deep muscle relaxation facilitated by EEG, EMG and sometimes skin temperature or GSR has been used with traditional systematic desensitization for phobias and reduction of general anxiety[11]. EMG is especially useful in training to replace the anxiety response to a stimulus with a relaxation response. Biofeedback for anxiety is always individually tailored to the client's specific concerns and goals.

Obsessive–compulsive disorder

EEG training to help manage obsessive–compulsive disorder has been reported by some trainers. The approach is to up-regulate alpha electrical brain activity, which is thought to produce a relaxed state. The client may then be less likely to perform their obsessive behaviors.

Insomnia

Although general relaxation training for insomnia may be beneficial, most biofeedback approaches will concentrate on learning purposefully to shift the body towards sleep. This protocol usually includes EMG training to relax muscles that are restless, and breath training to slow respiration. Once these techniques are managed, EEG training may be added with specific focus on regulating alpha and theta frequencies[11].

Asthma

The physiologically paired events of bronchial constriction with general relaxation make psychological management of asthma appropriate for preventive measures, and not acute attacks[11]. Common approaches for those with asthma include EEG, EMG and skin temperature training to facilitate relaxation. Guided imagery is often used to supplement biofeedback; the client is commonly asked to visualize a tree growing or expanding as a representation of the bronchioles. Asthma-specific benefits of biofeedback include exploring stressful triggers to avoid attacks and becoming more comfortable taking medications. Success of training is usually measured by a decrease in the number of attacks.

Fecal incontinence

A few research studies have examined biofeedback training to reduce fecal incontinence. However, the results have been difficult to generalize, since each study presents a different definition of biofeedback[52]. Four common methods of training are described in one systematic review article[52]. The first approach uses EMG for feedback of the success of anal sphincter exercises. Similarly, EMG can also be used in periodic sessions to monitor correct technique and progress when exercises are performed at home. Using a balloon system to train patients to contract the anal sphincter at lower and lower distention stimuli is a third approach. Last, a more general sensory awareness around the anus may be the focus of training. The majority of studies have used the number of incontinent episodes as the primary outcome measure, but there is wide variety in the reported success of training. Most studies observed at least 50% reduction in incontinent events, which led one set of authors to suggest that biofeedback should play a role in treatment of this condition. Specific situations where biofeedback may be useful include ileostomy closure and tertiary obstetric tear, although the long-term benefits are unclear[52]. Paying particular attention to sensory changes may be a key component of success[53]. As in all therapeutic applications, safety is a concern. No adverse outcomes have been reported for fecal incontinence biofeedback training, and training is unlikely to aggravate symptoms[52]. The safety of biofeedback suggests that training be a first-line treatment in adults before they undergo surgery of the anal sphincter.

In children, one study compared anal sphincter bio-feedback training, intensive medical therapy and expanded toilet training in children with chronic encopresis[54]. Increased toilet training was most effective at reducing the frequency of encopresis in the highest number of children, although similar results were seen 1 year after treatment with the biofeedback training and medical intervention groups.

Urinary incontinence

Treatment of urinary incontinence often includes pelvic floor muscle exercises. Although these are ultimately the responsibility of the patient to learn and perform, instruction and feedback can be useful. One study reported biofeedback and verbal instructions as beneficial for learning these exercises after radical prostatectomy[55]. In general, biofeedback is a safe and effective approach to dealing with urinary incontinence, especially if there is follow through with the training program. It is difficult to predict who is well suited for this type of biofeedback training. However, patients who initially are successful at keeping records of bladder activity for 1 week are more likely to finish their training program[56].

Sports, music performance, education and business

Biofeedback applications in sports, music performance, education and business are numerous and rapidly expanding, but are outside the medical scope of this chapter. Stress management protocols may be useful in these settings and the personalization of training allows for flexibility to address many issues over time or to be used only as needed. Along with visualization and other psychological approaches, biofeedback can be used in peak performance training for

Table 4 Common adjunctive procedures paired with biofeedback

Affirmations
Autogenic training
Cognitive/behavioral training
Home practice
Hypnosis
Meditation
Progressive relaxation
Quieting response
Relaxation response
Somatic exercises
Suggestion
Systematic desensitization
Visualization
Yoga

athletes and musicians at all competitive levels. Biofeedback is especially useful in learning to control arousal level, so that an individual may maintain appropriate awareness and not become 'over aroused' during key moments of a sports competition or musical performance[11]. Portable biofeedback has expanded sports and music applications, since training can take place while participating in these activities.

ADJUNCTIVE TECHNIQUES

Owing to the nature of the biofeedback practitioner's role and the goals of training, biofeedback sessions almost always include at least one type of additional technique (Table 4). Common approaches include suggestion, systematic desensitization, visualization, home practice and progressive relaxation. Additional methods employed are hypnosis, affirmations, autogenic training, the relaxation response, yoga, meditation, somatic exercises, the quieting response and cognitive/behavioral training[11]. The versatility and safety of biofeedback allow great flexibility. Adjunctive procedures are potentially limited only by the expertise and preference of client and trainer.

References

1. NCCAM. Minutes of the second meeting of the National Advisory Council for Complementary and Alternative Medicine (NCCAM). Available at: http://nccam.nih.gov/about/advisory/naccam/minutes/2000jan.htm. (Accessed 28 August 2002)

2. Straus S. Integrative medicine. Available online: http://nccam.nih.gov/about/offices/od/directortestimony/032800.htm#skipnav. (Accessed 28 August 2002)

3. Blanchard E. The definition of 'applied psychophysiology': a dangerous exercise in exclusivity. *Appl Psychophysiol Biofeedback* 1999;24:23–5, 43–54

4. Schwartz N, Schwartz M. *Biofeedback: a Practitioner's Guide*, 2nd edn. New York, NY: The Guilford Press, 1995

5. Folen R, James L, Earles J, Andrasik F. Biofeedback via telehealth: a new frontier for applied psychophysiology. *Appl Psychophysiol Biofeedback* 2001;26:195–204

6. Earles J, Folen R, James L. Biofeedback using telemedicine: clinical applications and case illustrations. *Behav Med* 2001;27:77–82

7. Brolinson P, Price J, Ditmyer N, Reis D. Nurses' perceptions of complementary and alternative medical therapies. *J Commun Health* 2001;26:175–89

8. Rooney B, Riocco G, Hughes P, Halter S. Provider attitudes and use of alternative medicine in a Midwestern medical practice in 2001. *WMJ* 2001;100:27–31

9. Thompson D. The national coverage decision for reimbursement for biofeedback and pelvic floor electrical stimulation for treatment of urinary incontinence. *J Wound Ostomy Continence Nurs* 2002;29:11–19

10. Middaugh S, Haythornthwaite J, Thompson B, *et al.* The Raynaud's treatment study: biofeedback protocols and acquisition of temperature biofeedback skills. *Appl Psychophysiol Biofeedback* 2001;26:251–78

11. Criswell E. *Biofeedback and Somatics: Toward Personal Evolution.* Novato, CA: Freeperson Press, 1995

12. Aikens J. Thermal biofeedback for claudication in diabetes: a literature review and case study. *Altern Med Rev* 1999;4:104–10

13. Kotchousbey B, Kubler A, Strehl U, Flor H, Birbaumer N. Can humans perceive their brain state? *Conscious Cogn* 2002;11:98–113

14. Kubler A, Neumann N, Kaiser J, Kotchoubey B, Hinterberger T, Birbaumer N. Brain–computer communication: self-regulation of slow cortical potentials for verbal communication. *Arch Phys Med Rehabil* 2001;82:1533–9

15. Lubar J. Electroencephalographic biofeedback methodology and the management of epilepsy. *Integr Physiol Behav Sci* 1998;33:176–207

16. Rosenfeld J. Applied psychophysiology: exclusions and inclusions. *Appl Psychophysiol Biofeedback* 1999;24:33–4, 43–54

17. Solomon, G. Chronic tension-type headache: advice for the viselike-headache patient. *Cleve Clin J Med* 2002;69:173–4

18. Marcus D. Pregnancy and chronic headache. *Expert Opin Pharmacother* 2002;3:389–93

19. Scharff L, Marcus D, Masek B. A controlled study of minimal-contact thermal biofeedback treatment in children with migraine. *J Pediatr Psychol* 2002;27:109–19

20. Grazi L, Andrasik F, D'Amico D, Leone M, Moschiano F, Bussone G. Electromyographic biofeedback-assisted relaxation training in juvenile episodic tension-type headache: clinical outcome at three-year follow-up. *Cephalalgia* 2001;21:798–803

21. McGrady A. Good news–bad press: applied psychophysiology in cardiovascular disorders. *Biofeedback Self Regul* 1996;21:335–46

22. Inoue Y, Sadamoto T. Effects of single trial of heart-rate biofeedback on the arterial blood pressure, ventilation volume, and oxygen consumption during ramp bicycling exercise. *Percept Mot Skills* 2002;94:106–18

23. Inoue Y, Sadamoto T. Effects of single trial heart-rate biofeedback during ramp bicycling exercise. *Percept Mot Skills* 2002;94:127–34

24. Goodie J, Larkin K. Changes in hemodynamic response to mental stress with heart rate feedback training. *Appl Psychophysiol Biofeedback* 2001;26:293–309

25. McCoy GC, Blanchard EB, Wittrock DA, *et al.* Biochemical changes associated with thermal feedback treatment of hypertension. *Biofeedback Self Regul* 1988;13:139–50

26. Patel C, Marmot M. Can general practitioners use training in relaxation and management of stress to reduce mild hypertension? *Br Med J* 1988;296:21–4

27. Pearce L, Engel B, Burton J. Behavioral treatment of isolated systolic hypertension in the elderly. *Biofeedback Self Regul* 1989;14:207–17

28. Jobe J, Beetham W, Roberts D, *et al.* Induced vasodilation as a home treatment for Raynaud's disease. *J Rheumatol* 1985;12:953–6

29. Mann C, Lubar J, Zimmerman A, Miller C, Muenchen R. Quantitative analysis of EEG in boys with attention-deficit-hyperactivity disorder: controlled study with clinical implications. *Pediatr Neurol* 1991;8:30–6

30. Arnold L. Some nontraditional (unconventional and/or innovative) psychosocial treatments for children and adolescents: critique and proposed screening principles. *J Abnorm Child Psychol* 1995;23:125–40

31. Brue A, Oakland T. Alternative treatments for attention-deficit/hyperactivity disorder: does evidence support their use? *Altern Ther Health Med* 2002:8:68–70

32. Egner T, Gruzelier J. Learned self-regulation of EEG frequency components affects attention and event-related brain potentials in humans. *Neuroreport* 2001;12:4155–9

33. Stevinson C, Ernst E. Complementary/alternative therapies for premenstrual syndrome – a systematic review of randomized controlled trials. *Am J Obstet Gynecol* 2001;185:227–35

34. Collins E, Langbein W, Fehr L, Maloney C. Breathing pattern retraining and exercise in persons with chronic obstructive pulmonary disease. *AACN Clin Issues* 2001;12:202–9

35. Nord S, Ettare D, Drew D, Hodge S. Muscle learning therapy – efficacy of a biofeedback based protocol in treating work-related upper extremity disorders. *J Occup Rehabil* 2001;11:23–31

36. Keren O, Reznik J, Groswasser Z. Combined motor disturbances following severe traumatic brain injury: an integrative long-term treatment approach. *Brain Inj* 2001;15:633–8

37. Guercio J, Ferguson K, McMorrow M. Increasing functional communication through relaxation training and neuromuscular feedback. *Brain Inj* 2001;15:1073–82

38. Deepak K, Behari M. Specific muscle EMG biofeedback for hand dystonia. *Appl Psychophysiol Biofeedback* 1999;24:267–80

39. Mauritz K. Gait training in hemiplegia. *Eur J Neurol* 2002;(Suppl 1):23–9

40. Petrofsky J. The use of electromyogram biofeedback to reduce Trendelenburg gait. *Eur J Appl Physiol* 2001;85:491–5

41. Glanz M, Klawansky S, Stason W, *et al*. Biofeedback therapy in poststroke rehabilitation: a meta-analysis of the randomized controlled trials. *Arch Phys Med Rehabil* 1995;76:508–15

42. Peterson H, Magnusson M, Johansson R, Fransson P. Auditory feedback regulation of perturbed stance in stroke patients. *Scand J Rehabil Med* 1996;28:217–23

43. Maulucci R. Eckhouse R. Retraining reaching in chronic stroke with real-time auditory feedback. *NeuroRehabilitation* 2001;16:171–82

44. Ramaratnam S, Baker G, Goldstein L. Psychological treatments for epilepsy. *Cochrane Database Syst Rev* 2001;4:CD002029

45. Fried R. Nonpharmacologic treatments in psychodermatology. *Dermatol Clin* 2002;20:177–85

46. Nielson W, Weir R. Biopsychosocial approaches to the treatment of chronic pain. *Clin J Pain* 2001;4(Suppl):S114–27

47. van Tulder MW, Koes BW. Low back pain. *Am Fam Physician* 2002

48. Newman D. Pelvic disorders in women: chronic pelvic pain and vulvodynia. *Ostomy Wound Manage* 2000;46:48–54

49. Van S, Bolwijn P, Verstappen F, *et al*. A randomized clinical trial comparing fitness and biofeedback training versus basic treatment in patients with fibromyalgia. *J Rheumatol* 2002;29:575–81

50. James L, Folen R. EEG biofeedback as a treatment for chronic fatigue syndrome: a controlled case report. *Behav Med* 1996;22: 77–81

51. Arnette J. Physiological effects of chronic grief: a biofeedback treatment approach. *Death Stud* 1996;20:59–72

52. Norton C, Kamm MA. Anal sphincter biofeedback and pelvic floor exercises for faecal incontinence in adults – a systematic review. *Aliment Pharmacol Ther* 2001;15:1147–54

53. Chiarioni G, Bassotti G, Stanganini S, Vantini I, Whitehead W, Stegagnini S. Sensory retraining is key to biofeedback therapy for formed stool fecal incontinence. *Am J Gastroenterol* 2002; 97;109–17

54. Borowitz S, Cox D, Sutphen J, Kovatchev B. Treatment of childhood encopresis: a randomized trail comparing three treatment protocols. *J Pediatr Gastroenterol Nutr* 2002;34:378–84

55. Floratos D, Sonke G, Rapidou C, *et al*. Biofeedback vs verbal feedback as learning tools for pelvic muscle exercises in the early management of urinary incontinence after radical prostatectomy. *Br J Urol Int* 2002;89:714–19

56. Kincade J, Peckous B, Busby-Whitehead J. A pilot study to determine predictors of behavioral treatment completion for urinary incontinence. *Urol Nurs* 2001;21:39–44

Further reading and resources

Biofeedback Certification Institute of America. www.bcia.org 10200 W 44th Ave, Suite 310, Wheat Ridge, CO 80033-2840. A tremendously useful website with resources including consumer information and a search tool to locate certified biofeedback practitioners in your area.

Criswell E. *Biofeedback and Somatics: Toward Personal Evolution*. Novato, CA: Freeperson Press, 1995. A concise and easy-to-read guide to biofeedback applications for both health-care providers and patients.

Schwartz N, Schwartz M. *Biofeedback: a Practitioner's Guide*, 2nd edn. New York, NY: The Guilford Press, 1995. Considered by many to be the handbook of choice for biofeedback trainers, this extensive reference contains sections addressing a majoring of the essential issues in applied psychophysiology.

Shared prayer 9

D. Schiedermayer

INTRODUCTION

Our deepest beliefs and fears surface during moments of severe illness. When we as physicians look upon the private terrors of our sick patients, we are often moved and humbled. Sometimes we just do not have enough in our black bags to help.

For example, when I do an inventory of my black bag, I find:

An old dissecting kit
a bottle
which contains a fingernail still on the skin tip
(I found it in a patient's bed
after she sloughed it from Stevens–Johnson
 syndrome)
Another bottle with
a little yellow and red
poisonous snake
preserved in formaldehyde.
Blue antibiotic pills.
A hundred feet
of no. 1 black silk non-absorbable
braided suture.
Tuning forks: 128 and 512 cps.
Tongue blades.
Pocket guidebooks.
Pens and pads.
A stethoscope
(with replacement bell and diaphragm
and earpieces).
A sphygmomanometer.
Ophthalmoscope and otoscope.
Reflex hammer.
Seems like enough, but
when I took care of the patient
dying slowly at home from a gaping sternal infection,

I was
rummaging with my hand
at the bottom of this bag[1].

KEEPING COMPANY

My point in this poem is that keeping company with the sick is a challenging notion in this era of technological tricks – often no other tools besides companionship exist, even in the intensive care unit (ICU). Sometimes our technology is an illusion, or even a desperate ploy, like 'rummaging . . . at the bottom of this bag'. Instead, what the patient may actually need is 'just' the caregiver's presence.

Presence always has a spiritual component. Since a patient's experience with sickness and death is somehow both shameful and endearing, degrading and ennobling, it takes us outside our normal framework. It can move us to pray.

In this chapter, which will by necessity be more personal than the rest, I am going to write about this spiritual task about keeping company with the sick. The reason for the personal-ness is that I am not going to write about how religion makes you live longer (if it does) or whether praying for far-away patients (distant or intercessory prayer) increases survival in the ICU (if it does). For those interested, there are studies on these topics[2–5].

METAPHYSICAL PROBLEMS WITH STUDIES OF PRAYER

Furthermore, I tend to agree with the thought-provoking essay of Chibnall, Jeral and Cerullo (a multi-religious and multi-disciplinary group) who argue that mixing experimental methods with faith degrades both concepts[6]. 'We do not need science to validate our spiritual beliefs, as we would never use faith to validate our scientific data', they note. 'In the major religious traditions, prayer that tests for a response from God in the way the intercessor requires would not be considered prayer at all because it requires no faith, leaves God no options, and is presumptuous regarding God's wisdom and plan. If distant (intercessory) prayer studies can make the results of prayer consistent, predictable, and replicable, then faith has become science'[6].

If I do not seek to use prayer (or God) for my own purposes, but rather to keep company with a praying patient, then prayer becomes part of the doctor–patient relationship. Prayer becomes part of the personal practice of medicine. Praying becomes part of sitting by the bedside.

A CLINICAL EXAMPLE OF SHARED PRAYER

Here is an example of how prayer is shared in the clinical setting. I have a patient who comes to see me at Family House, where I work in the central city of Milwaukee. She has hepatitis C and formerly used intravenous cocaine. She has now become a devout Christian believer, and is convinced that her faith is the cause of her changed life.

I see and examine her. She has a small breast mass. I think it is probably benign, but the right thing to do is order a mammogram, so I tell her that I will request it. Then, as we always do, we close the visit in prayer. The first time I saw her, I asked consent to pray with her, and she said, 'yes, please'.

So, here is my prayer: 'Dear Lord, I pray for Mrs Smith, that you would continue to be with her and bless her. Thank you for her life and what you have given her. I do pray for her family and her health. Thank you for her good blood pressure today. We do both pray for this lump in the breast, that you would help us find out what it is, and that if it is your will Lord, it would be alright. In Jesus' name, Amen.'

And she prays, 'Gracious Heavenly Father, thank you and bless your holy name for your many blessings

to me. We know that you are powerful and that you watch over us. Be with Dr Schiedermayer and strengthen him as he sees patients today. Be with his wife and family, Lord. Bless him and encourage him in his work. We know by your power you have promised us healing, and I thank you for your almighty presence this very day. We bless you and give you the praise, for in your name we pray, Jesus. Amen!'

So, that is the scene of a prayer. A white male doctor and an African-American female ex-addict pray together for each other, behind the closed doors, right in clinic. The breast lump is still there, but the patient feels better. I cannot tell you how much I appreciate her prayer for me.

PRACTICAL QUESTIONS ABOUT PRAYER

When we pray in the clinical setting, many practical and theological questions arise. First, what about various religious traditions? Some do not agree with praying for people outside their own faith tradition, which is why I always ask consent. No matter what the person's faith tradition (or spiritual focus/way of being) I am willing to pray for a patient if they are willing. I make it a practice not to interrogate a person on the fine points of his or her theology before I offer to pray. If we have to agree exactly on all doctrinal issues, we will never get to the helpful aspects of praying. I am willing to pray with people of any faith tradition, and have prayed with people of most religious faiths.

What if we are not praying to the same God? This is not a clinical question. It is a good theological question, but not a good clinical one. I pray in Jesus' name with Christians and will use, 'The God that Is' with people in other traditions or sometimes I just say Amen if it is unclear how to pray or the person's theology is unclear to me (or them!). I cannot be something I am not (I have my own faith and am praying to the God I know) but I can also pray with someone. If I do not understand what the patient needs in prayer I will sometimes just say, 'I will be with you if you would like to pray now'. Of course, I could also offer to pray later, but that would be intercessory prayer and outside the province of this chapter and my thesis that part of prayer is keeping company with the patient and with their relationship to their world/God.

If we agree that part of healing involves spiritual work in keeping company, then it makes sense that in certain situations prayer is part of it. I am not a theologian, and admit that I do not understand all the complexities of prayer, but I try to be united with my patient in prayer, in the sense that we are both seeking a spiritual element. We are both asking for help, and I, as a physician, am acknowledging that I am not God, and that there is an Other.

More than a few patients endow their health professionals with god-like powers, and more than a few doctors are willing to assume that mantle of power, but as a doctor I have discovered that:

When your patient dies
call the family
send a card
go to the funeral.
At the funeral
the patient's wife
will secretly become your patient.
She will call six months later
to say she's ready
to take care of herself now.
The patient's children
will do the same.
If you don't go to the funeral
chances are
you will never see any of them ever again.
When you go to the funeral
the family will see you
sitting in the back
and know in that moment
they can forgive you
for not being God[1].

RISKS OF PRAYER

Can prayer in the clinical setting decrease the risk of hubris? Perhaps, but a potential risk is that it might be coercive. I have a husband and wife who are having marital problems related to the husband's use of alcohol. He drinks several glasses of wine every night, and gets sleepy. When I pray with them, I pray, 'Lord, thank you for this marriage, and I pray that you may help this couple toward mutual respect and healing. Lord, I pray about this drinking situation. Give Tom strength and help, and be with him as he works on this. We are grateful for your love for them, In Jesus' name, Amen.'

I find this just on the edge of coercion. The coercion here would be if I were trying to insist to Tom through the prayer that he needs treatment. 'Be with him as he works on this' is as close as I get. I have told him in person, face to face, that he needs to deal with this, and I have suggested resources. It does not seem proper to ask God to make him get treatment or to ask God to help his wife get him treatment. That is up to Tom, not to God. My role is to pray for him, not to dictate to Tom or his wife with my eyes closed.

WHEN NOT TO PRAY

A last and very important layer, what if one does not really believe in God in the first place? What if one's sense of spirituality is related to a way of being in the world rather than related to a particular deity? The data show that, as a group, we physicians are less religious (or spiritual) than most of our patients. I have many patients who seem to me more deeply faithful or spiritual than I. Doctors and nurses and other providers are often working with patients who are more into prayer or mediation than we are, but the point in our discussion is that prayer may help a patient to verbalize their private terrors and fears, and perhaps the doctor or nurse could offer to hear the person's prayer and just be with them as they say it.

So, I am also offering the model of the patient praying with the doctor, or even for the doctor, not just the model of the doctor praying for the patient. For a patient whose spirituality is not 'religious' an offer to be present with the patient for some time of silent meditation may be appropriate.

For the patient who is not interested in prayer, traditional allopathic medicine is ready-made; in the purely 'medical world', at critical times in patient's lives, or at crucial decision-making points, information-related activities (such as providing statistics and obtaining informed consent) predominate over spiritual activities. These information-related activities are very important and vitally necessary, and should be provided to all patients. For the patient who is not spiritually oriented, these activities will virtually predominate. For the person who is spiritually oriented, informed consent can be supplemented with prayer.

PRAYING AT THE POINT OF NEED

For example, I had a patient with a large transitional cell cancer of the bladder. On ultrasound it was as big as a large plum. She had been informed by the urologist that she might have to have her bladder removed to eliminate all the cancer. I went to see her right before the operation. 'Dear Lord, please help Mrs Smith to do well during the surgery. Guide the doctor's hands and help him to do his best. We know that there is risk during the surgery. We know there is risk of anesthesia, even the risk of death. We know that she may lose her bladder as part of the cancer surgery, but we pray that you may be with her through all of this, that you would protect her, and that you would help her to get better.' Here the prayer acknowledges the likely possibility of losing the bladder, the less likely risk of death, but in the end offers more than statistical reassurance. Prayer offers this patient the sense that someone besides her doctor has her best interest at heart; that someone is the someone she believes in far more than she believes in doctors; that someone is her God. The timing of this prayer – right before surgery – is at her point of greatest need for prayer.

INFORMED CONSENT VS. PRAYER

Prayer differs from informed consent in both its object and its expectation. The object of prayer is God; the doctor and patient are asking God for a safe surgery, pleading, in a sense, for safe passage through what they both know is a dangerous situation. Granted, informed consent is far more effective than prayer

at imparting specific risk information, but the doctor's prayer is also informational in nature, because he or she prays about specific areas of protection. While both doctor and patient hear each other, their preoperative prayer is to God; this differs from preoperative informed consent, the object of which is solely in material. In the case of prayer, the patient is putting himself or herself finally in God's hands. In the case of informed consent, he or she is learning what risk there is in putting himself or herself finally in the doctor's hands. Of course, informed consent and prayer are not mutually exclusive, but there are fundamental differences behind the object of informed consent and prayer, the one materially based, the other spiritually based.

If the patient seeks only materially based assistance, and refuses or would be uncomfortable with additional spiritually based comfort, that is the patient's choice and I fully respect this wish. Those of us who pray with patients learn to respect these boundaries very early in our practice, by erring on both sides – not praying with those who desperately want it, or praying with those who vehemently reject it. We learn to discern, and if we are not clear, we learn to ask gently and obtain consent for prayer.

PRAYER VS. THE SPIRITUAL 'HISTORY'

Many ethicists argue that physicians should ask more detail about patients' spiritual and religious concerns near the end of life[7]. As Lo and colleagues point out[7], patients may make decisions based on their beliefs, or may be troubled by unresolved issues, or may refuse or insist on treatments for religious reasons. The authors note that if the patient asks about the doctor's religion, physicians should deflect the focus from their own faith and back to the patient's faith or spirituality, and especially back to why spirituality is or is not important to the patient. This approach seems both sensible and a good starting point. The next step would be to respect the patient's boundaries if he or she does not wish further spiritual discussions, and then (as I discuss in this chapter) also be willing to pray with the patient if needed. Lo and colleagues seem to relegate the role of prayer to others besides the physician, those more expert in prayer perhaps, but the fact is that the patient needs prayer right on the spot when they need it. Prayer is not about expertise, but about keeping spiritual company together.

In this sense most of the modern writers on spiritual issues are over-cautious to a fault. They want us as professionals to know many details about a patient's faith or spirituality but then to observe from a (knowledgeable) distance instead of keeping company in some sort of shared space (I argue for this as a more humane approach in the end).

CONCLUSION

To summarize, I keep prayers simple and targeted toward the patient's illness, the patient's overall well-being, the patient's family's well-being and coping, and the patient's community. I avoid prayers that would be coercive or proselytizing. I keep my own integrity as a person of a particular faith tradition, but I try to be as flexible as I know how to be in various modes of prayer. I try to pray at the point of the patient's need. I try to use prayer as an additional spiritual component of information and to the material, statistical world of informed consent. I do not pray with those who do not want prayer. If prayer is the right thing, the patient feels he or she has been involved; the doctor shares prayer as a fellow seeker, as a fellow human being, and not as a mighty professional. The doctor cares enough to ask for the best help anywhere – that which only God can give.

When faced with personal terror in our moments of illness, many of us seek prayer. I know I have spoken of prayer largely through my own experience and religious viewpoint, but I hope I have not been sectarian. Those of us who believe in prayer can be inclusive. We have a choice in the way we live our faith before God and each other. We are part of a pluralistic culture, but we can be more than sightseers. Perhaps the poem 'In Canterbury Cathedral' by E. W. Oldenburg puts it best:

> On a day sweet with April showers
> the safe tires of our tour bus
> had sung us south from London.
> Sightseer pilgrims, cameras slung,
> no need or time on patient plodding
> horses for long diverting tales.
> We stood at last at Beckett's shrine,
> lost in architecture and dates,
> confused by Norman and Gothic.
> Our ancient tiny guide seemed shrunk
> into his suit, dwarfed by his clothes
> as we all were dwarfed by time.
> His small precise English voice went on:
> pronounced 'Our Lord', and the words
> fell on us like a benediction.
> 'Our' – incredible assumption of union
> offered in passing to American strangers,
> mortar for diverse motley stones.
> Time and blood and history redeemed
> from meaningless: two words
> turned sightseers into pilgrims.

References

1. Schiedermayer D. *House Calls, Rounds, and Healings: A Poetry Casebook*. Tuscon, AZ: Galen Press, 1996
2. Dossey L. *Healing Words*. New York, NY: Harper Collins, 1993
3. Koenig HG. *Is Religion Good for Your Health?* Binghamton, NY: Haworth Press, 1997
4. Matthews DA, Clark C. *The Faith Factor – Proof of the Healing Power of Prayer*. New York, NY: Penguin Group, 1998
5. Harris WS, Gowda M, Kolb JW, *et al.* A randomized, controlled trial of the effects of remote, intercessory prayer on outcomes in patients admitted to the coronary care unit. *Arch Intern Med* 1999;159:2273–8
6. Chibnall JT, Jeral JM, Cerullo MA. Experiments on distant intercessory prayer: God, science, and the lesson of Massah. *Arch Intern Med* 2001;161:2529–36
7. Lo B, Ruston D, Kates L, *et al.* Discussing religious and spiritual issues at the end of life: a practical guide for physicians. *J Am Med Assoc* 2002;287:749–54

Acupuncture

10

Y. G. Wang

INTRODUCTION

Acupuncture is a medical therapy that uses the insertion of an acupuncture needle into the skin of certain points of the body, called acupuncture points, at different depths to treat a patient's syndrome or disease. Acupuncture dates back 4000 years in China since the Stone Age. It was adopted worldwide over the centuries: by Korea in AD 541, by Japan in AD 562 and by Europe in the 16th century[1]. The first person who introduced acupuncture into the USA is believed to be Dr Franklin Bache, grandson of Benjamin Franklin, in 1825[1]. However, acupuncture was not acknowledged by the USA until 1971, when, following China's ping-pong diplomacy, Henry A. Kissinger made his historical visit to Beijing. This not only resulted in President Nixon's visit to China the following year, but also introduced acupuncture to the USA through popular media and the medical profession. The story tells of Kissinger's visit, during which a staff member was treated with acupuncture when he suffered from post-surgical complications. When he returned from his trip, he wrote of his experience in the *New York Times*[2]. As a result, more and more doctors visited China to see it with their own eyes. Dr Rosenfield was one of them.

Parade Magazine carried Rosenfield's article 'Acupuncture goes mainstream (almost)' in 1998[3]. Accompanying the article was a color photograph taken on one of his hospital visits during the tour, which showed a wide-awake young woman in the middle of open-heart surgery under acupuncture anesthesia, smiling at the camera! Dr Rosenfield wrote, 'I first witnessed acupuncture at the University of Shanghai about 20 years ago. The patient was a 28-year-old woman about to have open-heart surgery. She was placed on the operation table, wide awake and smiling. Then to my astonishment, the surgeon proceeded to open her chest. Her only 'anesthetic' was an acupuncture needle in her right earlobe that was connected to an electrical source. She never flinched. There was no mask on her face, no intravenous needle in her arm. This account is not hearsay. I was there and took the photo on this page.'

Acupuncture has been accepted as conventional medical practice in most countries in the world for many years. The World Health Organization (WHO) listed more than 40 conditions for which acupuncture may be effective[4].

This chapter focuses on fundamental acupuncture issues. It covers the following topics:

- Acupuncture needles;

- Common meridians and most common acupuncture points;

- Auricular and scalp acupuncture;

- Acupuncture for common syndromes (including migraine headache, low back pain and insomnia) and indication of acupuncture therapy;

- Cautions in using acupuncture therapy;

- Who visits an acupuncturist?

- Physiological bases of acupuncture analgesia.

THE ACUPUNCTURE NEEDLE

Acupuncture involves a thin needle inserted into specific points of the body to stimulate its own natural system to treat the disease. The needle is called an acupuncture needle and the point is called an acupuncture point, or simply an acupoint.

Figure 1a shows the acupuncture needle, which mainly consists of two parts: the handle and the stem or needle body. Figure 1b shows the Chinese character for needle. The left side of the character means metal and the right side represents a sharp instrument. Therefore, an acupuncture needle is a sharp instrument made of metal, mostly stainless steel today. In the Stone Age, the acupuncture needle was made of stone. Figure 1c shows the Chinese word for stone puncture. The left part of the word means stone and the right side is the sound of the word, pronounced as '*bian*'.

In the USA, most acupuncturists use disposable needles, for a single acupuncture point only. The needle has a guide tube. The acupuncturist places it on a selected acupuncture point and taps the needle tail with the index finger to insert the needle. Acupuncture needles are not treated with any drug, which is why they are sometimes referred to as 'dry needles'.

Unlike a regular needle, in which there is a hollow channel for injecting drugs or withdrawing fluids, an acupuncture needle is solid and very fine. Most needles used in clinics measure 30 or 32 gauge in diameter. The length of the needle varies from half an inch (13 mm) to 5 inches (125 mm). Shorter needles are used in superficial areas, such as the head and face, and longer ones in

fleshy regions. The required depth of insertion is given with each formula point, but variations occur in different body types and the acupuncturist's own judgement should be used. Normally, when a needle reaches the desired depth, the patient will feel a sensation of fullness or radiating warmth (*De Qi* sensation). Because the tip of acupuncture needles is sharp and round, acupuncture needles do not normally cut or damage skin and muscles as regular needles do when they penetrate through them; therefore, they cause only slight bleeding and leave almost no needle holes afterwards.

MERIDIANS AND ACUPUNCTURE POINTS

The theoretical basis of acupuncture is the theory of the meridians, in which the *Qi* and blood of the human body are circulated. Meridians pertain to the *Zang-fu* organs interiorly and extend over the body exteriorly, forming a network and linking the tissues and organs into an organic whole. Meridians are divided into regular meridians and extra meridians. The 12 pairs of regular meridians constitute most of the meridian system. There are eight extra meridians. Twelve regular meridians plus two of the eight extra meridians, one running along the midline of the abdomen and chest and the other along the midline of the back, are the 14 meridians that fall into four groups.

Three *Yin* meridians of the hand

The lung meridian (LU), pericardium meridian (PC) and heart meridian (HT) run through the anterior aspect, midline and posterior aspect of the anterior side of the upper part of the body from the chest to the hands. They are collectively called the three *Yin* meridians of the hand (Figure 2).

The three *Yang* meridians of the hand

The large intestine meridian (LI), triple energizer meridian (TE) and small intestine meridian (SI) run through the anterior aspect, midline and posterior

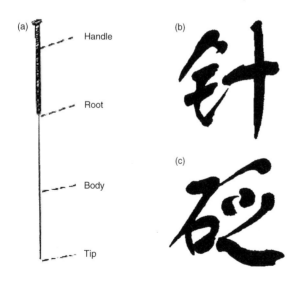

Figure 1 The acupuncture needle (a), the Chinese character for needle (b) and the Chinese character for stone puncture (c)

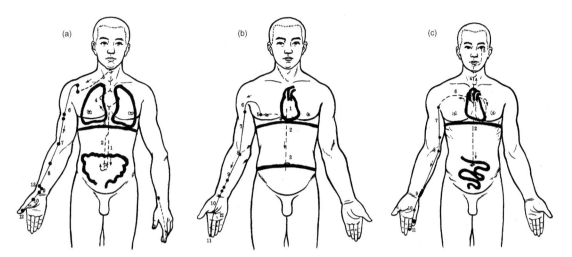

Figure 2 Three *Yin* meridians of the hand: the lung meridian (LU (a)) pericardium meridian (PC (b)) and heart meridian (HT (c))

aspect of the medial side of the upper body from the hands to the head. They are collectively called the three *Yang* meridians of the hand (Figure 3).

The three *Yin* meridians of the foot

The spleen meridian (SP), liver meridian (LR) and kidney meridian (KI) run respectively through the anterior aspect, midline and posterior aspect of the medial side of the lower limbs from the feet to the abdomen and the chest. They are collectively called the three *Yin* meridians of the foot (Figure 4).

The three *Yang* meridians of the foot

The stomach meridian (ST), gallbladder meridian (GB) and bladder meridian (BL) run from the head through the trunk to the feet along the anterior aspect, midline and posterior aspect of the lateral side of the lower limbs. They are collectively called the three *Yang* meridians of the foot (Figure 5).

Conception vessel and governor vessel

The extra meridian running along the meridian system of the abdomen and chest upward to the lower lip is called the conception vessel (CV). The extra

meridian running along the meridian system of the back upward to the top of the head and then downward to the middle of the face is called the governor vessel (GV) (Figure 6).

A total of 361 acupuncture points have been identified along the 14 meridians. The standard nomenclature of these points consists of the Chinese phonetic (*pinyin*) name followed by the alphanumeric code in parentheses. Apart from these, there are a number of acupuncture points with specific therapeutic properties not on the 14 meridians. They are called extraordinary points.

The acupuncture point and its action

Each acupuncture point has its own therapeutic action. For example, the point *Hegu* (LI 4), located between the first and second metacarpal bones, can sedate pain in the head and mouth, indicated for headache, toothache and sore throat (Figure 7). The point *Shenmen* (HT 7), located on the medial end of the transverse crease of the wrist, can induce tranquilization and remedy insomnia (Figure 8). *Yanglingquan* (GB 34) is located at the lateral aspect of the knee joint, in the depression anterior and inferior to the head of the fibula. It is indicated in the treatment of gallbladder diseases, shoulder pain and stiff neck (Figure 9). *Yinlingquan* (SP 9), located in the depression on the lower border of the medial condole of the tibia

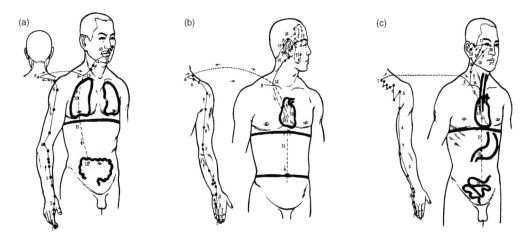

Figure 3 The three *Yang* meridians of the hand: the large intestine meridian (LI (a)) triple energizer meridian (TE (b)) and the small intestine meridian (SI (c))

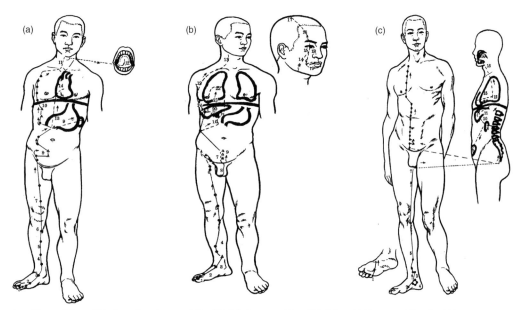

Figure 4 The three *Yin* meridians of the foot: the spleen meridian (SP (a)), liver meridian (LR (b)) and kidney meridian (KI (c))

(Figure 10), is indicated in the treatment of retention or incontinence of urine and seminal emission.

The *Ashi* point is any point where, when the doctor presses it, the patient groans with pain. 'A' is pronounced 'Ah' in Chinese and '*Shi*' means yes. It is the same as a trigger or tender point. Inserting an acupuncture needle directly into an *Ashi* point is recommended to treat pain. An *Ashi* point (trigger point) may be found outside abdominal muscles and in skin, scars, tendons, joint capsules, ligaments and periosteum. The cause of tenderness at trigger points may be poor

inactivation of calcium by muscle sarcoplasmic reticulum, which causes calcium to cross-link the actin and myosin, with ensuing permanent contraction[5]. How needling rectifies this problem, however, is unclear.

Anatomy of acupuncture points

Dung[6] listed ten structures in his review, which are found in the vicinity of acupoints. In decreasing order of importance they are listed as follows:

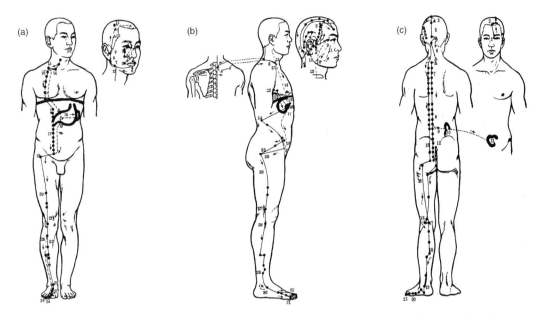

Figure 5 The three *Yang* meridians of the foot: the stomach meridian (ST (a)), gallbladder meridian (GB (b)) and bladder meridian (BL (c))

(1) Large peripheral nerves;

(2) Nerves emerging from a deep to a more superficial location;

(3) Cutaneous nerves emerging from deep fascia;

(4) Nerves emerging from bone foramina;

(5) Motor points of neuromuscular attachments (a neuromuscular attachment is the area where a nerve enters the muscle mass);

(6) Blood vessels in the vicinity of neuromuscular attachments;

(7) Nerves composed of fibers of varying sizes (diameters), more likely on muscular nerves than on cutaneous nerves;

(8) Bifurcation points of peripheral nerves;

(9) Ligaments (muscle tendons, joint capsule, fascial sheets, collateral ligaments), rich in nerve endings;

(10) Suture lines of the skull.

Heine[7] revealed that 80% of acupoints correlate with perforations in the superficia of cadavers. Through these holes, a cutanous nerve vessel bundle penetrates the skin. If replicated, this finding could be the morphological basis for acupoints.

Location of acupuncture points

Several experiments have shown that acupuncture needling of true acupoints produces marked analgesia for acute laboratory-induced pain in human subjects, while needling of sham points produces very weak effects[8–10]. Cho and co-workers[11,12] showed acupuncture needling on *Zhiyin* (UB 67), *Guangmin* (GB 37) and *Xiaxi* (GB 43), all located on the legs and toes, to treat eye disease. They are related to the eyes according to traditional meridian theory. Stimulating those points by acupuncture needles can surprisingly activate the vision cortex, which is detected by functional magnetic resonance imaging (fMRI). In contrast, stimulating the sham points on the same leg cannot activate the vision cortex. The results provided the first scientific evidence that acupuncture 'signals' are projected to neocortical areas of the brain for central processing. The data also demonstrated that accurately locating the true acupoints to treat

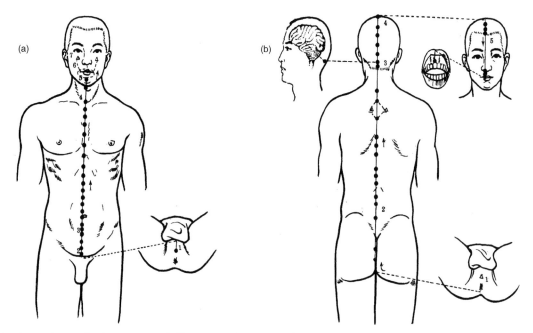

Figure 6 Conception vessel and governor vessel. The extra meridian running along the meridian system of the abdomen and chest upward to the lower lip is called the conception vessel (CV (a)). The extra meridian running along the meridian system of the back upward to the top of the head and then downward to the middle of the face is called the governor vessel (GV (b))

diseases could be important clinically, because sham points are not able to achieve effective results.

In order to locate acupoints accurately, the descriptions of the exact anatomical position must be followed, obviously the simplest method. Unfortunately, there are many acupoints that do not fall into an exact location. Their individual locations depend upon the dimensions of the patient. In order to account for variations in body size, the Chinese developed the 'human inch' called 'cun' as an acupuncture measuring unit (AMU). The AMU uses either the finger length of the patient as a unit (finger equivalent unit) or the bone length between joints of the patient as unit (bone equivalent unit).

Finger equivalent unit

As a variation of this finger equivalent unit, the width of the patient's thumb (not the medical provider's!) may be regarded as one *cun*. The combined breadth of index, middle, ring and little fingers of the hand at the level of the second metacarpophalangeal joints may be considered three *cun*. The distance between the

two creases of the interphalangeal joints of the patient's middle finger, when flexed, represents one *cun*. Figure 11 is an illustration of a modern version of the finger equivalent units.

Bone equivalent unit

A list of the proportional measurement is as follows:

- The bone equivalent unit of the head is calculated by one of the following measurements: midline of the anterior hairline to midline of the posterior hairline equals 12 *cun*; the distance between the anterior hairline and the glabella is 3 *cun*; the distance between the posterior hairline and the seventh cervical spinous process is 3 *cun* (Figure 12).

- The bone equivalent unit of the back is calculated by measuring the distance from the midline to the medial border of the scapula, which is 3 *cun*. The distance between the nipples is 8 *cun*, as is the lower end of the sternum to the umbilicus. The

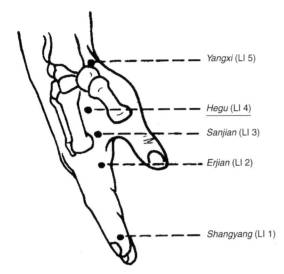

Figure 7 The location of the *Hegu* (LI 4) acupoint

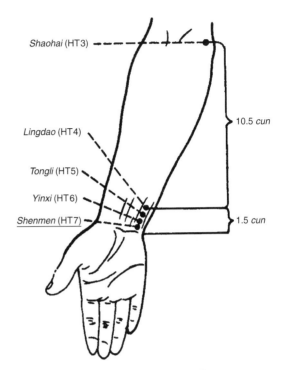

Figure 8 The location of acupoint *Shenmen* (HT 7)

distance between the umbilicus and the upper border of the symphasis pubis is 5 *cun* (Figure 13).

- The bone equivalent unit of the upper arm is calculated by measuring from the axillary fold to the cubital elbow crease, which is 9 *cun* (Figures 12 and 13).

- The bone equivalent unit for the upper leg is calculated by measuring from the proximal point of the greater trochanter to the lower aspect of the patella, a distance of 19 *cun*. The lower leg is calculated by measuring either the distance from the middle of the patella to the prominence of the lateral melleolus, which is 16 *cun*, or the distance from the medial condyle of the tibia to the prominence of the medial malleolus, which is 13 *cun* (Figures 12 and 13).

De Qi sensation

The results of acupuncture treatment eventually depend upon the response of the body to acupuncture stimulation. In a clinical setting, the efficacy of acupuncture therapy may rely on receiving *De Qi* sensation created by acupuncture needling, choosing acupoints and accurately locating them. *De Qi* is a kind of sensation to which the patient responds. In the

process of acupuncture needling, the patient feels numbness, fullness and sometimes soreness around the acupoint, or feels an electric sensation travelling to a certain area of the body. Similiarly, the acupuncture provider feels the acupuncture needle to be heavy, or as if 'a fish is biting the bait'. Chiang[13] showed that the essential correlate of acupuncture analgesia was a *De Qi* sensation. By injecting procaine (2%) into the acupoints LI 4 and LI 10 in humans, he determined that the subcutaneous injection did not block *De Qi* sensations, while intramuscular procaine abolished them. Moreover, whenever *De Qi* sensations were blocked, so was acupuncture analgesia. Perhaps the best experiment of all was performed on humans with direct microelectrode recordings from single fibers in the median nerve while acupuncture was performed distally[14]. They showed that when the *De Qi* sensation was achieved, type II muscle afferents produced numbness; type III gave sensations of heaviness, distension and aching; and type IV (unmyelinated fibers) produced soreness. As soreness is uncommon in *De Qi*, the main components of *De Qi* are carried by types II and III afferents (small myelinated afferents from muscles).

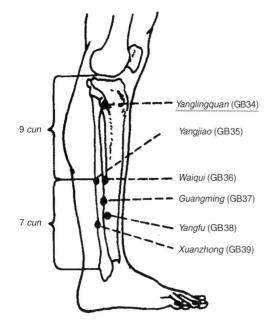

Figure 9 The location of the *Yanglingquan* (GB 34) point

MOXIBUSTION

In the clinic, an acupuncturist may use heat by burning a moxa made of an herb called *Ai* (dried leaves of *Artemesia vulgaris*), over the acupuncture point and the surrounding tissues, a technique called moxibustion, rather than inserting acupuncture needles. Some moxa are smokeless. Some clinics now use a heat source called a DTP light (Figure 14) to replace moxa. Moxibustion is usually used for the conditions caused by deficiency, weakness or 'cold'.

ELECTROACUPUNCTURE

In most circumstances, acupuncturists also connect the acupuncture needle to a mild electrical stimulator, a technique called electroacupuncture. The electrical pulses administered via the acupuncture needle stimulate the deep tissues. The intensity (1–3 mA), pulse width (0.2–1.0 ms) and frequency (1–500 Hz) can thus be precisely determined. Generally, low-frequency, high-intensity stimulation pulses of needling works through the endorphin system and acts in all three centers (spinal cord, midbrain and hypothalamus–pituitary) as mentioned below. The method produces

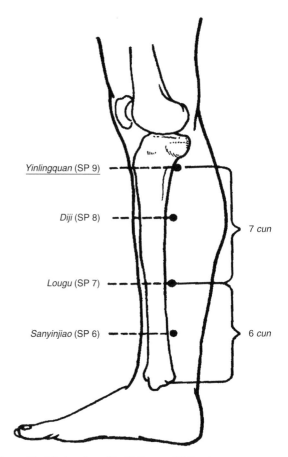

Figure 10 The location of the *Yinlingquan* (SP 9) point

analgesia of slower onset, but the analgesia lasts longer than fast-frequency stimulation and its effects are cumulative, improving increasingly after several treatments. In contrast, the high-frequency, low-intensity analgesia is rapid in onset but of very short duration and without cumulative effects.

Because low-frequency, high-intensity analgesia produces a cumulative effect, repeated treatment produces more and more benefit for the patient[15,16] or laboratory animal[17].

AURICULAR ACUPUNCTURE

Ear acupuncture or auricular acupuncture is stimulation achieved by inserting acupuncture needles into the acupoints located on the auricle.

The ear has the highest density of acupoints, comprising 10% of the acupoints of the whole

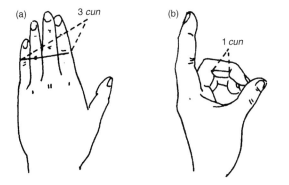

Figure 11   Finger equivalent units

body. There are 43 auricular points that have proven therapeutic values. The acupuncture points in the ear represent different body parts, including inner organs (Figure 15).

Because every part of the external ear is reflected through a microsystem to remote reflexes of every part of the body, a wide variety of health problems are relieved by auricular acupuncture therapy. Almost all health conditions can be affected to some degree by stimulating reactive ear points. The most commonly reported uses of auricular acupuncture therapy have been for the control of chronic pain, detoxification from addictive drugs, relief of nausea and reduction of hypertension.

SCALP ACUPUNTURE

Scalp acupuncture is acupuncture needling of the acupoints on the scalp, mainly over the cortical area, to treat diseases, for example, hemiplegia. The acupuncture needle is inserted at the area of the scalp over the motor cortex of the brain. Its efficacy needs further investigation, particularly for such self-limiting diseases as cerebral vascular accidents.

INDICATIONS FOR ACUPUNCTURE

List of the World Health Organization

In 1979, WHO listed more than 40 conditions for which acupuncture may be effective. Based on this list, conditions that we treat with acupuncture alone and which respond well include the following but are not limited to:

(1) *Neurological*: headache, migraine, neuralgia, postoperative pain, stoke residuals, Parkinson's disease and facial pain;

(2) *Emotional*: trauma, hypertension, insomnia, depression, anxiety, nervousness and neurosis;

(3) *Digestive*: abdominal pain, hyperacidity, chronic diarrhea, indigestion and constipation;

(4) *Musculoskeletal*: backache or pain, muscles cramping, localized traumatic injuries, sprains, strains, sports injuries, arthritis disc problems, sciatica, pain and weakness in the neck, shoulders, arms, hands, fingers, knees, legs and feet;

(5) *Ear, eye, nose, dental*: poor vision, tired eyes, tinnitus, nervous deafness, toothache, post-extraction pain and gum problems;

(6) *Respiratory*: sinusitis, common cold, tonsillitis, bronchitis, allergy and asthma;

(7) *Gynecological*: impotence, premenstrual syndrome, cramps, menopause syndrome and obstetrics;

(8) *Other benefits*: vitality and energy increase, stress reduction, deep relaxation, skin rejuvenation, weight control, smoking cessation and other addiction problems.

When to use acupuncture?

As an alternative medicine in the USA, the indication for acupuncture therapy could also be summarized as follows:

(1) Any properly diagnosed patient when conventional treatments have not worked, or conventional medicine is less effective or with more side-effects;

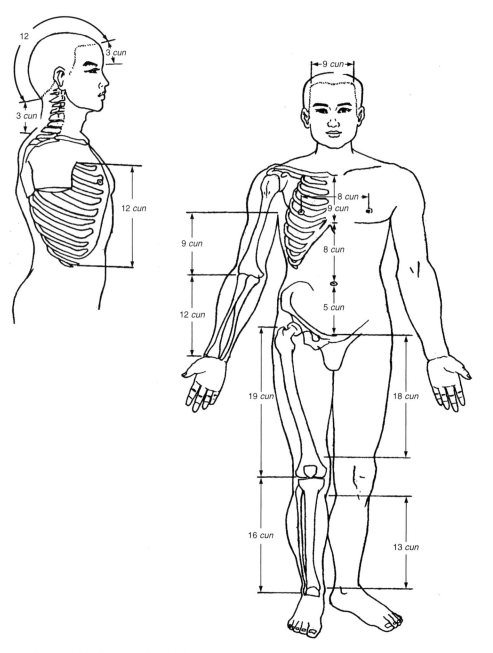

Figure 12 Bone equivalent units of the front and right side of the body

(2) Any patient feeling sick or abnormal when conventional diagnostic techniques show normal and/when or no conventional treatment is available;

(3) Used to increase the benefits of other medical care. For example, acupuncture for pain caused by cancer or for the side-effects of chemotherapy.

Principle of prescription and selection of acupoints

Before acupuncture treatment, the medical provider needs to decide how many acupoints to be selected and how to combine them for individual patients. Selection of acupoints and prescription of the combination

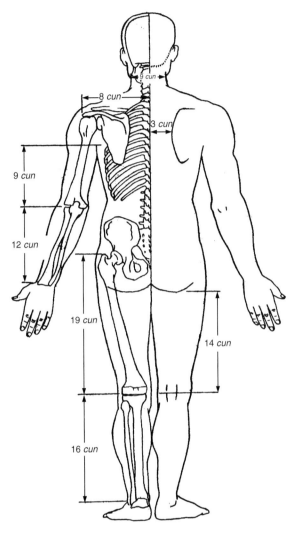

Figure 13 Bone equivalent units of the back of the body

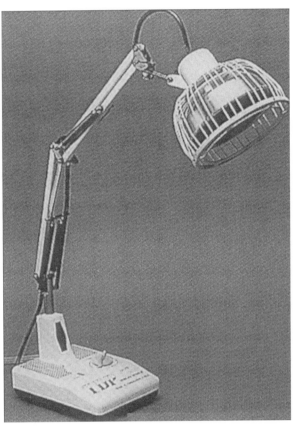

Figure 14 The DTP lamp

of acupoints are based on the theory of meridians, the actions of acupoints and the patient's symptoms or disease and their causes. The following is a brief introduction to the methods for selection of points and prescription.

Selection of acupoints on the diseased meridian

Acupoints are selected directly from the affected meridian. For example, *Zhonfu* (LU 1), *Chize* (LU 5) and other acupoints of the lung meridian are selected to treat a cough due to disease of the lung.

The combination of the exterior–interior acupoints

When a disease is on the *Yin* meridian, the prescription of acupoints could be selected from this *Yin* meridian itself. A *Yang* meridian is exteriorly–interiorly related to the *Yin* meridian, according to the theory of meridians. For example, the kidney meridian is a *Yin* meridian and related to the *Yang* bladder meridian in the leg. Thus, if the kidney meridian is affected, *Hunlun* (BL 60) and *Jinggu* (BL 64) of the bladder meridian are also selected to treat the kidney disease.

The combination of the anterior–posterior acupoints

Anterior is defined as the thoracic–abdominal region, belonging to *Yin*. Posterior is the lumbodorsal region, belonging to *Yang*. This method is also known as the combination of abdomen-*Yin* acupoints and back-*Yang* acupoints. Both acupoints on the anterior and posterior regions are selected to make up a prescription. For instance, selecting *Zhongwan* (Ren 12) on the abdomen and *Weishu* (BL 21) on the back to treat epigastric pain.

The combination of the distant–local acupoints

The selection of the acupoints on the diseased area and corresponding acupoints distant to the area simultaneously make up a prescription. For example, selecting *Jinming* (BL 1) near the eye and *Xingjian* (LR 2) distantly treats eye disease.

The combination of the left–right acupoints

According to the theory, the courses of the meridian cross each other. For example, select *Hegu* (LI 4) on the right side to treat facial paralysis on the left side and vice versa. Because of symmetrical distribution of the meridian, acupoints on both sides are selected in the treatment of diseases of the internal organs, in order to strengthen the co-ordinating effects. However, it has been found that acupoints on the healthy side and no acupoints on the diseased side are selected in practice, such as in the treatment of hemiparalysis, arthralgic pain, etc. with a certain theapeutic result.

TREATMENT OF COMMON DISEASES WITH ACUPUNCTURE

Acupuncture for lower back pain

In the USA, lower back pain was among the top five primary reasons adult patients visit office-based physicians, according to a National Ambulatory Medical Care Survey during 1980–90. Data show that 60–80% of adults have experience of lower back pain. Patients disabled from lower back pain increased by 168% from 1971 to 1986 and cost \$14 to \$20 billion

annually in treatment, according to the 1986 report of the National Center for Health Statistics. Surgery rates for lower back pain are five times higher in the USA than in England. Although operative procedures are frequently performed, 50–75% of the patients, unfortunately, continue to have disabling pain after the operation. Other conventional treatments are not very effective either. However, according to Liao[18], acupuncture treatment could relieve the disabling pain of the lower back of 85% of their patients for the first time in many years.

Causative factors

Causative factors are the retention of pathogenic wind, cold and damp in channels and collaterals; lumbar muscular strain, which is stagnation of *Qi* and blood in the lumbar region due to sprain or contusion; deficiency of *Qi* of the kidney due to excessive work; occupational sitting or standing for long periods of time; or excessive sexual activity causing loss of the essence of the kidney.

Select points

Select points are *Shenshu* (BL 23), *Weizhong* (BL 40) and a painful spot (i.e. *Ashi* point).

Acupuncture for headache

Headache is pain in the upper half of the head, excepting pain in the face. It is caused by many factors. Generally, it is divided into two main types: the diseases of inside the skull and outside the skull.

Causative factors

Factors causing pain are mainly cerebritis, meningitis and tumor. The disorders of the outside skull are mainly frontal sinusitis, teeth diseases, ear diseases, throat and pharyngohinitis, eye disease, as well emotional stress and hypertension.

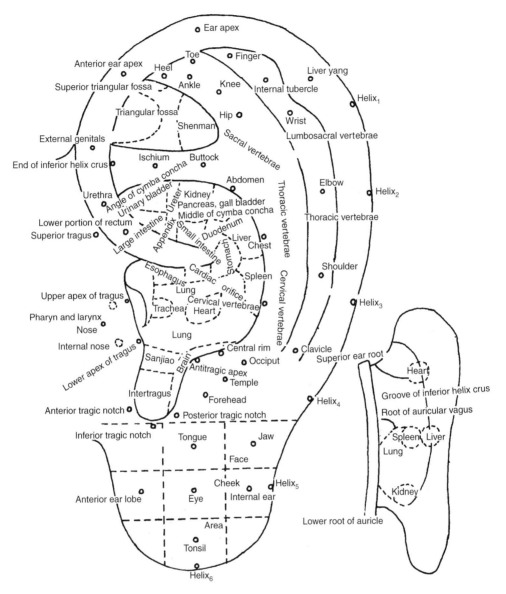

Figure 15 Ear acupoints

Select points

(1) *Migraine* (one-side headache): *Taiyang* (Extra 1), *Fengchi* (GB 20)

(2) *Forehead*: *Touwei* (ST 8), *Taiyang* (Extra 1)

(3) *Occipital region*: *Fengchi* (GB 20), *Dazhui* (DU 14), *Yintang* (Extra 2)

(4) *Whole potions*: *Yintang* (Extra 2), *Fengchi* (GB 20)

Acupuncture for stomachache

Stomachache is a symptom resulting from acute and chronic gastritis or peptic ulcer. Acute gastritis is expressed mainly as epigastric pain or upset, nausea and vomiting, and it is accompanied by diarrhea and fever. Chronic gastritis is mainly indicated as epigastric upset or dull pain, anorexia and postprandial distension. The peptic ulcer is rhythmic pain. The characteristic of pain includes anguish, distension, burning pain and hungry sensations.

Causative factors

The causative factors of this disease include irregular meals, overindulgence, a fatty diet and long-term alcohol intake, or it may arise from other *Zang-Fu* organ diseases. Some features of this disease are insidious onset, long incubation period or the result of acute attack of chronic pathogenic changes. Long-term treatment and watching one's diet are necessary.

Select acupoints

These are *Zusanli* (ST 36), *Zhongwan* (Ren 12), *Qimen* (LR 14, right), *Weishu* (BL 21, cupping) and *Liangqiu* (ST 34).

Acupuncture for arthritis

Arthritis is inflammation in the joints, as a result of various causes. The main clinical manifestation is arthralgia and a functional disturbance to different degrees. There are three main clinical types of arthritis: rheumatic arthritis, rheumatoid arthritis and osteoarthritis.

(1) *Rheumatic arthritis* occurs chiefly in adolescents. Before onset, it is commonly characterized by an upper respiratory infection. The acute stage is manifested as fever and profuse sweating. Characteristics are multiple with movement in large joints accompanied by acute inflammatory symptoms, such as redness, swelling, fever and pain, as well as functional disturbance. It is often a reoccurring attack.

(2) *Rheumatoid arthritis* occurs chiefly in the young and middle aged. The small joints of the hands and feet are the most commonly affected, usually symmetrically, but other large synovial joints (hip, knee and elbow) are often also involved. Onset is insidious and mainly chronic. Acute onset is uncommon. At onset, the syndromes of pathogenic joint changes are similar to rheumatic arthritis, and they may be accompanied by fever.

(3) *Osteoarthritis* is also named hypertrophied or denatured arthritis. The diseases usually presents in middle-aged persons (over 40 years of age). The joint lesions are chiefly at joints at dominant extremities, such as lumbar vertebra, hip, knee and finger. It is usually insidious in onset. Swelling is not present in the pathogenic joints.

Select points

(1) *Temporomandibular joint*: *Xiaguan* (ST 7), *Hegu* (LI 4)

(2) *Interspinal vertebrae joints*: Correspond with *Jiaji* points

(3) *Shoulder joints*: *Jianyu* (LI 15), *Jianliao* (SJ 14)

(4) *Elbow joints*: *Quchi* (LI 11), *Shaohai* (HT 3)

(5) *Wrist, metacarpophalangeal, digital joints*: *Waiguan* (SJ 5)

(6) *Lumbosacral joints*: *Yaoyangguan* (DU 3), *Ciliao* (BL 32)

(7) *Hip joints*: *Huantiao* (GB 30), *Fenshi* (GB 31)

(8) *Knee joints*: *Xiyan* (Extra 36), *Yanglingquan* (GB 34)

(9) *Ankle joints*: *Jiexi* (ST 41), *Kunlun* (BL 60)

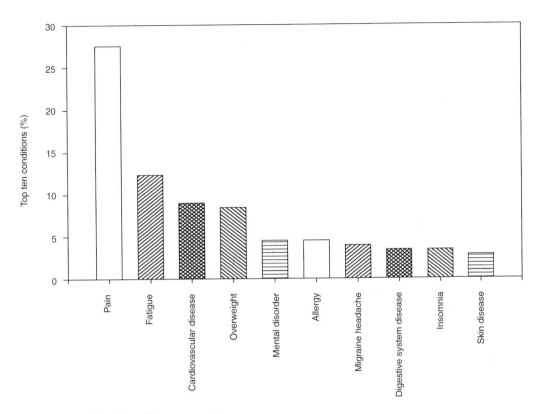

Figure 16 Top ten reasons why patients visit an acupuncturist

Table 1 How the patients heard about acupuncture

Year	Relative or friend		Website		Yellow pages		Doctor's referral	
	n	%	*n*	%	*n*	%	*n*	%
1998 (*n* = 40)	34	85	0	0	6	15	0	0
1999 (*n* = 40)	33	82.5	1	2.5	5	12.5	1	2.5
2000 (*n* = 40)	30	75	2	5	6	15	2	5
2001 (*n* = 40)	31	77.5	3	7.5	2	5	4	10

who learned from Yellow Pages which decreased each year from 15 to 5% (correlation coefficient, $r = -0.7502$). Patients learning from a website or following another medical practitioner's referral rose every year from 0 to 7.5% (correlation coefficient, $r = 1$) and 0 to 10% (correlation coefficient, $r = 0.9827$), respectively. We calculated the equation of the regression line of website information to be $y = 2.5x - 4995$ and a physician's referral is $y = 3.25x - 6494$. Based on those equations, we predicted that patients' visits to an acupuncturist through a physician's referral would increase to 12.5% and by

the website would increase to 10% in 2002. Figure 17 demonstrates how the patients obtained information about an acupuncturist in the consecutive 4 years, and the regression lines.

Before 2001 payment for acupuncture treatment was out of a patient's own pocket. The average cost for each visit was $68±27.16 (range $20–80, 95% confidence interval $68±8.42) in 1998; $71±23.43 (range $25–85, 95% confidence interval $71±7.27) in 1999; $76±18.80 (range $20–90, 95% confidence interval $76±5.83) in 2000; and $82.75±16.09 (range $30–120, 95% confidence interval $82.75±4.99) in

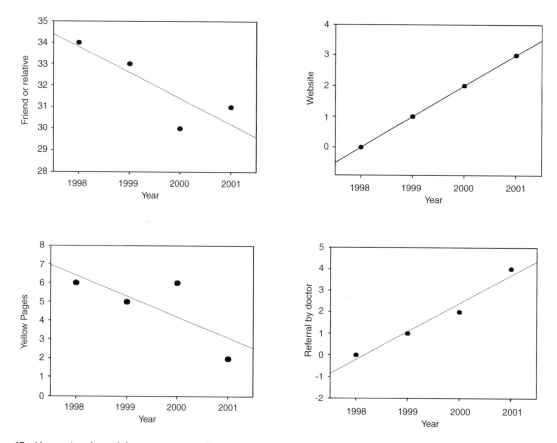

Figure 17 How patients learned about acupuncture in the years 1998–2001 in the author's experience

2001. In 2001, 12.5% of patients treated by acupuncture were covered by insurance fully or partially.

PHYSIOLOGICAL BASES OF ACUPUNCTURE ANALGESIA

Although acupuncture has been used in China for more than 4000 years and its efficacy has been proved by ample clinic experiences, its mechanisms of action are a recent focus of study. The facts of acupuncture anesthesia and its cures have astonished the modern medical field. The anesthesia produced by acupuncture is very different from that produced by drugs. First of all, consciousness is maintained, allowing the patient to eat, talk and co-operate with doctors during surgery. Second, stimulation of specific acupuncture points is essential to maintain analgesia.

Third, analgesia persists long after stimulation has been terminated, allowing the patient to move immediately or much earlier without pain postoperatively. Thus, the patient recovers from surgery sooner.

How can an acupuncture needle inserted in the hand possibly relieve toothache? Because such phenomena do not conform to accepted physiological concepts, scientists are puzzled and skeptical. They were confused by the way traditional Chinese medicine explained *Yin–Yang*, the five elements, the eight principles of diagnosis and the functioning of organs by *Zang-fu*. In 1973, Chinese scientists published the model of a cross-circulation experiment. The effect of acupuncture analgesia was transmitted from a donor rabbit, which received acupuncture, to a normal recipient. The pain threshold of both rabbits significantly increased. The experiment offered for the first time some evidence that acupuncture must have produced in the animals some kind of chemical substance or substances that potentially suppresses pain. It is now known that acupuncture may activate the endogenous systems of analgesia to be able to alleviate pain in the clinic.

According to Pomeranz[21], the mechanism of acupuncture analgesia is as follows: when an acupuncture needle penetrates an acupuncture point, the needle and electrical impulses stimulate nerve fibers in the muscle, which send impulses to the spinal cord and activate three centers (spinal cord, midbrain and hypothalamus/pituitary) to cause analgesia. The spinal site uses enkephalin and dynorphin to block incoming messages with low-frequency stimulation and other transmitters (perhaps γ-aminobutyric acid) at high-frequency stimulation. The midbrain uses enkephalin to activate the raphe-descending system, which inhibits spinal cord pain transmission by a synergistic effect of the monoamines serotonin and norepinephrine (noradrenaline). The midbrain also has a circuit, which bypasses endorphinergic links at high-frequency stimulation. Finally, at the third (hypothalamus/pituitary) center, the pituitary releases β-endorphin into the blood and cerebrospinal fluid to cause analgesia at a distance. The hypothalamus also sends long axons to the midbrain and activates the descending analgesia system via β-endorphin. This third center is not activated at high-frequency stimulation, but only at low frequencies.

The endorphin–acupuncture analgesia hypothesis is supported by the following:

(1) Naloxone, an endorphin antagonist, can antagonize acupuncture analgesia[22,23] and increasing the doses of naloxone produces increasing blockade, showing a dose–response curve[24].

(2) Acupuncture analgesia is enhanced by protecting endorphins from enzyme degradation[25–30].

(3) Lesions of the periaqueductal gray matter (site of endorphins) or the arcuate nucleus of the hypothalamus (the site of β-endorphins) abolishes acupuncture analgesia[31,32].

(4) The level of *c-Fos* gene protein, which measures increased neural activity, is elevated in endorphin-related areas of the brain during acupuncture analgesia[33–35].

(5) Rats deficient in endorphin show poor acupuncture analgesia[30,36].

(6) Mice genetically deficient in opiate receptors show poor acupuncture analgesia[37].

SUMMARY AND FUTURE PROSPECT

Patients who visit acupuncturists in the Chicago Metropolitan Area are similar to those who utilize other alternative medicines. The majority of patients are female, educated, white and middle aged. The top ten reasons for visiting an acupuncturist are pain, fatigue, cardiovascular disease, weight problems, mental disorder, allergy, migraine headache, digestive system disease, insomnia and skin disease. Our data indicate that more and more patients will find acupuncturists from websites and from their regular physician's referral, and that full and partial insurance coverage for acupuncture treatment is to be executed.

To enhance the acceptance of acupuncture in the USA the panel convened by the National Institutes of Health in 1997[38] suggested six points for the future: first, improvement of understanding between acupuncturists and the conventional health-care community; second, improvement of training and more uniform licensing, certification and accreditation of acupuncturists; third, full information for patients about their treatment options, prognosis, relative risks and safety practices; fourth, strengthened communication between health-care provider groups; fifth, coverage of acupuncture treatment by insurance; and sixth, identification of important areas for future acupuncture research.

References

1. Liao SJ, Lee MH, Ng LK. The historic background. In *Principles and Practice of Contemporary Acupuncture*. New York, NY: Marcel Dekker, 1994:8–41

2. Reston J. News about my operation in Peking. *New York Times*, 26 July 1971

3. Rosenfeld I. Acupuncture goes mainstream (almost). *Parade Magazine*, 16 August 1998:10

4. Bannerman RH. Acupuncture: the WHO view. *World Health* 1979; December: 27–8

5. Travell J, Sommons D. *Myofascial Pain and Dysfunction. The Trigger Point Manual*. Baltimore, MD: Williams and Wilkins, 1983

6. Dung HC. Anatomical features contributing to the formation of acupuncture points. *Am J Acupunct* 1984;12:139–43

7. Heine H. Akupunkturtherapie – Perforationen der oberflächlichen Körperfaszie durch hutane Gefäß- Nervenbndel. *Therapeutikon* 1988; 4:238–44

8. Stacher G, Wancura I, Bauer P, Lahoda R, Schulze D. Effect of acupuncture on pain threshold and pain tolerance determined by electrical stimulation of the skin: a controlled study. *Am J Chin Med* 1975; 3:143–6

9. Chapman CR, Chen AC, Bonica JJ. Effects of intrasegmental electrical acupuncture on dental pain: evaluation by threshold estimation and sensory decision theory. *Pain* 1977;3:213–27

10. Brockhaus A, Elger CE. Hypalgesic efficacy of acupuncture on experimental pain in men. Comparison of laser acupuncture and needle acupuncture. *Pain* 1990;43:181–5

11. Cho ZH, Chung SC, Jones JP, *et al*. New findings of the correlation between acupoints and corresponding brain cortices using functional MRI. *Proc Natl Acad Sci* 1998;95:2670–3

12. Cho ZH, Na CS, Wang EK, *et al*. Functional magnetic resonance imaging of the brain in the investigation of acupuncture. In Stux G, Hammerschlag R, eds. *Clinical Acupuncture, Scientific Basis*. Berlin: Springer, 2001: 83–95

13. Chiang CY, Chang CT. Peripheral afferent pathway for acupuncture analgesia. *Sci Sin* 1973;16:210–17

14. Wang K, Yao S, Xian Y, Hou Z. A study on the receptive field of acupoints and the relationship between characteristics of needle sensation and groups of afferent fibres. *Sci Sin* 1985;28:963–71

15. Martelete M, Fiori AM. Comparative study of the analgesic effect of transcutaneous nerve stimulation (TNS), electroacupuncture (EA), and meperidine in the treatment of postoperative pain. *Acupunct Electrother Res* 1985;10:183–93

16. Walker JB, Katz RL. Nonopioid pathways suppress pain in humans. *Pain* 1981;11:347–54

17. Pomeranz B, Warma N. Potentiation of analgesia by two repeated electroacupuncture treatments: the first opioid analgesia potentiates a second, nonopioid analgesia response. *Brain Res* 1988;452:232–6

18. Liao SJ, Lee MH, Ng LK. Acupuncture for chronic pain and surgical analgesia. In *Principles and Practice of Contemporary Acupuncture*. New York, NY: Marcel Dekker, 1994:290–326

19. Eisenbarg DM, Kessler RC, Foster C. Unconventional medicine in the United States – prevalence, costs and patterns of use. *N Engl J Med* 1993;328:246–52

20. Eisenberg DM, Davis RD, Ettner SL, *et al*. Trends in alternative medicine use in the United States, 1990–1997: results of a follow-up national survey. *J Am Med Assoc* 1998;280:1569–75

21. Pomeranz B. Acupuncture analgesia-basic research, In Stux G, Hammerschlag R, eds, *Clinical Acupuncture, Scientific Basis*. Berlin: Springer, 2001:1–28

22. Pomeranz B, Chiu D. Naloxone blocks acupuncture analgesia and causes hyperalgesia: endorphin is implicated. *Life Sci* 1976;19: 1757–62

23. Mayer DJ, Price DD, Raffii A. Antagonism of acupuncture analgesia in man by the narcotic antagonist naloxone. *Brain Res* 1977; 121:368–72

24. Cheng R, Pomeranz B. Electroacupuncture analgesia is mediated by stereospecific opiate receptors and is reversed by antagonists of type 1 receptors. *Life Sci* 1979;26:631–9

25. Zou K, Yi QC, Wu SX, *et al*. Enkephalin involvement in acupuncture analgesia. *Sci Sin* 1980;23:1197–207

26. Cheng R, Pomeranz B. Monoaminergic mechanisms of electroacupuncture analgesia. *Brain Res* 1981;215:77–92

27. Chou J, Tang J, Yang HY, Costa E. Action of peptidase inhibitors on methionine 5-enkephalin-arginine 6-phenylalanine 7 (YGGFMRF) and methionine 5-enkephalin (YGGFM) metabolism and on electroacupuncture antinociception. *J Pharmacol Exp Ther* 1984;230:349–52

28. Ehrenpreis S. Analgesic properties of encephalinese inhibitors: animal and human studies. *Prog Clin Biol Res* 1985;192:363–70

29. Hishida F, Takeshige C. Effects of D-phenylalanine on individual variation of analgesia and on analgesia inhibitory system in their separated experimental procedures [Japanese with English abstract]. In Takeshige C, ed. *Studies on the Mechanism of Acupuncture Analgesia Based on Animal Experiments*. Tokyo: Showa University Press, 1986:51

30. Murai M, Takeshige C, Hishida F, *et al*. Correlation between individual variations in effectiveness of acupuncture analgesia and those in contents of brain endogenous morphine-like factors. [Japanese with English summary]. In Takeshige C, ed. *Studies on the Mechanism of Acupuncture Analgesia Based on Animal Experiments*. Tokyo: Showa University Press, 1986:542

31. Wang Q, Mao L, Han J. The arcuate nucleus of hypothalamus mediates low but not high frequency electroacupuncture in rats. *Brain Res* 1990;513:60–6

32. Takeshige C, Zhao WH, Guo SY. Convergence from the preoptic area and arcuate nucleus to the median eminence in acupuncture and nonacupuncture stimulation analgesia. *Brain Res Bull* 1991;26: 771–8

33. Guo HF, Cui X. C-Fos proteins are not involved in the activation of preproenkephalin gene expression in rat brain by peripheral electric stimulation (electroacupuncture). *Neurosci Lett* 1996;207:163–6

34. Lee JH, Beitz AJ. The distribution of brainstem and spinal nuclei associated with different frequencies of electroacupuncture analgesia. *Pain* 1993;52:11–28

35. Pan B, Castro-Lopes JM, Coimbra A, *et al*. C-*fos* expression in the hypothalamic pituitary system induced by electroacupuncture or noxious stimulation. *Neuroreport* 1994;5:1649–52

36. Takahashi G, Mera H, Kobori M. Inhibitory action on analgesic inhibitory system and augmenting action on naloxone reversal analgesia of D-phenylalanine. [Japanese with English summary]. In Takeshige C, ed. *Studies on the Mechanism of Acupuncture Analgesia Based on Animal Experiments*. Tokyo: Showa University Press, 1986:608

37. Peets J, Pomeranz B. Studies of suppression of nocisensor reflexes using tail flick electromyograms and intrathecal drugs in barbiturate-anaesthetized rats. *Brain Res* 1987;416:301–7

38. National Institutes of Health. *Acupuncture,* NIH Consensus Statement, vol 15, Number 5. Bethesda, MD: NIH, 1997

Traditional Chinese Medicine   11

W. Xuan

INTRODUCTION

Traditional Chinese Medicine (TCM) is an ancient medical science in China. It originated thousands of years ago and came to maturity a few hundred years before Christ. The earliest classical book on TCM, *Huang Di Nei Jing*, was written in the 1st century BC during the Han Dynasty.

TCM is mainly composed of theory and therapeutic methods. Among these are Chinese materia medica (including Chinese herbal medicine, animal medicine and mineral medicine), acupuncture, moxibustion and naprapathy (*Tui Na*).

BASIC THEORY OF TRADITIONAL CHINESE MEDICINE

The theory of *Yin* and *Yang*

Yin/Yang, dating back to the Zhou Dynasty (approximately 1000-770 BC), was a symbolic representation of the universe that embodied the concept of patterns, process, change and relationships that can be seen graphically in the *Yin/Yang* symbol (Figure 1). The concept of *Yin/Yang* is the most important and distinctive theory in TCM. All Chinese medical physiology, pathology, diagnosis and treatment can eventually be reduced to the fundamental theory of *Yin/Yang*. *Yin/Yang* represents the opposite but also interdependence. Each could consume, but also support its opposite. *Yin* and *Yang* can be inter-transformed because *Yin* contains the seed of *Yang* and vice versa. Moreover, *Yin/Yang* can be further subdivided into another level of *Yin/Yang* and so on until infinity. From Table 1, it can be seen that *Yin* and *Yang* are essentially an expression of a duality and an alternation of two opposite stages in time.

Yin and *Yang* are related in that they are in opposite stages of a cycle, which constitutes the motive force of all the changes, development and decay of things. *Yin* and *Yang* are interdependent, although they are opposite, one cannot exist without the other. *Yin* and *Yang* are in a constant state of dynamic balance, which is maintained by a continuous adjustment of their relative levels. *Yin* and *Yang* transform into each other; *Yin* can change into *Yang* and vice versa. *Yin* and *Yang* within a human's body structure are shown in Table 2.

The Five Elements

The theory of the Five Elements, together with the theory of *Yin/Yang*, constitutes the basics of TCM theory. The five elements are Wood, Fire, Earth, Gold and Water. Each one has its own characteristic properties. The theory originally explained the composition and phenomena of the physical universe by concepts of 'Inter-Generating, Inter-Controlling, Over-Controlling and Inter-Insulting' relationships among the Five Elements. It was later used in TCM to expound the unity of the human body and the natural world. Clinically, this theory helps practitioners to identify the root cause of health problems.

Figure 2 illustrates different relationships among the Five Elements and those among internal organs. Interrelationships between the five elements and natural phenomena are shown in Table 3. In the Inter-Generating sequence, each element generates another and is generated by an element. In the Inter-Controlling sequence, each element controls another and is controlled by an element. In the Over-Controlling sequence, the same sequence is followe as the controlling one, but each element 'over-controls'

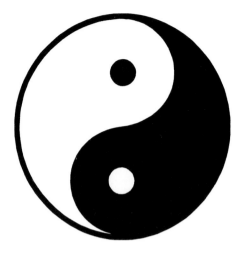

Figure 1   The symbol of *Yin* and *Yang*

Table 1   Indications for general identification of *Yin* and *Yang*

Yin	Yang
Darkness	Light
Moon	Sun
Shade	Brightness
Rest	Activity
Earth	Heaven
Flat	Round
Space	Time
West	East
North	South
Right	Left
Water	Fire
Cold	Hot
Quiet	Restless
Wet	Dry
Soft	Hard
Inhibition	Excitement
Slowness	Rapidity
Substantial	Non-substantial
Storage	Transformation
Sustaining	Change

Table 2   *Yin* and *Yang* within a human being's body structure

Yin	Yang
Inferior	Superior
Interior	Exterior
Anterior–medial surface	Posterior–lateral surface
Front	Back
Structure	Function
Body	Head
Organs	Skin/muscles
Below the waist	Above the waist
Blood and body fluids	*Qi*

another, so that it causes the other to decrease. In the Inter-Insulting sequence, the sequence takes place in the reverse order from the Controlling sequence.

The Five Elements are used in TCM physiology and pathology. The Inter-Generating and the Inter-Controlling sequences provide the basic model of physiological relationship among the internal organs. The Over-Controlling and the Inter-Insulting sequences provide a clinically useful pattern of pathological relationship among the internal organs. The Inter-Generating sequence can also give rise to pathological conditions when it is out of balance. The essence of the Five Element relationship is 'balance'. The Inter-Generating and the Inter-Controlling sequences keep a dynamic balance among the elements. When this balance is out of control for a prolonged period of time, disease occurs.

The Five Elements are used in TCM diagnosis. For example, a green color of the face indicates stagnation of the Liver-*Qi*; a red color of the face means Excess/Fullness of the Heart-Fire; a yellow or sallow complexion suggests Deficiency/Emptiness of the Spleen-*Qi*; a white color of the face implies Deficiency/Emptiness of the Lung-*Qi*; and a gray or black color recommends Deficiency/Emptiness of the Kidney-*Yang*.

The Five Elements are used in TCM treatment. Whenever the empty Liver-Blood is noted, the following (based on the relationships among the Five Elements) should always be considered: the Mother Element (Water/Kidney) fails to nourish the Son Element (Wood/Liver); Gold/Lung over-controls Wood/Liver; the Son Element (Fire/Heart) is drawing too much from the Mother Element (Wood/Liver); Earth/Spleen is insulting the Wood/Liver. It is necessary to keep all these relationships among the Five Elements in mind when determining treatment in TCM.

The Five Elements are also used in herbal and diet therapy. Diet therapy is partially based on the Five-Element model, and the principles underlying diet therapy are mostly the same as those in herbal

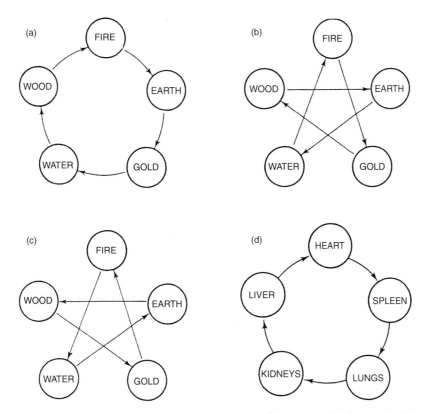

Figure 2 The Inter-Generating sequence (a); the Inter-Controlling and Over-Controlling sequence (b); the Inter-Insulting sequence (c); the Inter-Generating sequence among Internal Organs (d)

therapy. Each food or herb has a certain flavor that is related to one of the Elements, and is classified as having one of these flavors. The 'flavor' of a food or herb is not always related to its actual taste, although in most cases the two will coincide. For instance, lamb is classified as 'bitter' as is apple, which indicates that insomnia patients should avoid eating lamb and apple.

In addition, each of the flavors has a certain effect on the body. The sour flavor can generate body fluids and *Yin*, and control perspiration as well as diarrhea. The bitter flavor can clear away Heat, tranquilize and harden, and calm down restlessness and subdue rebellious *Qi*. The sweet flavor tones, balances and moderates. It is used to tone emptiness/deficiency, and to stop pain caused by Emptiness. The pungent flavor scatters, and is used to expel pathogenic factors. The salty flavor flows downwards and softens hardness, and is applied to treat constipation and swelling.

It is important to know that particular organs and systems might be affected by different flavors. The sour goes to the nerves and can upset the Liver, and it should be avoided for Spleen disease. The bitter goes to the bones, and it should be avoided for Lung disease. The sweet goes to the muscles, and it should be avoided for Kidney disease. The pungent scatters the *Qi*, and should be avoided for Liver disease. The salty dries the Blood, and should be avoided for Heart disease.

Qi, Blood and *Jin Ye*

TCM holds that *Qi*, Blood and *Jin Ye* (also known as body fluid) are fundamental substances in the human body to sustain normal vital activities. Together with the *Zang-Fu* organs and the Channels and Collaterals, they constitute the theoretical basis of human physiology.

Table 3   Introduction of natural phenomena to the Five Elements

	Wood (expansive/outward)	*Fire* (upward)	*Earth* (neutrality)	*Gold* (contractive/inward)	*Water* (downward)
Direction	East	South	Center	West	North
Season	Spring	Summer	Late summer	Autumn	Winter
Colors	green	red	yellow	white	black
Climate	wind	heat	dampness	dryness	cold
Tastes	sour	bitter	sweet	pungent	salty
Organs	Liver/GB	Heart/SI	Spleen/Stomach	Lungs/LI	Kidney/Bladder
Sense	eyes	tongue	mouth	nose	ears
Tissues	sinews	vessel	muscles	skin	bones
Grains	wheat	beans	rice	hemp	millet
Stage	birth	growth	transformation	harvest	storage

GB, Gallbladder; SI, Small Intestine; LI, Large Intestine

The concept of Qi in Traditional Chinese Medicine

The ancient Chinese scholars believed that *Qi* was the most basic substance of which the world was composed, and everything in the universe resulted from movement and changes of *Qi*. It was then introduced into the TCM field, and was gradually used to form the theory of TCM. Since TCM practitioners emphasize the interrelationship between the universe and human beings, they consider the human being's *Qi* as a result of the interaction of the *Qi* of Heaven and Earth. There is an old Chinese saying: '*Qi* is the root of a human being'. Generally speaking, the word *Qi* in TCM covers both substance and function. There are many different 'names' for *Qi*, which we can find from TCM books. However, all the various *Qi* are ultimately one *Qi*, merely manifesting in different forms. *Qi* varies by its names according to its source, location and function.

The Substantial *Qi*:

- Source *Qi* (*Yuan Qi*): also known as Congenital *Qi* as it is derived from the congenital essence of the parents;

- Pectoral *Qi* (*Zong Qi*): a combined *Qi* from the *Qi* essence of food and drink and the air inhaled, which serves as the dynamic force of respiration and blood circulation;

- Nutritive *Qi* (*Ying Qi*): transformed from the essence of food and drink, and flows with the blood in all 14 Channels and Collaterals;

- Defensive *Qi* (*Wei Qi*): also transformed from the essence of food and drink, but moves outside the Channels and Collaterals;

- Clean *Qi* (*Qing Qi*): the air inspired in the Lung;

- Waste *Qi* (*Zhuo Qi*): the air expired and the dense part of food.

The Functional *Qi*:

- Heart-*Qi*;

- Liver-*Qi*;

- Spleen-*Qi*;

- Lung-*Qi*;

- Kidney-*Qi*;

- Stomach-*Qi*.

The functions of *Qi* vary. First, *Qi* is of promoting action to activate the growth and development of the human body, and to speed up the formation and the circulation of the Blood. Second, *Qi* has a Warming Action as the main source to keep the body warm. Third, *Qi* guards the body surface against invasion of exogenous pathogenic factors, with a Defending Action. Fourth, *Qi* has a Holding Action, to hold, control and govern the secretion and excretion of liquid materials, such as sweat, urine and saliva, and to hold the internal organs in the abdominal cavity. Fifth, with a Transforming Action, *Qi* can metabolize fundamental substances, vital energy, Blood and *JinYe*.

The concept of Blood in Traditional Chinese Medicine

Blood in TCM has a different meaning from that in Western medicine. Blood itself is a form of *Qi*, and is inseparable from *Qi* itself. *Qi* infuses life into Blood, and without it, Blood would be an inert fluid. Blood is derived mostly from the Food-*Qi* produced by the Spleen. The Spleen then sends Food-*Qi* upward to the Lungs, and, through the pushing action of Lung-*Qi*, the Food-*Qi* is sent to the Heart, where it is transformed into Blood. Blood has the functions of nourishing and moistening the whole body, and it plays an important role in sustaining mental activity, as Blood provides the material foundation for the Mind (Figure 3).

The concept of JinYe in traditional Chinese medicine

JinYe is usually translated as body fluid in English. '*JinYe*' in TCM refers to the intracellular and the extracellular fluid in Western medicine. '*Jin*' indicates liquid that is diluted and moisturized, which is distributed under the skin and in muscles as well as pores/orifices of the body, while '*Ye*' means fluid that is sticky and hard to move, which infuses the joints, internal organs, and brain and marrow of the

body. *JinYe* originates from food and drink, which is transformed by the Stomach and transported by the Spleen. In addition, both the Small Intestine separating the clarity from the turbidity and the Large Intestine absorbing fluid from the waste are closely related to the transformation of *JinYe*. As for the distribution of *JinYe*, it is mainly completed by the Spleen's transmission and transportation, by the Lung's dispersing and descending, and by the Kidney's vaporization (Figure 4).

The Functions of *JinYe* are first, to moisturize and nourish the body; and second, to transform the Blood. *Jin* moisturizes the skin and hair, the muscles, the eyes, the nose and the mouth, etc., while *Ye* nourishes the internal organs, the brain and the marrow. In addition, *JinYe* joins the Blood through the Small Collaterals (*SunMai*) and becomes a component part of the Blood.

All *Qi*, Blood and *JinYe* derive from the essence of food and drink, but their properties and functions are different. Physiologically, they depend on each other, and they restrain and utilize each other. Pathologically, they also influence each other, and can cause imbalance of the other.

The relationship between Qi and the Blood

Theoretically, TCM holds that 'The *Qi* is the commander of the Blood while the Blood is the mother of the *Qi*'. To explain this we must look at how *Qi* acts on the Blood. First, *Qi* helps to transform the Blood. *Qi* is the primary power for transformation of the Blood. Therefore, insufficient *Qi* may lead to Blood

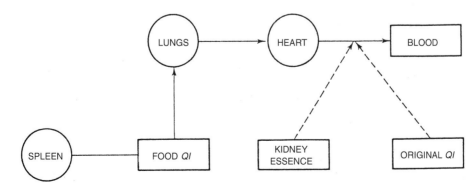

Figure 3   The origin of the Blood

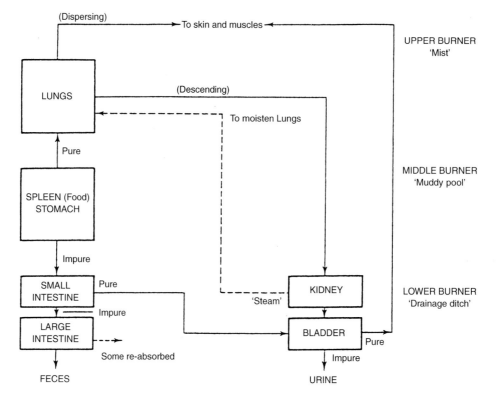

Figure 4 The origin, transformation and excretion of *JinYe*

Deficiency. Second, *Qi* drives the force to move the Blood. *Qi* is the driving power for circulation of the Blood, not only through its direct action, but also by means of relevant organs, such as the Heart-*Qi*'s pushing, the Lung-*Qi*'s dispersing or descending, and the Liver-*Qi*'s unrestraining. Consequently, *Qi*'s stagnation or deficiency often causes poor Blood circulation or even Blood Stasis. Third, *Qi* controls the movement of the Blood. *Qi* is able to keep the Blood circulated within the vessels, mainly through the Spleen-*Qi*. Whenever *Qi* becomes insufficient, various types of hemorrhage soon occur. Fourth, Blood carries the *Qi*. *Qi* exists in the Blood and is carried by the Blood. Last, Blood provides nutrients for *Qi*. *Qi* constantly receives nutrients provided by the Blood.

The relationship between Qi and JinYe

Qi transforms *JinYe*. *Qi* is the primary power for transformation of *JinYe* although *JinYe* is mainly transformed through the function of the Spleen and the Stomach. *Qi* promotes transportation of *JinYe*. *Qi* is the basic power for normal transportation and distribution of *JinYe*. *Qi* arrests excretion of *JinYe*. *Qi* is able to adjust and control excretion of *JinYe* so as to keep the balance between *JinYe*'s transformation and its excretion. *JinYe* is the carrier of *Qi* as *Qi* is always with *JinYe*. Therefore, loss of *JinYe*, such as profuse perspiring, frequent vomiting or diarrhea, often results in deficiency of *Qi*.

The relationship between the Blood and JinYe

Both the Blood and *JinYe* derive from the essence of food and drink, and are substances of the liquid state. Their main function is to nourish and moisturize the body. Since the Blood becomes *JinYe* when it extravasates the Collaterals and *JinYe* becomes a component of the Blood when it seeps into the Small Collaterals, both *JinYe* and Blood are believed to be from the same source. Therefore, insufficient Blood usually results in deficiency of *JinYe* and vice versa. In addition, the Blood and perspiration are also considered to come from the same source. Hence, TCM holds that 'Those who lose Blood cannot get themselves perspired, while those who perspire profusely will not have the same sufficiency of Blood as usual'.

The theory of *Zang-Fu*

Zang-Fu in TCM is equivalent to internal organs in Western medicine. The theory of *Zang-Fu* explains the physiological function and pathological changes of each internal organ and the mutual relationships among the organs. The theory also explains functional relationships that provide total integration of bodily functions, emotions, mental activities, tissues, sense organs as well as environmental influences. Although the name of each *Zang-Fu* used in TCM is basically the same as that of each internal organ used in Western medicine, their fundamental meanings are different, because the names of *Zang-Fu* not only indicate anatomic units, but also cover the physiological and pathological aspects of *Zang-Fu*. On the other hand, the names of internal organs used in Western medicine only point out the entities by means of anatomy.

In TCM, all internal organs of the human body are classified into three groups. They include: Five *Zang*, including the Heart (and the Pericardium), the Liver, the Spleen, the Lungs and the Kidney; Six *Fu*, containing the Gallbladder, the Stomach, the Large Intestine, the Small Intestine, the Urinary Bladder and the *SanJiao* (Triple *Jiao*); *QiHengZhiFu* also known as Extraordinary Organs, referring to the Brain, the

Table 4 The 12 *Zang-Fu* in Traditional Chinese Medicine

Zang (Yin)	*Fu (Yang)*	*Tissues*	*Sense organs*
Heart	Small Intestine	Blood vessels	Complexion
Liver	Gallbladder	Sinews/tendons	Nails
Spleen	Stomach	Muscles	Lips
Lung	Large Intestine	Skin and pores	Body hair
Kidney	Urinary Bladder	Bones	Hair
Pericardium	Triple *Jiao*		

Marrow, the Bone, Channels and Collaterals, the Gallbladder and the Uterus. The difference between *Zang* and *Fu* is that all *Zang* functionally stores vital substances, such as *Qi*, Blood and *JinYe*, while all of the *Fu* digests food and drink and transmits the essence.

There are 12 *Zang-Fu* in TCM. Among them, six are *Yin* and six are *Yang* (Table 4). The functions of each *Zang-Fu* follow.

Five Zang

(1) The Heart includes the Pericardium, and is considered the most important organ in the human body. It controls all the other organs' functions, and is therefore called the 'King of all the organs'. The Heart has three major functions. First, the Heart controls Blood circulation, and connects its vessels. It is believed that the Heart is connected with the Blood vessels to form a closed system, where the Blood is circulated by the Heart-*Qi*, which is considered as the motive power. Second, the heart houses the Mind. 'Mind' in TCM indicates the mental activities of the human body. TCM holds that the Heart controls mental/thinking activities as well as consciousness by way of 'Housing the Mind'. Third, the Heart opens into the Tongue and manifests in the complexion because the Collateral (*luo mai*) of the Heart Channel ascends to connect the Tongue and the Heart has its outward manifestation in the face. The Pericardium is the peripheral tissue of the Heart. It prevents the Heart from being directly invaded by exterior pathogenic factors.

(2) The Liver is divided into the Liver-*Yin* (Liver itself and the Blood stored in it) and the Liver-*Yang*, including the Liver-*Qi*. The Liver has four major functions. First, the Liver promotes the unrestrained and smooth flow of *Qi*. Ancient Chinese medical scholars believed that wood or a tree tended to spread out freely, as did the Liver, to correspond to this character, which is why the Liver is classified as 'wood' in the Five Elements of TCM. This is strongly associated with the Heart's function to sustain the normal mental

activities of human beings with the Spleen/ Stomach's function to keep normal digestion and absorption, and with keeping harmonious movement of both *Qi* and the Blood or removing any stagnated *Qi* within *SanJiao* so as to dredge or adjust the water passage. Second, the Liver stores the Blood and regulates the volume of the Blood according to physical activities at any time, which is a self-regulating process. Third, the Liver controls the sinews/tendons and manifests in the nails. The contraction and relaxation of the sinews/tendons depend on the nourishment of the Blood from the Liver, as does the nails. Finally, the Liver opens into the eye. The eye is a sensory organ, but connected to the Collateral of the Liver. It is the nourishment and moistening of the Liver-Blood that gives the eyes the capacity to see.

(3) The Spleen in TCM is believed to be located in the Middle *Jiao*. As a major organ in the digestive system, the Spleen has five main functions. First, the Spleen dominates the transformation and transportation of Food-*Qi*. The Spleen transforms Food-*Qi* from ingested food and drink, which have been digested by the Spleen and Stomach, and transports this Food-*Qi* and other refined parts of food and drink ('food essence') to the various organs and parts of the body to nourish them. In addition, the Spleen absorbs and transports water. Second, through its *Qi*, the Spleen keeps the Blood circulated within the Channels and Collaterals. Third, the Spleen controls the muscles and the four limbs because the muscles, the major components of the four limbs, are mainly nourished by the Food-*Qi*, which is transformed and transported by the Spleen. Fourth, the Spleen opens into the mouth and manifests in the Lips. When the Spleen's function is normal, the sense of taste is good, the lips are moist and rosy, and the action of chewing that prepares food for the Spleen to transform and transport its Food Essence is proper. Fifth, the Spleen raises the 'Clear' and keeps all the *Zang-Fu* at their locations. This means that the Spleen has an ability to send the Food Essence (Food-*Qi*) upward to the Lung, where the essence is distributed, and to keep all internal organs at their original locations.

(4) The Lung, believed in TCM to consist of the Lung-*Yin* and the Lung-*Qi*, has four main functions. First, the Lung governs *Qi*, which covers two aspects. The Lung controls respiration because the Lung is the main organ where the 'Clean *Qi*' from the environment and the 'Waste *Qi*' from the human body exchange. The Lung combines Food-*Qi* with inhaled Clean *Qi* to form Pectoral *Qi* (*ZongQi*), which is further spread all over the body to nourish tissues and to promote physiological processes. Second, the Lung controls the dispersion/descent and maintenance of water metabolism. The Lung can disperse or spread Defensive *Qi* and the essence of food and drink all over the body warmly to moisturize skin and muscles and to nourish the whole body. In addition, since the Lung is the uppermost organ in the body, the Lung-*Qi* must descend to communicate with the Kidney-*Qi*, and to push the water in upper *Jiao* downward to the Kidney and the Urinary Bladder. Third, the Lung connects the skin, perspiration glands, pores and hair, and is capable of spreading *JinYe* and Defensive *Qi* to the skin, perspiration glands, pores and hair to nourish and moisturize them so as to strengthen the body to fight against invasion of External Pathogenic Factors. Finally, the Lung opens into the nose, the gate of the Lung through which the fresh air enters and the 'Waste *Qi*' exhales. The major functions of the nose, ventilation and smelling, mainly depend on the Lung-*Qi*.

(5) The Kidney is often referred to as the Kidney Essence (Kidney-*Yin*) and the Kidney-*Qi* (Kidney-*Yang*). The former is derived from the parents and established at conception, while the latter is transformed from the former after birth. Since Kidney-*Yin* and Kidney-*Yang* are the foundation of the *Yin* and *Yang* for all the other organs, they are also called 'Original *Yin*' and 'Original *Yang*', respectively. Kidney-*Yin* is the fundamental substance for birth, growth and reproduction, while Kidney-*Yang* is the motive force of all physiological processes. The Kidney has various functions. A primary function of the Kidney is to store the essence. The Kidney stores both 'Inherited

Essence' and 'Acquired Essence', which are, respectively, born from the parents at conception and from refined essence extracted from food and drink through the transforming power of the other *Zang-Fu* (internal organs). The Inherited Essence determines the basic constitution, growth, sexual maturation, fertility, development, strength and vitality of the human body. The Acquired Essence is also known as 'Essence of Five *Zang* and Six *Fu*', part of which is stored in the Kidney in preparation for future needs. The second function of the Kidney is to dominate the regulation of water metabolism, which is to spread *JinYe* all over the body and to discharge the waste fluid produced by all the *Zang-Fu* from the body. The Kidney is like a gate that has the function of opening and closing. Under physiological conditions, a correct balance between Kidney-*Yin* and Kidney-*Yang* exists, resulting in the correct regulation of the opening and closing of the 'gate'. Opening the gate eliminates the water (urine), while closing the gate helps retain the water (*JinYe*) needed by the organs. The third function of the Kidney is to control the reception of *Qi* (air). TCM holds that, to make use of the 'Clear *Qi*' of the air, the Lung and the Kidney work together. The Lung has a 'Descending Action' on *Qi*, which is directed down to the Kidney that responds by 'holding' this *Qi* down. The fourth function of the Kidney is to produce the Marrow to nourish the bones and fill up the Brain. Kidney-Essence is the organic foundation for the production of the Marrow, which is stored in the bone cavity to supply the nourishment to bones. 'Marrow' in TCM means a substance that is the common matrix of bones, bone marrow, Brain and Spinal cord. Thus, the Kidney-Essence produces the Marrow, which generates the Spinal cord and 'fills up' the Brain. For this reason, the Brain has a physiological relationship with the Kidney in TCM. The fifth function of the Kidney is to manifest on the hair. The hair is nourished by the Blood, but originates from the Kidney-Essence, as it can transform the Blood. Therefore, the quality and color of the hair are related to the state of the Kidney-Essence. The final primary function of the Kidney is to

open into the ear and control the two lower orifices (Ear-*Yin*). The ears rely on nourishment from the Essence for their proper function and are therefore physiologically related to the Kidney. The two lower orifices mean the front and the rear private parts, which include the urethra, the genitalia and the anus. These orifices are functionally related to the Kidney.

Ming Men

Ming Men is often translated as 'The Gate of Vitality' in English. It first appeared in the classical *Huang Di Nei Jing* (475–221 BC), and many different explanations have been given since then. However, it is commonly believed that the real meaning of the term '*Ming Men*' is basically the same as that of the Kidney-*Yang*, and the term is only used to emphasize the importance of the Kidney-*Yang*.

Six Fu

(1) The Small Intestine dominates the reception of food content from the Stomach, absorbs and digests the food content and separates the useful/clarity from the waste/turbidity.

(2) The Gallbladder stores and excretes bile, and dominates decision-making and judgement.

(3) The Stomach receives food and drink, dominates the digestion of food, governs the transportation of the content of food/drink and directs Stomach-*Qi* downward.

(4) The Large Intestine dominates transportation of waste.

(5) The Urinary Bladder stores and eliminates urine.

(6) The Triple *Jiao* (*SanJiao*) has three components. The Upper *Jiao* (*ShangJiao*) controls respiration and dominates the Lung's dispersing function. It spreads nutrients and vital energy throughout

the whole body, which is why the Upper *Jiao* is referred to as a 'Sprayer'. The Middle *Jiao* (*ZhongJiao*), also referred to as a 'Fermentation Tank', dominates the digestion of food and the transformation of the 'Essence of Food and Drink'. The Lower *Jiao* (*XiaJiao*) controls the separation of the useful (clarity) from the waste (turbidity), and eliminates (to filter and drain off) the waste. It is often described as a 'Drainage Ditch'.

Extraordinary Organs

In addition to the regular *Yin* and *Yang* organs, there are also six Extraordinary Organs functioning like *Yin* organs (i.e. storing the Essence but not excreting anything), and having the shape of *Yang* organs (i.e. hollow). Functionally, all the six Extraordinary Organs are directly or indirectly related to the Kidney. The names of these organs are as follows: Brain, Marrow, Bones, Channels and Collaterals, Gallbladder and Uterus.

Since the Brain and the Uterus were not mentioned in the previous paragraphs, they are introduced here. The Brain is formed by the Marrow and is contained in the cranial cavity. As predicted by TCM, 'The Brain is a sea of the Marrow'. The Brain controls thinking activity of the human body and dominates the audio and visual senses. TCM also believes that the Uterus' functions in producing menses and conceiving pregnancy are mainly related to the functions of the Heart (controlling the Blood circulation), the Liver (storing the Blood), the Spleen (keeping the Blood flow within the vessels), the Kidney (retaining the reproductive essence) and the *Ren* Channel as well as the *Chong* Channel (both supplying the Blood to the Uterus). Therefore, the Uterus in TCM refers not only to the organ itself but also to the different internal systems.

The theory of the Channels and Collaterals

This theory describes the mutual relationship between the physiology and pathology of the Channels and Collaterals. It forms the basis for acupuncture and Naprapathy practitioners.

Channel means 'route' in Chinese, and is the main trunk distributed vertically in the whole system of Channels and Collaterals. The Collateral implies 'net', and is the branch of a channel in the system. Different Channels and Collaterals are linked with each other and distributed to cover the whole human body so that the superficial, interior, upper and lower portions of the body are connected into an organic whole.

The system of the Channels and Collaterals mainly consists of 20 Channels, their branches and their subsidiary parts. The Channels are divided into 12 regular and eight extra ones. The Collaterals, of which there are 15, are referred to as connective. Others may be superficial or small.

THE CAUSES OF DISEASES IN TRADITIONAL CHINESE MEDICINE

Identifying the root cause of the disease is a very important part in TCM practice. TCM stresses that balance is the key to a healthy body. Any long-term imbalance such as extreme climate change, overdue physical exercise, heavy workload, excessive rest, too frequent (or rare) sexual activity, unbalanced diet, unbalanced emotional changes, etc. can all be attributed to the cause of a disease. Therefore, various causes of disease in TCM mainly include Six Exogenous Factors, Epidemic Pathogenic Factors, parasites, internal imbalance caused by Seven Emotional Changes, Improper Diet, maladjustment between work/exercise and rest, trauma and the Phlegm/Fluid Retention and Blood Stasis.

In recognizing the cause of a disease, TCM practitioners focus on analyzing signs as well as symptoms, and identifying different patterns, in addition to understanding the objective conditions that might be possible factors in a disease, called 'Identifying the Pattern to work out the causes'. The causes of disease are discussed below.

Six Exogenous Factors

'Six Exogenous Factors' is a general term for the six climatic conditions in excess: Pathogenic Wind,

Pathogenic Cold, Pathogenic Summer Heat, Pathogenic Dampness, Pathogenic Dryness and Pathogenic Fire.

Pathogenic Wind prevails in the spring, but occurs in all the seasons. It has characteristics of being apt to move; tending to rise, disperse, and move upward and outward; being apt to migrate and change, leading to mobility; and causing all other diseases.

Pathogenic Cold prevails in winter, but also exists in other seasons. Its characteristics are quickly consuming the *Yang* of the human body; coagulating *Qi* and the Blood in Channels and Collaterals or even blocking circulation of both *Qi* and the Blood; and causing contraction of the skin, muscles, Channels and Collaterals, tendons and ligaments.

Pathogenic Summer Heat prevails in summer, with characteristics of a hot nature; quickly exhausting *Qi* and consuming *JinYe*; and often accompanying Pathogenic Dampness.

Pathogenic Dampness often occurs in late summer, a period of transition from summer to autumn. It always has characteristics of a heavy and turbid nature, of viscousness, lingering in nature, of going downward and of easily consuming the *Yang* of the human body.

Pathogenic Dryness prevails in autumn. It quickly consumes the *JinYe* of the human body, and easily impairs the Lung.

Pathogenic Fire is divided into External Fire and Endogenous Fire. It is hot in nature; capable of flaring up; quickly consuming *JinYe* and exhausting *Qi*; able to produce Endogenous Wind, resulting from over-consuming the Liver-*Yin*; causes various bleedings; easily causes carbuncles and sores; and frequently irritates the Heart and the Mind.

Epidemic Pathogenic Factor

Epidemic Pathogenic Factor is a kind of pathogen with very strong infectivity, and also a minute pathogenic substance, such as a pathogenic micro-organism, which usually invades the human body through the mouth and nose, and cannot be directly observed by the human sensory organs. Sudden onset, similar manifestations, strong infectivity and quick epidemicity

are characteristics in common for all diseases caused by Epidemic Pathogenic Factor.

Parasites

It was a long time ago when TCM started to demonstrate that parasites could cause diseases. The first discussion on treatment of Ascariasis of the Biliary Tract can be traced back to the book '*On Treatment of Diseases Caused by Pathogenic Wind and Cold*' (Shang Han Lun), written in the 3rd century AD. In the Sui dynasty, recognition of Oxyuriasis and Taeniasis was recorded in detail. Since then, it has been proved that Chinese herbs are safe and reliable in the treatment of parasitoses.

Internal imbalance caused by Seven Emotional Changes

Seven Emotional Changes in TCM refer to seven different kinds of emotional reactions, such as joy, anger, melancholy, over-thinking, grief, fright and shock. They are natural responses of the human body to environmental changes, and belong to the normal range of mental activities. However, Seven Emotional Changes become pathogenic factors when sudden/violent or persistent changes of the environment occur, and when it is beyond the human body's endurance.

If Joy becomes excessive excitement, the Heart has the potential to be harmed. Anger includes irritability, frustration and indignation, which affect the Liver. Melancholy/over-thinking indicates excessive mental work that weakens the Spleen. Grief includes sadness, which affects the Lung. Fright harms the Kidney and shock affects both the Kidney and the Heart.

Improper diet

Improper diet includes abnormal ingestion, contaminated food and food preference. Any of these gives rise to diseases, such as acid regurgitation, anorexia, vomiting and diarrhea.

Maladjustment between work/exercise and rest

Maladjustment includes physical over-strain, mental over-strain, sexual over-strain and excessive rest. Any of the above over-strains would result in a different type of disease due to 'Qi Exhaustion', 'Over-Consumption of the Heart–Blood/the Spleen-Qi' and 'Over-Consumption of the Kidney-Essence'. Excessive rest could give rise to poor circulation of Qi and the Blood, and thus cause further diseases.

Traumas

Traumas include gunshot or incised wounds; traumatic injuries (injuries by knife or spear, fall or stumble, contusion, stabbing and abrasion, and by sports); injuries by heavy load, twist, sprain or wrench; burns or scalds; and bites by insects or beasts. Any of the above would cause at least bleeding, swelling and pain, fractures or joint dislocation, internal bleeding and, at most, even death.

Phlegm/Fluid Retention and Blood Stasis

Both Phlegm/Fluid Retention and Blood Stasis derive from the pathological changes of the human body. When they are formed, they might, in turn, act directly or indirectly on some tissues or organs of the body to cause new diseases or different syndromes, in which Phlegm/Fluid Retention and Blood Stasis become another group of pathogenic factors.

Pathogenesis

Pathogenesis is the mechanism of the occurrence and the development of a disease. TCM believes that there are two major factors causing the occurrence of disease: the deficiency of the Vital-Qi, which refers to the physiological functions of the body, and the Pathogenic-Qi, which extensively covers any kind of pathogenic factor causing damage to the body. Basic pathogenesis includes Vital-Qi fighting against Pathogenic-Qi, an Imbalance between Yin and Yang and lack of control of Qi's ascending or its descending.

METHODS OF DIAGNOSIS IN TRADITIONAL CHINESE MEDICINE

TCM diagnosis is intimately related to 'Identification of Disease Patterns' as this provides the diagnostic tools necessary to identify the patterns, and is based on the fundamental principle that signs and symptoms reflect the condition of the internal organs. TCM uses not only symptoms and signs, but many other manifestations to form a picture of the disease pattern present in a particular person. Many of the so-called symptoms and signs would not be considered as such in Western medicine.

Over the centuries, TCM diagnosis has developed an extremely sophisticated system of correspondences between outward signs and internal organs. It includes four methods traditionally described with four words: observation, listening/smelling, inquiring and palpation.

Observation

Expression

This is the outward manifestation of the vital activities.

Body

The body consists of five different constitutional body shapes. The 'Wood type' is tall and slender. The 'Fire type' has a small pointed head and small hands. The 'Earth type' has a slightly fat body with a large head and belly, and wide jaw. The 'Gold type' has broad and square shoulders, a strongly built body and a triangular face. The 'Water type' has a round face and body with a long spine.

Hair

The state of the hair is related to the condition of the Blood/Kidney Essence.

Face color

Face color reflects the state of *Qi*/Blood and condition of the Mind.

Eyes

The eyes reflect the state of the Mind and the Essence.

Nose

If the tip of the nose is green/blue, abdominal pain is indicated. If the tip of the nose is yellow, Dampness is present. If the tip of the nose is white, Blood Deficiency is a concern. if the tip of the nose is red, Heat is present in the Lung and Spleen. If the tip of the nose is gray, an impairment of Water movement is indicated.

Ears

If the color of the ears is white, a Cold pattern exists. If they are black, pain is present. Dryness indicates extreme exhaustion of Kidney-*Qi*.

Mouth and lips

If the color of one's mouth and lips is very pale, Emptiness of Blood or *Yang* is suggested. If the color is deep red, Heat is present in the Spleen/Stomach. If the color is purple, Blood circulation is not functioning well. If the color is greenish, Stasis of Liver-Blood and Stagnation of Liver-*Qi* invading the Spleen could be problematic.

Teeth and gums

Teeth bright in color and dry like stone indicates Heat. A dry and gray (like bones) presentation indicates Empty-Heat. Bleeding, painful or swollen gums suggests extreme Heat in the Stomach. Swollen gums without pain indicate Empty-Heat. Very pale gums indicate Deficiency of Blood.

Throat

Pain, redness and swollen throat implies invasion of exterior Wind-Heat/Fire in the Stomach. Sore and dry throat reveals a 'Deficiency of Kidney-*Yin*' with Empty-Heat.

Limbs

If nails are pale, there is a potential suspect for Blood Deficiency. Stasis of the Blood produces a bluish color.

Skin

Deficiency of Liver-Blood will cause the skin to dry. Itchy skin is caused by the Wind. Edema produces swelling and is due to 'Emptiness of Kidney-*Yang*'. Yellow skin indicates jaundice.

Tongue

A normal tongue is of proper size, light red in color, free in motion and has a thin layer of white coating over the surface. It is neither dry nor over-moist. Tongue observation is based on the following:

(1) The tongue color indicates the conditions of Blood, Nutritive *Qi* and *Yin* organs.

   (a) A pale tongue indicates patterns of Empty-Cold, caused by 'Deficiency of *Yang*-*Qi*', 'Insufficiency of both *Qi* and Blood' and invasion by Exogenous Pathogenic Cold.

   (b) A red tongue indicates various patterns of Excess-Heat, due to invasion by Pathogenic Heat, and patterns of Empty-Heat resulting from over-consumption of *JinYe*.

   (c) A deep red tongue occurs in the severe stage of febrile disease in which the Pathogenic Heat has been transmitted to the inside body, and in patterns of Empty-Heat.

(d) A purplish tongue indicates 'Stagnation of both *Qi* and Blood' or 'preponderance of Endogenous Cold' due to 'Deficiency of *Yang*'.

(2) A flabby tongue indicates Deficiency of both *Qi* and *Yang* and 'Retention of Dampness' inside the body.

(3) A cracked tongue indicates over-consumption of *Jin Ye* by Excess-Heat, loss of Kidney-Essence and 'Hyperactivity of Empty-Fire'.

(4) A thorny tongue indicates 'Hyperactivity of Pathogenic Heat'.

(5) A rigid and tremulous tongue indicates invasion of Exogenous Heat and disturbance of the Mind by Damp-Heat, or consumption of the Liver-*Yin* due to 'Severe Endogenous-Heat Stirring up the Endogenous-Wind', or 'Obstruction of the Collaterals due to the Wind-Phlegm'.

(6) A deviated tongue indicates a typical 'Obstruction of the Collaterals due to the Wind-Phlegm'.

The tongue coating indicates the state of the *Yang* organs. The moisture indicates the state of the *Jin Ye*.

Channels

In regard to Channels, an observation of signs along the course of a Channel including redness, white streaks, purple spots and skin rashes is necessary.

Listening/Smelling

Listening to speech:

- Speaking feebly and in low tones indicates Patterns of Emptiness.

- Speaking lustily indicates Patterns of Excess/Fullness.

- Delirious speech indicates the Heart Collateral obstructed by Phlegm-Heat.

- Muttering or extreme verbosity indicates disturbance of the Mind.

- Stuttering suggests Collaterals obstructed by Wind-Phlegm.

Listening to breathing:

- A coarse and loud breathing sound indicates a Full Pattern.

- A weak and thin breathing sound indicates an Empty Pattern.

Listening to the cough:

- A loud cough suggests a Full Pattern, such as the Lung invaded by Wind-Cold or obstructed by Cold-Phlegm.

- A clear cough suggests a Full Pattern, but indicates the Lung invaded by Wind-Heat or obstructed by Heat-Phlegm.

- A dry cough with little sputum indicates the Lung invaded by Pathogenic Dryness or 'Deficiency of Lung-*Yin*' for a long time.

Smelling:

- A strong and foul scent is an indicator of Heat.

- An absence of scent indicates Cold.

- Foul breath indicates Heat in the Stomach.

Inquiring

It is necessary to listen attentively to the complaints of the patient, inquire about the onset and duration of the illness and record the medical history. To find out how the problem arose, TCM practitioners must inquire about the living conditions of the patient and his environment, both the emotional and familial environment. The most commonly used areas of questioning today are listed in Table 5.

Palpation

This mainly includes feeling the pulse and palpating Channels and points (Figure 5). When feeling for a pulse, three fingers should be placed above the wrist joint where the radial artery throbs. The area for feeling the pulse is divided into three regions, named *Cun*, *Guan* and *Chi*. The region opposite to the styloid process of the radius is known as *Guan*, that distal to *Guan* is *Cun* and that proximal to *Guan* is *Chi*. Finger force is exerted first lightly, then moderately and finally heavily to get a general idea of the depth, frequency, rhythm, strength and form of the pulse. The relationship between different regions of the pulse and internal organs is reflected in Table 6.

A normal pulse is of medium frequency (4–5 beats per breath) and regular rhythm. It must be even and forceful.

IDENTIFICATION OF DISEASE PATTERNS

TCM diagnoses diseases by using 'Identification of Disease Patterns'. Identification of Disease Patterns is not made from a list of symptoms and signs, but from a reflection on the pathogenesis of the disease. Over centuries of accumulated clinical experience, TCM has developed a comprehensive and extremely effective diagnostic system and symptomatology to identify disease patterns. There are several methods in identifying disease patterns. These methods are based on the following.

Eight Principles are based on the categories of Exterior/Interior, Cold/Hot, Full/Empty, and *Yin/Yang*, which are the foundation for all the other methods of disease pattern identification to identify the location and nature of the disease.

Qi, Blood and *JinYe*, also known as vital substances in TCM, indicate the basic disharmonies such as Deficiency, Stagnation, and Rebellion.

ZangFu is based on pathological changes occurring in the Internal Organs.

Pathogenic Factors are based on the pathological changes occurring when the body is invaded by factors such as Wind, Cold, Heat, Dampness, Dryness and Fire.

The Five Elements are based on the interpretation of clinical manifestations according to generating, over-controlling and insulting sequences.

The Channels, based on the courses of different Channels, is the oldest method that describes the symptoms and signs related to each Channel rather than the organs.

Table 5 Areas of inquiry

Chills and fever
Perspiration
Head and body
Thorax and abdomen
Food and taste
Stools and urine
Sleep
Deafness and tinnitus
Thirst and drink
Pain

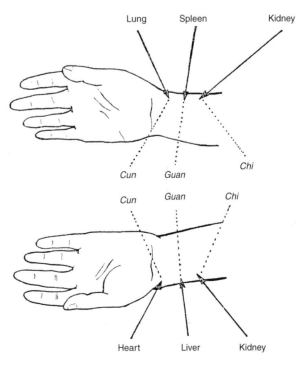

Figure 5 The Three Regions for Feeling the Pulse

Table 6 Relationship between Regions of the Pulse and Internal Organs

Pulse positions	Energy type	Triple Jiao	Organs (left/right)
Front/*Cun*	Qi	Upper	Heart/Lung
Middle/*Guan*	Blood	Middle	Liver/Spleen
Rear/*Chi*	*Yin*	Lower	Kidney/Gate of Vitality

The Reflections on Six Channels is utilized mainly for the diagnosis and treatment of diseases caused by Exterior-Cold, which was formulated by *Zhang, ZhongJing*. It has been the bible for Chinese doctors, especially in northern China, for about 16 centuries. Reflections on:

(1) *Tai-Yang Channel*: aversion to chills, headache, neck stiffness, superficial pulse and fever

(2) *Yang-Min Channel*: aversion to heat, perspiring, thirst, restlessness, abdominal pain aggravated by pressure and constipation

(3) *Shao-Yang Channel*: alternate chills and fever, full sensation in the chest, bitter taste and thirst

(4) *Tai-Yin Channel*: full abdomen, vomiting, diarrhea poor appetite, and weak and slow pulse

(5) *Shao-Yin Channel*: sleepiness, aversion to chills, cold limbs, diarrhea and very weak pulse

(6) *Ju-Yin Channel*: delirium, loss of consciousness, extremely cold limbs, thirst and poor appetite

The Four Stages are the most important and most widely used method, devised by Ye, TianShi (1667–1746), for the treatment of febrile infectious diseases that start with Invasion of the Exterior Wind-Heat:

(1) *Stage I*: *Wei*/Protective Level
    Fever, slight aversion to cold, headache, slight perspiring, slight thirst, superficial and fast pulse

(2) *Stage II*: *Qi*/Defensive Level
    Severe fever, aversion to heat, profuse perspiring, thirst, wheezing, scanty urine, constipation and strong pulse

(3) *Stage III*: *Yin* Level
    High fever (higher during nights), loss of consciousness, delirium, rashes, deep red tongue, yellow tongue coating, threadlike and rapid pulse

(4) *Stage IV*: Blood Level
    Delirium, coma, convulsion, mania, bleeding, and extremely deep red tongue

The Triple Jiao is combined with the Four Stages to make 'Identification of Disease Patterns' and to provide Treatment Principles for febrile infectious diseases starting with Invasion of the Wind-Heat.

TRADITIONAL CHINESE MEDICINE TREATMENT AND TREATMENT PRINCIPLES

Treatment is only provided when 'Treatment Principles' are established. The Treatment Principles are usually set up right after the disease pattern is identified. Since disease patterns are different, treatment principles for each pattern should vary accordingly, and so does treatment.

For example, in the view of Western medicine, cough is a symptom of many diseases, such as respiratory tract infection, bronchitis, bronchiectasis, pneumonia and pulmonary tuberculosis. However, in TCM, it can be identified by the following patterns:

(1) *Pattern A*: Wind-Cold attacking the Lung (*Feng-HanSuoFei*)
    Marked by cough with diluted sputum, profuse watery nasal discharge, chills, headache, stuffy nose, sneezing, thin and white tongue coating and superficial pulse

(2) *Pattern B*: Wind-Heat invading the Lung (*Feng-ReFanFei*)
    Manifested by cough with thick sputum, sore throat, thin and yellow tongue coating and rapid as well as superficial pulse

(3) *Pattern C*: Phlegm-Heat obstructing the Lung (*TanReYongFei*)

Demonstrated by cough with thick and yellow or blood-stained sputum, chest pain, dyspnea, red tongue with yellowish greasy coating and rapid rolling pulse

(4) *Pattern D*: Dryness–Heat over-consuming the Lung-*Yin* (*ZaoReShangFei*)
Marked by cough without sputum or with very sticky sputum, chest pain with severe coughing, dry mouth, red tongue tip, thin and yellow tongue coating without moisture and rapid but weak pulse

(5) *Pattern E*: Phlegm-Dampness blocking the Lung (*TanShiZuFei*)
Indicated by cough with whitish sputum, stuffy sensation in the chest, white and greasy tongue coating and rolling pulse

(6) *Pattern F*: Liver-Fire attacking the Lung (*GanHuo-FanFei*)
Manifested by dry cough caused by upward adverse flow of the Lung-*Qi*, hypochondriac pain with severe coughing, red complexion, dry throat, thin and yellow tongue coating with little moisture, and wiry or rapid pulse

(7) *Pattern G*: Deficiency of the Lung-*Yin* (*FeiYin-KuiXu*)
Indicated by dry cough or cough with little or blood-stained sputum, afternoon hot flush, night sweats, red tongue with little coating and rapid but weak pulse

Therefore, the Treatment Principles for each pattern mentioned above must be established and points selected as below:

(1) *Pattern A*: to Expel the Wind (*QuFeng*), disperse the Cold (*SanHan*) and Transform the Phlegm (*HuaTan*) to stop coughing (*ZhiKe*)
Points: LI 4 (*HeGu*), L 7 (*LieQue*), B 13 (*FeiShu*), G 20 (*FengChi*), S 40 (*FengLong*)

(2) *Pattern B*: to Expel the Wind, Clear away the Heat (*QingRe*) and Resolve the Phlegm (*HuaTan*) to stop coughing
Points: L 10 (*YuJi*), L 5 (*Chi Ze*), *TaiYang*, B 13 (*FeiShu*), G 20 (*FengChi*), S 40 (*FengLong*)

(3) *Pattern C*: to Clear away the Heat and Resolve the Phlegm to stop coughing
Points: L 5 (*Chi Ze*), S 40 (*FengLong*), L 10 (*YuJi*), LI 11 (*QuChi*)

(4) *Pattern D*: to Clear away the Heat from the Lung and Moisten the Dryness (*RunZao*) to stop coughing
Points: B 13 (*FeiShu*), L 5 (*Chi Ze*), CV 22 (*TianTu*), K 3 (*TaiXi*)

(5) *Pattern E*: to Strengthen the Spleen (*JianPi*) to Dispel the Dampness (*Huashi*), and to Transform the Phlegm to stop coughing
Points: B 13 (*FeiShu*), L 9 (*TaiYuan*), B 20 (*PiShu*), Sp 9 (*YinLingQuan*), S 40 (*FengLong*)

(6) *Pattern F*: to Reduce the Fire from the Liver (*QingxieGanHuo*) and Moisten the Lung (*RunFei*) to stop coughing
Points: B 13 (*FeiShu*), L 5 (*Chi Ze*), G 34 (*YangLingQuan*), LR 3 (*TaiChong*)

(7) *Pattern G*: to Tonify *Yin* (*YangYin*) to Distinguish the Empty-Fire in the Lung (*QingRe*) to stop coughing
Points: B 13 (*FeiShu*), L 5 (*Chi Ze*), L 7 (*LieQue*), K 7 (*FuLiu*), H 6 (*YinXi*), Sp 6 (*SanYinJiao*).

Bibliography

Maciocia, G. *The Foundations of Chinese Medicine, A Comprehensive Text for Acupuncturists and Herbalists.* Singapore: Churchill Livingstone, 1995

TCM Group. *The Foundation of Traditional Chinese Medicine.* Shanghai: Science-Technology Press, 1996

Wang, Z. *New Edition on Selection of Acupuncture Points in TCM Internal Medicine.* Beijing: Document Press of Science and Technology, 1995

Yang, Z. *Handbook of Practical Selection of Acupuncture Points.* Beijing: Jin Dun Press, 1990

Beijing College of Traditional Medicine. *Essentials of Chinese Acupuncture.* Beijing: Foreign Language Press, 1985

Chinese herbal medicine and formulation

12

B. Xu

CHINESE HERBAL MEDICINE

Chinese herbal medicine, as the major component of traditional Chinese medicine (TCM), has played a very important role in the promotion of health, prevention of disease and treatment of illnesses for Chinese people for several thousand years.

Nomenclature of Chinese herbs

China spans cold, warm and hot zones, and has a rich variety of medicinally used plants, animals and minerals which all fall into the umbrella of Chinese herbal medicine. Different Chinese herbs usually have different names. The herbal names may sometimes present confusion. However, there are some rules to follow in the nomenclature of Chinese herbs. Most Chinese herbs are named by one of the following rules:

(1) *Place of growth*. To stress the genuine medicinal materials, many Chinese herbs are named after the place where they are grown.

(2) *Growth property*. Different herbs have different growth properties. Therefore, some Chinese herbs are named after their corresponding growth properties.

(3) *Appearance, color or odor*. For intuitive reasons, some Chinese herbs are named after their appearance. Some are named after their color. Others are named after their characteristic odor.

(4) *Functions*. To stress the medicinal functions of herbs, some Chinese herbs are named after their chief therapeutic functions.

(5) *Medicinal parts*. Only a part of the original herb may be used for medicinal use. To stress the part that is used, some herbs are named after the corresponding medicinal part.

(6) *The discoverer*. To commemorate the discoverer of herbs, some Chinese herbs are named after the person who discovered the herb's medicinal function.

(7) *Translated name*. Some herbs originally were grown in other nations. To emphasize the original place from where the herb came, some herbs are named by translated names.

Properties of Chinese herbs

The properties of Chinese herbs are governed by the theory of the nature of TCM. Based on the theory, all Chinese herbs can be characterized by *Qi*, flavor, channel tropism and tendency.

Qi

The *Qi* is used to describe the cold, hot, warm and cool properties of herbs. They differ only by degree. Cold and cool herbs have the function of heat-clearing, fire-purging, detoxifying and removal of heat from the blood. Warm and hot herbs have the function of warming the middle-*jiao* to dispel cold, restore *yang* and invigorate the pulse.

Flavor

The flavor is used to describe the sour, bitter, sweet, acrid, salty and bland properties of herbs. Sour herbs have the property of astringency and astriction. They are used to treat sweating due to debility, diarrhea, seminal emission and leukorrhea. Bitter herbs have the property of purgation, drying and consolidation of the *Yin*. Bitter herbs are used to purge heat, relax the bowels, eliminate dampness and keep *Yin*. Sweet herbs have an invigorating property, regulating the stomach and producing respite. Sweet herbs are used to strengthen the body by means of tonics. Acrid herbs have the property of dispersing and moving. Acrid herbs are used to disperse exterior syndrome (caused by invasion of exopathogens in the muscle and skin, the effect of the defensive function by pathogens and the struggle between vital energy and the pathogenic factor), promote blood circulation and stop pain. Salty herbs have the property of softening a hard mass and purging. They are used to resolve hard lumps and relieve constipation. Bland herbs have the property of excreting dampness and diuresis. They are used to treat difficulty in micturition and edema.

The *Qi* and flavor of an herb are correlated with each other and act together to represent the property of the herb.

Channel tropism

Channel tropism represents the property of an herb to act selectively on a specific part of the body. It is employed to match the herbs selected and the organ affected.

Based on channel tropism, some herbs may act as a *medicinal guide*. A *medicinal guide* is a class of herbs meeting the following two criteria: they act on a specific organ; and they lead other herbs to act on this organ.

Tendency

Tendency represents the acting direction of an herb, including ascending, descending, floating and sinking. The ascending and floating herbs act upward and outward. The descending and sinking herbs act downward and inward.

Generally speaking, if the disease location is up and exterior, ascending and floating herbs are needed. If the disease location is low and interior, descending and sinking herbs are needed. If the disease trend is upward, descending herbs are needed. If the disease trend is downward, ascending herbs are needed. Tendency is correlated with herbal *Qi*, flavor, weight, processing and compatibility.

Compatibility of herbs

An herbal formula or prescription usually contains different herbs. The herbs in a formula are not randomly selected. There are close relationships between these herbs. These relationships are summarized as compatibility of herbs.

Generally speaking, there are seven types of compatibility in a formula:

(1) *Using a single herb*. This is the simplest case, in which only one herb is used.

(2) *Mutual reinforcement*. In this case, two herbs reinforce each other's functions.

(3) *Mutual assistance*. In this case, a herb (ministerial herb) can promote the function of another herb (monarch herb).

(4) *Mutual restraint*. In this case, one herb's side-effects and toxicity are reduced or eliminated by another herb.

(5) *Mutual detoxification*. In this case, one herb can reduce or eliminate another herb's toxicity or side-effects. This is in fact another expression of mutual restraint.

(6) *Mutual inhibition*. In this case, one herb reduces or nullifies another herb's function.

(7) *Antagonism*. In this case, the combination of two herbs causes adverse side-effects and toxicity. This is where the herbs can be toxic or dangerous if applied inappropriately.

Owing to current confusion and misunderstanding regarding herbs and herbal products, it is necessary to address the herbal safety issue further here. There are differences between the adverse side-effects of chemical drugs and the adverse side-effects of herbs[1]. The adverse side-effects of a chemical drug are experienced no matter whether the drug is applied appropriately or not. The side-effects of a chemical drug will be experienced even if the physician and the patient follow the correct directions. However, most adverse side-effects in Chinese herbal medicine arise from the inappropriate application of herbs.

The inappropriate applications of Chinese herbal medicine include: wrong diagnosis; inappropriate selection of herbs; inappropriate combination of herbs; inappropriate processing of herbs; inappropriate methods of administering herbs; inappropriately high dosage; inappropriately long application; and inappropriate administration of herbs with other drugs. Any one or more of the above inappropriate applications will lead to herbal adverse effects. Because only qualified TCM doctors are capable of avoiding the above situations, the public are not recommended to take Chinese herbs without supervision.

There are many contraindications in Chinese herbal medicine. If a Doctor of Chinese Medicine fails to observe these precautions, or if the public take herbs by their own choice, serious adverse effects or even fatal accidents may occur. There have been numerous lessons on the danger of herbs in TCM history.

Currently in the USA, herbs are classified as Food Dietary Supplements[2]. In this author's opinion, this classification is inappropriate and even misleading. It has sent a misleading message to the public that herbs are as safe as other dietary supplements. In fact, herbs are very different from other dietary supplements. Herbs can be very dangerous or even fatal if they are administered inappropriately. It is due to this safety consideration that we strongly recommended that the Food and Drug Administration (FDA) takes herbs out of the Food Dietary Supplement category, and classifies herbs into a new category[3].

Commonly used Chinese herbs

There are over 5000 documented Chinese herbs; it is beyond the scope of this chapter to cover them all. In this section, we introduce a few commonly used Chinese herbs.

Dan Shen (radix Salviae miltiorrhizae)

Properties Bitter and mild cold. Belonging to the heart, pericardium and liver channels.

Functions and indications

(1) Promoting blood circulation by removing blood stasis. *Dan Shen* is used to treat stasis due to blood-heat.

(2) Promoting blood circulation to subdue swelling. *Dan Shen* is used to treat carbuncles and boils.

(3) Nourishing the blood and tranquilizing. *Dan Shen* is used to treat insomnia, headache, dizziness and palpitations.

Dosage and directions Approximately 3–15 g/day. Used in decoction.

Dang Gui (radix Angelicae sinensis)

Properties Sweet, acrid and warm. Belonging to the liver, heart and spleen channels.

Functions and indications

(1) Enriching the blood and regulating menstruation. *Dang Gui* is used to treat blood deficiency.

(2) Promoting blood circulation to stop pain. *Dang Gui* is used to treat traumatic injury, carbuncles, boils, and arthralgia due to wind-dampness.

(3) Loosening the bowel to relieve constipation. *Dang Gui* is used to treat constipation of blood deficiency type.

Dosage and directions Approximately 6–15 g/day. Used in decoction. The body (the trunk of the herb) is used to enrich blood. The tail is used to promote blood circulation.

Du Huo (radix Angelicae pubescentis)

Properties Acrid, bitter and mild warm. Belonging to kidney and urinary bladder channels.

Functions and indications

(1) Expelling wind, removing dampness, and alleviating pain. *Du Huo* is used to treat arthralgia due to wind-cold-dampness.

(2) Dispelling cold and relieving exterior syndrome. *Du Huo* is used to treat effect of exopathogen with wind-cold-dampness.

Dosage and directions Approximately 3–9 g/day. Used in decoction.

Attention and contraindications *Du Huo* should not be applied in arthralgia with deficiency of *Qi* and blood.

Ma Huang (herba Ephedra)

Properties Acrid, mildly bitter and warm. Belongs to lung and urinary bladder channels.

Functions and indications

(1) Relieving superficies syndrome (similar to exterior syndrome but located more superficially) by means of diaphoresis. *Ma Huang* is used to treat the effect of wind-cold with aversion to cold, fever, headache, stuffy nose, anhidrosis, and floating and tense pulse.

(2) Facilitating the flow of lung-*Qi* to relieve asthma. *Ma Huang* is used to treat excess dyspnea due to attack of pathogenic wind-cold and obstruction of the lung-*Qi*.

(3) Inducing diuresis to alleviate edema. *Ma Huang* is used to treat excess edema with exterior syndrome, aversion to wind and general edema with fever.

Dosage and directions Approximately 3–10 g/day. Used in decoction. Raw *Ma Huang* is usually used for (1) and (3), and honey-fried *Ma Huang* is usually used for (2).

Attention and contraindications The dosage of *Ma Huang* should not be too large. Patients with lung deficiency, hyperhidrosis and cough with dyspnea should not take *Ma Huang*.

Mai Dong (radix Ophiopogonis)

Properties Sweet, mildly bitter and mildly cold. Belonging to the heart, lung and stomach channels.

Functions and indications

(1) Nourishing *yin* and reinforcing the stomach. *Mai Dong* is used to treat consumption of body fluid caused by heat.

(2) Moistening the lung and clearing away the heart-fire. *Mai Dong* is used to treat *yin* deficiency and dryness of the lung.

Dosage and directions Approximately 6–15 g/day. Used in decoction.

Attention and contraindications *Mai Dong* should not be applied to diarrhea with cold of insufficiency type and cough affected by wind-cold.

Ren Shen (radix Ginseng)

Properties   Sweet, mildly bitter and mildly warm. Belonging to the spleen and lung channels.

Functions and indications

(1) Invigorating *Qi* for emergency treatment of collapse. *Ren Shen* is used to treat collapse due to *Qi* deficiency.

(2) Invigorating *Qi* to strengthen the spleen. *Ren Shen* is used to treat lung, kidney and spleen deficiency.

(3) Promoting the production of body fluid to quench thirst. *Ren Shen* is used to treat febrile disease with thirst and sweating.

(4) Tranquilizing the mind and promoting mentality.

Dosage and directions   Approximately 3–9 g/day (maximum 30 g/day). Used in decoction.

Attention and contraindications   *Ren Shen* cannot be used for heat of excess type, hyperactivity of the liver-*yang* and retention of dampness with overabundance of heat. Incompatible with *Li Lu* (*Veratrum nigrum* L.). Antagonistic with *Wu Ling Zhi* (feces *Trogopterorum*).

Sheng Di (radix Rehmanniae)

Properties   Sweet, bitter and cold. Belonging to the heart, liver and kidney channels.

Functions and indications

(1) Removing pathogenic heat from blood. *Sheng Di* is used to treat epidemic febrile disease.

(2) Removing heat from the blood to stop bleeding. *Sheng Di* is used to treat various types of bleeding due to blood-heat.

(3) Nourishing *Yin* and promoting production of body fluid. *Sheng Di* is used to treat consumption of body fluid caused by febrile disease.

Dosage and directions   Approximately 6–15 g/day. Used in decoction. *Sheng Di* is used unprepared for (1) and is parched into charcoal for (2).

Attention and contraindications   Patients with water retention due to hypofunction of the spleen, abdominal distention and diarrhea should not use *Sheng Di*.

Yin Chen (herba Artemisiae capillaris)

Properties   Bitter and mild cold. Belonging to spleen, stomach, liver and gallbladder channels.

Functions and indications

(1) Clearing away heat, promoting diuresis and treating jaundice. *Yin Chen* is usually used to treat jaundice due to pathogenic damp-heat. It can also be applied to treat jaundice due to cold-dampness.

(2) Expelling ascaris and relieving itching. *Yin Chen* is used to treat biliary ascariasis.

Dosage and directions   Approximately 9–15 g/day (maximum 30 g/day). Used in decoction. Avoid boiling for too long.

CHINESE HERBAL FORMULATION

A formula, or a prescription, in Chinese herbal medicine is composed of a number of herbs. It is formed through careful selection of herbs based on diagnosis, differentiation of symptoms and signs, and treatment plan.

Principles of formulating a prescription

Generally speaking, a formula is composed of four kinds of herb: monarch herb, ministerial herb, adjuvant herb and conductant herb.

Monarch herb

The monarch herb is also called the principal herb. It is the herb in a formula that plays the major role in treating the chief complaint.

Ministerial herb

The ministerial herb is also called the subsidiary herb. It has two functions in a formula:

(1) Assisting the monarch herb to strengthen the treatment for the chief complaint;

(2) Playing a major role in treating accompanying diseases and symptoms.

Adjuvant herb

An adjuvant herb has three functions in a formula:

(1) *Assiting* To assist the monarch and ministerial herbs to strengthen the treatment function.

(2) *Balancing* To eliminate or restrain the toxicity or drastic action of monarch or ministerial herbs.

(3) *Corrigent* In some serious conditions, it is necessary to use a small dosage of corrigent herbs with a property opposite to that of the principal herbs in order to modify the action of the principal herb.

Conductant herb

A conductant herb has two functions in a formula:

(1) *Guiding* To lead other herbs in the formula to reach the diseased location.

(2) *Mediating* To mediate between various herbs in the formula.

In a formula, there is no specific requirement for the number of monarch and ministerial herbs. The rule is to be concise. In addition, not all formulae contain complete monarch, ministerial, adjuvant and conductant herbs. These depend on the disease condition.

Variations of formulae

In addition to the principle of formulating a prescription, some changes of the formula might be needed in application. There are four types of changes to a formula:

(1) *Changing medicinal ingredients.* In this situation, the ministerial herbs are changed and the monarch herb remains. Thus, the formula can be applied to treat different accompanying symptoms.

(2) *Changing the compatibility.* In this situation, the monarch herb is changed, and the formula's functions and indications are changed.

(3) *Modifying the dosage.* In this situation, no herbal component is changed; only the dosage of each component herb is changed. This may also lead to a change in the formula's functions and indications.

(4) *Changing the dosage form.* In this situation, only the dosage form is changed. For example, the decoction form is changed to pill or tablet form, etc. This change will also affect the formula's function and indications.

Dosage forms of formulae

There are many dosage forms in Chinese formulae. The following will introduce some of the commonly used dosage forms.

Decoction

A decoction is prepared by decocting prepared herbs in water or another solvent for a certain time. The decoction is kept as a soup. A decoction takes effect quickly and can be modified easily. It is the most widely used dosage form in TCM.

Pill

A pill is prepared by blending powdered herbs with honey, water or other excipient to make into a bolus. A pill takes effect slowly but lasts longer, and is applicable to chronic disease. It is convenient to administer, store and carry.

Powder

A powder is a preparation of herbs ground into granules for oral administration or external application. It can be easily absorbed, and is convenient to carry.

Medicinal extract

A medicinal extract is prepared by boiling herbs with water or vegetable oil to a concentrated state. It can be used for both oral administration and external application.

Pellet

A pellet is made of melted or sublimated minerals. It can be used for both oral administration and external application.

Tincture

A tincture is prepared by soaking herbs in alcohol for a number of days. It is used for deficiency conditions, pain due to wind–damp, or traumatic injury.

Medicinal tea

Medicinal tea is a brick tea-like preparation made of coarse powdered herbs (with or without tea leaves) and adhesive excipient. It is convenient to carry and administer.

Herbal distillate

An herbal distillate is a preparation obtained through the distillation process via a herb and water.

Commonly used formulae in traditional Chinese medicine

There are thousands of documented Chinese formulae. It is impossible to cover them in detail here. In the following, a few formulae will be discussed as examples of how Chinese formulae work.

An Shen Wan (sedative bolus)

Composition Huang Lian (rhizoma *Coptidis*) 4.5 g, *Zhu Sha* (*Cinnabaris*) 3 g, *Sheng Di* (radix *Rehmanniae*) 1.5 g, *Dang Gui Shen* (radix *Angelicae sinensis* body) 1.5 g, *Zhi Gan Cao* (radix *Glycyrrhizae preparata*) 1.5 g.

Directions Prepared as pills. Administer 9 g at bedtime. It also can be prepared as a decoction.

Functions Relieves palpitations and tranquilizes; replenishes *Yin* and removes heat.

Indications Heart-*Yin* deficiency and flaring-up of the heart-fire with palpitations and insomnias.

Bai Tou Weng Tang (radix Pulsatillae decoction)

Composition Bai Tou Weng (radix *Pulsatillae*) 15 g, *Huang Bai* (cortex *Phellodendri*) 12 g, *Huang Lian* (rhizoma *Coptidis*) 6 g, *Qin Pi* (cortex *Fraxini*) 9 g.

Directions Prepared as a decoction.

Functions Clears away heat and toxic materials, eliminates pathogenic heat from blood and treats diarrhea.

Indications Dysentery due to damp-heat pathogen with diarrhea, abdominal pain, tenesmus, bloody mucous stool, burning sensation of the anus, yellowish and greasy fur (on the tongue), slippery and rapid pulse.

Gui Zhi Tang (ramulus Cinnamomi decoction)

Composition Gui Zhi (ramulus *Cinnamomi*) 4.5–9 g, *Bai Shao* (radix *Paeoniae alba*) 4.5–9 g, *Gan Cao* (radix *Glycyrrhizae*) 3–6 g, *Sheng Jiang* (rhizoma *Zingiberis recens*) 2–4 g, *Da Zao* (fructus *Jujubae*) four pieces.

Directions Prepared as a decoction. Administer twice a day, and finish one unit per day. After administering the decoction, have the patient ingest a little warm gruel to produce mild sweating.

Functions Expels pathogenic factors from muscles and skin, and regulates *ying* and *wei*.

Indications Wind-cold exterior syndrome of deficiency with headache, fever, sweating, aversion to wind, arthralgia, myalgia, thin and white fur, and floating and moderate pulse.

Liu Wei Di Huang Wan (bolus of six drugs, including Rehmannia)

Composition *Shu Di* (radix *Rehmanniae preparata*) 24 g, *Shan Zhu Yu* (fructus *Corni*) 12 g, *Shan Yao* (rhizoma *Dioscoreae*) 12 g, *Ze Xie* (rhizoma *Alismatis*) 9 g, *Fu Ling* (*Poria*) 9 g, *Mu Dan Pi* (cortex *Moutan*) 9 g.

Directions Prepared as pills. Take 6–9 g one to two times a day. It can also be prepared as a decoction.

Functions Nourishes kidney-*Yin*.

Indications Kidney-*Yin* deficiency with lassitude in loin and leg, dizziness, tinnitus and deafness, night sweat, seminal emission, hectic fever, diabetes, red tongue, scanty fur (on tongue), thin and rapid pulse.

Ma Huang Tang (Ephedra decoction)

Composition *Ma Huang* (*Ephedra*) 4.5–9 g, *Gui Zhi* (ramulus *Cinnamomi*) 6 g, *Xin Ren* (bitter apricot seed) 9 g, *Gan Cao* (radix *Glycyrrhizae*) 3 g.

Directions Prepared as a decoction. After administering the decoction, cover the patient with a quilt to produce mild sweating.

Functions Relieves superficies syndrome by means of diaphoresis, and facilitates the flow of the lung-*Qi* to relieve asthma.

Indications Wind-cold exterior syndrome of excess type with aversion to cold, fever, headache, aching pain, anhidrosis, asthma, thin and white fur, and floating and tense pulse.

Si Wu Tang (decoction of four ingredients)

Composition *Shu Di* (radix *Rehmanniae preparata*) 12 g, *Dang Gui* (radix *Angelicae sinensis*) 9 g, *Bai Shao* (radix *Paeoniae alba*) 9 g, *Chuan Xiong* (rhizoma *Chuanxiong*) 6 g.

Directions Prepared as a decoction.

Functions Enriches the blood and regulates menstruation.

Indications Blood deficiency and stagnation with irregular menstruation, dysmenorrhea, scanty menstruation, blood stasis, metrorrhagia and metrostaxis; dizziness, palpitation, pale tongue, thin and small pulse.

Xiao Chai Hu Tang (minor decoction of Bupleurum)

Composition *Chai Hu* (radix *Bupleuri*) 9 g, *Huang Qin* (radix *Scutellariae*) 6 g, *Ban Xia* (rhizoma *Pinelliae*) 6 g, *Ren Shen* (radix *Ginseng*) 6 g, *Zhi Gan Cao* (radix *Glycyrrhizae preparata*) 3 g, *Sheng Jiang* (rhizoma *Zingiberis recens*) 6 g, *Da Zao* (fructus *Jujubae*) four pieces.

Directions Prepared as a decoction.

Functions Treats Shaoyang diseases.

Indications Shaoyang disease with alternate attacks of chills and fever, feeling of fullness and discomfort in the chest and hypochondria, bitter taste and dry throat, vexation and nausea, thin and white fur, and string pulse.

Yin Chen Hao Tang (Oriental Wormwood decoction)

Composition   *Yin Chen Hao* (herba *Artemisiae capillaris*) 18 g, *Zhi Zi* (fructus *Gardeniae*) 9 g, *Da Huang* (radix et rhizoma *Rhei*) 9 g.

Directions   Prepared as a decoction. Finish one unit per day. Continue taking several units after day 1.

Functions   Clears away heat, promotes diuresis and treats jaundice.

Indications   Jaundice due to damp-heat pathogen with skin and sclera as yellow or orange color, yellow and reddish urine, constipation, oppressed feeling in chest, thirst, greasy hair, and slippery and rapid pulse.

CONCLUSION

Traditional Chinese medicine, as an integral part of Chinese culture, is relatively new to most people in Western culture. The major component of TCM – Chinese herbal medicine – is used over ten times more frequently than acupuncture in China. For the best interest of patients and to protect the integrity of the TCM profession, this author has recommended that the US government regulates the profession of Chinese medicine[1]. For thousands of years, TCM has successfully treated and cured numerous diseases and saved millions or billions of lives. TCM can, should, and will benefit all human beings in the promotion of health, prevention of diseases and treatment of illnesses.

References

1. Xu B. Recommendation on Chinese Medicine in the United States of America to White House Commission on Complementary and Alternative Medicine Policy, December 2001 (www.chht.biz)
2. Food and Drug Administration. *Overview of Dietary Supplements*. US Food and Drug Administration, Center for Food Safety and Applied Nutrition. 3 January 2001 (www.fda.gov)
3. Xu B. Supplement of Recommendation on Chinese Medicine in the United States of America to White House Commission on Complementary and Alternative Medicine Policy, February 2002 (www.chht.biz)

Other forms of complementary and alternative medicine therapy 13

L. Dey, P. J. Barrett and C.-S. Yuan

CHIROPRACTIC MEDICINE

Chiropractic medicine is a healing approach that asserts that proper alignment of the spinal column is essential to health. Treatment is by improving the human body's natural ability to heal rather than by treating a specific disease. Although there are many references to spinal manipulation, dating as far back as Galen and Hippocrates[1], modern chiropractic medicine originated in 1895 after Daniel David Palmer performed his first spinal adjustment. Palmer, who was originally trained as a magnetic healer, believed in the body's inherent ability to heal itself, referred to as 'innate intelligence'. Palmer viewed surgery and drugs as invasive and unnatural, and believed that the most effective approach to healing was by restoring normal nervous system function. He is credited with developing spinal manipulations and making chiropractic medicine a profession[2].

Prevalence

Once considered to be unconventional, chiropractic medicine, since the 1970s, has quickly found itself in the mainstream of modern medicine, as the number of patients in the USA using chiropractors tripled from 3.6% to 11% during the 1980s to the late 20th century. Visits to chiropractors comprise about 30% (190 million patient visits) of all visits to complementary and alternative medicine (CAM) providers[3]. To meet the increasing demand, the number of chiropractors in the country, currently approximately 60000, is expected to grow to 100000 by 2010[4].

Since the 1970s, Medicare has paid for chiropractic services and currently approximately 50% of health maintenance organizations and 75% of private insurance companies cover costs[5]. Additionally, 65% of primary care physicians stated that they were 'moderately' or 'very' informed about chiropractic medicine, and that same percentage has referred patients to chiropractors[6]. Clearly, chiropractic medicine is widely utilized by many patients in the USA.

Training

Training to become a licensed chiropractor in the USA requires 4 years of professional education before qualifying for licensure examinations. Similar to allopathic medicine, those pursuing careers as chiropractors are required to spend about 30% of their time studying basic sciences and 70% in clinical courses, where they focus more on anatomy and physiology and less on public heath. Furthermore, little time is spent on surgery, pharmacology and critical care, and more is focused on learning manual treatment methods, biomechanics and musculoskeletal functions. There are also postgraduate opportunities to specialize in areas such as neurology, sports, rehabilitation, pediatrics and radiology[7].

Practice and treatment

Central to the practice of chiropractic medicine is spinal manipulation or adjustment. There are several different types of spinal adjustment techniques, but all utilize an applied force to a specific area of the body intending to be therapeutic. This force varies in intensity, duration, frequency and location, depending on the goal of treatment. Spinal adjustments have been associated with treating many problems including hypertension, musculoskeletal pain, migraines, asthma, carpal tunnel syndrome, infantile colic, enuresis, premenstrual syndrome, cervicogenic headache and muscle tension headache[8].

Chiropractors utilize a variety of approaches to heal, besides spinal adjustments. In addition to suggesting nutritional improvements and exercise regimens, many chiropractors use therapies such as heat, cold and electrical methods. The practice of chiropractic medicine also involves taking a history and performing a physical examination before treatment[8]. Use of advanced diagnostic techniques is rare except for plain film radiography, which corresponds to chiropractors' emphasis on knowledge of anatomy[9].

Mechanism and effectiveness

Spinal adjustments have been associated with physiological changes including attenuation of motor neuron activity[10], increased pain tolerance[11], changes in substance P levels[12] and β-endorphins[13], increased joint motion[14] and increased muscle strength[15]. Some randomized, controlled trials of chiropractic effectiveness in treating musculoskeletal pain have indicated that spinal adjustments appear to be useful in treating low-back pain, neck pain and headache. There are other studies, however, that have suggested that spinal adjustments have no effect on musculoskeletal problems[16–20].

Furthermore, anecdotal reports and case studies have suggested that chiropractic methods may help treat hypertension[21], chronic asthma[22], enuresis[23], premenstrual syndrome[24], infantile colic[25] and primary dysmenorrhea[26]. More studies are needed to investigate the effectiveness of chiropractic therapies.

Risks

Complications associated with chiropractic therapies include headache, fatigue and discomfort that subside after a few days[27]. Other, more serious, potential risks are cauda equina syndrome, resulting from lumbar manipulation and cerebrovascular artery dissection as a consequence of cervical manipulation. Complications from lumbar manipulations occur in one per 100 million cases[16] and cerebrovascular complications occur in about 1 of every 400 000 cervical manipulations[28].

Conclusion

Chiropractic medicine is utilized by many Americans and appears to be effective in treating many health problems. Although more studies are needed to demonstrate its effectiveness and role in modern medicine, it is evident that knowledge of chiropractic therapies will help physicians provide better care as this field continues to define itself, and moves from being considered an alternative approach to being a part of standard medical practice.

References

1. Anderson R. Spinal manipulation before chiropractic. In Haldeman S, ed. *Principles and Practice of Chiropractic*. Norwalk, CT: Appleton & Lange, 1992:3–14
2. Moore J. *Chiropractic in America. The History of a Medical Alternative.* Baltimore, MD: Johns Hopkins University Press, 1993
3. Eisenberg DM, Davis RB, Ettner SL, Appel S, Wilkey S, Van Rompay M. Trends in alternative medicine in the United States, 1990–1997: results of a follow-up national survey. *J Am Med Assoc* 1998;280:1569–75
4. Cooper RA, Stoflet SJ. Trends in the education and practice of alternative medicine clinicians. *Health Aff (Millwood)* 1996;15:226–38

5. Jensen GA, Mootz RD, Shekelle PG, Cherkin DC, Roychoudhury C, Cherkin DC. Insurance coverage of chiropractic services. In Cherkin DC, Mootz RD, eds. *Chiropractic in the United States: Training, Practice, and Research.* Rockville, MD: Agency for Health Care Policy and Research, 1997:39–47

6. Mainous AG, Gill JM, Zoller JS, Wolman MG. Fragmentation of patient care between chiropractors and family physicians. *Arch Fam Med* 2000;9:446–50

7. Coulter I, Adams A, Coggan P, Wilkes M, Gonyea M. A comparative study of chiropractic and medical education. *Altern Ther Health Med* 1998;4:64–75

8. Bergmann TF, Peterson DH, Lawerence DJ. *Chiropractic Technique: Principles and Procedures.* New York, NY: Churchill Livingstone, 1993

9. Christensen M. *Job Analysis of Chiropractic. A Project Report, Survey Analysis and Summary of the Practice of Chiropractic within the United States.* Greely, CO: National Board of Chiropractic Examiners, 2000

10. Dishman JD, Bulbulian R. Spinal reflex attenuation associated with spinal manipulation. *Spine* 2000;25:2519–24; discussion 2525

11. Terrett AC, Vernon H. Manipulation and pain tolerance. A controlled study of the effect of spinal manipulation on paraspinal cutaneous pain tolerance levels. *Am J Phys Med* 1984;63:217–25

12. Brennan PC, Triano JJ, McGregor M, Kokjohn K, Hondras MA, Brennan DC. Enhanced neutrophil respiratory burst as a biological marker for manipulation forces: duration of the effect and association with substance P and tumor necrosis factor. *J Manipulative Physiol Ther* 1992;15:83–9

13. Vernon HT, Dhami MS, Howley TP, Annett R. Spinal manipulation and beta-endorphin: a controlled study of the effect of a spinal manipulation on plasma beta-endophorin levels in normal males. *J Manipulative Physiol Ther* 1986;9:155–23

14. Mierau D. Manipulation and mobilization of the third metacarpophalangeal joint: a quantitative radiographic and range of motion study. *Manual Med* 1988;3:135–40

15. Keller TS, Colloca CJ. Mechanical force spinal manipulation increases trunk muscle strength assessed by electromyography: a comparative clinical trial. *J Manipulative Physiol Ther* 2000;25:585–95

16. Shekelle PG, Adams AH, Chassin MR, Hurwitz El, Brook RH. Spinal manipulation for low-back pain. *Ann Intern Med* 1992;117:590–8

17. Koes BW, Assendelft WJ, van der Heijden GJ, Bouter LM. Spinal manipulation for low back pain. An updated systematic review of randomized clinical trials. *Spine* 1996;21:2860–71; discussion 2872–3

18. Hurwitz EL, Aker PD, Adams AH, Meeker WC, Shekelle PG. Manipulation and mobilization of the cervical spine. A systematic review of the literature. *Spine* 1996;21:1746–59; discussion 1759–60

19. Aker PD, Gross AR, Goldsmith CH, Peloso P. Conservative management of mechanical neck pain: systematic overview and meta-analysis. *Br Med J* 1996;313:1291–6.

20. Anderson R, Meeker WC, Wirick BE, Mootz RD, Kirk DH, Adams A. A meta analysis of clinical trials of spinal manipulations. *J Manipulative Physiol Ther* 1992;15:181–94

21. Yates RG, Lamping DL, Abram NL, Wright C. Effects of chiropractic treatment on blood pressure and anxiety: a randomized, controlled trial. *J Manipulative Physiol Ther* 1988;11:484–8

22. Balon J, Aker PD, Crowther ER, Danielson C, Cox PG, O'Shaughnessy D. A comparison review of active and stimulated chiropractic manipulation as adjunctive treatment for childhood asthma. *N Engl J Med* 1998;339:1013–20

23. Reed WR, Beavers S, Reddy SK, Kern G. Chiropractic management of primary nocturnal enuresis. *J Manipulative Physiol Ther* 1994;17:596–600

24. Walsh MJ, Polus BI. A randomized, placebo-controlled clinical trial on the efficacy of chiropractic therapy on premenstrual syndrome. *J Manipulative Physiol Ther* 1999;22:582–5

25. Wiberg JM, Nordsteen J, Nilsson N. The short-term effect of spinal manipulation in the treatment of infantile colic: a randomized controlled clinical trial with a blinded oberserver. *J Manipulative Physiol Ther* 1999;22:517–22

26. Kokjohn K, Schmid DM, Triano JJ, Brennan PC. The effect of spinal manipulation on pain and prostaglandin levels in women with primary dysmenorrhea. *J Manipulative Physiol Ther* 1992;15:279–85

27. Senstad O, Leboeuf-Yde C, Borchgrevinck C. Frequency and characteristics of side effects of spinal manipulative therapy. *Spine* 1997;22:435–40; discussion 440–1

28. Dvorak J, Orelli F. How dangerous is manipulation of the cervical spine: case report and results of a survey. *Manual Med* 1985;2:1–4

Further reading

McGill L. *The Chiropractor's Health Book: Simple, Natural Exercises for Relieving Headaches, Tension, and Back Pain.* New York, NY: Crown Publishing, 1997

Rondberg TA, Feuling TJ. *Chiropractic: Compassion and Expectation.* Gardena, CA: SCB Distributors, 1999

Wardwell WI. *Chiropractic. History and Evolution of a New Profession.* St Louis, MO: Mosby-Year Books, 1992

MASSAGE THERAPY

Massage therapy is one of the oldest forms of treatment in the world, having been first described in China in the 2nd century BC and soon after in India and Egypt. The development of modern massage is attributed to the Swede Per Henrik Ling, who developed an integrated system consisting of massage and exercises, which was later termed 'Swedish massage'. In the middle of the 19th century it was introduced into the USA and was practiced predominantly by physicians until the early 20th century. The interest in massage therapy gradually declined, but increased again in the 1970s.

Massage therapy is a method of manipulating the soft tissue of whole body areas using pressure and traction. Touch is fundamental to massage therapy and allows the therapist to locate areas of muscle tension. The friction of the hands and the mechanical pressure exerted on cutaneous and subcutaneous structures affect the body. The circulation of blood and lymph is generally enhanced, resulting in an increased oxygen supply and facilitating the removal of waste products. Direct mechanical pressure and effects mediated by the nervous system beneficially affect areas of increased muscular tension. This is accompanied by the release of natural pain killers such as serotonin and natural killer cells, which enhance immune function. Conditions frequently treated are back pain and other musculoskeletal disorders, constipation, anxiety, depression, stress and many other conditions.

Swedish massage is usually given on a massage table, on the floor or on a special massage chair. Therapists often use oil to facilitate movement of their hands over the patient's body. The five fundamental techniques used in massage are effleurage (smooth stroking), pétrissage (kneading-type movements), friction, tapotement and vibration. Sometimes sessions are followed by other treatments, such as external heat application. Usually, one or two sessions per week for a treatment period of 4–8 weeks of 30 min duration would be initially recommended. Child sessions in the studies were performed by parents on a nightly basis for 15 min in a duration of 30 days.

Studies showed the beneficial effects of massage therapy in facilitating growth, increasing alertness and enhancing immune function, while reducing pain, stress, anxiety and depression. There is evidence that abdominal massage could be a promising treatment option for constipation[1]. Another systematic review[2] of controlled trials for the treatment of lower back pain concluded that it seemed to have some potential. Some evidence from controlled trials suggested positive effects of massage for anxiety in depressed adolescent mothers[3], in women with premenstrual syndrome[4] and in elderly institutionalized patients[5]. In patients with fibromyalgia, it has been suggested to relieve pain and depression and improve the quality of life[6]. Pain alleviation by massage therapy has often been attributed to the gate theory[7]. This theory suggests that pain can be alleviated by pressure or a cold temperature because pain fibers are shorter and less myelinated than pressure and cold temperature receptors. The pressure or cold temperature stimuli are received by the brain before the pain stimulus. The gate is closed and thus the pain stimulus is not processed.

Another possible theory explains the increased serotonin levels after massage therapy for both infants[8] and adults[9]. Serotonin may inhibit the transmission of noxious nerve signals to the brain. Quiet or restorative sleep may also be related to pain alleviation from massage therapy. During deep sleep, somatostatin is normally released[10]. Without this substance, pain is experienced. Substance P, which is notable for causing pain, is released when an individual is deprived of deep sleep[10]. Thus, when people are deprived of deep sleep, they may have less somatostatin and increased substance P, which results in greater pain. One of the leading theories for the pain associated with fibromyalgia syndrome, for example, is the production of substance P due to deep sleep deprivation[10]. Participants in the study with fibromyalgia syndrome experienced less pain following the massage therapy treatment period. The reason may be that they experienced less sleep disturbance after massage therapy.

There is evidence of increased peak air flow as noted in the asthma study[8], and decreased glucose levels as noted in diabetic children after massage therapy. In addition, anxiety, depression, stress hormones (cortisol) and catecholamines are decreased after massage therapy. Increased parasympathetic activity may be the underlying mechanism for these changes. The pressure stimulation associated with touch may increase vagal activity, which in turn lowers physiological arousal and stress hormones (cortisol levels). Decreased cortisol in turn leads to enhanced immune function. The pressure is critical because light stroking is generally aversive, and the above effects have not been noted for light stroking. Parasympathetic activ-

ity is also associated with increased alertness and better performance on cognitive tasks[11]. Since massage therapy alleviates stress, this alternative treatment may help reduce stress-related disease. However, lasting effects of massage therapy following the termination of treatment, and the contraindications for massage therapy have not been addressed in the literature.

References

1. Ernst E. Abdominal massage therapy for chronic constipation: a systematic review of controlled clinical trials. *Forsch Komplementärmed* 1999;6:149–51
2. Ernst E. Massage therapy for low back pain: a systematic review. *J Pain Symptom Manage* 1999;17:65–9
3. Field T, Grizzle N, Scafidi F, Schanberg S. Massage relaxation therapies' effects on depressed adolescent mothers. *Adolescence* 1996;31:903–11
4. Hernandez-Reif M, Martinez A, Field T, Quintero O, Hart S, Burman I. Premenstrual symptoms are relieved by massage therapy. *J Psychosom Obstet Gynecol* 2000;21:9–15
5. Fraser J, Kerr JR. Psychophysiological effects of back massage on elderly institutionalised patients. *Nursing* 1993;18:238–45
6. Brattberg G. Connective tissue massage in the treatment of fibromyalgia. *Eur J Pain* 1999;3:235–45
7. Melzack R, Wall PD. Pain mechanism: a new theory. *Science* 1965;150:971–9
8. Field T, Grizzle N, Scafidi F, Abrams S, Richardson S. Massage therapy for infants of depressed mothers. *Infant Behav Dev* 1996;19:109–14
9. Ironson G, Field T, Scafidi F, *et al.* Massage therapy is associated with enhancement of the immune systems cytotoxic capacity. *Int J Neurosci* 1996;84:205–18
10. Sunshine W, Field T, Schanberg S, *et al.* Massage therapy and transcutaneous electrical stimulation effects on fibromyalgia. *J Clin Rheumatol* 1997;2:18–22
11. Porges, SW. The integrative neurobiology of affiliation. *Ann NY Acad Sci* 1997;807:62–77

Further reading

Field TM. Massage therapy effects. *Am Psychologist* 1998;53:1270–81
Vickers A. *Massage and Aromatherapy: a Guide for Health Professionals.* Cheltenham, UK: Stanley Thornes, 1998
Vickers A, Ohlsson A, Lacey JB, Horsley A. Massage therapy for premature and/or low birth weight infants to improve weight gain and/or decrease hospital length of stay. *Cochrane Library*. Oxford: Update Software, 1998

AYURVEDIC MEDICINE

'Ayurveda' is a Sanskrit word meaning knowledge or science (*Veda*) of life (*Ayur*). Ayurvedic medicine is based on a 5000-year-old system from India. This medicine is the major East Indian traditional medicine system, utilizing a detailed system of diagnosis involving examination of the pulse, tongue, urine and physical features. Conditions frequently treated are arthritis, cancer, fever, hypertension, allergies, headache and peptic ulcer.

Ayurvedic medicine is based on the concept of metabolic body types or individual constitutions, which are known as *doshas*. Three types of *dosha* are *vata*, *pitta* and *kapha*. The key feature of *vata* is changeability, and *vata* types are active, energetic and thin. The key feature of *pitta* is intensity, and *pitta* types are of medium build, strong and with good endurance. The key feature of *kapha* is relaxation. *Kapha* types have a heavy solid build, are strong, sleep long and deeply, and tend to be slow to act and slow to anger.

Treatments of Ayurvedic medicine include diet, exercise, meditation, herbs, oil massages, sun and breathing.

Diet

Diet is prescribed according to *dosha* and season. The taste of the food and nature of the food are primary considerations.

Exercise

Vigorous exercise and yoga stretching are encouraged in Ayurveda to improve circulation, stimulate metabolism and sharpen the mind. Exercises are prescribed according to an individual's constitution.

Meditation

Meditation is considered a form of mental cleansing. It enhances self awareness of one's environment, family, friends and business.

Herbs

Ayurvedic physicians use an extensive number of herbs in treating conditions. Depending on their innate qualities, herbs are used to rebuild and rejuvenate the body and its various systems. Although many herbs are listed as Ayurvedic herbs, there is limited evidence for their effectiveness.

Herbal formulations containing Triphala, Sinhnad guggul, Gokshuradi guggul and Chandraprabha vati

One controlled trial assessed the effect of Ayurvedic herbal formulations on obesity[1]. They used *Triphala*, *Sinhnad guggul*, *Gokshuradi guggul* and *Chandraprabha vati* and placebo in four different groups of obese patients. The authors reported that patients in the treatment group experienced a significant weight loss compared with those in the placebo group.

Terminalia arjuna

The Ayurvedic herb *Terminalia arjuna* has been tested in a cross-over randomized controlled trial in patients suffering from congestive heart failure (New York Heart Association stage IV)[2]. The results showed that in the experimental phase of this study there was a significant improvement of all relevant signs and symptoms of congestive heart failure. After the trial, all patients received treatment for up to 28 months and the clinical improvement continued, including amelioration in quality of life.

Misrakasneham

A controlled trial assessed the effects of a liquid Ayurvedic herbal preparation (*Misrakasneham*) including *Clitoria ternatea*, *Curcuma longa* and *Vitis vinifera* as well as castor oil in the management of opioid-induced constipation[3]. Fifty cancer patients received either the Ayurvedic herbal preparation or up to 360 mg of purified senna extract daily for 14 days. Seventeen of 20 patients (85%) who completed the study in the

Ayurveda group had satisfactory bowel movements, as compared to 11 of 16 (69%) in the senna group. There were no significant intergroup differences.

Boswellia serrata

Boswellia (*Boswellia serrata*) is used in Ayurvedic medicine and has been shown to have anti-inflammatory activity by reducing leukotriene synthesis. One preliminary report of a controlled clinical trial showed that 3600 mg of extract daily was not effective in reducing pain or increasing function in 37 patients with rheumatoid arthritis[4].

Massage

In Ayurvedic treatment, herbal oils are used for massage. The medicated oils help to remove toxins from the system through absorption through the skin.

Sun

Ayurvedic philosophy states that sun improves circulation, increases absorption of vitamin D and strengthens the bones. Different lengths of time spent in the sun depend on three *dosha* constitutions. People should use sun block, and people with multiple moles should not lie in the sun for extended periods of time.

Breathing

Breathing exercises can be learned from an experienced teacher. It can bring peace and alleviate stress.

Recently, Ayurveda has been revived in accordance with the classical texts by Maharishi Mahesh Yogi and in collaboration with leading Ayurvedic scholars and physicians. This specific reformulation of Ayurveda is known as Maharishi Ayurveda. Hundreds of physicians worldwide have been trained in Maharishi Ayurveda and have incorporated its principles into their practice. In addition, Maharishi Ayurveda schools, institutions and universities are being opened all over the USA to train physicians, technicians and nurses to teach the general public about various areas of health-care management. Several medical institutions have also incorporated this teaching into their curriculums. More double-blind, randomized, placebo-controlled studies are required to assess various aspects of Ayurvedic medicine.

References

1. Paranjpe P, Patki P, Patwardhan B. Ayurvedic treatment of obesity: a randomized double-blind, placebo-controlled clinical trial. *J Ethnopharmacol* 1990;29:1–11
2. Bharani A, Ganguly A, Bhargava KD. Salutary effect of *Terminalia arjuna* in patients with severe refractory heart failure. *Int J Cardiol* 1995;49:191–9
3. Ramesh PR, Kumar KS, Rajagopal MR, Balachandran P, Warrier PK. Managing morphine-induced constipation: a controlled comparison of an Ayurvedic formulation and senna. *J Pain Symptom Manage* 1998;16:240–4
4. Sander O, Herborn G, Rau R. Is H15 (resin extract of *Boswellia serrata*, 'incense') a useful supplement to established drug therapy of chronic polyarthritis? Results of a double-blind pilot study. *Zeitschr Rheumatol* 1998;57:11–16

Further reading

Burton Goldberg Group. *Alternative Medicine: The Definitive Guide*. Fife, WA: Future Medicine Publishing, 1994

Micozzi MS, ed. *Fundamentals of Complementary and Alternative Medicine*. London: Churchill Livingstone, 2001

YOGA

Yoga, an integral part of Ayurvedic medicine, is an ancient practice deriving from Vedic traditions of East India. It is the practice of gentle stretching, breathing-control exercises and meditation as a mind–body intervention. The word 'yoga' is derived from the Sanskrit word *yuj*, which means 'to yoke', reflecting its purpose in joining mind and body in harmonious relaxation. Yoga practices mostly used in the West, called hatha yoga, create balance, physically and emotionally, by using postures (*asanas*), breathing techniques (*pranayama*) and meditation.

Physical benefits of regular yoga practice that have been described include bodily suppleness and muscular strength. Mental benefits include feelings of well-being and, possibly, reduction of sympathetic drive. Yoga breathing exercises counter the rapid breathing that accompanies the stress response, and may in addition reduce muscular spasm and expand the available lung capacity.

Conditions frequently treated by yoga are stress, insomnia, headaches, anxiety, premenstrual syndrome, arthritis, back pain and gastrointestinal, respiratory and cardiovascular problems. It is also used in pregnancy as preparation for childbirth. Yoga can also be used by healthy people to gain self-mastery. Yoga is used daily by enthusiastic adherents, and is probably best practiced more than once a week for maximum benefit. It should be regarded as a long-term commitment.

Controlled trials suggest that yoga may have a useful long-term effect in the treatment of hypertension[1] and asthma[2]. It may also have a role in reducing joint stiffness in osteoarthritis[3]. In a recent study, Yoga lifestyle intervention retarded progression and increased regression of coronary atherosclerosis in patients with severe coronary artery disease[4]. Another study indicated that regular hatha yoga practice could elicit improvements in health-related aspects of physical fitness[5].

References

1. Patel C. Twelve month follow-up of yoga and bio-feedback in the management of hypertension. *Lancet* 1975;1:62–4
2. Vedanthan PK, Kesavalu LN, Murthy KC, *et al.* Clinical study of yoga techniques in university students with asthma: a controlled study. *Allergy Asthma Proc* 1998;19:3–9
3. Garfinkel MS, Schumacher HR, Husain A, Levy M, Reshetar RA. Evaluation of a yoga based regimen for treatment of osteoarthritis of the hands. *J Rheumatol* 1994;21:2341–3
4. Manchanda SC, Narang R, Reddy KS, *et al.* Retardation of coronary atherosclerosis with yoga lifestyle intervention. *J Assoc Physicians India* 2000;48:687–94
5. Tran MD, Holly RG, Lashbrook J, Amsterdam EA. Effects of hatha yoga practice on the health-related aspects of physical fitness. *Prev Cardiol* 2001;4:165–70

Further reading

Collins C. Yoga: intuition, preventive medicine, and treatment. *J Obstet Gynecol Neonatal Nurs* 1998;September/October:563–8

Manocha R, Marks GB, Kenchington P, Peters D, Salome CM. Sahaja yoga in the management of moderate to severe asthma: a randomised controlled trial. *Thorax* 2002;57:110–15

RELAXATION THERAPY

Progressive muscle relaxation is one of the most common relaxation techniques modified over time, but still based on original principles. Conditions frequently treated are anxiety, headaches, stress disorders and musculoskeletal pain. Other relaxation techniques involve passive muscle relaxation, refocusing, breathing control and imagery.

With progressive muscle relaxation, in a typical treatment session, subjects usually lie on their back with arms to their side in a quiet environment without bright light. Occasionally, a sitting posture in a comfortable chair is adopted instead. Muscle groups are systematically contracted then relaxed in a predetermined order. In the early stages, an entire session will be devoted to a single muscle group. With practice it becomes possible to combine muscle groups, and then eventually relax the entire body all at once.

Progressive muscle relaxation has been shown to be effective in eliciting the relaxation response, resulting in normalizing blood supply to the muscles; decreasing oxygen consumption, heart rate, respiration and skeletal muscle activity; and increasing skin resistance and alpha brain waves. Applied relaxation, which is developed from progressive relaxation, is a coping technique that has been found to be effective for panic disorder, agoraphobia, social phobia and specific phobia. It was observed that applied relaxation and cognitive therapy yielded approximately the same effects.

Much clinical evidence suggests that relaxation therapies are useful in treating anxiety. Positive results from controlled clinical trials exist for relaxation in association with desensitization for agoraphobia, panic disorder[1,2] and anxiety, associated with serious conditions such as cancer[3] or in undergoing medical interventions such as radiation therapy[4]. Systematic reviews of controlled clinical trials in both acute[5] and chronic[6] pain have found only weak and contradictory evidence that relaxation is an effective form of treatment on its own. Relaxation therapy may contribute to the standard treatment of asthma in adult patients[7]. Promising evidence for other medical conditions by controlled clinical trials include depression[8–10], insomnia[11–13] and menopausal symptoms[14–16].

In addition, several controlled clinical trials have demonstrated the effectiveness of range of relaxation techniques, including visualization or music therapy[17], in reducing stress[18], pain[19] and irritable bowel syndrome[20]. Further research is required to determine the type of relaxation technique that is best for each type of patient, and to establish how these interventions compare with conventional treatments.

References

1. Ost LG, Westling BE, Hellstrom K. Applied relaxation, exposure *in vivo* and cognitive methods in the treatment of panic disorder with agoraphobia. *Behav Res Ther* 1993;31:383–94
2. Beck JG, Stanley MA, Baldwin LE, Deagle EA 3rd, Averill PM. Comparison of cognitive therapy and relaxation training for panic disorder. *J Consult Clin Psychol* 1994;62:818–26
3. Bindemann S, Soukop M, Kaye SB. Randomized controlled study of relaxation training. *Eur J Cancer* 1991;27:170–4
4. Kolcaba K, Fox C. The effects of guided imagery on comfort of women with early stage breast cancer undergoing radiation therapy. *Oncol Nurs Forum* 1999;26:67–72
5. Seers K, Carroll D. Relaxation techniques for acute pain management: a systematic review. *J Adv Nurs* 1998;27:466–75
6. Carroll D, Seers K. Relaxation for the relief of chronic pain: a systematic review. *J Adv Nurs* 1998;27:476–87
7. Ritz T. Relaxation therapy in adult asthma. Is there new evidence for its effectiveness? *Behav Modif* 2001;25:640–66
8. Reynolds WM, Coats KI. A comparison of cognitive–behavioral therapy and relaxation training for the treatment of depression in adolescents. *J Consult Clin Psychol* 1986;54:653–60
9. Broota A, Dhir R. Efficacy of two relaxation techniques in depression. *J Pers Clin Stud* 1990;6:83–90
10. Murphy GE, Carney RM, Knesevich MA, Wetzel RD, Whitworth P. Cognitive behaviour therapy, relaxation training and tricyclic antidepressant medication in the treatment of depression. *Psychol Rep* 1995;77:403–20
11. Greeff AP, Conradie WS. Use of progressive relaxation training for chronic alcoholics with insomnia. *Psychol Rep* 1998;82:407–12
12. Engle Friedman M, Bootzin R R, Hazlewood L, Tsao C. An evaluation of behavioural treatments for insomnia in the older adult. *J Clin Psychol* 1992;48:77–90
13. Hauri PJ. Can we mix behavioural therapy with hypnotics when treating insomniacs? *Sleep* 1997;20:1111–18

14. Irvin JH, Domar AD, Clark C, Zuttermeister PC, Friedman R. The effects of relaxation response training on menopausal symptoms. *J Psychosom Obstet Gynecol* 1996;17:202–7

15. Freedman RR, Woodward S. Behavioural treatment of menopausal hot flushes: evaluation by ambulatory monitoring. *Am J Obstet Gynecol* 1992;167:436–9

16. Germaine LM, Freedman RR. Behavioural treatment of menopausal hot flashes: evaluation by objective methods. *J Consult Clin Psychol* 1984;52:1072–9

17. Beck BB. The variety of relaxation techniques. *Pflege Aktuell* 1999; 53:222–5

18. Sloman R, Brown P, Aldana E, Chee E. The use of relaxation for the promotion of comfort and pain relief in persons with advanced cancer. *Contemp Nurse* 1994;3:6–12

19. Syrjala KL, Cummings C, Donaldson GW. Hypnosis or cognitive behavioral training for the reduction of pain and nausea during cancer treament: a controlled clinical trial. *Pain* 1992;48:137–46

20. Keefer L, Blanchard EB. The effects of relaxation response meditation on the symptoms of irritable bowel syndrome: results of a controlled treatment study. *Behav Res Ther* 2001;39:801–11

Further reading

Eppley K R, Abrams A I, Shear J. Differential effects of relaxation techniques on trait anxiety. *J Clin Psychol* 1989;45:957–74

Ost LG, Breitholtz E.. Applied relaxation vs. cognitive therapy in the treatment of generalized anxiety disorder. *Behav Res Ther* 2000;38:777–90

Paranjpe P, Patki P, Patwardhan B. Ayurvedic treatment of obesity: a randomised double-blind, placebo-controlled clinical trial. *J Ethnopharmacol* 1990;29:1–11

HYPNOSIS

The word 'hypnosis' is derived from the Greek word *hypnos*, meaning sleep. Hypnosis is the induction of a deeply relaxed state with increased suggestibility and suspension of critical facilities for behavior change or symptom relief[1]. Hypnotic techniques alter sensory awareness, perception, memory and behavior, and therefore have the potential to influence physiological functioning and the course of medical conditions.

Conditions frequently treated are anxiety disorders with a strong psychological component (such as asthma and irritable bowel syndrome), conditions that can be modulated by levels of arousal (such as pain), and psychosomatic conditions such as stress, anxiety, phobia and addiction.

Once patients are in a hypnotic state, they are given therapeutic suggestions to encourage changes in behavior or relief of symptoms. For example, in a treatment to stop smoking, a hypnosis practitioner might suggest that the patient will no longer find smoking pleasurable or necessary. Hypnosis for a patient with arthritis might include a suggestion that the pain can be turned down like the volume of radio. Some practitioners use hypnosis as an aid to psychotherapy. The rationale is that, in the hypnotized state, the conscious mind presents fewer barriers to effective psychotherapeutic exploration, leading to an increased likelihood of psychological insight.

A meta-analysis of 18 controlled trials[2] suggested that hypnotherapy enhanced the effects of cognitive–behavioral psychotherapy for various conditions, including anxiety, insomnia, pain, hypertension and obesity[3]. A systematic review of nine controlled clinical trials of smoking cessation[4] concluded that hypnotherapy was no more effective than controls or other interventions[5]. A meta-analysis of 18 studies of the analgesic effects of hypnosis[6] found a moderate to large positive effect in pain management. A review of clinical trials[7] suggested that there was reasonable evidence for the use of hypnosis in preparation for surgery, treatment of asthma, dermatological conditions, irritable bowel syndrome, hemophilia, nausea and emesis in oncology. In a controlled clinical trial[8], hypnotherapy was found to be effective for post-traumatic conditions[9]. A review of 15 controlled trials of hypnosis in children[10] also found promising results for pain, enuresis and chemotherapy-related distress.

Adverse effects may be seen after hypnotherapy. Recovering repressed memories can be painful and psychological problems may be exacerbated by retraumatizing those with post-traumatic disorder or by inducing false memories in psychologically susceptible individuals. Hypnosis should be avoided in patients with personality disorder, dissociative disorders, or with patients who have histories of profound abuse. Studies investigating negative consequences of hypnosis have concluded that, when practiced by a clinically trained professional, it is safe.

References

1. Vickers A, Zollman C, Payne DK. Hypnosis and relaxation therapies. *West J Med* 2001;175:269–72
2. Kirsch I, Montgomery G, Sapirstein G. Hypnosis as an adjunct to cognitive–behavioural psychotherapy: a meta-analysis. *J Consult Clin Psychol* 1995;63:214–20
3. Schoenberger NE. Research on hypnosis as an adjunct to cognitive–behavioural psychotherapy. *Int J Clin Exp Hypn* 2000;48:154–69
4. Abbot NC, Stead LF, White AR, Barnes J, Ernst E. Hypnotherapy for smoking cessation (Cochrane Review). In *Cochrane Library*. Oxford: Update Software, 1998
5. Green JP, Lynn SJ. Hypnosis and suggestion-based approaches to smoking cessation: an examination of the evidence. *Int J Clin Exp Hypn* 2000;48:195–224
6. Montgomery GH, Du Hamel KN, Redd WH. A meta-analysis of hypnotically induced analgesia: how effective is hypnosis? *Int J Clin Exp Hypn* 2000;48:138–53
7. Pinnell CM, Covino NA. Empirical findings on the use of hypnosis in medicine: a critical review. *Int J Clin Exp Hypn* 2000;48:170–94
8. Cardeña E. Hypnosis in the treatment of trauma: a promising, but not fully supported, efficacious intervention. *Int J Clin Exp Hypn* 2000;48:125–38
9. Brom D, Kleber RJ, Defares PB. Brief psychotherapy for post-traumatic stress disorders. *J Consult Clin Psychol* 1989;57:607–12
10. Milling LS, Costantino CA. Clinical hypnosis with children: first steps toward empirical support. *Int J Clin Exp Hypn* 2000;48:113–37

MAGNETIC FIELD THERAPY

Magnetic field therapy involves permanent or pulsed magnetic fields applied to the head or other parts of the body. The therapy is often used with acupuncture. Externally applied pulsed electromagnetic fields have been used in promoting the healing of non-union fractures. More recently, the use of static magnetic fields in the form of locally applied magnets has become popular in sports medicine, arthritis, back pain, fatigue, poor sleep and many other conditions. Static magnetic fields are produced by natural or artificial magnets, and pulsating magnetic fields are generated by electrical devices.

In a double-blind, randomized, controlled trial, the application of static magnets was found to be useful in reducing pain in patients with post-polio syndrome[1]. Suggested mechanisms included alteration of the flux of ions into and out of cells, affecting nerve tissue or neuropeptides because of the locally altered magnetic field, changes in circulation and clearance of local mediators of pain and inflammation. In another study, Pelka and colleagues observed that impulse magnetic field therapy had a beneficial effect on different types of headache and migraine[2]. The same investigators recently observed that patients with insomnia who received impulse magnetic field therapy experienced substantial or even complete relief of their complaints[3].

Some studies of the use of magnets have shown negative outcomes. Concerns have been expressed about noxious effects of magnets and magnetic fields. Some have suggested that positive magnets may stimulate cancer cells to grow *in vitro*, and that living near high-tension power lines may be associated with higher rates of certain childhood malignancies[4]. However, the Office of Alternative Medicine observed therapeutic potential of non-thermal, non-ionizing electromagnetic fields in bone repair, nerve stimulation, wound healing, treatment of osteoarthritis, electroacupuncture, tissue regeneration, immune system stimulation and neuroendocrine modulation[5].

References

1. Vallbona C, Hazlewood CF, Jurida G. Response of pain to static magnetic fields in postpolio patients: a double-blind pilot study. *Arch Phys Med Rehabil* 1997;78:1200–3
2. Pelka RB, Jaenicke C, Gruenwald J. Impulse magnetic-field therapy for migraine and other headaches: a double-blind, placebo-controlled study. *Adv Ther* 2001;18:101–9
3. Pelka RB, Jaenicke C, Gruenwald J. Impulse magnetic-field therapy for insomnia: a double-blind, placebo-controlled study. *Adv Ther* 2001;18:174–80
4. Bierman P, Peters J, eds. *Proceedings of the Scientific Workshop on the Health Effects of Electric and Magnetic Fields on Workers.* Cincinnati, OH: National Institute of Occupational Safety and Health (NIOSH) Report No. 91-111. NTIS Order No. PB-91-173-351/ A13. Springfield, VA: National Information Service, 1991
5. Workshop on Alternative Medicine, Chantilly, VA. *Alternative Medicine: Expanding Medical Horizons. A Report to the National Institutes of Health on Alternative Medical Systems and Practices in the United States.* Washington, DC: US Government Printing Office, 1992;50–61:134–46

Further reading

Segal NA, Toda Y, Huston J, *et al.* Two configurations of static magnetic fields for treating rheumatoid arthritis of the knee: a double-blind clinical trial. *Arch Phys Med Rehabil* 2001;82:1453–60

TAI CHI

Tai chi or tai chi chuan is a system of movements and postures. This form of martial arts in the Chinese culture is used to enhance mental and physical health. It has become increasingly popular in many Western countries. A number of different styles and forms were developed from the original 13 postures. The various forms of tai chi comprise a series of postures linked by gentle and graceful movements. Tai chi chuan is an exercise with moderate intensity, and is aerobic in nature.

The slow movement between different postures that are normally held for a short period of time are physical stimuli with effects on the cardiovascular and muscular systems. These stimuli, much like other physical exercise, result in muscular adaptation, which ultimately leads to increased muscle strength if performed regularly. In addition to adaptation processes at the level of the nervous system, these effects may produce better cardiovascular function, co-ordination and balance.

Conditions frequently treated are stress-related conditions, depression, osteoporosis and high or low blood pressure. Evidence from controlled clinical trials suggested beneficial effects of tai chi as an intervention to maintain balance and strength[1] and to reduce the risk of falls[2] in elderly individuals. The results of another controlled clinical trial suggested tai chi to be as effective as moderate walking exercise and alleviating induced anxiety[3]. It has also had beneficial effects on depression, anger and fatigue, muscle strength and on cardiorespiratory function in elderly individuals[4–6].

References

1. Wolfson L, Whipple R, Derby C, *et al*. Balance and strength in older adults: intervention gains and tai chi maintenance. *J Am Geriatr Soc* 1996;44:498–506
2. Wolf SL, Barnhart HX, Kutner NG, *et al*. Reducing frailty and falls in older persons: an investigation of tai chi and computerized balance training, Atlanta FISCSIT Group. *J Am Geriatr Soc* 1996;44:489–97
3. Jin P. Efficacy of Tai Chi, brisk walking, meditation, and reading in reducing mental and emotional stress. *J Psychosom Res* 1992;36: 361–70
4. Jin P. Changes in heart rate, noradrenaline, cortisol and mood during tai chi. *J Psychosom Res* 1989;33:197–206
5. Lai J-S, Wong M-K, Lan C, Chong C-K, Lien I-N. Cardiorespiratory responses of tai chi chuan practitioners and sedentary subjects during cycle ergometry. *J Formos Med Assoc* 1993;92:894–9
6. Lai J-S, Lan C, Wong M-K, Teng S-H. Two-year trends in cardiorespiratory function among older tai chi chuan practitioners and sedentary subjects. *J Am Geriatr Soc* 1995;43:1222–7

Alternative sports medicine

14

P. J. Barrett

INTRODUCTION

Sports are competitive by nature. Athletes and their coaches are constantly searching for ways to gain muscle, lose fat and improve athletic performance in order to beat the competition. There are numerous rewards for success in athletics, ranging from million-dollar salaries to college scholarships to adoration from peers. These prizes fuel athletes to seek methods to gain a competitive edge. The field of sports medicine has developed in order to meet the demands of athletes striving for improvement. Since 1976, sports medicine fellowship programs in the USA have trained physicians to help athletes maximize their physical potential and treat their injuries related to participating in sports.

Just as complementary and alternative medicine (CAM) therapies have found their way into other fields of medicine, CAM therapies are also popular in sports medicine. Since, in the USA, the rewards for success in athletics are tremendous, many athletes often utilize methods before their efficacy and safety have been established. As a result, physicians need to be aware of the type of CAM therapies athletes are using in order to help them avoid negative consequences.

Some commonly used CAM therapies used in sports medicine are nutritional supplements and mind–body methods. In the USA, the nutrition industry generated $48 billion in annual sales during 2001 and this figure is expected to grow by 6.2% by 2003. The sports nutrition market comprises 3% or $1.5 billion and some predict it will increase by 7.7% in 2003[1]. Clearly, sports nutrition is a significant market that is increasing in popularity.

Too often, without discussing it with their physicians, athletes take sports nutritional supplements based on information they learn from other athletes and media reports, hoping to experience an ergogenic effect (athletic performance enhancement). Often, contradictory information circulates, which leaves the athlete confused and unable to make educated decisions. Discussing nutritional sports supplements allows physicians to help athletes to make safe and effective choices and avoid harmful consequences. There are many different types of nutritional sports supplement, but the most widely used in the USA are creatine, protein (whey, glutamine and branched-chain amino acids), testosterone prohormones (androsteronedione, androsteronediol and dehydro-epiandrosterone (DHEA)), and fat loss products such as ephedrine/caffeine and chromium picolinate.

Other unconventional methods used to enhance performance are mind–body methods such as meditation, yoga and hypnosis. Although these approaches are not as common as nutritional supplementation, mind–body methods are increasing in popularity among athletes and, once incorporated into their training programs, they may hold promise for maximizing performance.

NUTRITIONAL SPORTS SUPPLEMENTS

During the summer of 1998, the race to beat the previously held home run record between professional baseball players Mark McGuire and Sammy Sossa captivated many Americans. Few other things are more sacred to Americans than professional baseball, so when news broke that Mark McGuire was taking the sports supplement androsteronedione to enhance his performance, many became outraged and accused the star of cheating. Androsteronedione, commonly known as 'andro', is a substance designed to increase testosterone levels and mimic the effects of anabolic steroids. Although 'andro' is banned by both the United States military and international sports communities, it is a legal substance. Despite the public criticism against McGuire, annual sales of androsteronedione had multiplied by a factor of five by the end of the summer of 1998.

Other nutritional sports supplements also have received media attention. Ephedrine, a sympathetic stimulate found naturally in some herbs, has been linked to deaths of high school and college athletes. Reports of these incidents have made many question the safety and legality of using sports nutritional supplements. Regardless of the type of attention, nutritional sports supplements are gaining in popularity and physicians and other health-care professionals should be familiar with them.

Creatine

Creatine is found naturally in meat and fish, and was first characterized early in the 20th century as a dietary element. When phosphorylated, creatine acts as a primary energy substrate and provides cells with adenosine triphosphate (ATP), the energy source in the body[2]. Since one of the primary limitations in strenuous exercise is depletion of ATP, creatine has been used recently as a dietary supplement to enhance athletic performance by increasing the amount of energy available.

Ergogenic effects

Many studies have demonstrated that short-term creatine supplementation improves athletic performance during resistance training and other short-term high-intensity activities in healthy adults. Consuming creatine (5–30 g/day) during weight training for 4–12 weeks increased muscular strength, fat-free mass and body mass, and enabled athletes to perform at higher intensity levels[3–6]. Although creatine supplementation has been shown to increase power output by approximately 30% during short sprints[7,8], it does not appear to enhance long-duration aerobic performance[3,8].

Creatine supplementation may elicit its ergogenic effect by increasing skeletal muscle fiber hypertrophy. Muscle fiber diameter significantly increased among individuals consuming 1.5 g of creatine each day for 1 year. Other studies have demonstrated that creatine decreases muscle recovery time following exercise by facilitating recovery. Men who participated in resistance training while consuming 25 g of creatine per day for 7 days, followed by a daily creatine intake of 5 g for 12 weeks, showed skeletal muscle cross-sectional area increases of 29–35%, approximately twice those observed in control subjects (6–15%)[6]. Creatine supplementation may work by increasing protein synthesis and/or decreasing protein degradation. Another possibility is that creatine enhances muscular growth by enabling users to lift heavier loads by providing more available energy in the form of ATP during resistance training, which inevitably increases muscle hypertrophy.

Creatine supplementation among sedentary adults provided some of the same benefits found among athletes; however, improvements were not as significant. After creatine loading (5-g doses four times a day for 5 days), maintaining (5-g dose once a day for 5 days) and cessation (no creatine for 7 days), isometric force production of muscle groups was measured. Results indicated that creatine supplementation did not increase muscle strength as it did among athletes. However, muscle recovery time did decrease, allowing participants to increase task performance frequency[9]. It appears that creatine supplementation needs to be coupled with resistance training to provide the maximum benefits.

Neuromuscular diseases

Since neuromuscular diseases are characterized by decreases in muscle strength, it has been proposed that creatine supplementation may alleviate symptoms among these individuals. In fact, decreases in phosphocreatine levels have been found in patients with muscular dystrophy, mitochondrial cytopathy and inflammatory myopathy. Subsequent creatine supplementation of 10 g daily for 5 days, followed by 5 days of 5 g daily in these individuals, significantly improved high-intensity muscle performance[10]. Creatine supplementation in combination with conventional therapies may offer patients with neuromuscular diseases better outcomes.

Long-term effects

The effects of chronic creatine supplementation on the body after several years of use is still unclear. One study in rats, however, showed that repeated creatine supplementation down-regulated the expression of the creatine transporter, a transmembrane protein that is responsible for cell uptake of creatine[11]. Thus, chronic creatine consumption may decrease the ability of cells to absorb creatine and thus decrease the ergogenic effect of the supplement. Taking periodic breaks in creatine consumption may prevent this down-regulation and provide the optimum benefit for users.

Potential adverse effects

Although it appears that creatine supplementation provides benefits for athletes, non-athletes and patients with neuromuscular diseases, some studies have suggested that there are harmful consequences to taking the supplement. The negative side-effects reported are diarrhea/indigestion[8], kidney problems[12], liver dysfunction[4] and muscle cramps[10]. These findings are based on case studies and anecdotal reports. Subsequent double-blind studies that investigated these claims did not support these findings and found that creatine supplementation did not cause deleterious side-effects. A more likely explanation of these reported problems with creatine is over-exertion or lack of proper hydration. Therefore, creatine supplementation does not seem to cause harmful side-effects in most situations when used properly.

Two side-effects of creatine supplementation, however, that appear to be verifiable and consistent are fluid retention and plasma volume changes. Wrestlers taking creatine were not able to lose weight before a competition at the rate of athletes who consumed glucose instead. Additionally, there was a small decrease in plasma volume found among wrestlers who took creatine[13]. These data suggest that creatine alters fluid homeostasis and therefore should be avoided when participating in sports activities performed in hot and humid environments.

Dosage

There is a great deal of dosage variability among creatine users. The majority of studies employ a loading period in which individuals use approximately four times the normal dose of creatine for 1 week. Subsequently, users reduce their use in order to maintain creatine levels in muscle. Typically, during the loading phase, individuals take 5–20 g/day followed by 2–5 g during the maintenance period[3,14,15]. The loading phase does not seem necessary to achieve the same results, however. One study demonstrated that the same creatine levels in muscle found among those who took 20 g/day were achieved by taking 3 g/day, although it took 30 days to reach the same creatine levels achieved in 5 days by individuals taking 20 g/day[3].

Interactions with other substances

Taking creatine with large quantities of simple carbohydrates significantly increases creatine muscle levels as compared with taking it alone. Ingesting 100 g of carbohydrates with every 5 g of creatine provides the optimum creatine accumulation in muscle. This process is mediated by insulin-stimulated creatine transport[16]. Although consuming that much carbohydrate with creatine provides the best results, it may not be feasible for users to consume that quantity of carbohydrate each day, especially if they are taking four doses a day of the supplement.

Other dietary combinations of creatine with other dietary substances are not as beneficial. Caffeine seems completely to negate any benefit from creatine supplementation. After taking creatine (0.5 g/kg body mass/day) with caffeine (5 g/kg body mass/day), subjects performed identically on strength tests to when they did not take creatine and significantly worse than when they consumed creatine alone[17]. Further studies demonstrated that, during muscle recovery, caffeine inhibited phosphocreatine resynthesis[5]. The data concerning creatine supplement interactions with other substances are limited, and therefore future research should be conducted.

Protein loading

During both anaerobic and aerobic exercise, protein synthesis decreases and degradation increases, resulting in a negative nitrogen balance and consequent decrease in lean body muscle mass[18,19]. This indicates that athletes could benefit from consuming more than the recommended daily allowances of 0.8 g/kg body weight of protein per day for adults currently suggested by the National Academy of Sciences[20]. This is commonly referred to as 'protein loading', the consumption of tremendous amounts of daily protein by many athletes, who often do not know the amount they need for their activity level and fitness goals.

During aerobic exercise, the body's glycogen stores are not sufficient to provide the necessary energy to maintain activity and thus the body relies on protein for approximately 10% of its total energy requirements. This reliance on protein as an energy source increases the likelihood of loss of lean muscle mass[21]. Consequently, endurance athletes should consume between 1.2 and 2.2 g of protein/kg body weight to prevent skeletal muscle degradation[22,23].

The protein requirements for strength-training athletes, however, are not as clear. One study suggested that strength-training athletes should consume 1.76 g protein/kg body weight per day in order to maintain a positive nitrogen balance and thus promote strength and muscle growth[24]. Further studies confirmed the benefit of increasing protein intake. Weight lifters consuming 1.0 g/kg body weight per day maintained nitrogen balance while those who took 2.77 g/kg body weight per day attained positive nitrogen balance, which was almost twice as much as the previous group[25].

Other studies, however, have indicated that strength-training athletes may need to consume only 0.82 g of protein/kg body weight per day in order to maintain nitrogen balance. More recent findings, however, support the increased need for protein consumption and suggest that 1.5–2.0 g protein/kg body weight per day provides the maximum benefit for strength-training athletes by maintaining a positive nitrogen balance[26]. The inconsistencies found among the data may be due to variations among intensity of workouts among research participants. Additional research may help to determine the exact protein amount needed to provide the optimum benefit. It is clear, though, that athletes require more protein than the recommended daily allowances.

Protein consumption timing, in addition to the quantity of protein ingested, also affects body composition. Elderly men (74 ± 1 year) who consumed 10 g of protein immediately following resistance training experienced greater benefits than comparable subjects who drank the same solution of 10 g of protein 2 h after exercising. Magnetic resonance imaging and dual energy X-ray absorptiometry used before and after a 6-week program revealed a mean quadriceps femoris increase of 3.7 cm^2 (6.7%) and mean muscle fiber area increase of 972 μm^2 (19.36%). No muscle size gains were reported for those who took protein 2 h after training[27].

The men who drank the protein drink immediately after exercising improved both their dynamic and their isokinetic strength significantly (46% and 15%, respectively) while the two post-training groups demonstrated a dynamic strength gain of only 36% without increasing their isokinetic strength. These results indicate that taking protein immediately following training may provide athletes with better results.

The confusion surrounding protein intake also extends to the forms of protein that will provide the greatest ergogenic effect. Many believe that whey protein provides the most significant muscle gains. Others swear by daily consumption of specific amino acids, such as glutamine and branched-chain amino acids, to enhance athletic performance. Some adhere to a more aggressive approach and take whey protein, glutamine and the branched-chain amino acids together on a daily basis.

Whey protein

There are many different sources of protein that athletes have consumed over the years, but it appears that whey protein may provide the most benefits. Whey proteins, which contain high levels of essential and non-essential amino acids such as lysine, methionine, cysteine and branched-chain amino acids, come from the fluid left over after the coagulation and removal of curd (i.e. casein protein) from milk during cheese production. The whey fluid is composed of 50% milk solids, 20–24% milk proteins and nearly all of the vitamins and minerals found in milk. The majority of whey is α-lactalbumin and β-lactoglobulin; together they comprise 70–80% of whey proteins. The remaining fractions contain immunoglobulins, phospholipoproteins, lactoferrin, bovine serum albumin, glycomacropeptides and enzymes[28,29].

When compared to other proteins, whey proteins seem to increase lean muscle mass and enhance athletic performance more than other sources. After 3 months of consuming either whey or casein proteins, athletes who ingested whey protein outperformed those who took casein proteins, in both peak cycling power and 30-s cycling work capacity (13.3% (whey) vs. 1.6% (casein) and 12.7% (whey) vs. 0.9% (casein), respectively). Most dramatically, lymphocyte glutathione levels increased by 35.5% among those who consumed whey proteins while the casein protein group of athletes experienced a 0.9% drop in their levels[30]. This is significant, because lymphocyte glutathione is an important antioxidant in the body, which decreases the concentration of free radicals. Increasing lymphocyte glutathione levels suggests that whey protein supplementation may help with muscle recovery, because hypertrophy of muscle increases free radicals, which slow repair.

Whey protein may also provide body compositional benefits. Athletes who consumed whey proteins over a 3-month period reduced their body fat by 4.8%, while the casein group experienced a 5.1% increase in body fat[30]. Additionally, there do not appear to be negative effects associated with whey protein supplementation. Patients with HIV/AIDS[31], cancer[32], cirrhosis[33] or cystic fibrosis[34] did not report any harmful effects associated with taking whey

protein supplements. Whey proteins appear to be a good and safe source of protein for athletes because of their high concentration of essential amino acids, their effect on performance and body composition and their lack of negative side-effects.

Currently, there have been few studies investigating the effect of combining supplements, which is surprising, since many athletes often combine products. One study investigated the effects of taking creatine with whey protein. Thirty-six male subjects, who did resistance training for 6 weeks, showed that consuming whey protein and creatine together enhanced the ergogenic effect over taking whey protein alone or placebo. Those who consumed 1.2 g of whey protein and 0.1 g of creatine/kg body weight improved their performance on the bench-press exercise as compared with those who took the identical amount of whey protein alone (15.2 kg (17%) for the whey/creatine group, while the whey-only group increased by 6.3 kg (7%)). Knee extension performance also improved more for the whey plus creatine group than for the athletes who took whey protein only (26.2 N m (10%) and 16.5 N m (7%), respectively)[35].

Average lean muscle mass gains for the whey protein/creatine subjects (4.0 kg, 6.5%) were greater than for the whey protein group (2.3 kg, 3.8%). Both groups exceeded the gains observed for the control group (0.9 kg, 1.5%). Subjects did not report any negative effects associated with taking the supplements together[35]. Apparently, taking creatine and whey protein together is safe, as well as effective, for improving strength and muscle mass.

Glutamine

Glutamine is a non-essential amino acid synthesized primarily in skeletal muscle tissues. Since there is evidence that indicates that glutamine is important in maintaining skeletal muscle protein, it has become one of the most popular nutritional supplements. It is synthesized by glutamine synthetase from glutamate, which is formed by the Krebs cycle intermediate α-ketoglutarate[36]. Glutamine supplementation may provide benefits to athletes because the body cannot produce the amount of glutamine it requires during exercise. Insufficient available glutamine may cause catabolism of skeletal muscle proteins; supplementing with glutamine may prevent this degradation from occurring[37,38].

Studies have indicated that glutamine supplementation does indeed prevent decreases in muscle mass during stress or illness. When compared to glycine, glutamine directly delivered to the intestine increased protein synthesis significantly more than glycine[39]. In addition to increasing the pool of amino acids available, glutamine may provide its ergogenic effect by increasing growth hormone levels[40] and/or by helping to maintain a positive nitrogen balance in the body[41].

Post-surgically, taking glutamine supplements appears to lessen skeletal muscle degradation. Undergoing elective abdominal surgery, a group of subjects received an amino acid solution with or without glutamine. Those who consumed 0.285 g of glutamine/kg body weight displayed improved nitrogen balance and decreased muscle loss[42]. Similar benefits were found among patients who had their gallbladders removed and consumed glutamine post-surgically[43]. Currently, there are few studies investigating glutamine supplementation for athletes; however, it is reasonable to conclude that, since increasing glutamine consumption helps to augment the strain of surgery on the body, it could possibly help to alleviate exercise-induced stress. Additionally, no harmful effects have ever been linked to glutamine supplementation, even after years of use, and therefore it appears to be safe.

Branched-chain amino acids

Valine, leucine and isoleucine are essential amino acids and make up the branched-chain amino acids. These serve as the primary amino acid fuel source in tissues other than the liver[44]. Since branched-chain amino acids provide nitrogen for glutamine synthesis in skeletal muscle, many athletes supplement their diets with branched-chain amino acids, hoping to increase lean muscle mass and improve strength.

Indeed, many studies have indicated that branched-chain amino acid supplementation provides body compositional benefits and enhances performance among individuals who exercise regularly. A double-blind, placebo-controlled study involving 16 mountain hikers over a 21-day trek showed that those who consumed 11.5 g of branched-chain amino acids (5.76 g leucine, 2.88 g isoleucine and 2.88 g valine) showed a 1.5% increase in lean muscle mass, while the placebo group did not change. Furthermore, the branched-chain amino acid group lost 11.7% of their body fat while controls lost 10.3%. Cross-sectional area of arm muscle mass did not change among the group of athletes taking branched-chain amino acids while the control group lost 6.8%. Additionally, athletes who consumed branched-chain amino acids experienced less decline in limb power versus the controls (2.4% vs. 7.8% decline, respectively)[45]. These results suggest that branched-chain amino acid supplementation may act anticatabolically in the body, and decrease protein degradation caused by strenuous exercise.

Another study involving marathon runners during a 30-km race also indicated that branched-chain amino acid supplementation may decrease muscle protein breakdown associated with exercise. Those who consumed 7.5–12 g of branched-chain amino acids experienced no change in amino acid concentration in their skeletal muscle while the placebo group of athletes showed 20–40% increase in free skeletal muscle tyrosine and phenylalanine levels[46]. The increase in free amino acids of skeletal muscle among controls suggested degradation of protein, and the lack of change in amino acid concentration in the amino acid group indicated that protein catabolism did not occur.

Similar beneficial results were reported among 25 calorie-restricted (28 kcal/kg body weight/day) wrestlers. After consuming branched-chain amino acids for 19 days, magnetic resonance imaging revealed that this group of wrestlers experienced the greatest fat loss. Interestingly, the branched-chain amino acid group of wrestlers had substantial visceral fat loss (34.4%)[47]. Since high levels of abdominal visceral fat contribute to cardiovascular disease, branched-chain amino acids may reduce the risk of heart problems, in addition to providing benefits to athletes. These studies indicate that branched-chain amino acid supplementation is an effective strategy for improving body composition, in addition to being safe, since no harmful health effects have ever been associated with their consumption.

Combining whey protein, glutamine and branched-chain amino acids appears to provide athletes with the maximum body composition and performance benefits. In one study, healthy adult male athletes took either whey protein (40 g/day) or whey protein (40 g/day) plus glutamine (5 g/day) and branched-chain amino acids (3 g/day). All participants consumed a total of 1.6 g protein/kg body weight per day while engaging in identical resistance training programs over the course of the 10-week study. Those who supplemented their diets with whey/glutamine/branched-chain amino acids performed an average of eight more bench presses and 9.13 more leg presses than before the study, while the whey group increased the number of repetitions of bench and leg presses by only 2.75 and 5.13, respectively. Additionally, the whey/glutamine/branched-chain amino acid group gained almost 1.6 kg on average of lean muscle mass, while the whey group gained approximately 0.5 kg of lean muscle mass over the 10-week period[48]. Clearly, athletes benefit from supplementing their diets with whey protein, glutamine and branched-chain amino acids.

Testosterone prohormones

Anabolic steroids have been widely used by athletes to increase physical size and strength for years. Despite their being illegal and the numerous harmful effects associated with their use, such as uncontrollable aggressive behavior and cardiac problems,

many individuals in sports continue to use these harmful substances. Taking advantage of public perception that legal, nutritional supplements are perceived to be safe, the nutritional sports industry has developed androgen prohormones or precursor supplements based on the premise that the body will form testosterone from these substances (Figure 1). The most popular testosterone precursor supplements are androstenedione, androstenediol and DHEA, which are widely used by athletes in the USA in spite of the fact that both the United States military and the international sports community have banned their use.

Androstenedione and androstenediol

Androstenedione, more commonly known as 'andro' among sports communities and the public, is the most popularly sold androgen supplement. Androstenediol is another type of androgen precursor that is similar to androstenedione since both can be directly converted to testosterone; therefore, they are often combined together in commercially available products. Despite their media attention and popularity, there are conflicting data concerning the efficacy of both of these types of androgen precursor supplement.

In one study involving seven healthy male subjects, consuming 100 mg androstenedione did not affect their free or total testosterone levels. Conversely, when subjects consumed 100 mg of androstenediol both free and total testosterone levels increased (29% and 40%, respectively) when measured 60 min after ingestion. The effect on test levels were more pronounced when measured 90 min after ingestion (43%

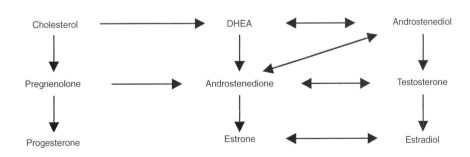

Figure 1   Testosterone synthesis pathway. DHEA, dehydroepiandrosterone

increase of free testosterone and 48% increase of total testosterone levels)[49].

Another study, however, found androstenedione and androstenediol supplementation to increase both free and total testosterone levels similarly when subjects consumed 200 mg[50]. Furthermore, taking a 150-mg supplement that contained various types of androstenedione and androstenediol increased total testosterone levels by 98%, 40 min post-ingestion. Testosterone levels, however, returned to normal 180 min after ingestion. The subjects who took the androstenedione/androstenediol supplement and controls performed similarly on certain athletic activities[49].

When the same researchers increased the androstenedione/androstenediol supplement dose to 450 mg from 150 mg, 4 weeks later the subjects improved their performance on the vertical jump by 9.3% (average increase of 5.1 cm); their vertical jump did not change after consuming only 150 mg of the same supplement. Additionally, the larger dose of the supplement also affected body composition, evidenced by fat reduction of an average of 1.8 kg, a 5.4-l (10.5%) increase in total body water and a 2.3-l (11.8%) increase in extracellular fluid volume[49]. Although the 450-mg dose of androstenedione/androstenediol supplement indeed reduced body weight, the benefits of the loss may be outweighed by the gain in fluid volume caused by the supplementation.

Other studies involving androstenedione have suggested different outcomes of supplement use. Twenty untrained men who consumed 300 mg per day of androstenedione over 8 weeks of resistance training had similar lean muscle mass, fat loss and testosterone levels to controls. Elevated estradiol concentrations and a 12% reduction in high-density lipoprotein (HDL)-cholesterol, however, were reported in the androstenedione supplement group[51]. The HDL drop suggests that androstenedione supplementation may cause cardiac problems by increasing arteriosclerosis, since HDL molecules are essential to plaque removal in arteries. Furthermore, increased estradiol levels have been associated with cardiovascular diseases and pancreatic cancer.

One of the major criticisms of the King study is that it involved men previously not in training and that androstenedione supplementation provides an ergogenic effect only when used by athletes. Several case studies, however, involving young, healthy bodybuilders who took androstenedione showed negative results as well, such as increases in body fat and decreases in lean muscle mass with only marginal strength improvements[52,53]. Evidently, more studies are needed to determine the effects of androstenedione and androstenediol supplementation before they are used.

Dehydroepiandrosterone

DHEA is another testosterone precursor with which many athletes supplement their diets in order to improve performance and strength. DHEA can be converted to androstenedione or androstenediol (and subsequently testosterone), which can be made into estrogen[54] (Figure 1). Despite its potential to become testosterone, the vast majority of data suggest that DHEA does not alter androgen blood levels or improve athletic performance and strength.

One study involving 19 young men (mean 23 years old) who consumed 150 mg DHEA per day during 8 weeks of resistance training did not show any difference in serum hormone levels or strength performance compared to the placebo group[55]. Similar studies showed that DHEA did not affect serum testosterone or estrogen levels either[56,57]. It appears that DHEA supplementation does not enhance strength and muscle power.

Wilson's review of several studies involving androgen precursor supplementation concluded that the efficacy of androgen precursor supplementation for athletic performance was unclear[58]. Since many androgens can cause harmful effects such as cardiovascular disease, pancreatic cancer, lipid density alterations as well as other negative consequences, athletes should avoid using them until additional studies are completed. Furthermore, it is not clear whether androgen supplementation is beneficial for athletes and it may even negatively affect their training by increasing body fat and decreasing lean muscle mass. Better and safer results can be expected by utilizing other methods for improving athletic performance, strength and body composition.

Fat reduction

In the USA, obesity is a major health problem and the second leading cause of preventable death. Despite the prevalence of low-fat foods, health clubs and billions of dollars spent annually on weight loss, the situation is getting worse. The number of overweight people in the USA has increased by approximately 10% over the past 20 years[59] and one out of every five adolescents is now considered obese, which is a 45% jump from a similar study carried in the early part of the 20th century[60]. Overweight individuals are not the only ones interested in fat loss, however. Bodybuilders and many other athletes actively seek ways to reduce their percentage of body fat in order to be able to meet weight requirements for certain competitions or to appear more muscular or 'defined'. Not surprisingly, approximately 400 dietary supplements are now available to consumers that purport to function by increasing fat breakdown, suppressing appetite, decreasing absorption, or utilizing a combination of these approaches.

Ephedrine and caffeine

Ephedrine, which mimics norepinephrine (noradrenaline) by acting as a β_2 agonist, is a sympathetic nervous system stimulator found in many dietary fatburning supplements. Typically, the ephedrine found in these supplements comes from *Ephedra* or Ma Huang herbs, which are composed of approximately 6% ephedrine[61]. Ephedrine enhances fat reduction by increasing fat metabolism, heart rate, heart contractility and glycolysis, and by suppressing the appetite. Since ephedrine has been shown to be more effective in fat reducing when combined with caffeine, the majority of ephedrine-containing supplements also have caffeine in them. Typically, users take 20 mg ephedrine and 200 mg caffeine 2–3 times per day[62].

Indeed, several studies have demonstrated that ephedrine/caffeine supplementation increases fat loss while decreasing lean muscle mass when people are placed on a calorie-restricted diet. In one study, obese patients who were placed on a restricted 1000-calorie/day diet consumed either caffeine, ephedrine, ephedrine plus caffeine, or placebo over 24 weeks. Those who took ephedrine plus caffeine lost approximately 17 kg, while the other individuals lost between 11 and 14 kg[62]. Another study showed that those who took ephedrine and caffeine lost 4.5 kg more fat and 2.8 kg less lean muscle mass than those taking a placebo over the course of 8 weeks[63].

Interestingly, one study showed the ephedrine/caffeine combination to be more effective in increasing fat burning than a formerly prescribed weight-loss medication called dexfenfluramine. After reports of cardiac complications due to use of dexfenfluramine, the Federal Food and Drug Administration (FDA) banned the serotonin agonist. Over the course of 15 weeks, patients who consumed ephedrine and caffeine daily lost more fat than those who took dexfenfluramine (8 kg vs. 7 kg, respectively). The combination of ephedrine and caffeine was even more effective as a fat burner than dexfenfluramine among obese patients (i.e. body mass index over 30 kg/m²). The ephedrine/caffeine subjects lost an average of 9 kg, while those in the dexfenfluramine group lost 7 kg[64,65]. These results indicate that ephedrine/caffeine-containing supplements enhance fat reduction.

Despite the media attention regarding the dangers associated with ephedrine supplementation, many studies have demonstrated that, when used properly by healthy individuals, ephedrine/caffeine-containing supplements are safe and cause relatively few and minor side-effects. One study found that individuals consuming ephedrine/caffeine supplements experienced tremors, dizziness and insomnia. These effects were temporary and disappeared after 8 weeks of use[62]. Headaches and arrhythmias have also been reported as side-effects[65].

Currently, over 800 adverse incidents and some deaths have been attributed to ephedrine-containing supplements, causing some states to ban the sale of ephedrine. In the majority of these cases, however, those who died had a pre-existing health condition or did not take the supplement properly, significantly exceeding the recommended dose. Some athletes did experience deleterious effects even when they used the supplement properly, however. People should be warned about potential consequences of taking ephedrine and the increased risks associated with exceeding the recommended dose.

It appears that ephedrine/caffeine-containing supplements effectively increase fat metabolism, as well as decreasing loss of lean muscle mass associated with exercise. Long-term studies investigating prolonged ephedrine use and possible ephedrine interactions with other substances need to be conducted in order to rule out significant complications associated with use. Until future research studies are conducted, athletes should avoid taking ephedrine-containing products.

Chromium picolinate

Chromium is a metal, which must be chelated to be able to be absorbed by cells. It is often chelated with picolinic acid, forming chromium picolinate, which is stable in the body[66]. Chromium picolinate has been shown to improve insulin sensitivity in patients with type 2 diabetes by increasing membrane fluidity and insulin internalization[67,68]. Since chromium picolinate has been shown to increase insulin sensitivity, some have proposed that it could be used as a sports supplement to increase muscle mass and decrease body fat by increasing the cellular transport of amino acids[69].

In fact, chromium picolinate is the active ingredient in many fat-reducing supplements, and is the most widely used. Unlike ephedrine-containing supplements, however, it appears that chromium picolinate supplements are not effective at increasing fat metabolism, and may cause harmful effects in the body.

Some studies have indicated that chromium picolinate did not help reduce fat among healthy adults when compared to individuals taking placebo[66,70–72]. However, one study reported that inactive obese women gained approximately 2 kg on average over the course of a 9-week controlled study[73]. Chromium picolinate appears not to be effective in fat reduction among athletes and sedentary adults.

Taking chromium picolinate supplements can have negative consequences as well. The stable properties of chromium picolinate allow it to accumulate in cells and cause damage. Since chromium enters cells via transferrin, the iron transport protein, it competes with iron for transport into cells. This can result in reduced cellular iron absorption, which can lead to a decrease in hemoglobin production and subsequent decrease in the oxygen-carrying capacity of blood. Indeed, chromium picolinate has been shown to decrease iron saturation of transferrin by 24%[66]. Additionally, there have been case reports of chromium picolinate supplementation causing kidney failure and rhabdomyolysis[74,75]. Furthermore, chromium picolinate supplements may alter DNA structure, especially when combined with vitamin C[76]. Based on available data, athletes and consumers should avoid chromium picolinate-containing supplements, because they do not appear to provide an ergogenic effect and may be harmful.

Table 1 summarizes the nutritional sports supplements discussed.

MIND–BODY METHODS FOR ENHANCING ATHLETIC PERFORMANCE

Phil Jackson, a Zen Buddhist and one of the most successful head coaches in the history of professional basketball, often receives media attention for his unconventional approaches to coaching. Before many practices, Jackson brings in instructors to teach his players meditation and yoga exercises. Many criticize his methods, while others have followed his lead, and have also experienced improved results. As a result of Phil Jackson and others in professional sports, there is a growing trend among athletes in the USA to utilize mind–body methods.

Meditation

Meditation is a mental technique practiced repeatedly to achieve 'pure consciousness', which is an experience characterized subjectively as restful, blissful, peaceful, silent and heightened awareness. Centuries ago, meditation originated either from Vedic, Buddhist or Taoist traditions[77,78]. Despite its long history and worldwide popularity, the physiological effects of meditation have begun to be studied only recently.

Table 1 Summary of nutritional sports supplements

Supplement	Erogenic effects?	Harmful effects?	Comments
Creatine	↑ muscle mass ↑ fat loss	↓ plasma volume fluid retention	caffeine negates its effect ↑ absorption with carbohydrates
Whey protein	↑ muscle mass ↑ fat loss	none	from milk; complete source of amino acids
Glutamine	↑ muscle mass ↑ fat loss	none	useful for post-surgical patients
BCAAs	↑ muscle mass ↑ fat loss	none	precursors to glutamine
Androsterone	inconsistent	inconsistent	commonly known as andro
Androsteronediol	inconsistent	inconsistent	direct testosterone prohormone
DHEA	inconsistent	inconsistent	precursor to androsterone and androsteronediol
Epehdrine and caffeine	↑ muscle mass ↑ fat loss	↑ dizziness ↑ heart rate	serious heath problems associated with use
Chromium picolinate	inconsistent	kidney failure rhabdomyolysis	combined with vitamin C, may damage DNA

BCAAs, branched-chain amino acids; DHEA, dehydroepiandrosterone

Studies have revealed that those who practice meditation have a decreased red blood cell count, a reduction in muscle and overall body metabolism, as well as decreased thyroid and adrenocortical serum hormone levels[79–83]. Additional effects include decreased oxygen consumption, redistributed brain circulation and increased coherence of heart rhythms[80,84–88]. Long-term practice of meditation enhances these effects, resulting in improved physiological efficiency. Reports of its benefits have prompted some to turn to meditation for enhanced athletic performance.

One study investigated meditation and its effects on shooting performance. Twenty-five elite shooters practiced daily meditation and improved their shooting accuracy. Conversely, the shooters did not improve when they utilized relaxation techniques[89]. The fact that relaxing did not improve shooting performance suggests that the efficacy of meditation is not limited to its ability to reduce tension.

Similarly, adult runners also improved their performance through the use of meditation over the course of 6 months. Those who practiced daily meditation had significantly lower blood lactic acid levels as compared with controls[90]. The decrease in lactic acid may be due to the reduction in red blood cell metabolism, associated with the practice of meditation[91]. The drop in lactate levels as a result of the decline in red blood

cell metabolism indicates an increase in fatty acid utilization, suggesting that meditation may improve athletes' ability to use fat as an energy source. Although limited, the initial data concerning meditation and sports performance are encouraging and warrant further investigation.

Yoga

Yoga is one of six Indian orthodox philosophies, based on the 2000-year-old teachings of Patanjali found in his work the *Yoga Sutras*. Derived from the Sanskrit root *yuj* meaning 'bind', 'join' and 'attach', the practice of yoga attempts to connect an individual's mind and body with the Supreme Universal Spirit (*Paramatma* or God) through both meditative and physical activities. The practice of yoga consists of correct breathing exercises, specific postures and certain gazing points in order to increase control of the senses and deepen self-awareness[92].

There have been many physical and mental benefits attributed to the practice of yoga. Those who consistently practice yoga techniques exhibit increased endurance[93] and better control of autonomic functions[94]. Similar to meditation, yoga has also been shown to reduce oxygen consumption[95] and improve

Textbook of Complementary and Alternative Medicine

cardiorespiratory efficiency[96]. Yoga exercises have also been known to improve muscular efficiency[97], increase aerobic power[98] and decrease both visual and auditory reaction time responses[99]. These studies indicate that yoga may improve athletic performance because of its mind and body benefits.

Many sports, such as figure skating and gymnastics, require the execution of precise, complicated movements which require the athlete to have a good sense of balance. The results of one study indicates that yoga improves balance, and thus may be advantageous for athletes engaged in sports. In one study, 18 medical students either practiced yoga or took either dextroamphetamine (10 mg) or lactose (placebo) 1 h prior to testing their balance using a balance board. Average balance time and error scores for ten trials showed that those who practiced yoga prior to testing outperformed controls by 27.8% while those who took dextroamphetamine peformed 40.6% worse than those taking placebo. Additionally, the yoga group progressively improved their balance over the course of the ten trials, which suggests that repeated, long-term practice of yoga could improve balance even further[100]. Incorporating yoga into an athletic training program could help improve co-ordination by enhancing balance.

Yoga may also improve dexterity and visual perception, abilities involved in many sports. Girls (12–16 years old) who practiced yoga daily for 6 months performed better on visual perception and dexterity tasks than comparable female adolescents who participated in other physical activities for 6 months[101]. Yoga may provide benefits that other forms of exercise cannot.

Another study compared the physiological effects of yoga with those of other physical activities. Athletes engaged in either judo and volleyball or yoga for 1 h daily over the course of a year. At the end of the study, both groups displayed physical improvements. Those who practiced yoga, however, had lower blood lactate levels, reduced oxygen consumption at rest and an increased work-load capacity compared to those who played volleyball and judo all year[102]. It appears that yoga affects the body differently from other physical activities.

For some people, yoga seems to provide psychological as well as physical benefits. Physical exercise has been shown to affect mood positively. In one study, those who either practiced yoga or swam reported experiencing more positive feelings than those who did not engage in physical activities. Furthermore, men who practiced yoga experienced even greater mood benefits than their male swimmer counterparts. There were, though, no differences reported between women swimmers and their yoga-practicing female counterparts[103]. Yoga may enhance feelings of wellness more than other physical activities.

There are many benefits, both physical and psychological, attributed to yoga. Athletes may be able to improve their performance in sports by incorporating yoga exercises into their training programs. Future studies will identify the specific atheletes and the sports in which they participate who might benefit most from yoga; however, all athletes seeking improvements in performance will benefit from practicing yoga.

Hypnosis

Hypnosis is a technique that attempts to turn the subconscious and conscious, which normally work independently, towards a single focal point. Health professionals sometimes use hypnosis to help precipitate changes in subjects' perceptions, sensations, thoughts, or behaviors. Undergoing hypnosis typically entails imagining pleasant experiences while being instructed to relax. Most people report hypnosis as a pleasant experience, although responses to it differ. Visualization is one method sometimes used in conjunction with hypnosis in order to help individuals improve their performance of a particular skill or activity, by having them mentally perform the task perfectly in their minds[104]. Hypnosis has been shown to improve the ability to imagine among athletes[105], and some have used it to help athletes perform better.

Gymnastics is a sport characterized by complex, precise movements that are difficult to perform. Often, a maneuver is hindered, not because of physical limitation on the part of the athlete, but rather owing to difficulties in mentally co-ordinating all of the movements. To see whether hypnosis could improve the mental capabilities of athletes in this regard, two gymnasts underwent hypnosis that utilized visualization.

The gymnasts were male college athletes who had been struggling with a particular task for several months.

The first gymnast initially was not able to complete a double back flip layout with a twist without error, even after a year of practice. Under hypnosis, he was instructed to speak his way through the maneuver step-by-step slowly. If he made a mistake in his mind, he was asked to start over. Initially, his response to the visualization was only verbal. Eventually, strong muscle reactions were observed as he mentally went through the movements. After he had perfected the maneuver visually in his mind, he was asked to repeat it five more times, while still under hypnosis. The very next day he performed the double back flip layout with a twist perfectly five consecutive times, and he continued to perform it accurately for days following the hypnosis session[105].

The next gymnast in the study had difficulty completing two tasks consecutively on the high bar, despite the fact that he could do each maneuver separately. After 2 years of practicing, he still was not able to complete them in combination. As was the case with the first gymnast, while under hypnosis, this gymnast was asked to perform the task verbally slowly, until he performed it perfectly mentally. Again, the gymnast repeated the visualization several times until he was comfortable with it. Immediately after the session, the gymnast performed each maneuver on the high bar consecutively without problems[105]. The gymnasts' experiences suggest that hypnosis may have an effective role in sports.

Hypnosis may additionally help athletes by reducing stress and performance anxiety. Often, athletes report difficulty accomplishing tasks during competitions where audiences are present. Excessive anxiety may cause their performance to be sub-optimal. Hypnosis may reduce stress and help athletes perform at their best.

In one study, a 16-year-old male tennis player who was hyperkinetic and taking Ritalin and had not won a major match for 6 years, was able to win a state doubles championship and a major regional singles tournament following hypnosis[106]. Other case studies showed similar benefits of hypnosis in sports. Twenty female gymnasts (8–16 years old) complained of excessive levels of stress during both practice and competitions. Following hypnosis, the athletes reported reduced fear, anxiety and stress levels. Their coach also indicated that he had observed improvements among his players after hypnosis. Eight of the 20 female gymnasts went on to qualify for a highly competitive meet[106]. These initial case studies suggest that hypnosis may reduce psychological barriers to athletic performance, although further studies are needed.

CONCLUSION

Many alternative sports medicine therapies are safe and effective in improving athletic performance. Based on available data, athletes who consume creatine, whey protein, glutamine and branched-chain amino acids will experience improved strength and body composition safely in a way that training alone cannot provide or can achieve only at a slower rate. Conversely, chromium picolinate and the testosterone prohormone supplements should be avoided, not only because they may be ineffective, but because they may cause harm to users. Although ephedrine and caffeine-containing supplements seem to promote fat reduction, athletes should be cautioned about the possible consequences of taking them and the risks associated with improper use. Currently, there is a lack of sufficient studies that have investigated long-term use of nutritional sports supplements and their possible interactions with other substances. Further studies need to be conducted. Regardless of the outcome of future research, athletes and physicians need to discuss supplements, and work together to make sure patients achieve the most benefits safely.

Although not as popular as sports nutritional supplements, mind–body methods in sports have also been shown to be effective in enhancing sports performance. While future studies are needed to demonstrate the athletes who could benefit from such techniques, initial data suggest that mind–body methods may contribute positively to training programs. Whether it is supplemental use or yoga exercises, discussing alternative sports medicine therapies with patients will improve physician and patient communication, and will enhance care.

References

1. Annual Report. *Nutr Bus J* 2001

2. Chanutin A. The fate of creatine when administered to man. *J Biol Chem* 1926;67:29–41

3. Balsom PD, Harridge SD, Soderlund K, *et al.* Creatine supplementation per se does not enhance endurance exercise performance. *Acta Physiol Scand* 1993;149:521–3

4. Kreider RB, Ferreira M, Wilson M, *et al.* Effects of creatine supplementation on body composition, strength, and sprint performance. *Med Sci Sports Exerc* 1998;30:73–82

5. Vandenberghe K, Goris M, Van Hecke P, Van Leemputte M, Vangerven L, Hespel P. Long-term creatine intake is beneficial to muscle performance during resistance training. *J Appl Physiol* 1997;83:2055–63

6. Volek JS, Kraemer WJ, Bush JA, *et al.* Creatine supplementation enhances muscular performance during high-intensity resistance exercise. *J Am Diet Assoc* 1997;97:765–70

7. Engelhardt M, Neumann G, Berbalk A, Reuter I. Creatine supplementation in endurance sports. *Med Sci Sports Exerc* 1998;30:1123–9

8. Vandebuerie F, Vanden Eynde B, Vandenberghe K, Hespel P. Effect of creatine loading on endurance capacity and sprint power in cyclists. *Int J Sports Med* 1998;19:490–5

9. Bemben MG, Tuttle TD, Bemben DA, Knehans AW. Effects of creatine supplementation on isometric force–time curve characteristics. *Med Sci Sports Exerc* 2001;33:1876–81

10. Tarnopolsky M, Martin J. Creatine monohydrate increases strength in patients with neuromuscular disease. *Neurology* 1999;52:854–7

11. Guerrero-Ontiveros ML, Wallimann T. Creatine supplementation in health and disease. Effects of chronic creatine ingestion *in vivo*: down-regulation of the expression of creatine transporter isoforms in skeletal muscle. *Mol Cell Biochem* 1998;184:427–37

12. Koshy KM, Griswold E, Schneeberger EE. Interstitial nephritis in a patient taking creatine. *N Engl J Med* 1999;340:814–15

13. Oopik V, Paasuke M, Timpmann S, *et al.* Effect of creatine supplementation during rapid body mass reduction on metabolism and isokinetic muscle performance capacity. *Eur J Appl Physiol Occup Physiol* 1998;78:83–92

14. Harris RC, Soderlund K, Hultman E. Elevation of creatine in resting and exercised muscle of normal subjects by creatine supplementation. *Clin Sci (Lond)* 1992;83:367–74

15. Greenhaff PL, Casey A, Short AH, *et al.* Influence of oral creatine supplementation of muscle torque during repeated bouts of maximal voluntary exercise in man. *Clin Sci (Lond)* 1993;84:565–71

16. Steenge GR, Lambourne J, Casey A, Macdonald IA, Greenhaff PL. Stimulatory effect of insulin on creatine accumulation in human skeletal muscle. *Am J Physiol* 1998;275:E974–9

17. Vandenberghe K, Gillis N, Van Leemputte M, Van Hecke P, Vanstapel F, Hespel P. Caffeine counteracts the ergogenic action of muscle creatine loading. *J Appl Physiol* 1996;80:452–7

18. Dohm GL, Kasperek GJ, Tapscott EG, Barakat H. Protein metabolism during endurance exercise. *Fed Proc* 1985;44:348–52

19. Lemon PWR, Nagel FJ. Effects of exercise on protein and amino acid metabolism. *Med Sci Sports Exerc* 1981;13:141–9

20. Food and Nutrition Board. *Recommended Dietary Allowances*, 10th edn. Washington, DC: National Academy of Sciences, 1989:30

21. Lemon PWR, Mullin JP. Effect of initial muscle glycogen levels on protein catabolism during exercise. *J Appl Physiol* 1980;48:624–9

22. Friedman JE, Lemon PWR. Effect of protein intake and endurance exercise on daily protein requirements. *Med Sci Sports* 1985;17:231

23. Tarnopolsky MA, MacDougall JD, Atkinson SA. Influence of protein intake and training status on nitrogen balance and lean body mass. *J Appl Physiol* 1988;64:187–93

24. Tarnopolsky MA, MacDougall JD, Atkinson SA. Evaluation of protein requirements for trained strength athletes. *J Appl Physiol* 1992;73:1986–95

25. Tarnopolsky MA, MacDougall JD, Atkinson SA. Dietary protein requirements for body builders verses sedentary controls. *Med Sci Sports Exerc* 1986;18:S64

26. Lemon PWR, Tarnopolsky MA, MacDougall JD, Atkinson SA. Protein requirements and muscle mass/strength changes during intensive training in novice bodybuilders. *J Appl Physiol* 1992;73:767

27. Esmarck B, Andersen JL, Olsen S, *et al.* Timing of postexercise protein intake is important for muscle hypertrophy with resistance training in elderly humans. *J Physiol* 2001;535:301–11

28. Smith G. Whey protein. *World Rev Nutr Diet* 1976;24:88–116

29. Smithers GW, Ballard FJ, Copeland AD, *et al.* New opportunities from the isolation and utilization of whey proteins. *J Dairy Sci* 1996;79:1454–9

30. Lands LC, Grey VL, Smountas AA. Effect of supplementation with a cysteine donor on muscular performance. *J Appl Physiol* 1999;87:1381–5

31. Bounous G, Baruchel S, Falutz J, Gold P. Whey proteins as a food supplement in HIV-seropositive individuals. *Clin Invest Med* 1993;16:204–9

32. Kennedy RS, Konok GP, Bounous G, Baruchel S, Lee TD. The use of whey protein concentrate in the treatment of patients with metastatic carcinoma: a phase I–II clinical study. *Anticancer Res* 1995;5:2643–50

33. Charlton CP, Buchanan E, Holden CE, *et al.* Intensive enteral feeding in advanced cirrhosis: reversal of malnutrition without precipitation of hepatic encephalopathy. *Arch Dis Child* 1992;67:603–7

34. Canciani M, Mastella G. Absorption of a new supplemental diet in infants with cystic fibrosis. *J Pediatr Gastroenterol Nutr* 1985;4:735–40

35. Burke DG, Chilibeck PD, Davidson KS, Candow DG, Farthing J, Smith-Palmer T. The effect of whey protein supplementation with and without creatine monohydrate combined with resistance training on lean tissue mass and muscle strength. *Int J Sport Nutr Exerc Metab* 2001;11:349–64

36. Newsholme EA, Leech AR. *Biochemistry for the Medical Sciences*. New York, NY: John Wiley & Sons, 1983:423–5

37. Rowbottom DG, Keast D, Morton AR. The emerging role of glutamine as an indicator of exercise stress and overtraining. *Sports Med* 1996;21:80–97

38. Hall JC, Heel K, McCauley R. Glutamine. *Br J Surg* 1996;83:305–12

39. Hankard RG, Haymond MW, Darmaun D. Effect of glutamine on leucine metabolism in humans. *Am J Physiol* 1996;271:E748–54

40. Welbourne TC. Increased plasma bicarbonate and growth hormone after an oral glutamine load. *Am J Clin Nutr* 1995;61:1058–61

41. Rosene MF, Finn KJ, Antonio J. Glutamine supplementation may maintain nitrogen balance in wrestlers during a weight reduction program. *Med Sci Sports Exerc* 1999;31:S123

42. Hammarqvist F, Wernerman J, Von Der Decken A, Vinnars E. Alanyl-glutamine counteracts the depletion of free glutamine and the postoperative decline in protein synthesis in skeletal muscle. *Ann Surg* 1990; 212:637–44

43. Peterson B, Von Der Decken A, Vinnars E, Wernerman J. Long-term effects of postoperative total parenteral nutrition supplementation with glycylglutamine on subjective fatigue and muscle protein synthesis. *Br J Surg* 1994;81:1520–3

44. Marks DB, Marks AD, Smith CM. *Basic Medical Biochemistry*. Baltimore, MD: Williams and Wilkins, 1996

45. Schena F, Guerrini F, Tregnaghi P, Kayser B. Branched-chain amino acid supplementation during trekking at high altitude: the effects on loss of body mass, body composition, and muscle power. *Eur J Appl Physiol* 1992;65:394–8

46. Blomstrand E, Newsholme EA. Effect of branched-chain amino acid supplementation on the exercise-induced change in aromatic amino acid concentration in human muscle. *Acta Physiol Scand* 1992;146:293–8

47. Mourier A, Bigard AX, de Kerviler E, Roger B, Legrand H, Guezennec CY. Combined effects of caloric restriction and branched-chain amino acid supplementation on body composition and exercise performance in elite wrestlers. *Int J Sports Med* 1997;18:47–55

48. Colker CM. Effects of supplemental protein on body compostion and muscular strength in healthy athletic male adults. *Curr Ther Res* 2000;61:19–28

49. Ziegenfuss TN, Lambert CP, Lowery LM. Oral administration of testosterone precursors elevates plasma androgens in men. Presented at *The International Conference on Weight Lifting and Strength Training*, Finland, 1998:abstr

50. Earnest CP, Olson MA, Broeder CE, Breuel KF, Beckham SG. *In vivo* 4-androstene-3,17-dione and 4-androstene-3 beta,17 beta-diol supplementation in young men. *Eur J Appl Physiol* 2000;81:229–32

51. King DS, Sharp RL, Vukovich MD, *et al*. Effect of oral androstenedione on serum testosterone and adaptations to resistance training in young men: a randomized controlled trial. *J Am Med Assoc* 1999;281:2020–8

52. Antonio J, Sanders M. Effects of self-administered androstenedione on a young male bodybuilder: a single-subject study. *Curr Ther Res* 1999;60:486–92

53. Antonio J, Sanders MS, Kalman D, Woodgate D, Street C. The effects of high-dose glutamine ingestion on weightlifting performance. *J Strength Cond Res* 2002;16:157–60

54. Longcope C. Dehydroepiandrosterone metabolism. *J Endocrinol* 1996;150(Suppl):S125–7

55. Brown GA, Vukovich MD, Sharp RL, Reifenrath TA, Parsons KA, King DS. Effect of oral DHEA on serum testosterone and adaptations to resistance training in young men. *J Appl Physiol* 1999;87:2274–83

56. Nestler JE, Barlascini CO, Clore JN, Blackard WG. Dehydroepiandrosterone reduces serum low density lipoprotein levels and body fat but does not alter insulin sensitivity in normal men. *J Clin Endocrinol Metab* 1988;66:57–61

57. Welle S, Jozefowicz R, Statt M. Failure of dehydroepiandrosterone to influence energy and protein metabolism in humans. *J Clin Endocrinol Metab* 1990;71:1259–64

58. Wilson JD. Androgen abuse by athletes. *Endocr Rev* 1988;9:181–99

59. Kuczmarki RJ, Flegal KM, Campbell SM, Johnson CL. Increasing prevalence of overweight among US adults. The National Health and Nutrition Examination Surveys, 1960 to 1991. *J Am Med Assoc* 1994;272:205–11

60. Must A, Jacques PF, Dallal GE, Bajema CJ, Dietz WH. Long-term morbidity and mortality of overweight among adolescents. A follow-up of the Harvard Growth Study of 1922 to 1935. *N Engl J Med* 1992;327:1350–5

61. Astrup A, Toubro S, Christensen NJ, Quaade F. Pharmacology of thermogenic drugs. *Am J Clin Nutr* 1992;55:246S–8S

62. Astrup A, Breum L, Toubro S, Hein P, Quaade F. The effect of safety of an ephedrine/caffeine compound compared to ephedrine, caffeine and placebo in obese subjects on an energy restricted diet: a double blind trial. *Int J Obes* 1992;16:269–77

63. Daly PA, Krieger DR, Dulloo AG, Young JB, Landsberg L. Ephedrine, caffeine and aspirin: safety and efficacy for treatment of human obesity. *Int J Obes* 1993;17:S73–8

64. Guy-Grand B, Apfelbaum M, Crepaldi G, Gries A, Lefebvre P, Turner P. International trial of long-term dexfenfluramine in obesity. *Lancet* 1989;2:1142–5

65. Breum L, Pedersen JK, Ahlstrom F, Frimodt-Moller J. Comparison of an ephedrine/caffeine combination and dexfenfluramine in the treatment of obesity: a double-blind multicentre trial in general practice. *Int J Obes* 1994;18:99–103

66. Lukaski HC, Bolonchuk WW, Siders WA, Milne DB. Chromium supplementation and resistance training: effects on body composition, strength, and trace elements status of men. *Am J Clin Nutr* 1996;63:954–65

67. Evans GW, Bowman TD. Chromium picolinate increases membrane fluidity and rate of insulin internalization. *J Inorg Biochem* 1992;46:243–50

68. Anderson RA, Cheng N, Bryden NA, *et al*. Elevated intakes of supplemental chromium improve glucose and insulin variables in individuals with type 2 diabetes. *Diabetes* 1997;46:1786–91

69. Hasten DL, Rome EP, Franks BD, Hegsted M. Effects of chromium picolinate on beginning weight training students. *Int J Sports Nutr* 1992;2:343–50

70. Clancy SP, Clarkson PM, DeCheke ME, *et al*. Effects of chromium picolinate supplementation on body compostion, strength, and urinary chromium loss in football players. *Int J Sports Nutr* 1994;4:142–53

71. Trent LK, Thieding-Cancel D. Effects of chromium picolinate on body composition. *J Sports Med Phys Fitness* 1995;35:273–80

72. Walker LS, Bemben MG, Bemben DA, Knehans AW. Chromium picolinate effects on body composition and muscular performance in wrestlers. *Med Sci Sports Exerc* 1998;30:1730–7

73. Grant KE, Chandler RM, Castle AL, Ivy JL. Chromium and exercise training: effects on obese women. *Med Sci Sports Exerc* 1997;29:992–8

74. Cerulli J, Grabe DW, Gauthier I, Malone M, McGoldrick MD. Chromium picolinate toxicity. *Ann Pharmacother* 1998;32:428–31

75. Martin WR, Fuller RE. Suspected chromium picolinate-induced rhabdomyolysis. *Pharmacotherapy* 1998;18:860–2

76. Vincent. Annual Chemical Society Meeting, 1999

77. Zimmer H. *Philosophies of India*. Princeton, NJ: Princeton University Press, 1951

78. Swami Prabhavananda. *The Eternal Companion*. Hollywood, CA: Vedanta Press, 1970

79. Michaels RR, Parra J, McCann DS, Vander AJ. Renin, cortisol, and aldosterone during transcendental meditation. *Psychosom Med* 1979;41:50–4

80. Jevning R, Wilson AF, Davidson JM. Adrenocortical activity during meditation. *Horm Behav* 1978;10:54–60

81. Werner O, Wallace RK, Charles B, Janssen G, Chalmers R. *Endocrine Balance and the TM-Sidhi Program. Scientific Research on the Transcendental Meditation Program: Collected Papers.* Vol. 2. Rheinweiler, Germany: MERU Press, 1993

82. Jevning R, Pirkle HC, Wilson AF. Behavioral alteration of plasma phenylalanine concentration. *Physiol Behav* 1977;19:611–14

83. Jevning R. Integrated metabolic regulation during acute rest states in man, similarity to fasting: a biochemical hypothesis. *Physiol Behav* 1988;43:735–7

84. Banquet JP, Sailhan M. EEG analysis of spontaneous and induced stress states of consciousness. *Rev Electroencephalogr Neurophysiol Clin* 1974;4:445–53

85. Badawi K, Wallace RK, Rouzere AM, Orme-Johnson D. Electrophysiological changes during periods of respiratory suspension in the transcendental meditation technique. *Psychosom Med* 1984;46:267–76

86. Herbert R, Lehmann D. Theta bursts: an EEG pattern in normal subjects practicing the transcendental meditation technique. *Electroencephalogr Clin Neurophysiol* 1977;42:397–405

87. Bagchi BK, Wenger MA. Electrophysiological correlates of some yogi exercises. *Electroencephalogr Clin Neurophysiol* 1957;7(Suppl):132–49

88. Benson H, Stewart RF, Greenwood MM, Klemchuk H, Peterson N. Continuous measurement of oxygen consumption and carbon dioxide elimination during a wakeful hypometabolic state. *J Hum Stress* 1975;1:37–44

89. Solberg EE, Berglund KA, Engen O, Ekeberg O, Loeb M. The effect of meditation on shooting performance. *Br J Sports Med* 1996;30:342–6

90. Solberg EE, Ingjer F, Holen A, et al. Stress reactivity to and recovery from a standardised exercise bout: a study of 31 runners practising relaxation techniques. *Br J Sports Med* 2000;34:268–72

91. Jevning R, Wilson AF, Pirkle H, O'Halloran JP, Walsh RN. Metabolic control in a state of decreased activation: modulation of red cell metabolism. *Am J Physiol* 1983;245:C457–61

92. Iyengar BKS, Menuhin Y. *Light on Pranayama the Yogic Art of Breathing.* The Crossword Publishing Company; 1995

93. Vakil RJ. Remarkable feat of endurance by a yogi priest. *Lancet* 1950;2:871

94. Kothari LK, Bordia A, Gupta OP. The yogic claim of voluntary control over heart beat: an unusual demonstration. *Am Heart J* 1973;86:282–4

95. Madan M, Rai UC, Balavital V, Thombre DP. Cardiorespiratory changes during savitri pranayam and shavasan. *Yoga Rev* 1983;3:25–34

96. Gopal KS, Bhatnagar OP, Subramanian N, Nishith SD. Effect of yogasanas and pranayamas on B.P., pulse rate and some respiratory functions. *Indian J Physiol Pharmacol* 1973;17:273–6

97. Ray US, Hegde KS, Selvamurthy W. Improvement in muscular efficiency as related to a standard task after yogic exercises in middle aged men. *Indian J Med Res* 1986;83:343–8

98. Balasubramanian B, Pansare MS. Effect of yoga on aerobic and anaerobic power of muscles. *Indian J Physiol Pharmacol* 1991;35:281–2

99. Madan M, Thombre DP, Balakumar B, et al. Effect of yoga training on reaction time, respiratory endurance and muscle strength. *Indian J Physiol Pharmacol* 1992;36:229–33

100. Dhume RR, Dhume RA. A comparative study of the driving effects of dextroamphetamine and yogic meditation on muscle control for the performance of balance on balance board. *Indian J Physiol Pharmacol* 1991;35:191–4

101. Raghuraj P, Telles S. Muscle power, dexterity skill and visual perception in community home girls trained in yoga or sports and in regular school girls. *Indian J Physiol Pharmacol* 1997;41:409–15

102. Raju PS, Madhavi S, Prasad KV, et al. Comparison of effects of yoga and physical exercise in athletes. *Indian J Med Res* 1994;100:81–6

103. Berger BG, Owen DR. Mood alteration with yoga and swimming: aerobic exercise may not be necessary. *Percept Mot Skills* 1992;75:1331–43

104. Bandura A. *Social Foundations of Thought and Action: A Social Cognitive Theory.* Englewood Cliffs, NJ: Prentice Hall, 1986

105. Liggett DR, Hamada S. Enhancing the visualization of gymnasts. *Am J Clin Hypn* 1993;35:190–7

106. Krenz EW. Improving competitive performance with hypnotic suggestion and modified autogenic training: case reports. *Am J Clin Hypn* 1984;27:58–63

Further reading

Aaserud R, Gramvik P, Olsen SR, Jensen J. Creatine supplementation delays onset of fatigue during repeated bouts of sprint running. *Scand J Med Sci Sports* 1998;8:247–51

Balasubramanian B, Pansare MS. Effect of yoga on aerobic and anaerobic power of muscles. *Indian J Physiol Pharmacol* 1991;35:281–2

Bell DG, McLellan TM, Sabiston CM. Effect of ingesting caffeine and ephedrine on 10-km run performance. *Med Sci Sports Exerc* 2002;34:344–9

Bellinger BM, Bold A, Wilson GR, Noakes TD, Myburgh KH. Oral creatine supplementation decreases plasma markers of adenine nucleotide degradation during a 1-h cycle test. *Acta Physiol Scand* 2000;170:217–24

Berglund B, Hemmingsson P. Effects of caffeine ingestion on exercise performance at low and high altitudes in cross-country skiers. *Int J Sports Med* 1982;3:234–6

Bermon S, Venembre P, Sachet C, Valour S, Dolisi C. Effects of creatine monohydrate ingestion in sedentary and weight-trained older adults. *Acta Physiol Scand* 1998;164:147–55

Boone T, Cooper R. The effect of massage on oxygen consumption at rest. *Am J Chin Med* 1995;23:37–41

Bosco C, Tihanyi J, Pucspk J, et al. Effect of oral creatine supplementation on jumping and running performance. *Int J Sports Med* 1997;18:369–72

Bosy TZ, Moore KA, Poklis A. The effect of oral dehydroepiandrosterone (DHEA) on the urine testosterone/epitestosterone (T/E) ratio in human male volunteers. *J Anal Toxicol* 1998;22:455–9

Brown GA, Vukovich MD, Reifenrath TA, *et al*. Effects of anabolic precursors on serum testosterone concentrations and adaptations to resistance training in young men. *Int J Sport Nutr Exerc Metab* 2000;10:340–59

Burke DG, Smith-Palmer T, Holt LE, Head B, Chilibeck PD. The effect of 7 days of creatine supplementation on 24-hour urinary creatine excretion. *J Strength Cond Res* 2001;15:59–62

Burke LM, Pyne DB, Telford RD. Effect of oral creatine supplementation on single-effort sprint performance in elite swimmers. *Int J Sport Nutr* 1996;6:222–33

Campbell WW, Joseph LJ, Davey SL, Cyr-Campbell D, Anderson RA, Evans WJ. Effects of resistance training and chromium picolinate on body composition and skeletal muscle in older men. *J Appl Physiol* 1999;86:29–39

Casey A, Constantin-Teodosiu D, Howell S, Hultman E, Greenhaff PL. Creatine ingestion favorably affects performance and muscle metabolism during maximal exercise in humans. *Am J Physiol* 1996;271:E31–7

Chaloupka EC, Kang J, Mastrangelo MA. The effect of flexible magnets on hand muscle strength: a randomized, double-blind study. *J Strength Cond Res* 2002;16:33–7

di Luigi L, Guidetti L, Pigozzi F, *et al*. Acute amino acids supplementation enhances pituitary responsiveness in athletes. *Med Sci Sports Exerc* 1999;31:1748–54

Felber S, Skladal D, Wyss M, Kremser C, Koller A, Sperl W. Oral creatine supplementation in Duchenne muscular dystrophy: a clinical and ^{31}P magnetic resonance spectroscopy study. *Neurol Res* 2000;22:145–50

Gill ND, Shield A, Blazevich AJ, Zhou S, Weatherby RP. Muscular and cardiorespiratory effects of pseudoephedrine in human athletes. *Br J Clin Pharmacol* 2000;50:205–13

Gopal KS, Anantharamn V, Nishith SD, Bhatnagar OP. The effect of yogasanas on muscular tone and cardio-respiratory adjustments. *Indian J Med Sci* 1974;28:438–43

Gotshalk LA, Volek JS, Staron RS, Denegar CR, Hagerman FC, Kraemer WJ. Creatine supplementation improves muscular performance in older men. *Med Sci Sports Exerc* 2002;34:537–43

Guber AJ, Pope HG Jr. Ephedrine abuse among 36 female weightlifters. *Am J Addict* 1998;7:256–61

Hemmings B, Smith M, Graydon J, Dyson R. Effects of massage on physiological restoration, perceived recovery, and repeated sports performance. *Br J Sports Med* 2000;34:109–14; discussion 115

Hespel P, Eijnde BO, Derave W, Richter EA. Creatine supplementation: exploring the role of the creatine kinase/phosphocreatine system in human muscle. *Can J Appl Physiol* 2001;26(Suppl):S79–102

Hespel P, Op't Eijnde B, Van Leemputte M, *et al*. Oral creatine supplementation facilitates the rehabilitation of disuse atrophy and alters the expression of muscle myogenic factors in humans. *J Physiol* 2001;536:625–33

Izquierdo M, Ibanez J, Gonzalez-Badillo JJ, Gorostiaga EM. Effects of creatine supplementation on muscle power, endurance, and sprint performance. *Med Sci Sports Exerc* 2002;34:332–43

Javierre C, Lizarraga MA, Ventura JL, Garrido E, Segura R. Creatine supplementation does not improve physical performance in a 150 m race. *Rev Esp Fisiol* 1997;53:343–8

Kanayama G, Gruber AJ, Pope HG Jr, Borowiecki JJ, Hudson JI. Over-the-counter drug use in gymnasiums: an underrecognized substance abuse problem? *Psychother Psychosom* 2001;70:137–40

Lemon PWR. Protein and amino acid needs of the strength athlete. *Int J Sports Nutr* 1991;1:127–45

Livolsi JM, Adams GM, Laguna PL. The effect of chromium picolinate on muscular strength and body composition in women athletes. *J Strength Cond Res* 2001;15:161–6

Lukaszewska JH, Obuchowicz-Fidelus B. Serum and urinary steroids in women athletes. *J Sports Med Phys Fitness* 1985;25:215–21

Maganaris CN, Maughan RJ. Creatine supplementation enhances maximum voluntary isometric force and endurance capacity in resistance trained men. *Acta Physiol Scand* 1998;163:279–87

McGavock JM, Lecomte JL, Delancy JS, Lacroix VJ, Hardy P, Montgomery DL. Effects of hyperbaric oxygen on aerobic performance in a normobaric environment. *Undersea Hyperb Med* 1999;26:219–24

McGuine TA, Sullivan JC, Bernhardt DT. Creatine supplementation in high school football players. *Clin J Sport Med* 2001;11:247–53

Metzl JD, Small E, Levine SR, Gershel JC. Creatine use among young athletes. *Pediatrics* 2001;108:421–5

Mujika I, Padilla S, Ibanez J, Izquierdo M, Gorostiaga E. Creatine supplementation and sprint performance in soccer players. *Med Sci Sports Exerc* 2000;32:518–25

Naylor AH, Gardner D, Zaichkowsky L. Drug use patterns among high school athletes and nonathletes. *Adolescence* 2001;36:627–39

Olivardia R, Pope HG Jr, Hudson JI. Muscle dysmorphia in male weightlifters: a case–control study. *Am J Psychiatry* 2000;157:1291–6

Op't Eijnde B, Vergauwen L, Hespel P. Creatine loading does not impact on stroke performance in tennis. *Int J Sports Med* 2001;22:76–80

Pope HG Jr, Gruber AJ, Choi P, Olivardia R, Phillips KA. Muscle dysmorphia. An underrecognized form of body dysmorphic disorder. *Psychosomatics* 1997;38:548–57

Preen D, Dawson B, Goodman C, Lawrence S, Beilby J, Ching S. Effect of creatine loading on long-term sprint exercise performance and metabolism. *Med Sci Sports Exerc* 2001;33:814–21

Prevost MC, Nelson AG, Morris GS. Creatine supplementation enhances intermittent work performance. *Res Q Exerc Sport* 1997;68:233–40

Rawson ES, Gunn B, Clarkson PM. The effects of creatine supplementation on exercise-induced muscle damage. *J Strength Cond Res* 2001;15:178–84

Ray TR, Eck JC, Covington LA, Murphy RB, Williams R, Knudtson J. Use of oral creatine as an ergogenic aid for increased sports performance: perceptions of adolescent athletes. *South Med J* 2001;94:608–12

Redondo DR, Dowling EA, Graham BL, Almada AL, Williams MH. The effect of oral creatine monohydrate supplementation on running velocity. *Int J Sport Nutr* 1996;6:213–21

Rico-Sanz J, Mendez Marco MT. Creatine enhances oxygen uptake and performance during alternating intensity exercise. *Med Sci Sports Exerc* 2000;32:379–85

Samenuk D, Link MS, Homoud MK, *et al*. Adverse cardiovascular events temporally associated with ma huang, an herbal source of ephedrine. *Mayo Clin Proc* 2002;77:12–16

Schedel JM, Terrier P, Schutz Y. The biomechanic origin of sprint performance enhancement after one-week creatine supplementation. *Jpn J Physiol* 2000;50:273–6

Smith LL, Keating MN, Holbert D, *et al.* The effects of athletic massage on delayed onset muscle soreness, creatine kinase, and neutrophil count: a preliminary report. *J Orthop Sports Phys Ther* 1994;19:93–9

Syrotuik DG, Game AB, Gillies EM, Bell GJ. Effects of creatine monohydrate supplementation during combined strength and high intensity rowing training on performance. *Can J Appl Physiol* 2001; 26:527–42

Tamarin FM, Conetta R, Brandstetter RD, Chadow H. Increased muscle enzyme activity after yoga breathing during an exacerbation of asthma. *Thorax* 1988;43:731–2

Theodorou AS, Cooke CB, King RF, *et al.* The effect of longer-term creatine supplementation on elite swimming performance after an acute creatine loading. *J Sports Sci* 1999;17:853–9

Thompson CH, Kemp GJ, Sanderson AL, *et al.* Effect of creatine on aerobic and anaerobic metabolism in skeletal muscle in swimmers. *Br J Sports Med* 1996;30:222–5

Viitasalo JT, Niemela K, Kaappola R, *et al.* Warm underwater water-jet massage improves recovery from intense physical exercise. *Eur J Appl Physiol Occup Physiol* 1995;71:431–8

Wells CL, Schrader TA, Stern JR, Krahenbuhl GS. Physiological responses to a 20-mile run under three fluid replacement treatments. *Med Sci Sports Exerc* 1985;17:364–9

Ziegler TR, Benfell K, Smith RJ, *et al.* Safety and metabolic effects of L-glutamine administration in humans. *J Parenter Enteral Nutr* 1990;14:137S–46S

Herbal, food and drug interactions

15

J. Moss

INTRODUCTION

Although potential interactions between drugs and foods have long been appreciated by pharmacologists, several highly publicized interactions between the two, and a trend toward the use of herbal medications, have made the subject a matter for public concern and discussion.

One example of a drug–food interaction is that between the monoamine oxidase inhibitors (MAOIs) and foods containing tyramine. Some 40 years ago, the interaction of tyramine with MAOIs was recognized as one of the most lethal adverse reactions in medicine. Tyramine, which is present in many foods including beer, wine and cheese, is usually degraded by intestinal monoamine oxidase (MAO). When an MAOI is administered, tyramine is absorbed systemically and transported into the presynaptic sympathetic nerve terminals[1], where it is converted to octopamine. The expected long-term consequence of the storage and release of octopamine is sympathetic inhibition. Because of the release of this relatively inactive biogenic amine, acute tyramine uptake or release can cause sympathetic excess. When MAO in the gut and liver is inhibited, excess dietary tyramine enters the circulation, causing precipitous release of norepinephrine (noradrenaline) with potential catastrophic cardiovascular consequences. Such a reaction was widely publicized in the Libby Zion case[2]. After Ms Zion, who was taking the MAOI phenalzine, was given meperidine by the resident who treated her, she suffered respiratory arrest and died. The development of linezolid antibiotics and selegiline-based antiepileptics has refocused interest on such interactions[3].

Although the interaction between tyramine and MAOIs is well recognized by both physicians and patients, the extent to which other dietary factors contribute to variability in patient response to drugs is less well appreciated. Most physicians in clinical practice acknowledge interpatient variability in responsiveness to drugs. Traditionally, the causes have been explained as pharmacokinetic, pharmacodynamic or pharmacogenetic. There is evidence, however, that some variability in response may be attributed to dietary factors. Two examples of the interaction between food and drugs reported in the literature are the effect of grapefruit juice on cytochrome P450 3A4 and the effect of solanaceous plants (potato, eggplant and tomato) on butyrylcholinesterase. Because of these interactions, several approved drugs have been withdrawn from the marketplace, and the strategy behind drug development has changed.

CYTOCHROME P450 3A4

Cytochrome P450 3A4, located in the liver and the small bowel, affects the metabolism of oral and parenteral drugs. Cytochrome P450 enzymes are the major degradative pathways for many drugs including alfentanil[4], midazolam, lidocaine and numerous antibiotics. The pharmacokinetic and pharmacodynamic effects of inhibition of cytochrome P450 3A4 have been reviewed by Dresser and co-workers[5]. Although the effect of inhibition may appear to be of academic interest only (extending half-lives of drugs, for example), inhibition has resulted in prolonged sedation or serious arrhythmias and rhabdomyolysis. Drugs such as cimetidine, which inhibits P450-mediated metabolism, also inhibit the breakdown of opioids such as morphine or fentanyl. In animals treated with cimetidine before they were given fentanyl, the half-life of fentanyl increased from 155 to 340 min[6]. In this instance, excessive sedation resulted from the drug interaction[7]. Ventricular arrhythmias (torsades de pointes) are other manifestations of the interaction when cisapride, astemizole, or terfenidine are co-administered with ketoconazole or erythromycin, potent cytochrome P450 inhibitors. Hypotension is associated with the interaction between the isoenzyme CYP 3A4 and the calcium channel antagonists or sildenifil. Finally, fatal rhabdomyolysis has been associated with co-administration of some of the co-enzyme A reductase inhibitors (statins) and some cytochrome 3A4 inhibitors. Drug-induced inhibition of cytochrome P450 is so well documented that there have been attempts to exploit inhibition of this pathway to reduce the dosage (and thereby decrease the cost) of concomitantly administered drugs such as cyclosporin.

Natural products in the diet may have the same effect as drug–drug interaction on cytochrome P450 3A4. The inhibitory effect of grapefruit juice on drug metabolism was discovered accidentally during studies of the calcium channel receptor antagonist felodipine. After grapefruit juice was added to mask the taste of the drug, investigators noticed a doubling of the drug's peak concentration in plasma[8]. In a subsequent trial, drinking 200 ml of grapefruit juice or double-strength grapefruit juice increased the felodipine mean area under the plasma concentration–time curve by 185% and 234%, respectively[9]. The interaction was tested with similar and then with other drugs also dependent on this route for metabolism[10–13]. That grapefruit juice could alter drug concentrations became widely known during the Phase-IV monitoring studies of the best-selling antihistamines terfenadine and astemizole, which ultimately led to their removal from the marketplace. Sudden death (defined by prolonged Q-T interval) and torsades de pointes were associated with patients who were taking both the antihistamines and antifungal drugs or erythromycin.

The mechanism for this unusual arrhythmia was inhibition of the cytochrome P450 isozyme CYP 3A4. Normally, the presystemic metabolism of oral terfenedine (Seldane®) by CYP 3A4 is so efficient that unmetabolized terfenedine is not detectable in plasma, protecting the patient against its potentially cardiotoxic effects (prolonged Q-T interval, torsades de pointes). In a study of six subjects in whom unmetabolized terfenedine had accumulated, grapefruit juice increased plasma terfenedine concentrations and aggravated Q-T prolongation[14]. In a follow-up study, when 11 healthy volunteers received a single dose of amiodarone along with three glasses of grapefruit juice on the same day, metabolism was inhibited completely and PR and QTc intervals changed[15].

CYP 3A4 inhibition is more important with orally than intravenously administered drugs. Although CYP 3A4 is predominantly found in the liver and intestine, its clinically important inhibition occurs in the small bowel. In a study of the interaction between grapefruit juice and midazolam in humans, subjects received either intravenous or oral midazolam (5 and 15 mg, respectively) after pretreatment with water or grapefruit juice. The investigators hypothesized that, because midazolam does not undergo significant enterohepatic circulation, some of the oral midazolam might be metabolized by the intestinal enzyme during the absorption phase. With inhibition of the intestinal enzyme, a higher level of midazolam would reach the circulation. The pharmacokinetics and pharmacodynamics of intravenous midazolam were unchanged by ingestion of grapefruit juice, but oral midazolam with grapefruit juice versus water increased peak plasma concentration by 56%[16]. Similar effects of grapefruit juice on triazolam (Halcion®) concentrations were found in ten young subjects[17]. The altered pharmacokinetics were manifested by increased drowsiness.

In addition to interaction with prescription medications, foods can also interact with over-the-counter or herbal medications. For example, drinking grapefruit juice may make caffeine levels rise. Grapefruit juice decreased the metabolism and increased the area under the plasma concentration–time curve of caffeine by 28% and prolonged its half-life by 31%. On the other hand, when herbals (e.g. St John's wort) induce the cytochrome P450 3A4 enzyme, peak levels of a drug are decreased. Decrease in peak levels has been demonstrated for warfarin, theophylline, cyclosporine, birth control pills and other drugs[18–21].

Although the effects of grapefruit juice on CYP 3A4 are known, the component in it and the mechanism that produces inhibition are unknown. The first candidate studied for inhibition was naringin, a bioflavonoid that gives grapefruit juice its bitterness. Several studies demonstrated that naringonen, the human metabolite of naringin, inhibits the CYP 3A4 enzyme. Recently, however, another candidate for the natural inhibitor in grapefruit juice has emerged[22]. Bergamottin, a citrus psoralen[23], inactivates cytochrome P450 3A4[24] and increases P-glycoprotein-mediated ATP hydrolysis more than two-fold. In animals, bergamottin inhibited the metabolism of nifedipine[25]. In healthy volunteers who received 40 mg of simvastatin, inhibition dissipated 3–7 days after ingestion of the last dose of grapefruit juice.

BUTYRYLCHOLINESTERASE

Acetylcholinesterase and butyrylcholinesterase are closely related enzymes. Acetylcholinesterase is predominant in the neuromuscular junction and terminates the action of cholinergic transmission. Butyrylcholinesterase, which is present in plasma, has an unknown action[26]. A desire to minimize paralysis time in patients undergoing surgical procedures was the impetus for the development of short-acting drugs degraded by endogenous enzymes. Drugs such as succinylcholine and mivacurium are highly dependent upon butyrylcholinesterase for their metabolism[27,28].

Although the natural role of butyrylcholinesterase is unknown, the mutation that substitutes glycine for aspartate at position 70 'pseudocholinesterase' prevents hydrolysis of succinylcholine and a variety of other drugs. In individuals expressing the genetic mutation for butyrylcholinesterase, the action of these drugs is prolonged. The genetic mutation is rare enough that drugs such as mivacurium were designed with this enzyme as a specific metabolic pathway. Variation of the butyrylcholinesterase gene has been

explored[29]. While the true biological function of butyrylcholinesterase remains unknown[30], studies in Israel suggest that the perpetuation of the ASP 70 mutation in humans is based on diet. Many naturally occurring butyrylcholinesterase mutants exist, but few are of clinical importance.

As with cytochrome P450, there is an important drug–drug interaction with butyrylcholinesterase. That non-depolarizing muscle relaxants inhibit cholinesterase has been known since the 1950s. In a more recent study, inhibition of butyrylcholinesterase by the neuromuscular antagonist pancuronium prolonged neuromuscular block by mivacurium[31].

We and others have focused on a possible interaction of the enzyme with diet. The interaction between food and butyrylcholinesterase is complex. Naturally occurring cholinesterase inhibitors, solanadine and chaconine, are found in solanaceous plants such as potato, eggplant and tomato. It is believed that they developed as natural insecticides. The ASP 70 mutation in butyrylcholinesterase confers resistance to these natural insecticides[32]. Solanaceous glycoalkaloids inhibit butyrylcholinesterase *in vitro*, and the atypical enzyme is much less sensitive to this inhibition. This hypothesis is confirmed by the geographical overlap between the frequency of the mutation and the distribution of solanaceous plants.

The function and inhibition of acetylcholinesterase have also been studied. The history of direct toxicity from potatoes and solanaceous plants is significant[33–35]. The symptoms of toxicity are consistent with cholinergic overdose (acetylcholinesterase inhibition), and sometimes toxicity has resulted in fatalities. Symptoms appear approximately 2–24 h after ingestion of potatoes[34]. In a well-documented outbreak of potato poisoning that involved 78 British school children, the most severely affected child recovered only after 1 week of hospitalization. Butyrylcholinesterase concentrations in 10 of 17 children analyzed were abnormally low 6 days after exposure. In all but one child, levels had returned to normal after 4–5 weeks, suggesting that solanaceous glycoalkaloids persist in the body. The level of circulating glycoalkaloids associated with an ordinary serving of potatoes can significantly alter butyrylcholinesterase activity in plasma.

To ascertain the interaction between solanaceous glycoalkaloids and certain anesthetic drugs, we demonstrated that solanaceous glycoalkaloids inhibit human butyrylcholinesterase at concentrations similar to those found in the serum of individuals who have eaten a serving of potatoes (Figure 1)[36]. After co-application of anesthetic drugs with neuromuscular-blocking drugs and cholinesterase inhibitors, inhibition of cholinesterase was additive. When rabbits treated with solanaceous glycoalkaloids were paralyzed with mivacurium, which depends upon butyryl-cholinesterase for its metabolism, mivacurium levels persisted. Because mivacurium metabolism had been inhibited, time for recovery from mivacurium-induced paralysis was prolonged (149±12% of control, Figure 2). Our *in vivo* and *in vitro* findings suggest that solanaceous glycoalkaloids in a normal diet could significantly impair the metabolism of anesthetic drugs.

SUMMARY

The effect on drug metabolism of common foods such as cheese, grapefruit juice and potatoes has been demonstrated in a variety of pre-clinical and clinical studies. Patients immediately recognized that food–drug interactions exist; perhaps their recognition will eventually have the greatest impact on pharmaceutical manufacturers. Increasingly, pharmaceutical companies have become aware of potential drug interactions such as those described above, because of both safety issues and the economic impact of these interactions. There is already evidence that food–drug interactions have altered the process for the development of new entities. For example, new muscle relaxants under development do not utilize butyrylcholinesterase to facilitate rapid and predictable metabolism but rather rely on organic degredation. Similarly, drugs that bypass cytochrome P450 metabolism have already

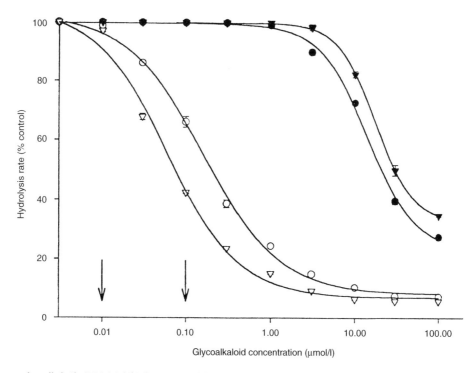

Figure 1 Solanaceous glycoalkaloids (SGAs) inhibit human acetylcholinesterease (AChE) and butyrylcholinesterase (BuChE). The effects of varied SGA concentrations on the hydrolytic activity of human AChE (solid symbols) and BuChE (open symbols) are shown. Substrate hydrolysis activity was normalized and is presented as percentage of control. Inhibition by both α-solanine (circles) and α-chaconine (triangles) was concentration-dependent. Arrows denote the range of serum SGA levels after potato consumption. Data points are mean±standard error of the mean of at least five experiments for each concentration. Determinations within each experiment were carried out in triplicate. Error bars not visible are within symbol size. Reprinted with permission from reference 36

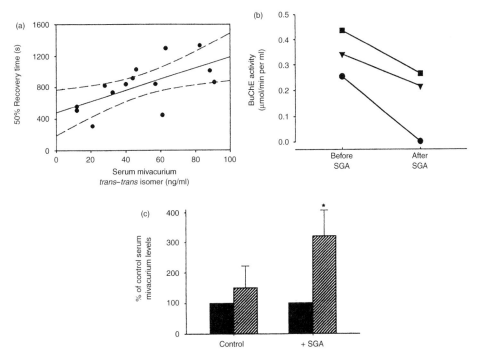

Figure 2 Serum mivacurium levels correlate with neuromuscular blockade. Solanaceous glycoalkaloid (SGA) administration inhibits serum cholinesterase and increases serum mivacurium levels. (a) Levels of the *trans–trans* isomer of mivacurium were determined in 14 rabbits. Each value is the mean of
triplicate determinations. Mivacurium levels are plotted versus the time needed for 50% recovery of twitch amplitude after mivacurium administration.
Animals with higher mivacurium levels showed longer recovery times ($r^2 = 0.39$; dashed lines show 95% confidence interval; $p < 0.05$). (b) Three animals
with measurable serum cholinesterase activity showed decreases after SGA administration. Blood samples from two other animals had basal cholinesterase
activity near the lower limit of detection (not shown). (c) Mivacurium *trans–trans* isomer levels were determined in blood samples collected after two consecutive mivacurium administrations (10 min after each mivacurium infusion). All data were normalized to the serum levels after the first mivacurium
administration. Hatched bars indicate the percentage change in mivacurium levels after the second administration under control conditions (left) and with
coadministration of SGA (right; $\star p < 0.05$ relative to initial determinations, paired t test; $n = 7$ animals). Reprinted with permission from reference 36

replaced older drugs that utilize that pathway. While
physicians and consumers ultimately bear the responsibility for recognition of potential interactions, the

downstream effects will be keenly perceived by
pharmaceutical manufacturers in the development of
new drugs.

References

1. Brown C, Taniguchi G, Yıp K. The monoamine oxidase inhibitor–
   tyramine interaction. *J Clin Pharmacol* 1989;29:529–32
2. Asch DA, Parker RM. The Libby Zion case. One step forward or
   two steps backward? *N Engl J Med* 1988;318:771–5
3. Humphrey SJ, Curry JT, Turman CN, Stryd RP. Cardiovascular
   sympathomimetic amine interactions in rats treated with monoamine oxidase inhibitors and the novel oxazolidinone antibiotic
   linezolid. *J Cardiovasc Pharmacol* 2001;37:548–63
4. Yun CH, Wood M, Wood AJ, Guengerich FP. Identification of
   the pharmacogenetic determinants of alfentanil metabolism:

cytochrome P-450 3A4. An explanation of the variable elimination
clearance. *Anesthesiology* 1992;77:467–74
5. Dresser GK, Spence JD, Bailey DG. Pharmacokinetic–pharmacodynamic consequences and clinical relevance of cytochrome P450 3A4
   inhibition. *Clin Pharmacokinet* 2000;38:41–57
6. Borel JD, Bentley JB, Nenad RE, Sipes IG. Cimetidine alteration of
   fentanyl pharmacokinetics in dogs. *Proceedings of the International
   Anesthesia Research Society 56th Congress*, San Francisco, CA; 1982:149
7. Hiller A, Olkkola KT, Isohanni P, Saarnivaara L. Unconsciousness
   associated with midazolam and erythromycin. *Br J Anaesth*
   1990;65:826–8

8. Bailey DG, Spence JD, Munoz C, Arnold JM. Interaction of citrus juices with felodipine and nifedipine. *Lancet* 1991;337:268–9

9. Edgar B, Bailey D, Bergstrand R, *et al*. Acute effects of drinking grapefruit juice on the pharmacokinetics and dynamics of felodipine – and its potential clinical relevance. *Eur J Clin Pharmacol* 1992;42:313–17

10. Fuhr U, Harder S, Lopez-Rojas P, *et al*. Increase of verapamil concentrations in steady state by coadministration of grapefruit juice. *Naunyn Schmiedebergs Arch Pharmacol* 1994;349(Suppl):R134(abstr)

11. Soons PA, Vogels BA, Roosemalen MC, *et al*. Grapefruit juice and cimetidine inhibit stereoselective metabolism of nitrendipine in humans. *Clin Pharmacol Ther* 1991;50:394–403

12. Fuhr U, Maier A, Blume H, *et al*. Grapefruit juice increases oral nimodipine bioavailability. *Eur J Clin Pharmacol* 1994;47:A100 (abstr)

13. Bailey DG, Arnold JM, Strong HA, *et al*. Effect of grapefruit juice and naringin on nisoldipine pharmacokinetics. *Clin Pharmacol Ther* 1993;54:589–94

14. Honig P, Wortham D, Lazarev A, Cantilena LR. Pharmacokinetics and cardiac effects of terfenadine in poor metabolizers receiving concomitant grapefruit juice. *Clin Pharmacol Ther* 1995;57:185(abstr)

15. Libersa CC, Brique SA, Motte KB, *et al*. Dramatic inhibition of amiodarone metabolism induced by grapefruit juice. *Br J Clin Pharmacol* 2000;49:373–8

16. Kupferschmidt HH, Ha HR, Ziegler WH, *et al*. Interaction between grapefruit juice and midazolam in humans. *Clin Pharmacol Ther* 1995;58:20–8

17. Hukkinen SK, Varhe A, Olkkola KT, Neuvonen PJ. Plasma concentrations of triazolam are increased by concomitant ingestion of grapefruit juice. *Clin Pharmacol Ther* 1995;58:127–31

18. Barone GW, Gurley BJ, Ketel BL, *et al*. Drug interaction between St. John's wort and cyclosporine. *Ann Pharmacother* 2000;34:1013–16

19. Moore LB, Goodwin B, Jones SA, *et al*. St. John's wort induces hepatic drug metabolism through activation of the pregnane X receptor. *Proc Natl Acad Sci USA* 2000;97:7500–2

20. Izzo AA, Ernst E. Interactions between herbal medicines and prescribed drugs: a systematic review. *Drugs* 2001;61:2163–75

21. Wang Z, Gorski JC, Hamman MA, *et al*. The effects of St John's wort (*Hypericum perforatum*) on human cytochrome P450 activity. *Clin Pharmacol Ther* 2001;70:317–26

22. Wang EJ, Casciano CN, Clement RP, Johnson WW. Inhibition of P-glycoprotein transport function by grapefruit juice psoralen. *Pharm Res* 2001;18:432–8

23. He K, Iyer KR, Hayes RN, *et al*. Inactivation of cytochrome P450 3A4 by bergamottin, a component of grapefruit juice. *Chem Res Toxicol* 1998;11:252–9

24. Kane GC, Lipsky JJ. Drug–grapefruit juice interactions. *Mayo Clin Proc* 2000;75:933–42

25. Mohri K, Uesawa Y. Effects of furanocoumarin derivatives in grapefruit juice on nifedipine pharmacokinetics in rats. *Pharm Res* 2001;18:177–82

26. Cooper JR. Unsolved problems in the cholinergic nervous system. *J Neurochem* 1994;63:395–9

27. Savarese JJ, Ali HH, Basta SJ, *et al*. The clinical neuromuscular pharmacology of mivacurium chloride (BW B1090U). A short-acting nondepolarizing ester neuromuscular blocking drug. *Anesthesiology* 1988;68:723–32

28. Cook DR, Freeman JA, Lai AA, *et al*. Pharmacokinetics of mivacurium in normal patients and in those with hepatic or renal failure. *Br J Anaesth* 1992;69:580–5

29. Whittaker M. Cholinesterase. In Beckman L, ed. *Monographs in Human Genetics*, vol 11. Basel: Karger, 1986:45–85

30. Cooper JR. Unsolved problems in the cholinergic nervous system. *J Neurochem* 1994;63:395–9

31. Erkola O, Rautoma P, Meretoja OA. Mivacurium when preceded by pancuronium becomes a long-acting muscle relaxant. *Anesthesiology* 1996;84:562–5

32. Neville LF, Gnatt A, Loewenstein Y, *et al*. Intramolecular relationships in cholinesterases revealed by oocyte expression of site-directed and natural variants of human BCHE. *EMBO J* 1991;11:1641–9

33. Harris FW, Cockburn T. Alleged poisoning by potatoes. *Analyst* 1918;43:133–7

34. Morris SC, Lee TH. The toxicity and teratogenicity of Solanaceae glycoalkaloids, particularly those of the potato (*Solanum tuberosum*): a review. *Food Technol Aust* 1984;36:118–24

35. Hansen A. Two fatal cases of potato poisoning. *Science* 1925;61:340–1

36. McGehee DS, Krasowski MD, Fung DL, *et al*. Cholinesterase inhibition by potato glycoalkaloids slows mivacurium metabolism. *Anesthesiology* 2000;93:510–19

Evidence-based herbal pharmacology: an example using ginseng

16

A. S. Attele and J.-T. Xie

INTRODUCTION

Ginseng is a slow-growing perennial herb that belongs to the family Araliaceae. It is an aromatic plant with a short rhizome with a fleshy white root and a simple aerial stem bearing one to six leaves. The root system of ginseng consists of the primary root and its branches, and some adventitious roots develop from the rhizome. The ginseng root has been used for over 2000 years, and is believed to be a panacea, promoting longevity. As described in Chinese traditional medicine textbooks, its effectiveness reaches mythical proportions. Ginseng's genus name *Panax* is derived from the Greek *pan* (all) and *akos* (cure), meaning cure-all[1-3].

The efficacy of ginseng was known in the West by the 18th century, although the study of ginseng dates back further. Ginseng is one of the most popular herbal remedies in the USA and a number of health claims are made to support it[4,5]. There is a renewed interest in investigating ginseng pharmacology using biochemical and molecular biological techniques. Pharmacological effects of ginseng have been demonstrated in the central nervous, cardiovascular, endocrine and immune systems. The great diversity of pharmacological properties attributed to ginseng root suggest that it might act in a unique and fundamental way on the body. In fact, its activity often appears to be based on whole-body effects, rather than on particular organs or systems[6]. In addition, ginseng and its constituents have been ascribed antineoplastic, antistress and antioxidant activities. It is an herb with many active components, and there is evidence from numerous studies that ginseng has beneficial effects[7,8].

Seven major species of ginseng are distributed throughout East Asia, Central Asia and North America. Most studies of ginseng, including those cited in this commentary, have utilized constituents from three common species, *Panax ginseng* (Asian ginseng), *Panax quinquefolius* (American ginseng) and *Panax japonicus* (Japanese ginseng)[5,9].

Active constituents found in most ginseng species include ginsenosides (or panaxosides), polysaccharides, peptides, polyacetyleinic alcohols and fatty acids[7,10,11]. There is wide variation (2–20%) in ginsenoside content in different species of ginseng. Ginsenosides belong to a chemical group called saponins, which are similar in composition and structure to steroids[5,12]. Moreover, pharmacological differences within a single species cultivated in two different locations have been reported. For example, the potency of extracts from *Panax quinquefolius,* cultivated in the USA, for modulating neuronal activity was significantly higher than for the same species cultivated in China[13].

There is extensive literature on the beneficial effects of ginseng and its constituents. This chapter aims to review evidence-based pharmacological effects of ginseng and ginsenosides, and their possible mechanisms of action.

PHARMACOLOGICAL EFFECTS

Previous studies have demostated that ginseng and its constituents possess multiple pharmacological actions, within the central nervous system (CNS), cardiovascular system, endocrine system and immune system. It is also known that ginseng has anti-stress, anti-fatigue, antiviral, antifungal, antineoplastic, anti-ischemia–reperfusion and antihyperglycemic effects. Most pharmacological actions of ginseng are attributed to ginsenosides[5,14]. More than 20 ginsenosides have been isolated[8], and novel structures continue to be reported, particularly from *Panax quinquefolius* and *Panax japonicus*[15]. Figure 1 illustrates the structures of some ginsenosides.

Effects on the central nervous system

Ginseng has both stimulatory and inhibitory effects on the CNS[16], and may modulate neurotransmission. Ginsenosides Rb_1 and Rg_1 play a major role in these effects[17,18].

Memory, learning and neuroprotection

Results of several animal studies have shown that Rb_1[19], Rg_1[20] and Re[21] prevent scopolamine-induced memory deficiencies. Central cholinergic systems have been implicated in mediating learning and memory processes[22]. Rb_1 was shown to increase the uptake of choline in central cholinergic nerve endings[18], and to facilitate the release of acetylcholine from hippocampal slices[19]. Both Rb_1 and Rg_1 appear partially to reverse scopolamine-induced amnesia by increasing cholinergic activity. Results from these investigations suggest that ginsenosides may facilitate learning and memory and are able to enhance nerve growth[23,24]. In fact, the total effect of the ginseng root is stimulatory, but diols, such as Rb_1, are sedative, and triols, such as Rg_1, are stimulatory. A previous study

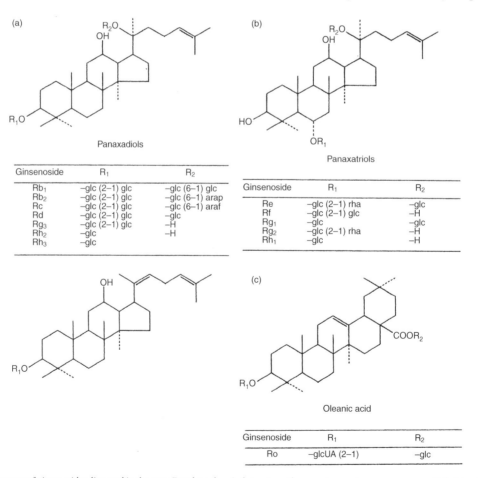

Figure 1 Structures of ginsenosides discussed in the text. Based on chemical structure, there are two major groups, panaxadiols (a) and panaxatriols (b). Rh_3, as shown in the lower part of (a), differs from other panaxadiols at the side chain. Ginsenoside Ro, a non-steroidal saponin, is shown in (c)

showed that, with the 'shuttle-box' method for active avoidance, the most pronounced effect on learning and memory was obtained by 10 mg/kg. With the 'step-down' method for passive avoidance, the dose of 30 mg/kg significantly improved retention. These results show that ginseng at appropriate doses improves learning, memory and physical capabilities[6].

Ginsenosides may also possess the ability to protect neurons from ischemic damage. Rb_1 was shown to rescue hippocampal neurons from lethal ischemic damage[25], and to delay neuronal death from transient forebrain ischemia *in vitro*[26]. In another *in vivo* experiment, total saponins of ginseng were shown to possesses protective effects against ischemia–reperfusion in the rat brain[27]. In addition, Rg_1 was shown to increase the membrane fluidity of cortical cells from 27-month-old rats[28]. Rb_1 increased the fluidity of synaptosomal membranes impaired by $FeSO_4$–cystein[29]. Both Rb_1 and Rg_1 significantly decreased hippocampal $[Ca^{2+}]_i$ level that was found to increase in aged rats[30].

Neurotransmitter modulation

Results of *in vitro* studies have shown that ginsenosides may modulate nerve transmission by decreasing the availability of neurotransmitters. Tsang and colleagues[17] demonstrated that ginseng extract concentration-dependently inhibited the uptake of γ-aminobutyric acid (GABA), glutamate, dopamine, noradrenaline (norepinephrine) and serotonin in rat brain synaptosomes. Ginsenosides competed with agonists for binding to $GABA_A$ and $GABA_B$ receptors[31]. Yuan and co-workers[32] demonstrated that *Panax quinquefolius* extracts interact with the ligand binding of $GABA_A$ receptors in brainstem neurons, which suggests that regulation of GABA-ergic neurotransmission may be an important action of ginseng.

Other central nervous system effects

An *in vivo* study that explored effects of ginsenosides on drug-induced sleep showed that a mixture of Rb_1,

Rb_2 and Rc prolonged the hexobarbital sleeping time in mice and decreased exploratory activity[33], suggesting a CNS-depressing effect. Other studies demonstrated that ginseng may ameliorate some adverse effects of morphine. Rats sensitized to morphine developed dopaminergic hyperfunction[34]. Kim and associates[35] showed that total saponin of ginseng prevented the development of dopamine receptor supersensitivity induced by the chronic administration of morphine. Ginsenosides may also possess antinociceptive properties. Ginseng total extract and Rf were shown to inhibit Ca^{2+} channels on primary sensory neurons to the same degree as opioids[36]. In addition, pretreatment of rats with ginsenosides inhibited substance P-induced pain behaviors[37].

Recently, ginseng effects on actions induced by opioids and psychostimulants were evaluated. Analgesic effects of opioids, such as morphine and U-50,488H, were blocked by ginseng in a non-opioid-dependent manner. Ginseng inhibited the tolerance to and dependence on morphine, and prevented the suppressive effect on the development of morphine tolerance caused by co-exposure to foot-shock stress but not psychological stress. These results provide evidence that ginseng may be useful clinically for the prevention of abuse and dependence of opioids and psychostimulants[38]. In addition, oral administration of *Panax notoginseng* reduced grooming episode duration and number and increased inner crossing in open field. The experiments suggested that notoginsenosides can modulate emotional responses in rats[39].

Ca^{2+} is an important regulator for many neuronal functions, including exocytosis and excitability. Voltage-dependent Ca^{2+} channels play a key role in control of free cytosolic Ca^{2+}. It is also known that there are at least more than five different subtypes of voltage-dependent Ca^{2+} channels in the nervous system, such as L-, N-, P-, O- and T-type of Ca^{2+} channels. Recent data showed that ginsenosides are negatively coupled to three types of Ca^{2+} channel in bovine adrenal chromaffin cells. Thus, the selective regulation of voltage-dependent Ca^{2+} channel subtypes by ginsenosides in bovine adrenal chromaffin cells could be the cellular basis of the anti-stress effect by ginseng[36,40].

Data from our laboratory indicated that American ginseng aqueous extract tonically and reversibly blocked the Na^+ channels in a concentration- and voltage-dependent manner using whole-cell patch clamp techniques. Ginsenoside Rb_1, a major constituent of the American ginseng extract, produced a similar effect. The data suggest that Na^+ channels are blocked by ginseng extract and Rb_1, primarily owing to interaction with the inactive state of the channel. Inhibition of Na^+ channel activity by American ginseng extract may contribute to its neuroprotective effect during ischemia[41].

Effects on the cardiovascular system

Effects on blood pressure

Cardiovascular effects of ginseng root and individual ginsenosides have been studied extensively. Human studies suggested that ginseng may decrease systolic blood pressure[42] and enhance the efficacy of digoxin in class IV heart failure[43], and that the prolonged hypotensive effect is probably due to a Ca^{2+} channel blocking effect and interference with Ca^{2+} mobilization into vascular smooth muscle cells[5]. Ginsenoside Rb_1 decreased blood pressure in animal experiments[44], perhaps owing to relaxation of smooth muscle. However, ginsenoside Rb_1 has also been reported to have hypertensive effects[45]. Sung and associates[46] noted that, in hypertensive subjects treated with Korean red ginseng, forearm blood flows after infusion of acetycholine or bradykinin were higher than those of non-treated hypertensive subjects. Similar results have been reported in *in vivo* animal studies. A crude saponin fraction of Korean red ginseng decreased systolic blood pressure in hypertensive rats[47], while the hypotensive effect of the saponin-free fraction was minimal. Lee and co-workers[48], working with anesthetized dogs, noted that intravenous administration of an ethanol or ether extract of ginseng (40 mg/kg) decreased total peripheral resistance and caused vasodilatation and bradycardia, while a similar dose of an aqueous extract increased total peripheral resistance. These discrepancies could reflect differences in ginsenoside content due to the method of extraction. On the other hand, it was shown that ginsenoside potentiated nitric oxide (NO)-mediated neurogenic vasodilatation of monkey cerebral arteries[49].

Anti-ischemia–reperfusion effects

The preventive effects of ginseng and ginsenoside on myocardial ischemia and reperfusion damage have been shown in both animal experiments and clinical trials[50–52]. *Panax ginseng* extract significantly limited the increase in left ventricular end-diastolic pressure and coronary perfusion pressure in rats responding to hyperbaric oxygen compared to untreated rats. The results indicated that ginseng prevented myocardial ischemia–reperfusion injury and impairment of endothelial function induced by reactive oxygen species arising from hyperbaric oxygen exposure, through an antioxidant intervention. In a clinical trial, both total ginsenosides and ginsenoside Rb showed protective effects on myocardial ischemic and reperfusion injuries in open heart surgery. In addition, ginsenosides possess protective effects against cultured vascular endothelial cell damage induced by oxygen free radicals *in vitro*.

Nitric oxide-related activities

Many reports have described vasodilator actions mediated by NO release. Results of *in vitro* studies using vascular ring preparations suggested that the vasodilator actions of ginseng reflect the interaction of ginseng with an endogenous vasoactive substance[53], subsequently identified as NO. Total ginseng root extract did not alter basal vascular tone in ring preparations of vessels from rabbits, dogs and humans, but relaxed vessels precontracted with norepinephrine or prostaglandin $F_2\alpha$[53]. Endothelium-dependent relaxation of the isolated rat aorta by ginsenoside Rg_3 was 100-fold more potent than by ginsenoside Rg_1[54].

Other studies reported that the NO-mediated vasorelaxation induced by ginsenosides may involve Ca^{2+}-activated K^+ channels[55] and tetraethylammonium-sensitive K^+ channels[54]. The ability of ginseng to release NO from the corpus cavernosum and cause concentration-dependent relaxation may contribute to the mechanism of penile erection[56]. The adrenergic nervous system has also been implicated in the complex cardiovascular effects of ginseng[57]. It was reported that panaxatriols, particularly Rg_2, reduced acetylcholine-evoked release of catecholamines from adrenal chromaffin cells[58].

Much evidence points to a close link between damaging action, oxygen free radicals and many forms of human disease[59,60], including cardiopulmonary pathology and reperfusion ischemia in the heart and lung. It is interesting that ginseng, an important component of a traditional Chinese mixture of herbs used to treat coronary artery disease and myocardial infarction[61], has well-recognized antioxidant actions[62,63]. Antioxidant effects have been demonstrated in neonatal rat cardiomyocyte preparations in which ginseng reduced lactic acid dehydrogenase release[61]. In an *in vivo* animal experiment, *Panax ginseng* extract prevented myocardial ischemia–reperfusion damage and impairment of endothelial function induced by reactive oxygen species arising from hyperbaric oxygen exposure through an antioxidant intervention[51,64].

The vascular endothelial cell of the circulatory system is an early target of free radical injury. The protective action of ginseng against endothelial cell injury caused by a variety of reduced oxygen species generated by brief electrolysis of the medium was reported in a pulmonary model[8,65]. Such treatment decreases the synthesis of NO and reverses the normal vasodilator response to acetylcholine in lungs precontracted with a thromboxane analog U46619[65,66]. Ginsenoside prevented these vascular effects and reduced the pulmonary edema that followed free radical injury[67]. Ginsenoside-induced vascular effects were reversed by nitro-L-arginine, an inhibitor of NO release. An aqueous extract of ginseng root inhibited iron-mediated peroxidation of arachidonic acid, and hydroxyl radical formation from added hydrogen peroxide[68].

Red ginseng was found to promote the proliferation of vascular endothelial cells, and inhibit the production and promote the decomposition of endothelin, which is known to constrict blood vessels and raise blood pressure[69].

Oxidized low-density lipoprotein is believed to be involved in the pathogenesis of atherosclerosis. *Panax quinquefolius* saponins were reported to reduce lipid peroxide levels in cultured rat cardiomyocytes[70]. The cardioprotective action of ginseng against ischemia–reperfusion injury has been demonstrated in patients undergoing cardiopulmonary bypass for mitral valve surgery. Total ginseng extract enhanced recovery of cardiac hemodynamic performance and significantly lowered mitochondrial swelling during the period of ischemia[51]. Treatment of rats with a standardized ginseng extract for 7 days resulted in cardioprotective effects. After exposure to hyperbaric hypoxia (100%, 2.5 atm for 6 h), the hearts of rats in the ginseng-treated group showed less coronary vasoconstriction in response to angiotensin II.

It is recognized that NO, as well as being an important cell-signaling molecule, is an antioxidant[71]. NO-releasing agents protected lung fibroblasts from oxygen-radical damage caused by hypoxanthine/xanthine oxidase[72]. Several observations have suggested that release of NO by ginseng may underlie its antioxidant effects. In bovine aortic endothelial cells, ginseng extract and Rg_1 enhanced the conversion of $[^{14}C]$L-arginine to $[^{14}C]$L-citrulline[67]. Under conditions that simulated oral ingestion, ginseng extract dilated preconstricted perfused lung and preserved acetylcholine dilatation following free radical injury[66]. Superoxide dismutase converts superoxide radical to hydrogen peroxide, which, in turn, is broken down to water and oxygen by catalase. Thus, superoxide dismutase and catalase constitute the first co-ordinated unit of defense against oxygen free radicals. Recent reports[73,74] indicate that Rb_1 and Rb_2 enhanced expression of the Cu,Zn-superoxide dismutase gene, probably mediated by the AP2 transcription factor. Rb_2 was reported to be the major inducer of the catalase gene[74]. If demonstrated to occur in vascular endothelial cells, this effect may be thought to contribute to the antioxidant activity of ginseng.

Antineoplastic and immunomodulatory effects

Considerable interest has been shown by researchers in how ginseng might prevent or assist in the treatment of cancer. Ginsenosides have been shown to exert anticarcinogenic effects *in vitro* through different mechanisms. Several ginsenosides show direct cytotoxic and growth inhibitory effects against tumor cells[6,75,76]. Others have been shown to induce differentiation and inhibit metastasis[77,78].

Tumor cell growth inhibition and apoptosis

Ginsenoside Rh_2 inhibited growth and stimulated melanogenesis[75], and arrested cell cycle progression at the G_1 stage[79] in B16-BL6 melanoma cells. In association with G_1 arrest, there was a suppression of cyclin-dependent-kinase-2 (Cdk2) activity. Ginsenosides Rb_1, Rb_2 and Rc are metabolized by intestinal bacteria after oral administration to a modified ginsenoside named M1[80,81]. Wakabayashi and associates[76] reported that M1 inhibited the proliferation of B16-BL6 mouse melanoma cells, and at a higher concentration induced cell death within 24 h by regulating apoptotis-related proteins. Ginsenosides from *Panax notoginseng* (Sanchi ginseng) also showed effects in a two-stage mouse skin model with 7,12-dimethylbenz[a]anthracene (DMBA) and in lung carinogensis induced by 4-nitroquinilin-1-oxide. Anticardinogenic effects of majonoside from Vietnamese ginseng have also been shown in two-stage tests of mouse skin[3].

It has been reported that orally administered and subcutaneously injected Rh_2 inhibited the growth of human ovarian cells transplanted into nude mice, and significantly prolonged their survival times[82]. Intravenously or orally administered Rg_3 led to a decrease in lung metastasis of B16-BL6 melanoma cells[77]. Several studies which utilized medium-term and long-term anticarcinogenesis models of mice showed that ginseng extracts had a tumor inhibitory effect in mice that were exposed to chemical carcinogens[83,84]. Results of a cohort study showed that ginseng consumers had a lower risk for gastric and lung cancers, suggesting that ginseng may have a non-organ-specific anticarcinogenic effect[85]. It seems that a large-scale, controlled clinical study is needed to validate this result.

Antimitogenic activity

Sister chromatid exchange is regarded as a sensitive indicator of DNA damage[86], and significantly correlates with the mutagenic activities of many chemicals[87]. Rh_2 significantly suppressed both the baseline and induced sister chromatid exchanges in human lymphocytes[88]. In addition, ginseng may enhance the proofreading activity of eukaryotic DNA polymerase. Cho and colleagues[89] showed that total ginseng extracts activated both polymerase and exonuclease activities of DNA polymerase δ.

Differentiation, and inhibition of metastasis

In vitro studies have demonstrated that Rh_2 and Rh_3 induced differentiation of promyelocytic leukemia HL-60 cells into granulocytes, possibly by modulating protein kinase-C isoforms[78]. Total ginseng extract was shown to induce differentiation of cultured Morris hepatoma cells[90]. In addition, Mochizuki and co-workers[77] showed that Rg_3 significantly inhibited the adhesion and invasion of B16-BL6 cells into reconstituted basement membranes, and inhibited pulmonary metastasis.

Immunomodulatory effects

In general, immunomodulatory and anticarcinogenic activities of ginsenosides are discussed together. However, few investigations have viewed these two events as sequential steps. Yun and co-workers[91] followed the natural killer (NK) cell activity and the incidence of lung adenoma in mice treated with urethane or benzopyrenes. In mice administered ginseng, the NK activity was depressed for 4–24 weeks, and then returned to control levels. Concurrently, in animals treated with ginseng, a lower incidence of lung adenoma was reported. Kim and colleagues[92] evaluated multiple immune system components in mice subchronically exposed to cyclophosphamide. This study also revealed that ginseng possesses some immunomodulatory properties, primarily associated with NK cell activity. In fact, ginseng may also prevent cancer through effects on the immune system. The effects of long-term oral administration of ginseng extract (30 and 150 mg/kg per day) on levels of immunoglobulin types were studied in mice. Serum levels of γ-globulin decreased dose-dependently after ginseng administration. Among the immunoglobulin isotypes, only serum IgG_1 decreased. The researchers suggested that, since IgG_1 is rarely involved in killing cancer cells and can act as a blocking antibody, this effect of ginseng may be beneficial for the prevention and inhibition of cancer. Experiments have also shown that the anticarcinogenic activity of ginseng may be related to the augmentation of NK cell activity[6].

An experiment *in vivo* showed that oral administration of ginseng extract for 4 consecutive days enhanced the activities of B and T lymphocytes and NK cells in mice and increased production of interferon following an interferon inducer. In another animal experiment, ginseng extract was found to be effective against Semliki forest viral infection in mice[6]. Ginsenoside Rg_1 was shown to increase both humoral and cell-mediated immune responses. Kenarova and co-workers[93] reported that spleen cells, recovered from ginsenoside-treated mice injected with sheep red cells as the antigen, showed a significantly higher plaque-forming response and hemagglutinating antibody titers. In addition, Rg_1 increased the number of antigen-reactive T helper cells, T lymphocytes and NK cells. Recently Park and associates[94] observed that the acidic polysaccharide isolated from *Panax ginseng* possesses immunomodulating activities, mediated by the production of NO.

As described above, ginseng extracts and several ginsenosides have been shown to possess some anticarcinogenic and immunomodulatory effects. It would be interesting to see whether their efficacy could be observed in double-blind, randomized, placebo-controlled clinical studies.

Effect on human immunodeficiency virus

Cho and colleagues[95] observed that $CD4^+$ T-cell counts in human immunodeficiency virus (HIV)-1-infected patients treated with Korean red ginseng were maintained or even increased during 24 months of therapy. Their data also suggested that the maintenance of $CD4^+$ T-cell counts by zidovudine and Korean red ginseng intake for a prolonged period might be indirectly associated with delayed development of resistance to zidovudine by the ginseng intake.

Antihyperglycemic effects

Historical records reveal that, in traditional medical systems, a disease corresponding to type 2 diabetes was treated with plant extracts[96]. Pharmacological activity evaluations of ginseng root on blood sugar levels started early last century. Between 1921 and 1932, Japanese scientists reported that ginseng root decreased baseline blood glucose and reduced hyperglycemia caused by adrenaline (epinephrine) or high-concentration glucose administration[97,98]. Ginseng root has since been used to treat diabetic patients[2,5,99]. Since the 1980s, the number of published studies on ginseng root in treating diabetes increased remarkably, including both *in vitro* studies[100,101] and *in vivo* experiments[102–105]. Ginseng root has been shown in clinical studies to have beneficial effects in both insulin-dependent and non-insulin-dependent diabetic patients. Oral administration of ginseng tablets (2000 mg daily for 8 weeks) to 36 non-insulin-dependent patients elevated mood, improved physical performance, reduced fasting blood glucose and serum aminoterminal propeptide of type III procollagen concentrations, and lowered glycated hemoglobin level[106–108]. Other clinical trials have also supported the notion that ginseng root possesses antihyperglycemic activity[109,110].

Recently, we have observed that *Panax ginseng* berry extract, which has a distinct ginsenoside profile compared to the profile of the root, has the ability to reduce hyperglycemia and body weight in C57BL/6J (*ob/ob*) mice and in C57BL/KsJ (*db/db*) mice as well[111,112]. Furthermore, the data also demonstrated that ginsenoside Re, a major constituent of the ginseng berry, plays a significant role in anti-hyperglycemic action. This anti-diabetic effect of ginsenoside Re was not associated with body weight changes, suggesting that other constituents in the berry extract have distinct pharmacological mechanisms on energy metabolism. In addition, we also observed that another constituent, the polysaccharide fraction, obtained from American ginseng berry extract, possesses an anti-hyperglycemic effect in both adult *ob/ob* and *db/db* mice. The polysaccharide fraction, however, did not affect body weight changes in diabetic mice.

WHY ARE THERE SO MANY DIVERSE EFFECTS?

Ginseng contains over 20 ginsenosides, and single ginsenosides have been shown to produce multiple effects in the same tissue. Furthermore, the variety of ginsenosides may produce diverse pharmacological effects[17,113,114]. A recent study showed the influence of centrally administered ginsenoside by *in situ* hybridization histochemistry in the rat brain on the regulation of mRNA levels of the family of N-methyl-D-aspartare (NMDA) receptor subtypes. The ginsenosides Rc and Rg[1], the major components of ginseng saponin, differentially modulate NMDA receptor subunit mRNA levels. The results show that structure differences of ginsenosides may diversely affect the modulation of expression of NMDA receptor subunit mRNA after infusion into the cerebroventricle in rats[114]. In addition, non-ginsenoside constituents of ginseng also exert pharmacological effects. Thus, it is not surprising that the overall activity of the herb is complex.

Ginsenosides and steroids

Ginsenosides (except Ro) belong to a family of steroids named steroidal saponins[75,78,115]. They have been named ginsenoside saponins, triterpenoid saponins, or dammarane derivatives under previous classifications[116,117]. Ginsenosides possess a rigid four *trans*-ring steroid skeleton, with a modified side chain at C-20[118]. The classical steroid hormones have a truncated side chain (progesterone, cortisol and aldosterone) or no side chain (estradiol and testosterone)[115,119]. Many steroids have a β-OH group at C-3; ginsenosides (Rb[1], Rb[2], Rc and Rd, etc.) usually have a sugar residue attached to the same site[5,118]. Sugar moieties are cleaved by acid hydrolysis during extraction, or by

endogenous glycosidases to give the aglycone[5,115,118]. Steroidal saponins, which share structural features with steroid hormones, have been used in the industrial synthesis of progesterone and pregnanolone[115].

Steroids possess numerous physiological activities, partly due to the nature of the steroid skeleton. The *trans*-ring junctions of the skeleton allow substituent groups, which interact with receptors, to be held in rigid stereochemically defined orientations[115]. In addition, the steroid skeleton endows a favored structure for the whole molecule to allow, for example, insertion into membranes[120]. Reports showed that Rg[1] is a functional ligand of the nuclear glucocorticoid receptor (GR)[121,122].

Structural diversity of ginsenosides

As illustrated in Figure 1, ginsenosides exhibit considerable structural variation. They differ from one another by the type of sugar moiety, their number and site of attachment. The sugar moieties present are glucose, maltose, fructose and saccharose. They are attached to C-3, C-6 or C-20. The binding site of the sugar has been shown to influence biological activity. Rh[1] and Rh[2] are structurally similar, except for the binding site of the β-D-glucopyranosyl group. In Rh[1] the sugar is at C-3, and in Rh[2], at C-6. Ginsenoside Rh[2] decreased growth of B16-BL6 melanoma cells, and stimulated melanogenesis and cell-to-cell adhesiveness. On the other hand, Rh[1] had no effect on cell growth and cell-to-cell adhesiveness but stimulated melanogenesis[113]. Significantly, only Rh[2] was incorporated in the lipid fraction of the B16-BL6 melanoma cell membrane.

Ginsenosides also differ in their number and site of attachment of hydroxyl groups. Polar substituents interact with phospholipid head groups in the hydrophilic domain of the membrane. Consequently, the insertional orientation of ginsenosides into membranes would be influenced by the number and site of polar OH groups. Differences in the number of OH groups were shown to influence pharmacological activity. Ginsenoside Rh[2] and Rh[3] differ only by the presence of an OH group at C-20 in Rh[2]. Although both Rh[2] and Rh[3] induced differentiation of promyelocyte leukemia HL-60 cells into morphological and functional granulocytes, the potency of Rh$_2$ was higher[78].

Stereoisomerism

Another factor that contributes to structural differences between ginsenosides is stereochemistry at C-20. Most ginsenosides that have been isolated are naturally present as enantiomeric mixtures[115,123]. Since the modules with which they react in biological systems are also optically active, stereoisomers are considered to be functionally different chemical compounds[124]. Consequently, they often differ considerably in potency, pharmacological activity and pharmacokinetic profile. Both 20(*S*) and 20(*R*) ginsenoside Rg$_2$ inhibit acetylcholine-evoked secretion of catecholamines from cultured bovine adrenal chromaffin cells[125]. However, the 20(*S*) isomer showed a greater inhibitory effect.

(*S*)-Ganodermic acids are steroidal saponins which share structural features with ginsenosides[126]. Twelve compounds of (*S*)-ganodermic acid are either paired stereo or positional isomers, and show differential activation of human phospholipase C and A$_2$ by infiltrating into platelet membranes[127]. In this regard, the stereochemistry of the substituent was found to be the most important structural characteristic.

Structural alterations in the gut after oral administration also contribute to diversity. Certain ginsenosides, such as Rb$_1$ and Rg$_1$, are poorly absorbed after ingestion[128]. Rb$_1$ was hydrolyzed to compound K by intestinal flora[81]; this was shown to increase the cytotoxicity of antineoplastic drugs[129] and induce apoptosis in B16-BL6 melanoma cells[76].

WHAT ARE THE UNDERLYING MECHANISMS OF ACTION?

Ginsenosides are amphiphilic in nature[115], and have the ability to intercalate into the plasma membrane. This leads to changes in membrane fluidity, and thus affects membrane function, eliciting a cellular response. There is evidence to suggest that ginsenosides interact directly with specific membrane proteins. Moreover, like steroid hormones, they are lipid-soluble signalling molecules, which can traverse the plasma membrane and initiate genomic effects. Figure 2 illustrates possible sites of action of ginsenosides, which are discussed below.

Ginsenosides and the plasma membrane

Cellular membranes may exist under conditions of curvature stress, being close to the hexagonal phase transition[130]. Consequently, the physicochemical properties of these membranes are sensitive to changes in membrane components and lipophilic agents, which may modulate curvature stress[131].

It has become increasingly evident that the lipid environment of membrane proteins, including ion channels, transporters and receptors, plays an important role in their function[120]. In artificial and biological membranes, cholesterol, a major membrane lipid, is organized into structural and kinetic domains or pools[132]. Membrane proteins are thought to be selectively localized in cholesterol-rich domains (acetylcholine receptor) or in cholesterol-poor domains (the sarcoplasmic Ca^{2+}-ATPase)[132]. Therefore, the biophysical properties of the different domains, rather than the bulk lipid, may selectively influence transmembrane protein function and mimic specificity at the effector level.

Ginsenosides may interact with the polar heads of membrane phospholipids and the β-OH of cholesterol through their OH groups. Moreover, their hydrophobic steroid backbone could intercalate into the hydrophobic interior of the bilayer. Both of these effects may contribute to altering the lipid environment around membrane proteins. Cholesterol is an intrinsic membrane lipid, which shares the steroid backbone and amphipathic nature of ginsenosides. Cholesterol enrichment has an inhibitory effect on the function of many membrane ATPases[120], and it may directly interact with the boundary lipids of ATPase and alter the intermolecular hydrogen bonds of the protein[133]. In contrast, ginsenoside Rb$_1$ has been shown to increase Na$^+$–K$^+$-ATPase and Ca^{2+}–Mg^{2+}-ATPase activity in neurons[29]. It is possible that some ginsenosides interact with membrane cholesterol and displace it from the immediate

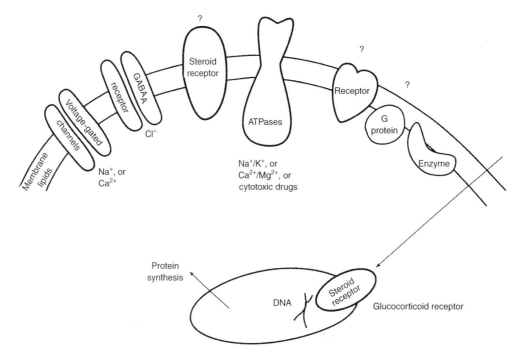

Figure 2   Drawing to illustrate potential sites of action of ginsenosides on plasma membrane and nuclear membrane. '?' indicates hypothetical sites

environment of ATPases. Since removal of cholesterol will lead to an increase in membrane fluidity[134], conformational changes that ATPases undergo during their transport cycle[135] may be facilitated.

Non-genomic action by steroids has only recently been widely recognized. Evidence for these rapid effects is now available for steroids of all classes[136]. In many of these cases, the steroid effect occurs at the membrane level and is not associated with entry into the cell. Several mechanisms for these effects have been proposed, including changes in membrane fluidity and activity of steroid hormones on plasma membrane receptors[137]. Ginsenosides may also modify membrane protein structure by changing membrane dynamics and modulating the activity of ion channels, membrane-bound receptors and enzymes. Consequently, a single ginsenoside may be capable of interacting with multireceptor systems.

Ginsenosides and membrane channels

Ginsenoside effects on membrane channels show similarities to those of steroid hormones including progesterone, estrogen and vitamin D metabolites, which modulate rapid Ca^{2+} influx in several tissues[137]. Several ginsenosides inhibit Ca^{2+} influx through voltage-gated Ca^{2+} channels in adrenal chromaffin cells[78]. Of the five ginsenosides that were tested (Rb_1, Re, Rf, Rg_1 and Rc), the inhibitory potency was highest for Rc. Tachikawa and associates[58] showed that, in bovine adrenal chromaffin cells, Rg_2 inhibited Na^+ influx through nicotinic receptor-gated cation channels, possibly by binding to the receptor-operated Na^+ channel. It is likely that the resulting decrease in catecholamine secretion may contribute to the anti-stress effects of *Panax ginseng*. Ginsenosides can also regulate Na^+ channels on nerve cells. Using standard patch clamp techniques, we recently observed that extracts of *Panax quinquefolius* and ginsenoside Rb_1 reversibly inhibited Na^+ channels in a concentration- and voltage-dependent manner[41], caused partial inhibition of neuronal Na^+ channels during activation and inactivation states (unpublished data).

Ginsenoside activity on membrane pumps is not limited to ion transporters. P-glycoprotein is a membrane ATPase pump that actively exports cytotoxic compounds, and contributes to anticancer multidrug resistance[138]. Several ginsenosides, including 20(S)Rh$_2$, inhibit the transport function of P-glycoprotein and increase sensitivity to cancer chemotherapeutics in resistant cells[129].

Ginsenosides and GABA receptors

Several ginsenosides (Rb$_1$, Rb$_2$, Rc, Re, Rf and Rg$_1$)[31] and total ginseng extracts[32] modulated the binding of the GABA$_A$ agonist muscimol. Ginseng extract and Rc decreased the affinity of GABA$_B$ agonist baclofen binding[31]. Like ginsenosides, steroidal compounds regulate GABA-ergic neurotransmission in the brain. Several endogenous steroids such as progesterone, androsterone, neurosteroids and their metabolites stimulate GABA$_A$-mediated chloride ion flux[136].

Ginsenosides and other membrane proteins

Agents that modify the physical properties of the phospholipid bilayer, such as its fluidity, can modulate the activity of membrane-bound G proteins in the absence of the receptors[139]. Some Ca^{2+} channels in sensory neurons are linked to G protein-coupled receptors[36]. Ginsenoside Rf was shown to produce antinociception by inhibiting Ca^{2+} channels on sensory neurons through a pertussis toxin-sensitive G protein[140]. However, whether Rf binds to the receptor or directly modulates G protein activity is not known.

One target molecule that may account for the anticancer effects of ginsenoside Rh$_2$ is Cdk2[79], an intracellular cell cycle regulating enzyme. It is not known whether Rh$_2$ directly inhibits Cdk2 activity. However, Cdk2 can also be indirectly suppressed via modulating signalling cascades originating at the cell membrane[141]. Rh$_2$ was shown to be incorporated in membranes to a level comparable to that of steroids[75]. Its ability to change membrane fluidity, adhesiveness and cell-surface sugar structures further demonstrates that Rh$_2$ targets membrane components[75].

Some pharmacological effects of ginsenosides may be mediated by binding to steroid hormone receptors.

Both neural and non-neural membrane steroid receptors have been reported, and in most cases, steroids bind to membrane receptors with specificity and modest affinity[137]. The differential effects of various ginsenosides on the lipid bilayer argues against a non-specific activity. In contrast, these effects suggest a specific interaction between the ginsenoside and specific membrane proteins.

Membrane-associated enzymes sensitive to curvature strain such as protein kinase C (PKC) are highly responsive to perturbations of membrane structure[142]. Recent work has shown that the synergism exhibited by diacylglycerol and fatty acids in activating PKC is due to the synergistic effect of these molecules in inducing curvature strain in bilayers[131]. It was shown that ginsenosides Rh$_2$ and Rh$_3$ induced differentiation of human promyelocytic leukemia HL-60 cells into morphological and functional granulocytes by modulating PKC activity[78]. PKCs directly phosphorylate a number of intracellular proteins and regulate important cellular functions, including cell growth and cell differentiation[143]. Coincidently, with the differentiation of HL-60 cells by ginsenoside Rh$_2$ there was an increase in PKC activity[78]. It is possible that ginsenosides Rh$_2$ and Rh$_3$ modulate PKC activity by altering curvature strain of the lipid bilayer. The ability of ginsenosides independently to target multiple plasma membrane-anchored proteins may account for the variety of responses that can be triggered.

Genomic effects of ginsenosides

As discussed earlier, ginsenosides belong to a family of steroids and share their structural characteristics[115]. Like steroids, they can freely traverse cell membranes. Moreover, their presence has been demonstrated within cells, particularly in the nucleus[76]. According to the classical theory of steroid hormone action, steroids, which bind nuclear receptors, are thought primarily to affect the transcription of mRNA and subsequent protein synthesis[136]. Intracellular steroid-binding proteins present possible attractive targets for ginsenosides.

A recent study showed the biological effects resulting from structural similarities between ginsenosides and steroids. Lee and co-workers[121] showed that Rg_1 is a functional ligand of the GR. In this regard, the binding of the synthetic glucocorticoid dexamethasone to the GR was competitively inhibited by Rg_1, although the affinity of Rg_1 for the GR was lower than for dexamethasone. Ligand-occupied GR, when complexed with specific DNA sequences named glucocorticoid response elements (GRE), regulated the transcription of target genes[144]. Subsequent to ligand binding, Rg_1 activated GRE-containing reporter plasmids in a dose-dependent manner. Moreover, the GR-mediated transactivation and growth inhibition of FTO2B cells by dexamethasone and Rg_1 were inhibited by the specific glucocorticoid antagonist RU486. Rg_1 exhibits many other features of a glucocorticoid, such as synergistic activation of gene transcription by cAMP and the ability to down-regulate the GR content of cells[122].

After oral administration, ginsenosides Rb_1 and Rb_2 are metabolized by intestinal bacteria to compound K, also known as M1[81], which induces apoptosis of tumor cells[76]. Compound K was shown to have a nucleosomal distribution[76]. This, together with the observation of up-regulation of the CDK inhibitor p27 and the down-regulation of c-Myc and cyclin D1, suggest that the modification of apoptosis-related proteins by compound K is induced by transcriptional regulation[76]. Another investigation showed the binding of Rb_2 to transcription factor AP2[73]. The subsequent genomic event was shown to be the induction of the *SOD1* gene (Cu–Zn superoxide dismutase), a key enzyme in the metabolism of oxygen free radicals.

SUMMARY

Ginseng is a highly valued herb in the Far East, and has gained popularity in the West during the past decade. The major active components of ginseng are ginsenosides, a diverse group of steroidal saponins, which demonstrate the ability to target a myriad of tissues, producing an array of pharmacological responses. However, many mechanisms of ginsenoside activity still remain unknown. Since ginsenosides and other constituents of ginseng produce effects that are different from one another, and a single ginsenoside initiates multiple actions in the same tissue, the overall pharmacology of ginseng is complex. The ability of ginsenosides independently to target multi-receptor systems at the plasma membrane, as well as activate intracellular steroid receptors, may explain some pharmacological effects.

Structural variability of ginsenosides, structural and functional relationship to steroids, and potential targets of action are discussed in this chapter. It seems that ginsenoside effects may be initiated at the cell membrane, as well as via intracellular protein binding. Consequently, ginsenosides may follow a dual model of action.

One pathway of ginsenoside activity involves binding to membrane receptors that trigger changes in electrolyte transport systems and activating signalling pathways. In this regard, differences in lipophilicity between the ginsenosides, and the cholesterol content of membrane domains, may be important. Future studies should be carried out to demonstrate the partitioning of ginsenosides in membranes, and to determine whether they induce changes in the structure of membrane proteins. Another possible mechanism by which ginsenosides produce pharmacological effects is by binding to plasma membrane steroid receptors. Research in this area is still in its infancy, although there is a growing interest in non-genomic signalling by steroids.

The second pathway of ginsenoside activity involves binding to intracellular steroid receptors, where the ligand–receptor complex acts as a transcription factor in the nucleus. The demonstration of ginsenoside Rg_1 as a functional ligand of the nuclear glucocorticoid receptor[121,122] supports this view. More studies should be directed to show that other ginsenosides may function as steroid receptor agonists, and to quantitate their binding. In this regard, computer-based images of functional groups on ginsenosides for the construction of pharmacophore models[145] would be useful. Future research should also focus on whether there is interaction between the two pathways of ginsenoside action, both of which may occur in the same cell. Therefore, the initial rapid response via membrane phenomena may be augmented by the delayed genomic response.

Two factors may contribute to the multiple pharmacological effects of ginseng. The first is the structural and stereoisomerism exhibited by ginsenosides, which increase their diversity. The second is the ability of ginsenosides to target membrane-anchored receptors and ion channels, as well as nuclear receptors. Certainly, the argument can be raised that evidence for most pharmacological effects of ginseng have been obtained from *in vitro* studies, many of which have not been confirmed *in vivo*. Nevertheless, the view that ginsenosides may initiate effects at the plasma membrane by interacting with multireceptor systems, and that they also freely traverse the membrane and produce genomic effects, complements the intriguing pharmacology of ginseng.

References

1. Hu SY. A contribution to our knowledge of ginseng, *Am J Chin Med* 1977;5:1–23
2. Blumenthal M, Goldberg A, Brinckmann J. Ginseng root. In *Herbal Medicine*. Newton, MA: Integrative Medicine Communications, 2000:170–7
3. Yun TK. *Panax ginseng* – a non-organ-specific cancer preventive? *Lancet Oncol* 2001;2:49–55
4. Vogler BK, Pittler MH, Ernst E. The efficacy of ginseng. A systematic review of randomised clinical trials. *Eur J Clin Pharmacol* 1999;55:567–75
5. Huang KC. Herbs with multiple actions. In *The Pharmacology of Chinese Herbs*. Boca Raton, FL: CRC Press, 1999:17–51
6. Mills S, Bone K, Corrigan D, Duke JA, Wright JV. Ginseng (*Panax ginseng* C. Meyer). In *Principles and Practice of Phytotherapy. Modern Herbal Medicine*. Edinburgh: Churchill Livingstone, 2000:418–32
7. Lee FC. *Facts about Ginseng, the Elixir of Life*. Elizabeth, NJ: Hollyn International, 1992
8. Gillis CN. *Panax ginseng* pharmacology: a nitric oxide link? *Biochem Pharmacol* 1997;54:1–8
9. Morgan A, Cupp MJ. *Panax ginseng*. In Cupp MJ, ed. *Toxicology and Clinical Pharmacology of Herbal Products*. Totowa, NJ: Humana Press, 2000:141–53
10. Harkey MR, Henderson GL, Gershwin ME, Stern JS, Hanchman RM. Variability in commercial ginseng products: an analysis of 25 preparations. *Am J Clin Nutr* 2001;73:1101–6
11. Li WK, Fitzloff JF. Determination of 24(*R*)-pseudoginenoside F_{11} in North American ginseng using high performance liquid chromatography with evaporative light scattering detection. *J Pharm Biomed Anal* 2001;25:257–65
12. Sierpina VS. Ginseng. In *Integrative Health Care*. Philadelphia, PA: FA Davis Company, 2001:134
13. Yuan CS, Wu JA, Lowell T, Gu M. Gut and brain effects of American ginseng root on brainstem neuronal activities in rats. *Am J Chin Med* 1998;26:47–55
14. Ng TB, Wang H. Panaxagin, a new protein from Chinese ginseng possesses anti-fungal, translation-inhibiting and ribonuease actions. *Life Sci* 2001;68:736–49
15. Yoshikawa M, Murakami T, Yashiro K, *et al*. Bioactive saponins and glycosides. XI. Structures of new dammarane-type triterpene oligoglycosides, quinquenosides I, II, III, IV, and V, from American ginseng, the roots of *Panax quinquefolium* L. *Chem Pharm Bull* 1998;46:647–54
16. Saito H, Tsuchiya M, Naka K, Takagi K. Effect of *Panax ginseng* root on conditioned avoidance response in rats. *Jpn J Pharmacol* 1977;27:509–16
17. Tsang D, Yeung HW, Tso WW, Peck H. Ginseng saponins: influence on neurotransmitter uptake in rat brain synaptosomes. *Planta Med* 1985;3:221–4
18. Benishin CG. Actions of ginsenoside Rb_1 on choline uptake in central cholinergic nerve endings. *Neurochem Int* 1992;21:1–5
19. Benishin CG, Lee R, Wang LCH, Liu HJ. Effects of ginsenoside Rb_1 on central cholinergic metabolism. *Pharmacology* 1991;42:223–9
20. Yamaguchi Y, Haruta K, Kobayashi H. Effects of ginsenosides on impaired performance induced in the rat by scopolamine in a radial-arm maze. *Psychoneuroendocrinology* 1995;20:645–53
21. Yamaguchi Y, Higashi M, Kobayashi H. Effects of oral and intraventricular administration of ginsenoside Rg_1 on the performance impaired by scopolamine in rats. *Biomed Res* 1996;17:487–90
22. Perry EK. The cholinergic hypothesis – ten years on. *Br Med Bull* 1986;42:63–9
23. Takemoto Y, Ueyama T, Saito H, *et al*. Potentiation of nerve growth factor-mediated nerve fiber production in organ cultures of chicken embryonic ganglia by ginseng saponins: structure–activity relationship. *Chem Pharm Bull* 1984;32:3128–33
24. Salim KN, McEwen BS, Chao HM. Ginsenoside Rb_1 regulates ChAT, NGF and trkA mNRA expression in the rat brain. *Mol Brain Res* 1997;47:177–82
25. Lim JH, Wen TC, Matsuda S, *et al*. Protection of ischemic hippocampal neurons by ginsenoside Rb_1 a main ingredient of ginseng root. *Neurosci Res* 1997;28:191–200
26. Wen TC, Yoshimura H, Matsuda S, Lim JH, Sakanaka M. Ginseng root prevents learning disability and neuronal loss in gerbils with 5 minute forebrain ischemia. *Acta Neuropathol* 1996;91:15–22
27. Zhang YG, Liu TP. Protective effects of total saponins of *P. ginseng* on ischemia–reperfusion injury in rat brains. *Chin J Pharmacol Toxicol* 1994;8:7–12
28. Li JQ, Zhang JT. Effects of age and ginsenoside Rg_1 on membrane fluidity of cortical cells in rats. *Acta Pharm Sin* 1997;32:23–7
29. Jiang XY, Zhang JT, Shi CZ, Mechanism of action of ginsenoside Rb_1 in decreasing intraceullar Ca^{2+}. *Acta Pharm Sin* 1996;31:321–6
30. Min L, Juntian Z. Effects of ginsenoside Rb_1 and Rg_1 on synaptosomal free calcium level, ATPase, and calmodulin in rat hippocampus. *Chin Med J* 1995;108:544–7

31. Kimura T, Saunders PA, Kim HS, Rheu HM, Oh KW, Ho IK. Interactions of ginsenosides with ligand-bindings of GABA$_A$ and GABA$_B$ receptors. *Gen Pharm* 1994;25:193–9

32. Yuan CS, Attele AS, Wu JA, Liu D. Modulation of American ginseng on brainstem GABAergic effects in the rat. *J Ethnopharmacol* 1998;63:215–22

33. Takagi K, Saito H, Tsuchiya M. Pharmacological studies of *Panax ginseng* root: pharmacological properties of a crude saponin fraction. *Jpn J Pharmacol* 1972;22:339–46

34. Bhargava HN. Cyclo (Leu-Gly) inhibits the development of morphine induced analgesic tolerance and dopamine receptor supersensitivity in rat. *Life Sci* 1980;27: 117–23

35. Kim HS, Kang JG, Oh KW. Inhibition by ginseng total saponin of the development of morphine reverse tolerance and dopamine receptor supersensitivity in mice. *Gen Pharmacol* 1995;26:1071–6

36. Nah SY, Park NJ, McCleskey EW. A trace component of ginseng that inhibits Ca^{2+} channels through a pertussis toxin-sensitive G protein. *Proc Natl Acad Sci USA* 1995;92:8739–43

37. Yoon SR, Nah JJ, Shin YH, *et al.* Ginsenosides induce differential antinociception and inhibit substance P induced-nociceptive response in mice. *Life Sci* 1998;62:319–25

38. Tokuyama S, Takahashi M. Pharmacological and physiological effects of ginseng on actions induced by opioids and psychostimulants. *Jpn J Pharmacol* 2001;117:195–201

39. Cicero AFG, Bandieri E, Arletti R. Orally administered *Panax notoginseng* influence on rat spontaneous behaviour. *J Ethnopharmacol* 2000;73:387–91

40. Choi S, Jung S-Y, Kim C-H, Rhim S-C, Nah S-Y. Effect of ginsenosides on voltage-dependent Ca^{2+} channel subtypes in bovine chromaffin cells. *J Ethnopharmacol* 2001;74:75–81

41. Liu D, Li B, Liu Y, Attele AS, Kyle JW, Yuan CS. Voltage-dependent inhibition of brain Na$^+$ channels by American ginseng. *Eur J Pharmcol* 2001;413:47–54

42. Han KH, Choe SC, Kim HS, Sohn DW, Nam KY, Oh BH. Effect of red ginseng on blood pressure in patients with essential hypertension and white coat hypertension. *Am J Chin Med* 1998;26:199–209

43. Ding DZ, Shen TK, Cui YZ. Effects of red ginseng on the congestive heart failure and its mechanism. *Zhongguo Zhongxiyi Jiehe Zazhi* 1995;15:325–7

44. Kaku T, Miyata T, Sako I, Kinoshita A. Chemico-pharmacological studies on saponins of *Panax ginseng*. *Arzneim Forsch* 1975;25: 539–47

45. Awang DVC. The anti-stress potential of North American ginseng. *J Herb Spices Med Plants* 1998;6:87–91

46. Sung J, Han KH, Zo JH, Park HJ, Kim CH, Oh BH. Effects of red ginseng upon vascular endothelial functions in patients with essential hypertension. *Am J Chin Med* 2000;28:205–16

47. Jeon BH, Kim CS, Kim HS, Park JB, Nam KY, Chang SJ. Effect of Korean red ginseng on blood pressure and nitric oxide production. *Acta Pharmacol Sin* 2000;21:1095–100

48. Lee DC, Lee MO, Kim CY, Clifford DH. Effect of ether, ethanol and aqueous extracts of ginseng on cardiovascular function in dogs. *Can J Comp Med* 1981;45:182–7

49. Toda N, Ayajiki K, Fujioka H, Okamura T. Ginsenoside potentiates NO-mediated vasodilation of monkey cerebral arteries. *J Ethnopharmacol* 2001;76:109–13

50. Facino RM, Carini M, Aldini G, *et al. Panax ginseng* administration in the rat prevents myocardial ischemia-reperfusion damage induced by hyperbaric oxygen: evidence for an antioxidant intervention. *Planta Med* 1999;65:614–19

51. Zhan Y, Xu XH, Jiang YP. Effects of ginsenosides on myocardial ischemia/reperfusion damage in open-heart surgery patients. *Med J China* 1994;74:626–8

52. Mei B, Wang YF, Wu JX, Chen WZ. Protective effects of ginsenosides on oxygen free radical induced damages of cultured vascular endothelial cells *in vitro*. *Acta Pharmacol Sin* 1994;29:801–8

53. Chen X, Gillis CN, Moalli R. Vascular effects of ginsenosides *in vitro*. *Br J Pharmacol* 1984;82:485–91

54. Kim ND, Kang SY, Park JH, Schini-Kerth VB. Ginsenoside Rg$_3$ mediates endothelium-dependent relaxation in response to ginsenosides in rat aorta: role of K$^+$ channels. *Eur J Pharmacol* 1999;367:41–9

55. Li Z, Chen X, Niwa Y, Sakamoto S, Nakaya Y. Involvement of Ca^{2+}-activated K$^+$ channels in ginsenosides-induced aortic relaxation in rats. *J Cardiovasc Pharmacol* 2001;37:41–7

56. Chen X, Lee TJ-F. Ginsenosides-induced nitric oxide-mediated relaxation of the rabbit corpus cavernosum. *Br J Pharmacol* 1995;115:15–18

57. Zhang FL, Chen X. Effects of ginsenosides on sympathetic neurotransmitter release in pithed rats. *Acta Pharmacol Sin* 1987; 8:217–20

58. Tachikawa E, Kudo K, Kashimoto T, Takahashi E. Ginseng saponins reduce acetylcholine-evoked Na$^+$ influx and catecholamine secretion in bovine adrenal chromaffin cells. *J Pharm Exp Ther* 1995;273:629–36

59. Cross C. Oxygen radicals and human disease. *Ann Intern Med* 1987;107:526–45

60. Das DK. Cellular, biochemical, and molecular aspects of reperfusion injury. *Ann NY Acad Sci* 1994;723:116–27

61. Chen X. Cardiovascular effects of ginsenosides and their nitric-oxide mediated antioxidant actions. In Packer L, Traber MG, Xin W, eds. *Proceedings of the International Symposium on Natural Antioxidants*. Champaign, IL: AOCS, 1996:485–98

62. Han BH, Han YN, Park MH. Chemical and biochemical studies on antioxidant components of ginseng. In Chang HM, Yeung HW, Tso WW, Koo A, eds. *Advances in Chinese Medicinal Materials Research*. Singapore: World Scientific Press, 1995:485–98

63. Kitts DD, Wijewickreme AN, Hu C. Antioxidant properties of a North American ginseng extract. *Mol Cell Biochem* 2000;203: 1–10

64. Maffei FR, Carini M, Aldini G, Berti F, Rossoni G. *Panax ginseng* administration in the rat prevents myocardial ischemia–reperfusion damage induced by hyperbaric oxygen: evidence for an antioxidant intervention. *Planta Med* 1999;65:614–19

65. Chen X, Gillis CN. Effect of free radicals on pulmonary vascular response to acetylcholine. *J Appl Physiol* 1991;71:821–5

66. Rimar S, Gillis CN. Nitric oxide and experimental lung injury. In Zapol WM, Bloch KD, eds. *Nitric Oxide and the Lung*. New York, NY: Marcel Dekker, 1997:165–83

67. Kim H, Chen X, Gillis CN. Ginsenosides protect pulmonary vascular endothelium against free-radical induced injury. *Biochem Biophys Res Commun* 1992;189:670–6

68. Zhang D, Yasuda T, Yu Y, *et al.* Ginseng extract scavenges hydroxyl radical and protects unsaturated fatty acids from decomposition caused by iron-mediated lipid peroxidation. *Free Radic Biol Med* 1996;20:145–50

69. Nakagima S, Uchiyama Y, Yoshida K, Mizukawa H, Haruki E. The effects of ginseng radix rubra on human vascular endothelial cells. *Am J Chin Med* 1998;26:365–73

70. Jiping L, Min H, Hee T, Man Tıcky YK. *Panax quinquefolium* saponins protect low density lipoproteins from oxidation. *Life Sci* 1999;64:53–62

71. Patel RP, McAndrew J, Sellak H, *et al*. Biological aspects of reactive nitrogen species. *Biochim Biophys Acta* 1999;1411:385–400

72. Wınk DA, Hanbauer I, Krishna MC, DeGraff W, Gamson J, Mitchell JB. Nitric oxide protects against cellular damage and cytotoxicity from reactive oxygen species. *Proc Natl Acad Sci* 1993;90:9813–17

73. Kim YH, Park KH, Rho HM. Transcriptional activation of the Cu, Zn-superoxide dismutase gene through the AP2 site by ginsenoside Rb$_2$ extracted from a medicinal plant, *Panax ginseng*. *J Biol Chem* 1996;271:24539–43

74. Chang MS, Lee SG, Rho HM. Transcriptional activation of Cu/Zn superoxide dismutase and catalase genes by panaxadiol ginsenosides extracted from *Panax ginseng*. *Phytother Res* 1999;13:641–4

75. Ota T, Fujikawa-Yamamoto K, Zong ZP, *et al*. Plant-glycoside modulation of cell surface related to control of differentiation in cultured B16 melanoma cells. *Cancer Res* 1987;47:3863–7

76. Wakabayashi C, Murakami K, Hasegawa H, Murata J, Saiki I. An intestinal bacterial metabolite of ginseng protopanaxadiol saponins has the ability to induce apoptosis in tumor cells. *Biochem Biophys Res Commun* 1998;246:725–30

77. Mochizuki M, Yoo YC, Matsuzawa K, *et al*. Inhibitory effect of tumor metastasis in mice by saponins, ginsenoside-Rb$_2$, 20(*R*)- and 20(*S*)-ginsenoside-Rg$_3$, of red ginseng. *Biol Pharm Bull* 1995;18:1197–202

78. Kim YS, Kim DS, Kim SI. Ginsenoside Rh$_2$ and Rh$_3$ induce differentiation of HL-60 cells into granulocytes: modulation of protein kinase C isoforms during differentiation by ginsenoside Rh$_2$. *Intl J Biochem Cell Biol* 1998;30:327–38

79. Ota T, Maeda M, Odashima S, Ninomiya-Tsuji J, Tatsuka M. G$_1$ phase-specific suppression of the Cdk2 activity by ginsenoside Rh$_2$ in cultured murine cells. *Life Sci* 1997;60:39–44

80. Hasegawa H, Sung J, Matsumiya S, Uchiyama M. Main ginseng saponin metabolites formed by intestinal bacteria. *Planta Med* 1996;62:453–7

81. Karikura M, Miyase T, Tanizawa H, Taniyama T, Takino Y. Studies on absorption, distribution, excretion and metabolism of ginseng saponins. VII. Comparison of the decomposition modes of ginsenoside-Rb$_1$ and -Rb$_2$ in the digestive tract of rats. *Chem Pharm Bull* 1991;39:2357–61

82. Tode T, Kikuchi Y, Kita T, Hirata J, Imaizumi E, Nagata I. Inhibitory effects by oral administration of ginsenoside Rh$_2$ on the growth of human ovarian cancer cells in nude mice. *J Cancer Res Clin Oncol* 1993;120:24–6

83. Yun TK, Kim SH, Lee YS. Trial of a new medium-term model using benzo(a)pyrene induced lung tumor in newborn mice. *Anticancer Res* 1995;15:839–45

84. Yun TK. Experimental and epidemiological evidence of the cancer-preventive effects of *Panax ginseng* C.A. Meyer. *Nutr Rev* 1996;54:S71–81

85. Yun TK, Choi SY. Preventive effect of ginseng intake against various human cancers: a case study on 1987 pairs. *Cancer Epidemiol Biomarker Prev* 1995;4:401–8

86. Perry P, Evans HJ. Cytological detection of mutagen–carcinogen exposure by sister chromatid exchange. *Nature (London)* 1975;258:121–5

87. Nishi Y, Hasegawa MM, Taketomi M, Ohkawa Y, Inui N. Comparison of 6-thioguanine-resistant mutation and sister chromatid

exchanges in Chinese hamster V79 cells with forty chemical and physical agents. *Cancer Res* 1984;44:3270–9

88. Zhu JH, Takeshita T, Kitagawa I, Morimoto K. Suppression of the formation of sister chromatid exchanges by low concentrations of ginsenoside Rh$_2$ in human blood lymphocytes. *Cancer Res* 1995;55:1221–3

89. Cho SW, Cho EH, Choi SY. Ginsenosides activate DNA polymerase from bovine placenta. *Life Sci* 1995;57:1359–65

90. Odashima S, Nakayabu Y, Honjo N, Abe H, Arichi S. Induction of phenotypic reverse transformation by ginsenosides in cultured Morris hepatoma cells. *Eur J Cancer* 1979;13:885–92

91. Yun YS, Moon HS, Oh YR, Jo SK, Kim YJ, Yun TK. Effect of red ginseng on natural killer cell activity in mice with lung adenoma induced by urethan and benzo(a)pyrene. *Cancer Detect Prev* 1987;1:301–9

92. Kim JY, Germolec DR, Luster MI. *Panax ginseng* as a potential immunomodulator: studies in mice. *Immunopharmacol Immunotoxicol* 1990;12:257–76

93. Kenarova B, Neychev H, Hadjiivanova C, Petkov VD, Immunomodulating activity of ginsenoside Rg$_1$ from *Panax ginseng*. *Jpn J Pharmacol* 1990;54:447–54

94. Park KM, Kim YS, Jeong TC, *et al*. Nitric oxide is involved in the immunomodulating activities of acidic polysaccharide from *Panax ginseng*. *Planta Med* 2001;67:122–6

95. Cho YK, Sung H, Lee HJ, Joo CH, Cho GJ. Long-term intake of Korean red ginseng in HIV-1-infected patients: development of resistance mutation to zidovudine is delayed. *Int Immunopharmacol* 2001;1:1295–305

96. Ackerknecht EH. *A Short History of Medicine*. Baltimore, MD: Johns Hopkins University Press, 1982

97. Wang CN. Advances in study of pharmacology of ginseng. *Acta Pharm Sin* 1965;12:477–586

98. Wang CN. Recent advances in study of pharmacology of ginseng. *Acta Pharm Sin* 1980;15:312–20

99. Bensky D, Gamble A. Ginseng. In *Chinese Herbal Medicine Materia Medica*. Seattle, WA: Eastland Press, 1993:314–17

100. Kimura M. Hypoglycemic component in ginseng radix and its insulin release. *Proceedings of the 3rd International Ginseng Symposium*, Korean Ginseng Research Institute, Seoul, Korea, 1980

101. Kimura M, Waki I, Chujo T, *et al*. Effect of hypoglycemic components in ginseng radix on blood insulin level in alloxan diabetic mice and insulin release from perfused rat pancreas. *J Pharm Dyn* 1981;4:410–17

102. Kimura M, Waki I, Tanaka O, Nagai Y, Shibata S. Pharmacological sequential trials for the fractionation of components with hypoglycemic activity in alloxan diabetic mice from ginseng radix. *J Pharm Dyn* 1981;4:402–9

103. Kimura M, Suzuki J. The pattern of action of blended Chinese medicine to glucose tolerance curves in genetically diabetic KK-CA^y mice. *J Pharm Dyn* 1981;4:907–15

104. Yokozawa T, Kobayashi T, Oura H, Kawashima Y. Studies on the mechanism of the hypoglycemic activity of ginsenoside-Rb$_2$ in streptozotocin-diabetic rats. *Chem Pharm Bull* 1985;33:869–72

105. Kimura I, Nakashima N, Sugihara Y, Fu-Jun C, Kimura M. The antihyperglycemic blend effect of traditional Chinese medicine Baykko-ka-ninjin-to on alloxan and diabetic KK-CA^y mice. *Phytother Res* 1999;13:484–8

106. Kwan HJ, Wan JK. Clinical study of treatment of diabetes with power of the steamed insam (ginseng) produced in Kaesong, Korea. *Tech Inf* 1994;6:33–5

107. Sotaniemi EA, Haapakoski E, Rautio A. Ginseng therapy in non-insulin-dependent diabetic patients. *Diabetes Care* 1995;18:1373–5

108. World Health Organization. Radix ginseng. In *WHO Monographs on Selected Medicinal Plants*, vol 1. Geneva: WHO, 1999:168–82

109. Vuksan V, Sievenpiper JL, Koo VYY, *et al*. American ginseng (*Panax quinquefolius* L) reduces postprandial glycemia in nondiabetic subjects and subjects with type 2 diabetes mellitus. *Arch Intern Med* 2000;160:1009–13

110. Vuksan V, Stavro MP, Sievenpiper JL, Beljan-Zdravkovic U, Leiter LA, Josse RG, Xu Z. Similar postprandial with escalation of dose and administration time of American ginseng in type 2 diabetes. *Diabetes Care* 2000;23:1221–6

111. Attele AS, Zhou YP, Xie JT, *et al*. Anti-diabetes effects of *Panax ginseng* berry extract and ginsenoside Re. *Diabetes* 2002;51:1851–8

112. Xie JT Zhou Y-P, Dey L, *et al*. Ginseng berry reduces blood glucose and body weight in *db/db* mice. *Phytomedicine* 2002;9:254–8

113. Odashima S, Ota T, Kohno H, *et al*. Control of phenotypic expression of cultured B16 melanoma cells by plant glycosides. *Cancer Res* 1985;45:2781–4

114. Kim HS, Hwang SL, Oh S. Ginsenoside Rc and Rg$_1$ differentially modulate NMDA receptor subunit mRNA levels after intracerebroventricular infusion in rats. *Neurochem Res* 2000;25:1149–54

115. Banthorpe DV. Terpenoids. In *Natural Products*. Essex: Longman Scientific and Technical, 1994:331–9

116. Ourisson G, Crabbe P, Rodic OR. *Tetracyclic Triterpenes*. San Francisco, CA: Holden-Day Publishers, 1964

117. Boar RB. *Terpenoids and Steroids*. Dorking, UK: Bartholomew Press, 1983

118. Shibata S, Tanaka O, Shoji J, Saito H. Chemistry and pharmacology of *Panax*. In Wagner H, Hikino H, Farnsworth NR, eds. *Economic and Medicinal Plant Research*, vol 1. New York, NY: Academic Press, 1985:217–84

119. Heftmann E, Mosettig E. *Biochemistry of Steroids*. London: Reinhold Publishing Corporation, 1960

120. Bastiaanse EM, Höld KM, Van der Laarse A. The effect of membrane cholesterol content on ion transport processes in plasma membranes. *Cardiovasc Res* 1997;33: 272–83

121. Lee YJ, Chung E, Lee KY, Lee YH, Huh B, Lee SK. Ginsenoside-Rg$_1$, one of the major active molecules from *Panax ginseng*, is a functional ligand of glucocorticoid receptor. *Mol Cell Endocrinol* 1997;133:135–40

122. Chung E, Lee KY, Lee YJ, Lee YH, Lee SK. Ginsenoside-Rg$_1$ down-regulates glucocorticoid receptor and displays synergistic effects with cAMP. *Steroids* 1998;63:421–4

123. Soldati F, Sticher O. HPLC separation and quantitative determination of ginsenosides from *Panax ginseng*, *Panax quinquefolium* and from ginseng drug preparations. *Planta Med* 1980;39:348–57

124. Islam MR, Mahdi JG, Bowen ID. Pharmacological importance of stereochemical resolution of enantiomeric drugs. *Drug Safety* 1997;17:149–65

125. Kudo K, Tachikawa E, Kashimoto T, Takahashi E. Properties of ginseng saponin inhibition of catecholamine secretion in bovine adrenal chromaffin cells. *Eur J Pharm* 1998;341:139–44

126. Shiao MS, Lin LJ. Two new triterpenes of the fungus *Ganoderma lucidum*. *J Nat Prod* 1987;50:886–91

127. Wang CN, Chen JS, Shiao MS, Wang CT. Activation of human platelet phospholipases C and A$_2$ by various oxygenated triterpenes. *Eur J Pharm* 1994;267:33–42

128. Odani T, Tanizawa H, Takino Y, Studies on the absorption, distribution, excretion and metabolism of ginseng saponins. III. The absorption, distribution and excretion of ginsenoside Rb$_1$ in the rat. *Chem Pharm Bull* 1983;31:1059–66

129. Hasegawa H, Sung JH, Matsumiya S, *et al*. Reversal of daunomycin and vinblastine resistance in multidrug-resistant P388 leukemia *in vitro* through enhanced cytotoxicity by triterpenoids. *Planta Med* 1995;61:409–13

130. Rilfors L, Hauksson JB, Lindblom G. Regulation and phase equilibria of membrane lipids from *Bacillus megaterium* and *Acholeplasma laidlawii* strain A containing methyl-branched acyl chains. *Biochemistry* 1994;33:6110–20

131. Goldberg EM, Zidovetzki R. Synergistic effects of diacylglycerols and fatty acids on membrane structure and protein kinase C activity. *Biochemistry* 1998;37:5623–32

132. Schroeder F, Jefferson JR, Kier AB, *et al*. Membrane cholesterol dynamics: cholesterol domains and kinetic pools. *Proc Soc Exp Biol Med* 1991;196:235–52

133. Mas-Oliva J, Santiago-Garcia J. Cholesterol effect on thermostability of the (Ca^{2+}–Mg^{2+})-ATPase from cardiac muscle sarcolemma. *Biochem Int* 1990;21:233–41

134. Kirkwood A, Prichard JR, Schwartz SM, Meadow MS, Stemerman MB. Effects of low density lipoprotein on endothelial cell membrane fluidity and mononuclear cell attachment. *Am J Physiol* 1991;260:C43–9

135. Pederson PL, Carafoli E. Ion motive ATPases. Ubiquity, properties, and significance to cell function. *Trends Biochem Sci* 1987;12:146–50

136. Wehling M. Specific, nongenomic actions of steroid hormones. *Annu Rev Physiol* 1997;59:365–93

137. Brann DW, Hendry LB, Mahesh VB. Emerging diversities in the mechanism of action of steroid hormones. *J Steroid Biochem Mol Biol* 1995;52:113–33

138. Pastan I, Gottesman MM. Multidrug resistance. *Annu Rev Med* 1991;42:277–86

139. Gudi R, Nolan JP, Frangos JA. Modulation of GTPase activity of G proteins by fluid shear stress and phospholipid composition. *Proc Natl Acad Sci USA* 1998;95:2515–19

140. Mogil JS, Shin YH, Mccleskey EW, Kim SC, Nah SY. Ginsenoside Rf, a trace component of ginseng root, produces antinociception in mice. *Brain Res* 1998;792:218–28

141. Sherr CJ. G$_1$ phase progression: cycling on cue [review]. *Cell* 1994;79:551–5

142. Zidovetzki R, Lester DS. The mechanism of activation of protein kinase C: a biophysical perspective [review]. *Biochim Biophys Acta* 1992;1134:261–72

143. Nishizuka Y. The role of protein kinase C in cell surface signal transduction and tumour promotion. *Nature (London)* 1984;308:693–8

144. McEwan IJ, Almlöf T, Wıkström A, Dahlman-Wright K, Wright AH, Gustafsson J. The glucocorticoid receptor functions at multiple steps during transcription initiation by RNA polymerase II. *J Biol Chem* 1994;269:25629–36

145. Rohrer DC. 3D molecular similarity methods: in search of a pharmacophore. In Codding PW, ed. *Structure-based Drug Design*. Norwell, MA: Kluwer Academic Publishers, 1998:65–76

Is ginseng free from adverse effects?

17

J.-T. Xie, S. Mehendale and S. A. Maleckar

INTRODUCTION

Ginseng is a deciduous perennial plant belonging to the araliaceous family (Araliaceae). Respected as a 'king herb' in the East, ginseng has been one of the most widely used in traditional Chinese medicine for several thousand years[1,2]. In oriental countries, ginseng has been used as a general tonic and to maintain, restore or increase health, vitality and longevity. It was reported that Marco Polo was aware of Chinese ginseng, and the plant was brought to Europe possibly with the silk trade; it is certain that the Arabs brought back ginseng from China in the 9th century[3]. Currently, ginseng is also one of the most commonly used herbal medications in the West[4,5].

Research data have demonstrated that ginseng and its major active components, ginsenosides, have a complex constitution and multiple pharmacological actions[6]. Ginseng and ginsenosides influence the central nervous system (including learning, memory and behavior), as well as cardiovascular, gastrointestinal, endocrine and immune systems[2,6,7]. It is commonly accepted that ginseng administration, in general, is safe when used appropriately[8,9]. However, like all other herbal medications, ginseng contains a number of identified and unidentified chemical constituents with or without pharmacological activities. We have studied the beneficial effects of ginseng in different organ systems[6,7,10–17]. In this chapter, we will discuss potential adverse effects of ginseng, especially when ginseng was consumed inappropriately or abused (e.g. ginseng abuse syndrome), or due to the lack of quality control in ginseng products[18–24]. Ginseng animal toxicity data are also reviewed.

TOXIC EFFECTS IN ANIMAL STUDIES

Acute toxic effect

Data have indicated that the LD_{50} of ginseng root extract in mice was 5 g/kg after oral administration[25]. In another report, the LD_{50} of the root was 10–30 g/kg in mice[26]. The LD_{50} of ginseng leaf and stem extract was approximately 625 mg/kg with intraperitoneal injection in mice[27], and the LD_{50} of the crude saponin fraction and saponins of ginseng leaf was 381 and 299 mg/kg, respectively, after intravenous injection. Behavioral changes observed after intraperitoneal administration of lethal doses showed that the crude saponin fraction produced extended posture with the abdomen of the mice touching the floor and abnormal gait after a few minutes. Approximately 10 min later, swimming convulsions appeared and mice died after 15–25 min. The LD_{50} was approximately 300 mg/kg[28]. Variable ginseng extracts contribute to the inconsistent LD_{50} data, making direct comparison impossible.

Our laboratory also evaluated the acute toxicity of ginseng berry extract in *ob/ob* mice. No adverse effects were observed in six animals that received 500 mg/kg daily by intraperitoneal injection for 12 days, while the maximum daily therapeutic dose used in other studies was 150 mg/kg[17]. However, all four *ob/ob* mice died within 24 h after receiving a single intraperitoneal dose of the extract at 1500 mg/kg (Yuan and colleagues, unpublished data).

Subacute toxic effect

In rats, ginseng leaf and stem extract at intraperitoneal doses up to 80 mg/kg for 21 days did not affect blood cells, hemoglobin levels or renal function[27]. In another subacute study, there were significant increases in body weight and food consumption in rats, while the brain, heart, lung, liver, spleen, kidneys, stomach and testis/ovaries were normal in both gross and histopathological examination[29].

Chronic toxic effect

No toxic effects were noted in rats following ingestion of ginseng extract at a daily dose of 105–210 mg/kg for 25 weeks[30]. Aphale and co-workers[29] found no toxicity after 90 days of ginseng administration. Chronic treatment of mice, rats, rabbits and dogs has shown very few observable signs of toxicity. No evidence of toxicity was observed in male and female beagle dogs fed ginseng extract for 90 days at daily doses up to 15 mg/kg. The study showed that there were no treatment-related changes in body weight or blood chemistry[31]. A long-term safety investigation of ginseng product was performed in rats. Intake of the product during a 6-month period at a dose of 0.75 ml/kg did not show any unfavorable effects on integral, morphological, biochemical or hematological parameters. In addition, two generations of rats that received ginseng product did not exhibit embryotoxic, gonadotoxic or teratogenic effects, or a negative effect on the growth and development of their offspring[32].

ADVERSE EFFECTS IN HUMANS

General

No significant adverse effects have been reported in ginseng clinical trials. However, several studies have observed that ginseng's side-effect profile includes insomnia, headache, nausea and vomiting, diarrhea, epistaxis and skin eruption. Although the incidence of the individual symptoms was not clear, these symptoms usually occurred after inappropriate ginseng dose and its long-term use[9,33,34]. In addition, nervousness and gastrointestinal upset have also been reported after prolonged high doses of ginseng (e.g. up to 15 g/day for 2 years)[35]. Clinically, 'ginseng abuse syndrome' was described by Siegel[18]; 10% of subjects experienced hypertension together with nervousness, sleeplessness, skin eruption and morning diarrhea. Edema was also seen in five subjects[18,21]. However, since this study did not differentiate between the species of ginseng used, its reliability was questioned by Mills and Bone[36]. Moreover, symptoms described in the study may also be attributable to significant caffeine intake in most of the subjects[37].

Significant ginseng adverse effects can be found in a limited number of cases. Stevens–Johnson syndrome was noted in a 27-year-old man following the intake of two ginseng tablets for 3 days, resulting in moderate infiltration of the dermis by mononuclear cells. The patient recovered completely after 30 days[19,22]. More seriously, agranulocytosis was induced after taking a Chinese ginseng product for relief of arthritis and back pain[30]. It is possible that some patients are very sensitive to ginseng administration.

Cardiovascular effects

Several clinical reports have demonstrated that ginseng and its products may cause cardiovascular adverse effects. A 39-year-old Czech man who had taken various ginseng products for 3 years manifested hypertension, dizziness, a loud palpable fourth heart sound and 'thrusting' apical pulse. Shortness of breath and inability to concentrate were also noted[19,22,38]. Another report showed that hypertension is a contraindication to ginseng administration[39]. Therefore, use of ginseng requires caution in patients with cardiovascular conditions, agitation, diabetes and psychosis[40]. In contrast, animal studies have shown that ginseng has a hypotensive effect and this effect may be related to the ginseng saponin fraction. Future studies are needed to address the inconsistent cardiovascular effects of ginseng.

Endocrine effects

There have been several clinical reports concerning endocrine adverse effects induced by high-dose ginseng or ginseng preparations. Several of ginseng's estrogen-like effects were reported. A post-menopausal woman who had used pills and topical creams containing ginseng experienced an estrogen-like effect of mastalgia and vaginal bleeding[41]. Another case reported that swelling and tenderness of the breasts were induced by ginseng in a menopausal woman. Likewise, another clinical case indicated postmenopausal bleeding in a 44-year-old woman who applied a topical ginseng face cream[42]. Oshima and colleagues[43] believed that the estrogen-like effects were not unexpected, since small quantities of estrone, estradiol and estriol are present in ginseng root. However, the major active constituents of ginseng are ginsenosides, which are structurally similar to steroids such as testosterone, estrogen and adrenocorticotropic hormone (ACTH)[40].

Based on the cases described above, pregnant, menopausal and elderly women should be advised to use ginseng prudently, and patients receiving hormonal therapy should avoid ginseng completely[3,33,37,40]. Additionally, patients who have spontaneous nose bleeding and excessive menstrual bleeding should take ginseng prudently.

Other adverse effects

Ginseng may induce diuretic resistance in some patients[44], although the possible ginseng–drug interaction mechanism is unknown. Ginseng may also interact with warfarin, an anticoagulant with a narrow therapeutic index. A case report showed that a man with a mechanical heart valve, stabilized with warfarin administration over 5 years, became destabilized following administration of a ginseng product[45]. The patient's International Normalized Ratio (INR) decreased from 3.1 to 1.5 after 2 weeks of ginseng

intake. Following the discontinuation of ginseng therapy, the INR returned to 3.3 within 2 weeks. In this patient, ginseng use appeared to be associated with a significant decrease in warfarin anticoagulation since no other changes in medicine and foods could be found to be responsible. Biochemical analysis did not detect vitamin K in ginseng[46]. The mechanism for this interaction has not been identified.

Although only one case report of ginseng–warfarin interaction has been reported, its impact on clinical medicine cannot be overestimated. In a number of recently published drug handbooks (e.g. *Mosby's Drug Guide*[47], *Drug Interaction Facts*[48] and *Handbook of Herbs and Natural Supplements*[49]) and herbal review articles published in widely read medical journals[9,23], a possible ginseng–warfarin interaction is discussed, indicating that the issue has received the medical community's attention. In addition, ginseng can inhibit platelet aggregation as seen in *in vivo* and *in vitro* animal experiments. Furthermore, potential bleeding caused by ginseng is a concern for surgical patients[23].

To date, most ginseng adverse effects have been reported from animal study data and individual clinical case reports. Controlled clinical studies are urgently needed to determine ginseng's potential adverse effects. Because long-term, high-dose ginseng use may be responsible for the reported adverse events, it is recommended that the daily ginseng dose should be 0.5–2.0 g dry root, or the equivalent extract, for short-term treatment[9]. Ginseng should not be used in children under the age of 2 years.

POSSIBLE REASONS FOR THE ADVERSE EFFECTS

Inappropriate use or abuse

As a 'king herb' in the Orient, the fame of ginseng has led to abuse or misconceptions in its use, thus inducing adverse effects, such as 'ginseng abuse syndrome'. Consumers may assume that, because ginseng is a natural product, it must be safe. Although the daily recommended ginseng dose is not over 2 g[9], a daily dose of 59 g was reported to achieve behavioral stimulation[18]. A large ginseng dose may result in sleeplessness, depression and nervous system disorder; long-term ginseng users may suffer from chronic insomnia, nervousness and loose stools, among other problems[18].

Variability in commercial preparations

Wide variability exists among ginseng products, and non-standardized pseudoginseng preparations are commercially available. In addition, some ginseng products have been adulterated with prescription medications, including ephedrine or pseudoephedrine[3,20].

Cui and colleagues[50] examined 50 commercial ginseng products sold in 11 countries. Each preparation was blindly analyzed in triplicate. In 44 of these preparations the concentration of ginsenosides varied from 1.9% to 9.0% (w/w). The ginsenoside concentration in several commercial products was very low. Surprisingly, six products from three different countries (the USA, UK and Sweden) did not contain any ginsenosides. Another study that analyzed 25 commercially available ginseng products demonstrated that the ginseng products were correctly labeled as to the plant content. However, the analyzed marker compound concentrations varied significantly from those reported on the labels. Also, the total ginsenoside content varied by 15- and 36-fold in tablets and liquid preparations, respectively, when compared to those reported. Ginseng preparations that listed specific concentrations of active ingredients contained as little as 11% and as much as 328% of the labeled concentration[51,52]. This variability may lead to a wide range of pharmacological activities or adverse effects. Standardization of ginseng products should be a primary focus for quality assurance[51].

Different ginseng species

There are up to six recognized species of the genus *Panax*, depending on the particular botanical authority. Most botanists currently recognize three medicinal species, i.e. *Panax ginseng* (Chinese or Korean ginseng), *Panax quinquefolius* (American ginseng) and *Panax japonicus* (Japanese ginseng)[3,6,53]. Chemical analysis results indicate that there are various components in different ginseng species, and each ginseng species has its own distinct ginsenoside profile. Even within a single species, the length of growth, cultivation conditions (such as soil, temperature, moisture) and harvest season affect the make-up of ginsenoside contents[24,54]. Siberian ginseng, on the other hand, is distinct from *Panax ginseng*, and does not contain any ginsenosides. Rather, its active constituents are eleutherosides, which are glycosides with aglycons and are chemically related to aridac glycosides, such as digoxin.

To compare the composition of ginsenosides in different ginseng samples, our laboratory measured six ginsenosides of Wisconsin-cultivated and Illinois-cultivated American ginseng by using high-performance liquid chromatography (HPLC) analysis. Our data showed remarkable variability in these specimens, in terms of ginsenoside profile and total ginsenoside concentration. In addition, the length of cultivation also influenced the content of ginsenosides[7,24]. Furthermore, distribution of ginsenosides varies between different parts of the ginseng plant in the same species[16,55]. The multiformity of ginseng species and variability of ginsenoside concentrations among different species may also contribute to variable pharmacological effects and adverse effects.

Ginseng–drug interaction

Co-administration of ginseng and prescription medications may cause adverse herb–drug interactions[23,56]. Ginseng may interact with a number of medications, such as warfarin, digoxin and vitamin C, possibly leading to adverse effects. It is suggested that concomitant use of ginseng with warfarin, heparin, aspirin and non-steroidal anti-inflammatory drugs should be avoided[33,57].

In addition to possible ginseng–warfarin interactions discussed earlier, another potential adverse interaction exists between ginseng and digoxin[58]. A 74-year-old male patient taking a constant dose of digoxin for many years was found to have an elevated serum digoxin level. Common causes of elevated serum digoxin were ruled out, yet the patient's digoxin level remained high. The patient revealed that he was taking Siberian ginseng. Soon after he stopped taking Siberian ginseng, his serum digoxin returned to an acceptable level and digoxin therapy resumed. The patient resumed taking Siberian ginseng several months later and the digoxin level rose again. Digoxin therapy was maintained at a constant daily dose while the ginseng was stopped once more, and the serum digoxin levels again returned to the therapeutic range. Although it is still unclear why Siberian ginseng changed the digoxin level, physicians should be aware that the drug interactions may exist between Siberian ginseng and digoxin.

Not all ginseng–drug interactions are detrimental. A report indicated that ginseng saponins at concentrations of 0.25–1.0 mg/ml significantly protected against oxidation of low-density lipoprotein *in vitro*. The presence of vitamin C (1–10 μmol/l) markedly enhanced the protective effects of ginseng[59].

SUMMARY

Herbal medications play an important role in our daily health-care maintenance. Ginseng is one of the most commonly used herbs in China, Japan and Korea, as well as in the USA. Although it is generally considered safe to use, adverse effects associated with ginseng use have been reported. Inappropriate ginseng use, such as high-dose administration, may cause insomnia, headaches and diarrhea, as well as cardiovascular and endocrine disorders. Other factors that may contribute to adverse effects of ginseng include the variety of ginseng species, variability in commercial ginseng preparations and potential ginseng–drug interactions. To minimize possible adverse effects of ginseng, consumers should be advised to use it appropriately, and the herbal industry has a responsibility to provide standardized ginseng preparations. Future investigations are needed to clarify both the beneficial and the adverse effects of ginseng, and their underlining mechanisms of action.

References

1. Keum YS, Park KK, Lee JM, *et al*. Antioxidant and anti-tumor promoting activities of the methanol extract of heat-processed ginseng. *Cancer Lett* 2000;150:41–8

2. Kim YK, Guo Q, Packer, L. Free radical scavenging activity of red ginseng aqueous extracts. *Toxicology* 2002;172:149–56

3. Phillipson JD, Anderson, LA. Ginseng – quality, safety and efficacy? *Pharmacol J* 1984;232:161–5

4. Vogler BK, Pittler MH, Ernst E. 1999. The efficacy of ginseng. A systematic review of randomised clinical trials. *Eur J Clin Pharmacol* 1999;55:567–75

5. Kaufman DW, Kelly JP, Rosenberg L, Anderson TE, Mitchell AA. Recent patterns of medication use in the ambulatory adult population of the United States. *J Am Med Assoc* 2002;287:337–44

6. Attele AS, Wu JA, Yuan CS. Multiple pharmacological effects of ginseng. *Biochem Pharmacol* 1999;58:1685–93

7. Yuan CS, Wang X, Wu JA, Attele AS, Xie JT, Gu M. Effect of *Panax quinquefolius* L. on brainstem neuronal activities: comparison between Wisconsin-cultivated and Illinois-cultivated roots. *Phytomedicine* 2001;8:178–83

8. Singh B, Saxena AK, Chandan BK, Gupta DK, Bhutani KK, Anand KK. Adaptogenic activity of a novel, withanolide-free aqueous fraction from the roots of *Withania somnifera* Dun. *Phytother Res* 2001;15:311–18

9. Ernst E. The risk–benefit profile of commonly used herbal therapies: ginkgo, St John's wort, ginseng, echinacea, saw palmetto, and kava. *Ann Intern Med* 2002;136:42–53

10. Yuan CS, Wu J, Lowell TK, Gu M. Gut and brain effects of American ginseng root on brainstem neuronal activities in the rat. *Am J Chin Med* 1998;26:G47–55

11. Yuan CS, Attele AS, Wu JA, Liu, D. Modulation of American ginseng on brainstem GABAergic effects in the rat. *J Ethnopharmacol* 1998;62:215–22

12. Yuan CS, Wu JA, Attele AS, Liu D. American ginseng affects brain neuronal activity. *Am J Compreh Med* 1999;1:27–33

13. Liu D, Li B, Attele AS, Kyle JW, Yuan, CS. Voltage-dependent inhibition of brain Na$^+$ channels by American ginseng. *Eur J Pharmacol* 2001;413:47–54

14. Yuan CS, Dey, L. Multiple effects of American ginseng in clinical medicine. *Am J Chin Med* 2001;29:567–9

15. Attele AS, Zhou YP, Xie JT, *et al*. Anti-diabetic effects of *Panax ginseng* berry extract and identification of its active component. *Diabetes* 2002;51:1851–8

16. Xie JT, Zhou YP, Dey L, *et al*. *Panax ginseng* berry extract reduces blood glucose and body weight in *db/db* mice. *Phytomedicine* 2002;9:254–8

17. Xie JT, Wang X, Attele AS, Yuan CS. Effects of American ginseng berry extract on blood glucose levels in *ob/ob* mice. *Am J Chin Med* 2002;30:187–94

18. Siegel R. Ginseng abuse syndrome. Problems with the panacea. *J Am Med Assoc* 1979;241:1614–15

19. Dega H, Laporte JL, Frances C, Herson S, Chosidow O. Ginseng as a cause for Stevens–Johnson syndrome. *Lancet* 1996;347:1344

20. Faleni R, Soldati F. Ginseng as cause of Stevens–Johnson syndrome? *Lancet* 1996;348:267

21. Nocerino E, Amato M, Izzo A. The aphrodisiac and adaptogenic properties of ginseng. *Fitoterapia* 2000;71:S1–5

22. Morgan A, Cupp MJ. *Panax ginseng*. In Cupp MJ, ed. *Toxicology and Clinical Pharmacology of Herbal Products*. Totowa, NJ: Humana Press, 2000:145–53

23. Ang-Lee MK, Moss J, Yuan C-S. Herbal medicines and perioperative care. *J Am Med Assoc* 2001;286:208–16

24. Yuan CS, Wu JA, Osinski J. Ginsenoside variability in American ginseng samples. *Am J Clin Nutr* 2002;75:600–1

25. Huang KC. *The Pharmacology of Chinese Herbs. Herbs with Multiple Actions*. Boca Raton, FL: CRC Press, 1999:17–51

26. Brekhman II, Dardymov IV. New substances of plant origin which increase nonspecific resistance. *Annu Rev Pharmacol* 1969;9:419–30

27. Wang BX, Cui JC, Liu AJ. The action of ginsenosides extracted from the stems and leaves of *Panax ginseng* in promoting animal growth. *Acta Pharma Sin* 1982;17:899–903

28. Saito H, Morita M, Takagi K. Pharmacological studies of *Panax ginseng* leaves. *Jap J Pharmacol* 1973;23:43–56

29. Aphale AA, Chhibba AD, Kumbhakarna NR, Mateenuddin M, Dahat SH. Subacute toxicity study of the combination of ginseng (*Panax ginseng*) and ashwagandha (*Withania somnifera*) in rats: a safety assessment. *Indian J Physiol Pharmacol* 1998;42:299–302

30. Popov IM, Goldwag WJ. Review of the properties amd clinical effects of ginseng. *Am J Chin Med* 1973;1:263

31. Hess FG, Parent RA, Stevens KR, Cox GE, Becci P. Effect of subchonic feeding of ginseng extract G115 in beagle dogs. *Food Chem Toxicol* 1983;21:95–7

32. Sorokina E, Asdiuk IN, Kirpatovskaia NA, Levitskaia AB. Experimental animal study of the safety of biological active food supplement obtained from ginseng root. *Vopr Pitan* 2000;69:53–6

33. Miller LG. Herbal medicinals: selected clinical considerations focusing on known or potential drug–herb interactions. *Arch Intern Med* 1998;158:2200–11

34. Awang DVC. Clinical trials of ginseng. *Altern Ther Wom Health* 2002;4:17–24

35. Gillis CN. *Panax ginseng* pharmacology: a nitric oxide link? *Biochem Pharmacol* 1997;54:1–8

36. Mills S, Bone K. *Principles and Practice of Phytotherapy. Modern Herbal Medicine*. New York, NY: Churchill Livingstone, 2000;418–32, 534–41

37. Bucci LR. Selected herbals and human exercise performance. *Am J Clin Nutr* 2000;72:624S–36S

38. Hammond TG, Whitworth JA. Adverse reactions to ginseng. *Med J Aust* 1981;1:492

39. Carabin IG, Burdock GA, Chatzidakis C. Safety assessment of *Panax ginseng*. *Int J Toxicol* 2000;19:293–301

40. Sierpina VS. *Integrative Health Care. Complementary and Alternative Therapies for the Whole Person*. Philadelphia, PA: F. D. Davis Company, 2001:134–5

41. Greenspan EM. Ginseng and vaginal bleeding. *J Am Med Assoc* 1983;249:2018

42. Hopkins MP, Takahashi M, Otake K, *et al.* Isolation and hypoglycemic activity of eleutherans A, B, C, D, E, F, and G: glycans of *Eleutherococcua senticosus* roots. *J Nat Prod* 1986;49:293–7

43. Oshima Y, Sato K, Hikino H. Isolation and hypoglycemic activity of quinquefolans A, B, and C, glycans of *Panax quinquefolium* roots. *J Nat Prod* 1987;50:188–90

44. Becker BN, Greene J, Evanson J, Chidsey G, Stone, WJ. Ginseng-induced diuretic resistance. *J Am Med Assoc* 1996;276:606–7

45. Janetzky K, Morreale AP. Problem interation between warfarin and ginseng. *Am J Health Syst Pharm* 1997;54:692–3

46. Zhang GD. Recent advances in chemical analysis of ginseng. *Acta Pharma Sin* 1980;15:375–84

47. *Mosby's Drug Guide*, 4th edn. Philadelphia, PA: Mosby, 2001

48. Tatro DS, ed. *Drug Interaction Facts*. St Louis, MO: Wolters Kluwer Company, 2001:98

49. Skidomore-Roth L. *Handbook of Herbs and Natural Supplements*. St. Louis, MO: Mosby, 2001

50. Cui J, Garle M, Eneroth P, Björkhem I. What do commercial ginseng preparations contain? *Lancet* 1994;344:134

51. Harkey MR, Henderson GL, Gershwin ME, Stem JS, Hanckman RM. Variability in commercial ginseng products: an analysis of 25 preparations. *Am J Clin Nutr* 2001;73:1101–6

52. Ang-Lee MK, Moss J, Yuan C-S. Use of herbal medicines before surgery. *J Am Med Assoc* 2001;286:2543–4

53. Awang DVC. Maternal use of ginseng and neonatal androgenization. *J Am Med Assoc* 1991;265:1828

54. Liu CX, Xiao PG. Recent advances on ginseng research in China. *J Ethnopharmacol* 1992;36:27–38

55. Zhang GD, Zhou ZH, Wang MZ, Gao, FY. Analysis of ginseng II. *Acta Pharma Sin* 1980;15:175–81

56. Windrum P, Hull DR, Morris TCM. Herb–drug interactions. *Lancet* 2000;355:1019–20

57. Vaes LPJ, Chyka PA. Interactions of warfarin with garlic, ginkgo, or ginseng: nature of the evidence. *Drug Inf Rounds* 2000;34:1478–82

58. McRae S. Elevated serum digoxin levels in a patient taking digoxin and Siberian ginseng. *CMAJ* 1996;155:293–5

59. Li J-P, Huang M, Teoh H, Man RYK. Interactions between *Panax quinquefolium* saponins and vitamin C are observed *in vitro*. *Mol Cell Biochem* 2000;204:77–82

A new medical vision: on the possibility of reconceptualizing 'conventional' medicine

18

S. Pessin

We differ not only because we select different objects out of the same world but because we see different worlds...

Murdoch

People only see what they are prepared to see.

Emerson

We cannot see anything until we are possessed with the idea of it, take it into our heads, – and then we can hardly see anything else...

Thoreau

In this chapter, various ways are examined in which a study of complementary and alternative medicine (CAM) can improve the possibilities for patient healing. The focus is most particularly on how CAM can do this not only by providing us with new medical information, tools and techniques, but additionally by affording us an opportunity to examine and reorient some of our most fundamental ideas about medicine, some of our most foundational conceptions about patients, care and healing, and some of the most deeply rooted presumptions and attitudes at the core of our 'conventional' medical vision.

INTRODUCTION: THREE BENEFITS OF COMPLEMENTARY AND ALTERNATIVE MEDICINE

In order to appreciate how CAM help improve the chances for patient wellness, we begin by distinguishing three distinct benefits of studying CAM.

New information

CAM can provide medical professionals with new medical information. This new information can improve the success rate of diagnoses, preventive medical care and treatment. An example of CAM's providing new information can be found in the link between omega−3 fatty acids and cardiovascular health, as well as in the role of green tea in the prevention of prostate cancer and other testosterone-related disorders.

New tools and techniques

CAM can offer medical professionals new tools and techniques, improving the comprehensive capacity to treat patients. Examples of new tools and techniques can be found in the study of meditation and acupuncture.

New ways of seeing

CAM can offer medical professionals new ways of thinking about the foundations of health and healing. Different from merely providing new information and techniques, CAM in this sense provides us with fresh insights into and perspectives on the nature of care and wellness, of patients and sickness, of bodies and minds, of pain and suffering, and thus helps us to re-examine and vigilantly improve our deepest sense of the underlying methodologies and overarching goals of medicine itself.

It is clear how CAM contributes to improved patient care in providing doctors with new information and new tools and techniques. It might be less obvious, though, how CAM contributes to improved patient care by asking doctors to reconsider the foundations of medicine itself. The goal of the current chapter is to explain how the conceptual business of reconsidering some of the basic presumptions at the heart of our medical practice has direct implications for patient healing.

We begin by distinguishing two different categories of CAM, and explaining how each can help us somewhat differently towards the goal of re-evaluating the foundations of our medical practices. We then turn in the remainder of the chapter to a better understanding of how re-evaluating the foundations of medicine directly impacts on patient healing.

TWO DIFFERENT SORTS OF COMPLEMENTARY AND ALTERNATIVE MEDICINE

In order to understand how CAM can help us re-examine our most basic medical presumptions, it is important to begin by distinguishing two distinct varieties of CAM.

Group A

The first group (group A) of CAM therapies works with the conventional Western medical conceptions of patients, bodies, health, disease and care. The efficacy of group A CAM therapies can be explained within the confines of conventional medical conceptual space.

Examples of group A CAM include Liao's and Sorrentino's respective biochemical analyses (in this volume) of the efficacy of green tea against prostate cancer and omega—3 fatty acids against heart disease. These are examples of CAM of the first sort, in that they are explicable in terms of conventional medical ideas (in this case, biochemistry). Borrowing from the above three-part distinction of goals of studying CAM, group A CAM most clearly provides us with new information and new tools and techniques, although, as will be seen below, even a study of group A CAM can help us re-examine the foundations of our medical vision.

Group B

The second group (group B), on the other hand, does not fit clearly into the space of our Western medical model. Examples of group B CAM include acupuncture and homeopathy. These are examples of therapies whose efficacy – hinging on regulating and balancing energy-flows – is arguably not fully explicable in terms of conventional biochemistry or solely in terms of the physiological pathways and systems at play in the current conventional medical model. While group B CAM contributes new information, tools and techniques, as we will see, group B CAM invites us to consider utterly new ways of seeing the entire space of health and healing. By essentially providing us with new fundamental orientations towards health and healing, the nature of this group of CAM therapies urges us to reconsider the foundations of 'conventional' medicine.

TWO DIFFERENT SORTS OF RE-EVALUATIONS OF 'CONVENTIONAL' MEDICINE

Having distinguished these two categories of CAM, we can now examine how each inspires us to re-examine the foundations of our current practice of medicine in slightly different ways.

Group B: blatant impetus for a new medical vision

Starting with group B, there are certain CAM therapies that very obviously invite us to reconsider the foundations of our medical beliefs and conceptions, providing us with essentially new conceptual frameworks in which to pursue medicine. One such example is the case of acupuncture. The study of acupoints by doctors within a Chinese medical context signals more than just a difference in practice from Western-trained medical practitioners. While the acupuncturist has a different set of practices from his or her Western-trained counterpart (here, we must look no further than the contents of their respective medical bags), this difference in practice signals deep differences in the way a practitioner within the Chinese tradition envisions patients, their bodies, health, disease and care. While the fullness of this difference can be arrived at only through a careful study of the Chinese medical tradition, for an initial way to see this difference, consider the acupuncturist's method of 'gazing upon *se*'. *Se*, literally meaning 'color' (with the sense here of the color of a patient's skin), has come, within the Chinese medical tradition, to mean also 'facial expression' and, by extension, to signify the overall disposition of a person.

This methodological commitment may appear to a Western reader to signal a serious engagement with the patient's surface symptomology, a commitment that is certainly shared by Western medicine. But the Chinese method of 'gazing upon *se*' signals something more. It signals a radically different medical model in which patients are encountered and treated as products of larger-ranging physical and mental states, as persons with deep-seated dispositions and practices, all of which are directly relevant when evaluating and caring for even a localized pain or symptom.

That the view of a patient (and hence, of bodies, health, disease and care) at play in this model signals significant differences from the Western medical way of seeing is drawn out in a marvelous study by

Shigehisa Kurriyama[1], who investigates the thoroughgoing conceptual divide between Chinese and Western medical models – and consequent conceptions of health, bodies, selves and care – in terms of a comparative analysis of the Chinese commitment to 'gazing upon *se*' on the one hand, versus the Greek (and Western) method of 'envisioning muscularity' on the other.

Group A: subtle impetus for a new medical vision

Group A CAM, too, can be invaluable in our quest for an overall improved medical vision if, in studying it, we use it as an opportunity to think and rethink the larger issues. In studying group A CAM, we must question not just which chemical will cause which metabolic change, or which technique will best fix which bodily ailment, but how all of that fits into what we take to be the larger aims of medicine, how and whether we do justice to those aims when ministering care to patients and, at the heart of all these questions, what we mean – or should mean – by the notions of health and healing.

To summarize, in our study of CAM – group B as well as group A – we have an opportunity to do more than simply learn new information, tools and techniques. We have, rather, an invitation to think about and critically evaluate the conceptual frameworks within which our current Western tradition of medicine operates and against which it defines the terms of health and healing. Such considerations, when properly engaged, can serve as the groundwork for critically re-evaluating our current framework, enabling us to begin making changes towards the goal of better patient care.

In working through a textbook on CAM, we serve our patients' interests best when we learn not only new information and new tools and techniques for their care, but when we consider entirely new ways of seeing – of seeing patients, bodies, illness, wellness, care, the notions of health and healing, and what we take the goals of medicine itself to be. In what follows, we turn to explaining how reconceptualizing the foundations of medicine in this way can improve patient care by directly improving patients' chances to heal.

THE IMPORTANCE OF RE-EVALUATING THE FOUNDATIONS OF WESTERN MEDICINE

We have shown how each of group A and group B CAM can be helpful conduits for re-evaluating the foundations of our practice of medicine. We have not, though, yet said why such a re-evaluation is important towards the goal of improved patient healing. In what follows, we offer two kinds of answers to this question. First, we explain just how patients' health is directly tied into doctors' views about medicine, and how those views can unwittingly prevent patients from healing. Next, we point to two particular flaws at the heart of our current medical practice that stand in the way of patient healing. Both sets of considerations help explain why it is so important for doctors to be ever-vigilant about questioning and seeking to improve the foundations of their medicine, being ever-vigilant to re-examine what they understand by the most basic notions of patients, care and healing.

Opening the space of patient health and healing

While the valuable contributions of our current Western medical practices are not in question, what must be in question is whether some of the foundational ideas underlying those practices unwittingly block some important and legitimate ideas about health and healing, with the unintentional but real result of preventing patients from healing in ways not currently invited by the Western medical practitioner. The limited ways in which doctors have been trained to understand the nature of persons and the notion of health, and, subsequently, how they have come to minister care to patients, limits the space in which patients are allowed to heal. In seeing things in certain limited way, doctors – unintentionally but undeniably – limit the possibilities for patient healing.

To make this point clear, it is helpful to consider briefly some phenomena at play in the placebo effect. Before proceeding, let me be explicit on one point: I do not mean to suggest that the benefits for patient healing presented by embracing new fundamental medical conceptions are cases of placebo responses. This said, there is, nonetheless, an important phenomenon that emerges from studies of placebo responses that can help impress upon us how doctors' understanding of basic underlying notions of persons, care and healing can directly limit – or expand – patients' chances for wellness.

In placebo studies, we find that patients who have their symptoms cured by placebo responses can revert back to their starting symptoms simply upon coming to learn that their current healthy state was 'merely' a placebo response[2]. Here we see that a patient's state of health can be affected by the way the doctor sees health, i.e. by the concepts his or her doctor employs to describe that state of health and the subsequent orientation which the doctor has towards that state of health. In the case of current Western medicine, doctors (and hence, patients) are virtually invited to see 'cure by placebo' as a hoax of some sort, and doctors (and hence, patients) are forced to have a negative, 'delegitimizing' attitude towards what is a perfectly wonderful outcome, namely a state of health! This is a fascinating fact for all sorts of reasons, but, for our current purposes, it can serve as a useful case in point of the larger claim we are interested in (larger, because not just a claim about placebo responses), namely, that our starting concepts – our medical 'way of seeing' such basic things as persons, care and healing – will shape, ground and limit the capacity for patients to heal and be healed.

This phenomenon – in which patient's bodies and health conform to and change to meet the limits of a doctor's medical concepts – can be seen in a variety of cases. One example is the case of 'snake sickness'. A medical tradition that has 'snake sickness' as a legitimate part of its medical model opens up a space for persons within the reach of that tradition to experience 'snake sickness' and to do so manifesting physical symptoms. Among Native Americans of Apache descent, crossing a path left by a snake can result in facial sores for members of that community – sores, furthermore, that can be alleviated only through the healing inter-mediation of a traditional 'snake doctor'[3,4].

Another example involves the experience of pain. A medical tradition that views pain as something entirely alien tacitly legitimates pain as something to be experienced with a great deal of fright, and opens the space for patients within the care of that tradition to experience and report severely disorienting reactions to pain, as compared with those from other traditions who do not report experiencing that same level of severe fear and disorientation in their own experiences of pain[4–6].

Finally, consider the phenomen of self-healing. A medical tradition that views wellness as something that is, for the most part, best left to doctors and pills, tacitly wrests control out of a patient's hands and can prevent the possibility for self-healing within that population. Recall the afore-mentioned case of those who, after being relieved of their symptoms, reverted to their sickness after learning that they had essentially healed themselves[2]. Here we might also recommend considering those authors who advocate the need to replace what in our current medical paradigm is mostly relegated to the 'placebo effect' with a notion of 'self-healing' or some other more positively reinforcing notion that supports – instead of delegitimizes – a patient's capacity to be cured without conventional drug interventions[7–9].

Although not itself best understood as a placebo response, the point that we can nonetheless carry over from certain phenomena at play in placebo responses is that patients are limited in how they can experience themselves, pain, care, disease and health, depending on how those concepts are defined and regarded within the medical community in which they have those experiences. In other words, the way in which the Western medical tradition and, hence, a health-care professional within that tradition, understands the complexity of persons, will serve as a lens through which doctors and patients can talk about, experience and cure disorders that afflict persons. The way in which the Western medical tradition understands the notion of care will serve as a lens through which doctors and patients can, respectively, minister and benefit from care. The way in which the Western medical tradition understands pain, disease and health

will serve as a lens through which doctors and patients can talk about and experience pain, disease and health. And so on for any of the basic medical concepts at play within the space of our medical discourse.

The exciting – and yet potentially frightening – implication is that what the medical community embraces (even if only tacitly) as legitimate medicine and legitimate conceptions of such things as selves, bodies, mind–body interactions, care, suffering, health and healing sets the ground-rules (the capacity and possibility) for patient healing.

In effect, our starting conceptual schemas not only dictate what we see but also how we are. In deeply shaping the world that we encounter, our starting beliefs and commitments affect not only what we understand by 'health' and 'body', but also our actual experience of health and body, including the way our bodies react. Starting assumptions about patients, cure and healing on the part of our doctors dictate not only what we see when we encounter the world and what we understand by bodies and health, but also how our bodies react to that world and to our doctors' attempts to heal us. Not only germs and bacteria, but even our ways of seeing ourselves, cure and healing (themselves influenced by our medical community's conceptions) can generate physiological results, and can dictate the space of wellness.

To summarize, the way doctors envision patients, cure and healing can directly limit patients' possibilities of being healed. The medical community must be ever-vigilant about examining and re-examining its assumptions at the most basic levels. Is it possible, for example, that the Chinese medical way of envisioning care (discussed above in our analysis of acupuncture) allows a better space for patient healing? Questions of this sort are essential; after all, it is the health of our patients that is directly at stake.

Of course, if it turns out that our current Western medical approach is perfect in its ability to provide patients with a space for healing, then we have nothing to worry about. In this next section, however, we point to two particularly deep flaws at the heart of the Western medical vision, flaws about which we should certainly worry and in light of which we should certainly take seriously the call to

re-examine and reorient some of our most fundamental medical ways of seeing.

Two flawed ways of seeing

In spite of its huge successes, the 'conventional' Western approach to medicine reveals crucial flaws that
can be traced back to two particularly faulty ways of
seeing – ways of seeing about which, it should be
stressed, a given doctor might not even be consciously
aware, but which, nonetheless, deeply impact both
the doctor's way of doing medicine and the possibilities left open for patient health and healing. There
are at least two deeply flawed conceptions underlying
the current state of Western medicine, and these are
first, seeing persons in terms of sharp mind/body
dualism and second, arguably related to this, seeing
medical care primarily in terms of fixing patients'
bodies. We turn to each of these two flawed conceptions in turn.

Ways of seeing persons: the limitation of stark mind/body dualism

Many authors stress that any attempt to envision
proper patient care is deeply hampered by the overly
sharp mind/body dualism at the heart of our current
Western medical paradigm[7,10]. Gordon and Fadiman[10], in their call for an 'integral medicine', note
that 'distinctions between body, mind and spirit are
peculiar to the last several hundred years of Western
thought and that all states of disease and health are at
once physical, mental and spiritual'. Hardcastle argues
that the medical tradition cannot hope to alleviate pain
if it continues to have wrong-headed ideas about
pain as essentially a 'subjective state of mind', itself
an outgrowth of the erroneous mind/body dualistic
presumptions at play in our current medical discourse[11].

Ways of seeing care: failing to make a genuine connection

Others worry that the Western tradition envisions
medical care primarily as 'fixing patients' bodies'. In
this picture, a doctor is very much like a plumber,
one fixes bodies, one fixes sinks. This picture of what
doctors do contrasts quite sharply from a picture in
which a key part of the doctor's job is to enter into a
moment of presence with the patient, in an attempt
to alleviate the patient's suffering. Since alleviating
suffering is more than just alleviating physical pain,
the job of the doctor in this approach involves more
than simply knowing the patient's physical symptomology and pathology. Here, 'fixing the body'
remains a crucial component of the doctor's job, but
it is contextualized as part of a more phenomenologically responsible engagement with a living
person experiencing a very personal moment of
suffering. In this spirit, a variety of authors focus on
the need for doctors to wrestle with the phenomenology of their patients' illness and suffering – to come to
reflect upon, be moved by and address the illness and
suffering as it is experienced in the individual human
life before them – if they are to be at all successful in
ministering care[12–16].

Identifying phenomenology as the perspective that
can locate illness 'within the larger context of the
human condition'[15], the suggestion is that a health-
care professional needs to reflect deeply upon 'the
experience of illness as it is lived through by the
patient' if, that is, 'his or her practice is to convey
more than simply an adequate technical comprehen-
sion of bodies and persons'[15].

Pellegrino and colleagues expand on this idea, adding that to heal is 'to make whole again', which entails
confronting and ameliorating the ways illness
wounds the humanity of the one who is ill[17]. They
call ultimately for a 'balance between competence and
compassion – interpreted here as the capacity to feel
something of the experience of illness with the
patient'[17].

Along similar lines, Bishop and Scudder, in their
study of nursing ethics, call for a 'caring presence', a
phenomenologically sensitive involvement with the
patient that allows for a moment of personal contact
and which tacitly works against any conception of
patients as mere bodies with pathologies[18].

We might also note that Cassell, who, stressing that
'the relief of suffering is the fundamental goal of medicine' (reference 15, p. 249) highlights the privacy,

uniqueness and complexity of every individual patient's individual suffering, and urges a re-examined sense of the nature and goals of physician care that must arise from such considerations (including a greater attention to patient wishes, an engagement with the human subject in place of an unbalanced focus on bodily illness alone, and a sustained commitment to enabling a patient's individual life-goal, as opposed to merely sustaining life).

To summarize, the above two categories of critique point not to problems in the details of our medical knowledge *per se*, but to problems that arguably lie deeper, in the foundation of our current medical practice, in our way of seeing persons, care and healing. These limitations can distort what we as a medical community take ourselves to be doing when we engage in the business of health and healing, and can limit patients' own capacity for genuine wellness.

Our consideration of two particular flaws at the heart of current medical practice, together with our above reflections on the intimate link between doctors' medical presumptions and patients' capacity to heal, should make clear why it is so important for doctors to re-examine their most fundamental medical ideas. As we have suggested, hopefully a study of CAM can afford us an opportunity for just this sort of reflection.

CONCLUSION

We have argued for the importance of re-evaluating our most basic medical conceptions of and orientations to health and healing, and we have additionally suggested how a study of CAM can be instrumental in helping us with this re-evaluative task. We end, then, with one brief concern about the term 'CAM' and, finally, with a closing insight from the tale, '*The Six Blind Men and the Elephant*'.

Worrying about the terms 'complementary' and 'alternative'

We end with a worry about terminology and, in particular, a worry about how one might be misled by the terms 'complementary' or 'alternative' medicine. The first thing to note is that any description of an area of medicine under either of these two terms tends to go along with a description of 'our own' (i.e. Western) tradition of medicine as the 'conventional' model. The second thing to note is that this way of carving things up can run the risk of making us feel as if our approach to medicine is the 'normal' or 'proper' or even 'main' approach, with other approaches being necessarily subordinate.

There are two worries here. First, philosophically speaking, even granting the successes within Western medicine, there are no grounds for asserting that our Western way of doing medicine is the 'right' one to the exclusion of other approaches; and second, practically speaking, the tendency to downplay the potential efficacy of other medical approaches (revealed in the terminology of 'complementary', 'alternative' and 'conventional') is a hazard to patient welfare as it (as we have seen) limits the space within which a patient is 'allowed' to heal. This worry then ought to alert us to the importance of remaining open to the possibility that, in these 'complementary' and 'alternative' medical ideas, we might find not only new information, tools and techniques to 'supplement' our own practice of medicine, but also ideas that can help us question and reorganize the foundations of how we practice medicine. We might, that is, find in CAM grounds for rethinking some of our most deep-seated conceptions of and orientations towards patient care and the art of healing. The point, then, is to be careful to ensure that the terminology of 'complementary' and 'alternative' never blinds us to this possibility.

Lessons from the six blind men

We end our discussion with the famous fable, '*The Six Blind Men and the Elephant*', a story which truly drives home the importance of always searching for new and better ways of seeing. In that tale, we are reminded that sometimes our 'way of seeing' the world is too limited, and that failing to recognize this involves a short-sightedness (or blindness) that can get us into trouble, making it difficult – if not impossible – to get things right. In the fable, each of six blind men in turn tell us what they think an elephant is, based on what the reader knows to be their limited engagement with the great beast. So, one blind man, passing his hands over the tusk of the elephant, concludes that an elephant is very much like a pointy spear. Another, groping at the thick leg of the animal, claims that an elephant is like a tree trunk. Yet another, feeling the tail of the creature, maintains, on the contrary, that an elephant is like a rope, and so on for each of the six investigators. None of them comes close to identifying what an elephant is, nor can any one of them hope to discover the truth of elephants by continuing to investigate only the circumscribed part of the elephant that they have set as their object of inquiry.

Reflecting on this story can hopefully help make us more sensitive to our own tendencies towards 'blind-ness'. When our own ways of seeing the world are too limited, and when we close our minds to new information and ideas that differ from our own, we run the risk of suffering the very same fate as each of our six blind men. When we are not careful about evaluating and re-evaluating our most basic ways of seeing the world, we minimize our chances of getting things right.

In the spirit of avoiding the fate of the six blind men, let us agree to use our own study of the CAM therapies in this book as a fruitful opportunity to check and re-examine our medical ways of seeing, our most basic and fundamental (and often tacit) conceptions of and orientations towards patients, care and healing. In this way, we can best ensure that, as a medical community, we provide a space for complete health and healing, responsibly ministering care towards the noble aim of enabling true wellness for each uniquely individual patient.

References

1. Kurriyama S. *The Expressiveness of the Body and the Divergence of Greek and Chinese Medicine.* New York, NY: Zone Books, 1999
2. Leuchter AF. [Study on placebo effects], cited in *Chicago Tribune*, Sunday April 14, 2002, Section 2, p. 6
3. Opler ME. The concept of supernatural power among the Chiricahua and Mescalero Apaches. *Am Anthropologist* 1935;37:65–70
4. Morris DB. Placebo, pain and belief: a biocultural model. In Harrington A, ed. *The Placebo Effect: An Interdisciplinary Exploration.* Cambridge, MA: Harvard University Press, 1997:187–207
5. Engel GL. 'Psychogenic' pain and the pain-prone patient. *Am J Med* 1959;26:899–918
6. Fordyce WE. Pain viewed as a learned behavior. In Bonica JJ, ed. *Advances in Neurology*, vol 4. New York: Raven Press, 1974:415–22
7. Weil A. *Spontaneous Healing: How to Discover and Enhance Your Body's Natural Ability to Maintain and Heal Itself.* New York, NY: Knopf, 1995
8. Benson H. *Timeless Healing: The Power and Biology of Belief.* New York, NY: Simon and Schuster/Fireside (reprint), 1997
9. Rudebeck CE. The doctor, the patient and the body. *Scand J Prim Health Care* 2000;18:4–8.
10. Gordon JS, Fadiman J. Toward an integral medicine. In Gordon JS, Jaffe DT, Bresler DE, eds. *Mind, Body and Health: Toward an Integral Medicine.* New York: Human Sciences Press, 1984:3–13
11. Hardcastle VG. *The Myth of Pain.* Cambridge, MA: MIT Press, 1999
12. Balint M. *The Doctor, His Patient, and the Illness.* London: Pitman Medical, 1964
13. Baron RJ. An introduction to medical phenomenology: I can't hear you while I'm listening. *Ann Intern Med* 1985;103:606–11
14. Cassell EJ. *The Nature of Suffering, and the Goals of Medicine.* New York, NY: Oxford University Press, 1991
15. Kestenbaum V. The experience of illness. In Kestenbaum V, ed. *The Humanity of the Ill.* Knoxville, TN: University of Tennessee Press, 1982:3–38
16. Zaner RM. *The Context of Self: A Phenomenological Inquiry Using Medicine as a Clue.* Athens, OH: Ohio University Press, 1981
17. Pellegrino ED, Thomasana DC. *A Philosophical Basis of Medical Practice: Toward a Philosophy and Ethic of the Healing Professions.* New York, NY: University of Oxford Press, 1981
18. Bishop AH, Scudder JR Jr. *Nursing Ethics: Therapeutic Caring Presence.* Boston, MA: Jones and Bartlett Publishers, 1996

Further reading

Foucault M. *The Birth of the Clinic: An Archaeology of Medical Perception.* New York, NY: Vintage Books, 1975

Foucault M. *The Care of the Self,* vol 3 of *The History of Sexuality.* New York, NY: Pantheon, 1986

Foucault M. The ethic of care for the self as a practice of freedom. In Brenauer J, Rasmussen D, eds. *The Final Foucault.* Cambridge, MA: MIT Press, 1988

Gastaldo D. Is health education good for you? Re-thinking health education through the concept of bio-power. In Peterson A, Bunton R, eds. *Foucault: Health and Medicine.* London: Routledge, 1997:113–33

Kuhn TS. *The Structure of Scientific Revolutions.* Chicago, IL: University of Chicago Press, 1962

Johnson TS. Contradictions in the cultural construction of pain in America. In Hill CS Jr, Fields WS, eds. *Advances in Pain Research and Therapy,* vol 11. New York, NY: Raven Press, 1989:27–37

Lupton D. Foucault and the medicalisation critique. In Peterson A, Bunton R, eds. *Foucault: Health and Medicine,* London: Routledge, 1997:94–112

Nettleton S. Governing the risky self: how to become healthy, wealthy and wise. In Peterson A, Bunton R, eds. *Foucault: Health and Medicine.* London: Routledge, 1997:207–22

Pellegrino ED. Being ill and being healed: some reflections on the grounding of medical morality. In Kestenbaum V, ed. *The Humanity of the Ill.* Knoxville, TN: University of Tennessee Press, 1982:157–66

Sacks O. To see and not see. *The New Yorker,* May 10, 1993:59–73

SECTION II

CAM therapies for common medical conditions

Prevention and treatment of cardiovascular disease using complementary and alternative medical therapies

19

M. J. Sorrentino

INTRODUCTION

Coronary artery disease is the number one killer of both men and women in the USA. Recognition of both traditional and emerging cardiovascular risk factors and effective treatment to modify these risk factors has the potential for marked reduction of cardiovascular events. The National Cholesterol Education Program Adult Treatment Panel III[1] recommends therapeutic lifestyle changes as an essential first step to reduce the risk for coronary artery disease. Complementary and alternative medical therapies can be incorporated into a lifestyle program to help further modify risk. Once heart disease has developed, therapies are needed to prevent the complications of the disease, such as a myocardial infarction and sudden cardiac death (secondary prevention). This chapter focuses on therapies to prevent the early development of atherosclerosis (antioxidants), prevention of a myocardial infarction by preventing thrombus formation (folic acid and B vitamins), and prevention of sudden cardiac death, especially in myocardial infarction survivors (omega−3 fatty acids).

THE DEVELOPMENT OF ATHEROSCLEROSIS

It has long been recognized that cholesterol levels are related to the development of coronary heart disease. The Multiple Risk Factor Intervention Trial[2] showed a clear relationship between cholesterol levels and death rate due to coronary artery disease. Pathological studies verified that cholesterol particles are involved in the formation of atherosclerotic plaque in the subendothelium of arteries. Primary prevention studies have focused on therapies to lower cholesterol levels, especially low-density lipoprotein (LDL) cholesterol, in an attempt to prevent the development of atherosclerosis.

The atherosclerotic process begins with damage to the endothelial cell layer of the coronary artery. There are many possible etiological agents responsible for endothelial damage including cigarette smoking, hypertension, diabetes mellitus and high LDL-cholesterol levels, and many emerging factors including markers of inflammation (high-sensitivity C-reactive protein (hsCRP)) and infectious agents, such as chlamydia (Table 1). Once endothelial damage has occurred, LDL-cholesterol particles are taken up by endothelial cells and transported to the subendothelial layer in an unregulated fashion. Macrophages in the subendothelial layer can then take up the LDL-cholesterol, forming foam cells. These cells release a number of cytokines, attracting further macrophages and T lymphocytes to the area, beginning the development of the atherosclerotic plaque. Macrophages take up LDL-cholesterol via the scavenger receptor, but this receptor recognizes only modified LDL particles. Oxidation is probably the most important LDL particle modification, and is thought to be a crucial step in the development of foam cells and plaque formation.

Oxidized LDL-cholesterol particles have many potentially deleterious effects on the coronary artery (Table 2). Oxidized LDL-cholesterol particles are recognized by the scavenger receptor on macrophages and form foam cells. Oxidized LDL is a chemoattractant for further macrophages and other inflammatory cells to accumulate in the growing plaque. Oxidized LDL can directly affect the coronary artery, leading to inappropriate vasoconstriction, which can be cytotoxic to endothelial cells. This further damages the artery, leading to further LDL-cholesterol accumulation. Oxidized LDL may also increase the thrombotic risk by increasing platelet aggregation and increasing the secretion of tissue factor.

Table 1 Known and emerging cardiovascular risk factors

Known risk factors
Increased total and low-density lipoprotein-cholesterol
Low high-density lipoprotein-cholesterol
Cigarette smoking
Hypertension
Diabetes mellitus
Age and male sex
Family history of premature heart disease
Left ventricular hypertrophy
Sedentary lifestyle

Emerging risk factors
Lipoprotein(a)
Homocysteine
C-reactive protein
Fibrinogen
Chlamydia infection
Oxidative stress
Postmenopausal estrogen deficiency

Table 2 Effects of oxidized low-density lipoprotein-cholesterol on coronary atherosclerotic plaque

Foam cell formation via the scavenger receptor
Cytotoxicity to endothelial cells
Monocyte and macrophage chemoattractant
Enhancement of monocyte binding to endothelial cells
Inhibition of macrophage migration
Endothelial dysfunction and inappropriate vasoconstriction
Increased platelet aggregation
Increased tissue factor secretion

Since oxidation of LDL particles appears to be a crucial early step in the development and the progression of atherosclerotic disease, there has been growing interest in antioxidant therapies as a primary and secondary preventive treatment of coronary artery disease. It is possible that antioxidants may prevent foam cell formation and be an effective early treatment to prevent plaque development. Once atherosclerosis is well established, antioxidants may lead to improvement in endothelial function and decrease the risk for thrombus formation.

VITAMIN E

Vitamin E is a fat-soluble antioxidant that has the potential to act as an effective treatment to prevent the oxidation of LDL-cholesterol particles. There has been increased interest in this vitamin since only small amounts are available in an average diet. A well-balanced diet can supply about 8–12 IU/day of vitamin E. Studies have typically used between 50 and 1000 IU of this vitamin as a therapeutic treatment.

Vitamin E is a fat-soluble vitamin contained in vegetable oils. After absorption through the gastrointestinal tract about 90% of the vitamin is transported in LDL-particles[3]. Therefore, the vitamin is present in the particles that it can potentially modify. Vitamin E has been shown to inhibit the oxidation of LDL particles *in vitro*. It is not known whether the same process occurs *in vivo* in the coronary artery.

Epidemiological studies have suggested that vitamin E may have a protective effect against the development of coronary disease. The Nurses' Health Study reported vitamin E use by over 80 000 nurses who completed a nutrition survey[4]. The lowest risk of coronary events was found in the group of nurses taking the largest amount of vitamin E daily. The Health Professionals' Follow-up Study found a similar reduction in coronary heart disease in over 39 000 male health professionals who took at least 100 IU/day of vitamin E[5].

There is very little completed primary prevention data available for vitamin E, although a number of large studies, including the Physicians Health Study

II, are ongoing. The α-tocopherol, β-carotene cancer prevention study was a Finnish study of over 27 000 male smokers designed to determine whether vitamin E (50 mg) or β-carotene (20 mg) would reduce the risk of lung cancer[6]. Vitamin E decreased the incidence of a first coronary event by 4% and fatal coronary disease by 8%, although these reductions did not achieve statistical significance. β-Carotene, another potential antioxidant, was found to have no benefit.

The Primary Prevention Project (PPP) was a trial designed to test whether treatment with aspirin and vitamin E reduces cardiac events in individuals 50 years of age or more with at least one major cardiovascular risk factor[7]. The study was stopped prematurely because of the emerging evidence for the benefit of aspirin. At the time of study termination, there was no documented benefit for cardiovascular endpoints with vitamin E, although the incidence of peripheral vascular disease was found to be lower in the vitamin E-treated individuals. The investigators of the study were concerned that the inadequate power of a prematurely stopped trial may obscure the findings for vitamin E. Ongoing primary prevention studies are investigating larger doses of vitamin E for longer periods of treatment to determine whether this antioxidant can prevent the early development of coronary disease and a first cardiac event.

Secondary prevention trials are designed to treat and prevent coronary events in individuals with known coronary heart disease. The Cambridge Heart Antioxidant Study (CHAOS) investigated 400–800 IU of vitamin E in over 2000 patients with angiographically documented coronary artery disease[8]. The primary endpoint (death and non-fatal myocardial infarction) was reduced 47% in the vitamin E group.

The positive results of the CHAOS study, however, have not been reproduced in larger more recently completed studies. The Heart Outcomes Prevention Evaluation (HOPE) study evaluated over 9000 men and women at high risk for cardiac events[9]. Patients received 400 IU of vitamin E from natural sources for a mean of 4.5 years. There was no decrease in the number of deaths, myocardial infarctions, strokes or hospitalizations in the vitamin E group.

The GISSI-Prevention trial randomized individuals with a recent myocardial infarction to vitamin E (300 mg of synthetic α-tocopherol)[10]. As with the HOPE trial, vitamin E had no effect on cardiovascular endpoints. The recently reported results of the Heart Protection Study, using a combination of vitamin E, β-carotene and vitamin C, likewise showed no antioxidant benefit[11].

Recommendations

Secondary prevention trials have failed to show a benefit with vitamin E supplementation. It is possible that, by the time atherosclerotic disease is well established, prevention of oxidation of LDL-cholesterol will have little impact on acute coronary events. Some subgroups of patients may still achieve some benefit from antioxidant therapy. There may be a decrease in peripheral vascular disease with vitamin E supplementation[7]. A small study of hemodialysis patients receiving 800 IU of vitamin E showed a reduction in the combined endpoint of myocardial infarction, stroke peripheral vascular disease and unstable angina[12]. Chronic hemodialysis patients have a high cardiovascular mortality that is thought to be caused, in part, by high oxidative stress. Further studies of high-risk subgroups, such as end-stage renal failure patients, are warranted.

Antioxidants have greater potential as an early preventive treatment, but we need to await the completion of the ongoing primary prevention studies for definitive proof of benefit. Since oxidation of LDL-cholesterol is an early step in the development of atherosclerosis, antioxidant therapy may have a role in inhibiting early plaque formation. The American Heart Association recommends a diet rich in fruits and vegetables that contain many natural vitamins and antioxidants. Supplementing the diet with nuts and vegetable oils can supply a higher intake of vitamin E. For example, a quarter cup of almonds, hazelnuts or pecans can add over 12 mg of vitamin E to the diet[13]. Individuals who cannot maintain a diet high in vitamin-containing foods can supplement with vitamin E (400 IU/day is a reasonable dose based on the epidemiological surveys).

THROMBUS FORMATION AND FOLIC ACID

Once atherosclerotic disease is present, acute events most often occur as a result of plaque rupture and thrombus formation. Medications such as aspirin that decrease clot production have been shown to reduce the risk of acute cardiovascular events. Folic acid, by lowering homocysteine levels, may decrease the risk of thrombus formation and reduce acute cardiovascular events.

Homocysteine is an amino acid produced by the metabolism of protein. Retrospective case–control studies first showed an association between elevated plasma homocysteine levels and cardiovascular disease. Malinow summarized 11 studies totaling more than 2000 patients and showed that homocysteine levels were higher in patients with coronary artery, cerebrovascular and peripheral vascular disease[14]. A meta-analysis of homocysteine studies indicated that homocysteine is an independent risk factor for vascular disease[15]. A prospective study of 587 patients with documented coronary artery disease showed a strong and graded relationship between homocysteine levels and total and coronary mortality[16]. This relationship was confirmed by the British United Provident Association Study, where men who died of coronary heart disease had higher homocysteine levels[17].

Administration of folic acid can reduce homocysteine levels by promoting the remethylation of homocysteine to methionine. To date there are no prospective clinical trials completed showing that folic acid supplementation can reduce coronary events. There is some emerging evidence, however, that the risk of thrombus formation may be reduced with folic acid therapy. A recent study found that the rate of restenosis of a coronary lesion following successful coronary angioplasty was found to be significantly decreased with a combination of folic acid, vitamin B_{12} and pyridoxine[18]. It is not known whether the folic acid helped to prevent thrombus formation in the recently treated artery or whether homocysteine can directly promote cell proliferation and restenosis.

Observational studies such as the Nurses' Health Study also suggested a preventive benefit of folic acid and vitamin B_6 supplementation[19]. The risk of coronary heart disease was found to be reduced among women with the highest intake of folic acid and vitamin B_6. Prospective randomized trials are needed to prove the protective effects of folic acid supplementation.

Recommendations

Both dietary and supplemental folic acid are effective in lowering homocysteine levels. For most individuals 400 μg/day should bring about a 5–6 μmol/l decrease in homocysteine levels[20]. Cereal-grain products are fortified with folic acid (140 μg per 100 g of cereal) to prevent congenital neural tube defects in newborns. Food sources of folic acid include spinach, asparagus and beans, which can supply over 100 μg per average serving.

FISH OILS AND PREVENTION OF SUDDEN CARDIAC DEATH

Once a myocardial infarction has occurred, patients are at increased risk for future ischemic events and sudden cardiac death. Sudden cardiac death can occur in a patient with known ischemic disease by the sudden onset of ventricular arrhythmias, such as ventricular tachycardia and ventricular fibrillation. Nearly half of myocardial infarct survivors may die suddenly. Prevention of sudden cardiac death has focused on the use of antiarrhythmic drugs and implantable cardiac defibrillators. There is a need for better therapies. There is increasing evidence that a diet rich in omega–3 fatty acids may help reduce cardiac mortality and sudden cardiac death.

Fish oils, both as a supplement and as a part of a Mediterranean diet, have been found to have multiple beneficial effects on the cardiovascular system (Table 3). Recently, there has been a renewed interest in the use of fish oils with the completion of well-designed studies indicating a clinical benefit.

The impact of fish oils on lipoproteins has been well documented. An average intake of 4 g/day of omega–3 fatty acids will reduce triglycerides

Table 3 Potential benefits of fish in the diet

Lipoprotein effects – reduction in triglycerides
Improved endothelial function
Decrease thrombosis by decreasing platelet aggregation
Lower blood pressure
Antiarrhythmic effect – prevention of ischemia-induced ventricular
   arrhythmias

between 25 and 34%[21]. Total LDL-cholesterol may increase slightly with increased omega−3 intake, but there is emerging evidence that LDL particles change from small, dense atherogenic particles to less dense, less dangerous particles as triglyceride values decrease to normal. Small, dense LDL particles are more likely to become oxidized and enter into the subendothelial space even if the LDL-cholesterol concentration is low. Strategies to reduce the prevalence of small, dense LDL particles may reduce the incidence of coronary events.

Fish oils may improve vascular endothelial function. In hyperlipidemic individuals, 3 months of fish oil supplementation was shown to improve the endothelial function of small arteries[22]. This benefit appeared to be independent of the lipoprotein effects of fish oils.

Fish oils will reduce platelet aggregation, prolong bleeding time and thereby reduce the risk of thrombus formation. Dietary effects of fish oils on platelet aggregation were found to be greater when combined with a diet low in saturated fat[23].

A diet rich in fish oils may lower blood pressure. A meta-analysis of 31 trials showed a small but significant reduction in blood pressure of about 3 mmHg with omega−3 fatty acid supplementation[24].

Finally, fish oils may have an antiarrhythmic effect in ischemic heart disease. Experimental studies have shown that the administration of omega−3 fatty acids could prevent malignant ventricular arrhythmias in an animal model of ischemic heart disease[25]. This benefit may be mediated through an effect of omega−3 fatty acids on sodium channels.

Clinical studies seem to support the experimental data. The Physicians' Health Study of over 20 000 United States male physicians showed that those individuals who had a diet high in fish consumption had a reduced risk of sudden cardiac death and total mortality[26]. This benefit became evident with one or more fish meals per week. The reduction in sudden cardiac death supports the possibility that fish oils may have an antiarrhythmic effect.

The GISSI prevention trial is the largest secondary prevention trial to evaluate the role of fish oil supplementation for the prevention of cardiac events[10]. Patients were randomized to a daily dose of fish oil capsules, in addition to a Mediterranean diet containing fish, as well as antioxidants from fruits and vegetables. The primary endpoint of death, non-fatal myocardial infarction and stroke was significantly reduced in the treated subjects.

The Mediterranean diet has also been investigated in the Lyon Diet Heart Study[27]. This trial was a randomized single-blind secondary prevention trial comparing a Mediterranean diet to a Western-style diet in individuals following their first myocardial infarction. The combined outcome of cardiac death and non-fatal myocardial infarction was significantly reduced in the individuals on the Mediterranean diet. This trial was not designed to determine which factor in the diet gave cardiac protection. The diet was high in omega−3 fatty acids, supporting a role for this supplement.

Recommendations

Omega−3 fish oils appear to have a substantial protective effect against cardiac complications, especially in individuals who have already suffered a myocardial infarction. Fish oils may have an antiarrhythmic action and decrease the incidence of sudden cardiac death in individuals prone to ischemia. As little as one fish meal per week may give benefit. The GISSI trial is the first major trial to indicate that fish oil capsules (at a reasonable dose of less than 1 g/day) may give the same benefit as fish in the diet. The Lyon Diet Heart Study suggests that a diet rich in omega−3 fatty acids and high in antioxidant vitamins from fruits and vegetables may give substantial benefit especially to myocardial infarction survivors.

There are many potential food sources of omega−3 fatty acids (Table 4)[28]. A Mediterranean diet rich in omega−3 fatty acids is the preferred therapy, because

Table 4 Food sources of omega–3 fatty acids

Food	Omega–3 (g/100 g)
Mackeral	2.5
Sardines	1.7
Salmon	1.2
Bass	0.8
Trout	0.5–1.0
Tuna	0.3

Table 5 Possible adverse effects of fish oil capsules. From reference 29

Gastrointestinal upset, fishy odor
Increased bleeding time and possible bleeding complications
Increased caloric intake/weight gain
Mild increase in low-density lipoprotein-cholesterol
Possible decrease in immune response
Possible contamination of certain fish oil products by pesticides
Vitamin A and D toxicity with some preparations

additional dietary elements, such as antioxidant vitamins, may give a further protective effect. Fish oil capsules at a dose of about 1 g/day may also be used. There are, however, some possible adverse effects of fish oil capsules that will need to be considered, including a decreased palatability compared to fish in the diet (Table 5)[29].

CONCLUSIONS

Cardiovascular disease is the number one killer of men and women in the USA. Treatment modalities need to focus on early prevention as well as the reduction in acute coronary events once clinical disease has become evident. A lifestyle program with a diet rich in antioxidants and omega–3 fatty acids can give early benefit and may help prevent sudden cardiac death in myocardial infarction survivors. This type of diet should be recommended to all individuals at increased risk for heart disease. In addition, the use of folic acid supplementation should be used in individuals who are at increased risk of thrombus formation. These modalities have the potential significantly to reduce the incidence of heart disease in individuals at increased risk.

References

1. Expert Panel on Detection, Evaluation, and Treatment of High Blood Cholesterol in Adults. Executive summary of the third report of the National Cholesterol Education Program (NCEP) expert panel on detection, evaluation, and treatment of high blood cholesterol in adults (Adult Treatment Panel III). *J Am Med Assoc* 2001;285:2486–97
2. Neaton JD, Wentworth D. Serum cholesterol, blood pressure, cigarette smoking, and death from coronary heart disease: overall findings and differences by age for 316,099 white men. Multiple Risk Factor Intervention Trial Research Group. *Arch Intern Med* 1992;152:56–64
3. Sorrentino M. Vitamin E and protection against coronary disease. *Alternative Med Alert* 1998;1:20–3
4. Stampfer MJ, Hennekens CH, Manson JE, Colditz GA, Rosner B, Willett WC. Vitamin E consumption and the risk of coronary disease in women. *N Engl J Med* 1993;328:1444–9
5. Rimm EB, Stampfer MJ, Ascherio A, Giovannucci E, Colditz GA, Willett WC. Vitamin E consumption and the risk of coronary heart disease in men. *N Engl J Med* 1993;328:1450–6
6. Virtamo J, Rapola JM, Ripatti S, *et al.* Effect of vitamin E and beta carotene on the incidence of primary nonfatal myocardial infarction and fatal coronary heart disease. *Arch Intern Med* 1998; 158:668–75
7. Collaborative Group of the Primary Prevention Project (PPP). Low-dose aspirin and vitamin E in people at cardiovascular risk: a randomised trial in general medicine. *Lancet* 2001;357:89–95
8. Stephens NG, Parsons A, Schofield PM, *et al.* Randomised controlled trial of vitamin E in patients with coronary disease: Cambridge Heart Antioxidant Study (CHAOS). *Lancet* 1996;347:781–6
9. The Heart Outcomes Prevention Evaluation Study Investigators. Vitamin E supplementation and cardiovascular events in high-risk patients. *N Engl J Med* 2000;342:154–60
10. GISSI-Prevenzione Investigators. Dietary supplementation with *n*−3 polyunsaturated fatty acids and vitamin E after myocardial infarction: results of the GISSI-Prevenzione trial. *Lancet* 1999;354:447–55
11. MRC/BHF Heart Protection Study Collaborative Group. MRC/BHF Heart Protection Study of cholesterol-lowering therapy and of antioxidant vitamin supplementation in a wide range of patients at increased risk of coronary heart disease death: early safety and efficacy experience. *Eur Heart J* 1999;20:725–41
12. Boaz M, Smetana S, Weinstein T, *et al.* Secondary prevention with antioxidants of cardiovascular disease in endstage renal disease (SPACE): randomised placebo-controlled trial. *Lancet* 2000;356:1213–18
13. Sorrentino M. Vitamin E for primary and secondary prevention of heart disease. *Alternative Med Alert* 2001;4:49–52

14. Malinow MR. Hyperhomocyst(e)inemia. A common and easily reversible risk factor for occlusive atherosclerosis. *Circulation* 1990;81:2004–6

15. Boushey CJ, Beresford SAA, Omenn GS, *et al*. A quantitative assessment of plasma homocysteine as a risk factor for vascular disease. *J Am Med Assoc* 1995;274:1049–57

16. Nygard O, Nordrehaug JE, Refsum H, *et al*. Plasma homocysteine levels and mortality in patients with coronary artery disease. *N Engl J Med* 1997;337:230–6

17. Wald NJ, Watt HC, Law MR, *et al*. Homocysteine and ischemic heart disease: results of a prospective study with implications regarding prevention. *Arch Intern Med* 1998;158:862–7

18. Schnyder G, Roffi M, Pin R, *et al*. Decreased rate of coronary restenosis after lowering of plasma homocysteine levels. *N Engl J Med* 2001;345:1593–600

19. Rimm EB, Willett WC, Hu FB, *et al*. Folate and vitamin B6 from diet and supplements in relation to risk of coronary heart disease among women. *J Am Med Assoc* 1998;279:359–64

20. Sorrentino MJ. Folic acid for the secondary prevention of heart disease. *Alternative Med Alert* 1999;2:49–52

21. Harris WS. *n*−3 fatty acids and serum lipoproteins: human studies. *Am J Clin Nutr* 1997;65(Suppl):1645S–54S

22. Goode GK, Garcia S, Heagerty AM. Dietary supplementation with marine fish oil improves *in vitro* small artery endothelial function in hypercholesterolemic patients: a double-blind placebo-controlled study. *Circulation* 1997;96:2802–7

23. Mori TA, Beilin LJ, Burke V, *et al*. Interactions between dietary fat, fish, and fish oils and their effects on platelet function in men at risk of cardiovascular disease. *Arterioscler Thromb Vasc Biol* 1997; 17:279–86

24. Morris MC, Sacks F, Rosner B. Does fish oil lower blood pressure? A meta-analysis of controlled trials. *Circulation* 1998;88:523–33

25. Kang JX, Leaf A. Antiarrhythmic effects of polyunsaturated fatty acids: recent studies. *Circulation* 1996;94:1774–80

26. Albert CM, Hennekens CH, O'Donnell CJ, *et al*. Fish consumption and the risk of sudden cardiac death. *J Am Med Assoc* 1998;279:23–8

27. De Lorgeril M, Salen P, Martin J-L, *et al*. Mediterranean diet, traditional risk factors, and the rate of cardiovascular complications after myocardial infarction: final report of the Lyon Diet Heart Study. *Circulation* 1999;99:779–85

28. Sorrentino M. Eating fish to prevent sudden death. *Alternative Med Alert* 2000;3:25–8

29. Stone NJ. Fish consumption, fish oil, lipids, and coronary heart disease. *Circulation* 1996;94:2337–40

Complementary and alternative medicine therapies in the management of lipid disorders: a review of current evidence

20

P. O. Szapary

INTRODUCTION

Hypercholesterolemia is an established risk factor for atherosclerotic cardiovascular disease (CVD)[1]. The bulk of observational and intervention studies have supported the validity of serum cholesterol as a surrogate marker for the development of atherosclerotic CVD[1]. The National Cholesterol Education Program (NCEP) has recognized the importance of serum cholesterol since 1988 and recently updated its recommendations for the evaluation and treatment of hypercholesterolemia[1,2]. According to the latest NCEP guidelines, an estimated 100 million Americans qualify for treatment of their hypercholesterolemia[1]. Of these, 65 million could be managed with diet and exercise alone, referred to as therapeutic lifestyle changes by the NCEP panel[1].

I propose that, in this group of patients, effective, safe and palatable complementary and alternative medicine (CAM) might be a useful adjunct to our armamentarium. In fact, the NCEP has already recognized the importance of diet and certain CAM therapies in the management of dyslipidemia by incorporating soluble fiber such as psyllium and plant-based stanol esters as part of therapeutic lifestyle changes[2]. The hope is that more research will shed light on which CAM therapies are safe and effective and could be incorporated into future cholesterol guidelines.

In this chapter, I comment on the state of the current evidence for commonly used CAM therapies in the management of dyslipidemia, focusing primarily on therapies aimed at reducing low-density lipoprotein (LDL)-cholesterol. However, the list of potentially useful CAM therapies is quite long and cannot adequately be covered. Table 1 lists many of these therapies organized by their primary effect and by the quality of the published literature.

THERAPIES AIMED AT LOW-DENSITY LIPOPROTEIN-CHOLESTEROL LOWERING

Of all the major lipoprotein fractions, LDL is the most important. Lowering LDL has consistently been associated with improved cardiovascular outcomes, making LDL one of the most potent surrogate markers of atherosclerotic CVD and the primary target of both lifestyle modification and pharmacotherapy[1]. When looking at the diverse world of what might be considered a CAM therapy, available therapies are divided into food-based therapies, also known as functional foods, and supplement-based therapies. While the definition of a functional food is the subject of some debate, for the purposes of this review, they are defined as those therapies which are primarily eaten as part of a diet. On the other hand, supplement-based CAM therapies are more like traditional drugs in that they are refined extracts ingested as pills, even though some come from foodstuff.

Table 1 Complementary and alternative therapies for hypercholesterolemia based on level of evidence. Adapted with permission from the Natural Standard Research Collaboration, 2002 Database of Herbs and Supplements, www.naturalstandard.com

	Grade A (solid scientific evidence)	Grade B (fair scientific evidence)	Grade C (insufficient scientific evidence)
LDL-cholesterol lowering	niacin plant sterols and stanols soluble fiber* red yeast rice policosanols soy protein flaxseed powder tocotrienols	inositol hexaniacinate garlic guggul extracts pantethine (vitamin B₅) artichoke extract	chromium turmeric extract hydroxymethylbutyrate
Triglyceride lowering	fish oils	flaxseed oil	L-carnitine
HDL-cholesterol raising	niacin	inositol hexaniacinate policosanols pantethine	guggul

LDL, low-density lipoprotein; HDL, high-density lipoprotein; Grade A, statistically significant evidence from ≥ 3 properly randomized trials or meta-analysis, with supporting evidence in basic science, animal studies, or theory; Grade B, statistically significant evidence from one properly randomized trial or > 1 cohort/case–control/non-randomized trial, with supporting evidence in basic science, animal studies, or theory; Grade C, unclear, conflicting, or lack of compelling scientific evidence; * soluble fiber includes psyllium, fenugreek, pectins, guar gum and hydroxypropylmethylcellulose

Food-based therapies

Plant sterols and stanols

Since the 1950s, it has been recognized that adding the phytosterol β-sitosterol to the diet of cholesterol-fed chickens and rabbits lowered their cholesterol levels[3]. Since then, more than 100 reports have been published in over 18 000 human subjects, describing the cholesterol-lowering efficacy of plant sterols and stanols[3]. In fact the NCEP now recommends including stanol esters as part of the second tier of therapeutic lifestyle changes[2]. The primary mode of action by which sterols and stanols reduce serum cholesterol is by decreasing cholesterol absorption from the small intestine[4]. Both these agents have a higher affinity than cholesterol for mixed bile salt micelles formed in the small bowel. By displacing cholesterol from these micelles, sterols and stanols decrease cholesterol absorption and, subsequently, serum cholesterol as well[4].

Phytosterols are found in trees (especially pine), soybeans, corn (maize), squash, vegetable oils and grains. Currently, the largest source of commercial sterols comes from 'tall oil', a by-product of the paper pulping industry. While initial studies used large doses of naturally occurring plant sterols, more recent studies have focused on lower doses of processed sterols called stanols and their esters. Both esterified sterols and stanols have been incorporated into fatty foods such as mayonnaise, margarine and salad dressing, and have been extensively tested and approved first in Europe and more recently in the USA.

These fortified spreads consistently lower LDL by 10–15% in patients with a wide range of cholesterol levels[5–7]. These spreads are palatable, have no side-effects and do not interact with many commonly prescribed drugs. There are a few reports of a small reduction in serum β-carotene during sustained use of stanol ester spreads[8], but most studies find that levels of all antioxidant vitamins are unchanged during treatment[7,9]. Phytosterols have also been used in conjunction with statins and appear to enhance their effect[10]. Phytosterols are available both in pill form and as food. In the USA, there are two available sterol spreads: Benecol® (McNeil Consumer Products, Fort Washington, PA) and TakeControl® (Unilever United States, Englewood, NJ). Substituting these high-calorie spreads into a low-fat diet can significantly reduce LDL by up to 15%. The problem is that incorporating the necessary two to three daily servings can lead to increased caloric intake, and thus, these spreads are not ideal for those hypercholesterolemic patients needing to lose weight. For those trying to avoid the calories, phytosterols also come in pill form and need to be taken three times daily with meals. In conclusion, the burden of evidence strongly suggests that plant sterols and stanols are modestly effective at reducing serum cholesterol and safe in a wide variety of patients, including those already treated with lipid-lowering agents.

Soluble fiber

Soluble fiber represents a broad class of foods and supplements, some of which have been shown as a class to reduce serum cholesterol by modest amounts. Dietary fiber is composed of both soluble (also known as viscous) and insoluble fiber. The viscous component of fiber is believed to interfere with dietary absorption of cholesterol and fat[11]. Other mechanisms of action of soluble fiber include enhanced gastric emptying, altered transit time, interference with bulk phase diffusion of fat and increasing the excretion of bile acids[11]. Soluble fiber is found primarily in fruits, vegetables and grains, as well as several dietary supplements such as psyllium, guar gum, fenugreek, flaxseed and pectins. Regardless of the type of soluble fiber, both randomized trials and meta-analyses suggest a mild hypocholesterolemic effect[12]. The majority of studies have been done with psyllium husk powder, which can be baked into food or mixed into beverages. One recent study found that adding 5.1 g psyllium powder (Metamucil®, Proctor & Gamble, Cincinnati, OH) twice daily for 26 weeks reduced LDL by 7% without affecting high-density lipoprotein (HDL)-cholesterol or triglycerides[13]. In that double-blind, randomized, placebo-controlled clinical trial (RCT) of 200 patients with mild hypercholesterolemia, there was no difference in the rate of gastrointestinal side-effects. More recently, an RCT aimed at comparing a high-fiber diet (8 g soluble fiber/day from various food types) to a low-fat diet found that, by incorporating four servings of soluble fiber a day, LDL could be only mildly reduced, by 2% ($p = 0.064$). While this had borderline statistical significance, the authors pointed out that, when applied to Framingham risk calculations of cardiovascular risk, the high-fiber diet could significantly reduce the 10-year risk of a cardiovascular event by 4% ($p = 0.003$ vs. low-fat diet)[14]. Aside from its small effect on lipids, fiber has also been shown to reduce postprandial glucose absorption in diabetics[15] and to produce slightly lower systolic blood pressure[16], factors that could also favorably impact on cardiovascular risk.

According to the NCEP guidelines, hypercholesterolemic patients should be counselled to eat 10–20 g of soluble fiber daily. This should first be accomplished by increasing dietary intake of fresh fruits and vegetables (five servings/day) and whole grains (6–11 servings/day). However, this amount of soluble fiber is very difficult to obtain in a typical Western diet. Some patients should therefore consider adding soluble fiber supplements to their diet. Psyllium powder at a dose of one serving twice daily before meals is the most efficient form of fiber therapy. The powder should be mixed in at least 8 oz (225 ml) of fluid, drunk quickly and followed by another 8 oz of liquid. This avoids the possibility of esophageal or gastric obstruction which has been associated with some forms of fiber therapy. I strongly suggest avoiding guar gum, since it is highly viscous and has been associated with multiple reports of intestinal obstruction[17,18]. All fiber supplements should be taken 1 h before or 2 h after taking prescription medications, to avoid problems with drug absorption. More research is needed to investigate whether certain types of soluble fiber such as fenugreek or flaxseed, which contain other phytonutrients, offer additional benefits over psyllium. In conclusion, soluble fiber at a dose of at least 4.5 g/day can produce small, but clinically significant, changes in LDL, and thus improve cardiovascular risk.

Phytoestrogens

Phytoestrogens, a diverse class of estrogenic compounds found in plants, bind to the estrogen receptor and act as partial agonists. In this capacity, phytoestrogens have been shown to reduce serum cholesterol as well as improving vascular function[19]. There are three major classes of phytoestrogens: isoflavones, lignans and coumestans. Only isoflavones from soy protein and lignans from flaxseed have been studied with regard to their lipid effects.

Soy protein Soy protein and particularly isoflavones have been extensively studied in modifying both lipids and other surrogate markers of atherosclerotic CVD. The most studied isoflavones are genistein and daidzein. Both in normal and in diseased animals and humans, concentrated soy protein has been shown to reduce serum LDL. An often-quoted meta-analysis pooled the results from 38 RCTs, and found that, on average, 47 g soy protein daily could reduce LDL-cholesterol by 12.9%, while not affecting triglycerides or HDL[20]. Interestingly, soy protein was effective only if the starting LDL-cholesterol level was > 160 mg/dl. Additionally, a recent RCT found that a soy protein shake (25 g soy protein) containing 62 mg of isoflavones administered once daily could decrease LDL more modestly by 6% in patients with starting LDL-cholesterol level of > 140 mg/dl[21]. This study confirmed that more realistic doses of soy protein had a lipid-lowering effect even in patients with modest LDL elevations. Interestingly, it appears that isolated isoflavones from soy or red clover given as supplements do not lower serum cholesterol, but do improve endothelial function and stabilize bone density[22,23]. The long-term safety of isoflavone ingestion is not known. Some worry about estrogenic stimulation, but epidemiological studies have suggested that Asian populations that consume large quantities of soy protein are protected against hormonally mediated cancers[24]. The Food and Drug Administration (FDA) has accepted the labeling claim that 25 g of soy protein as part of a diet low in saturated fat and cholesterol can reduce the risk of heart disease[25]. I suggest that hypercholesterolemic patients incorporate soy protein into their diet by substituting soy protein for animal protein. Practically, this means at least three servings per day of soy-based foods to reach the FDA target. This amount can also be accomplished with one serving of a soy protein-based powder mixed into a beverage. I would not, however, recommend isolated isoflavone supplements, as these have never been shown to reduce serum cholesterol.

Flaxseed Flaxseed (linseed) and flaxseed oil have emerged as popular functional foods for everything from cancer prevention to arthritis to heart disease. Flaxseed contains several lignans, and is the richest source of the main mammalian lignan precursor, secoisolariciresinol (SDG)[26]. In addition to lignans, flaxseed contains soluble fiber as well as α-linolenic acid (ALA), a cardioprotective omega-3 polyunsaturated fatty acid ($n-3$ PUFA)[27]. The bulk of the evidence from nine clinical trials suggests that flaxseed can modestly reduce total cholesterol and LDL-cholesterol by 5–15% without an effect on HDL-cholesterol or triglycerides[28]. One RCT found that 38 g of flaxseed powder baked into muffins or bread reduced LDL by 14% and lipoprotein(a) by 7% in 38 postmenopausal women[29]. It is not known whether the reduction in LDL can be attributed solely to the lignan component or to the combination of lignans and soluble fiber. There are no published studies on the lipid effects of isolated SDG supplements. The FDA allows inclusion of up to 12% (by weight) flaxseed in foods, but flaxseed and cold-pressed flaxseed oil have not attained GRAS (generally recognized as safe) status. Human studies using up to 50 g flaxseed/day for up to 1 month revealed no adverse effects and were well tolerated in one study, but the long-term effect of flaxseed consumption is not known[30]. Additionally, the small whole flaxseeds could theoretically precipitate a bout of diverticulitis and probably should be avoided in patients with known diverticular disease. Grinding the seeds should remove this theoretical risk, as well as increasing the bioavailability of both the lignans and ALA. Flaxseed powder at a dose of 2–4 tablespoons per day (25–35 g) can modestly reduce LDL, but much more research is needed to define the role of this potentially very useful nutraceutical.

Tree nuts

Data are now emerging that tree nuts may have lipid-lowering effects. The tree nuts almonds, walnuts, pecans, hazelnuts, pistachios and macadamias have all been shown in clinical trials to produce modest reduction of serum cholesterol. These nuts are a rich source of fiber, vitamin E and both mono- and polyunsaturated oils. Recently, an RCT compared a Mediterranean diet and a walnut-rich diet in which patients replaced their olive oil with 8–11 whole, shelled walnuts[31]. In the 55 patients, all with LDL between 130 and 250 mg/dl, the walnut diet reduced LDL by 6%, while men also had a 6% decrease in lipoprotein(a). The mechanism of action is unclear, but may be related to a replacement of saturated fat with monounsaturated fat. Before recommending tree nuts, clinicians should be aware of the high incidence of undiagnosed, life-threatening tree nut allergy[32]. Again, as with any energy-dense food, substitution and not addition is important, so as not to gain weight. This is especially important with nuts, as they tend to be eaten in large quantities.

Supplement-based therapies

Garlic

Garlic is the most popular botanical specifically taken in the USA for its purported cholesterol-lowering benefit. A recent meta-analysis by Stevinson and colleagues has confirmed a previous meta-analysis, which found a consistent benefit of garlic powder 300 mg orally three times daily over placebo in reducing total cholesterol by 8%[33]. However, a subset of six high-quality studies published up to 1998 found that the benefit was attenuated to 2–3% reduction in total cholesterol – which was *not* statistically significant[33]. Since then, two more RCTs have been published, both finding a negative result[34,35]. If these latest trials were to be figured into the analysis, the benefit of garlic powder on serum lipids would probably vanish. A systematic review by Ackermann and co-workers concurred with that of Stevinson and associates, stating that, while there seemed to be a modest LDL-lowering effect detectable at 1 and 3 months of use, there was no garlic-specific effect by 6 months[36]. There is still the question of whether garlic offers non-lipid benefits such as an antiplatelet, antioxidant, hypoglycemic or blood pressure-lowering effect[37]. Several studies have documented antiplatelet[38–40] and antioxidant[41–43] effects of garlic products. The antihypertensive effect of garlic pre-

parations is mixed and the data are inconclusive to date[36]. While there are no data with hard endpoints on garlic, one study did evaluate the effect of long-term consumption of garlic powder on carotid and femoral atherosclerosis as measured by ultrasound[44]. In that study, 280 adults were randomized to garlic powder 900 mg/day vs. placebo and treated for up to 4 years. Only 152 completed the full protocol and had carotid or femoral ultrasound scans that could be evaluated. Despite incomplete follow-up and lack of a standardized technique, subjects in the garlic group had evidence of plaque stabilization and some regression compared to placebo[44]. There was no mention of lipid changes in this large study, strongly suggesting the lack of a lipid-modulatory effect.

One reason for the recent number of disappointing trials with garlic may be the types of preparation used in the studies. There are many different types of garlic supplement, including dehydrated powder, garlic oil, garlic oil macerate and aged garlic extract. Additionally, the purported major bioactive constituent, allicin, is volatile. Thus, product standardization, processing and delivery are especially important when considering garlic.

As far as side-effects are concerned, garlic is well known to cause malodorous breath and dyspepsia. Another concern is the theoretical risk of bleeding from the antiplatelet effects. Bleeding has been seen in case reports but has not been reported in clinical trials of garlic supplements[45,46]. Another issue is the possibility of drug–supplement interaction. Notably, garlic powder has recently been shown to reduce saquinavir levels[47]. This clinically relevant interaction is important to know about, since patients with HIV-associated dyslipidemia frequently treat themselves with garlic supplements and thus may be reducing the efficacy of their antiretroviral regimens.

In conclusion, while it has been extensively studied, garlic supplements do not seem to provide a lasting and meaningful LDL-lowering effect. However, garlic may be more useful for its non-lipid effects, especially its antiplatelet and antioxidant properties. Its exact role in the contemporary management of cardiovascular risk is yet to be determined and awaits further study.

Red yeast rice

Red yeast rice (RYR) is the product of red yeast (*Monascus purpureus*) grown on rice. Red yeast is traditionally used as a food coloring, condiment or preservative in Asian cuisine. The use of RYR in China was first documented in the Tang Dynasty in AD 800[48]. A detailed description of its manufacture is found in the ancient Chinese pharmacopeia, Ben Cao Gang Mu-Dan Shi Bu Yi, published during the Ming Dynasty (1368–1644)[48]. In this text, RYR is proposed to be a mild aid for blood circulation and spleen and stomach health. RYR produces a family of natural substances called monacolins, which have hydroxymethylglutaryl coenzyme A (HMG-CoA) reductase inhibition properties similar to those of commonly prescribed statin drugs. In fact, monacolin K is structurally identical to the pharmaceutical compound known as mevalonin or lovastatin (Mevacor®, Merck & Co., Inc., Whitehouse Station, NJ). RYR can also be processed in a manner that enhances the monacolin content, yielding a red yeast rice extract (RYRE), which can be ingested in capsule form and used therapeutically to lower cholesterol. RYRE contains a full range of up to ten monacolins as well as some plant sterols and polyunsaturated fatty acids[48,49]. In the USA, a RYRE known as Cholestin™ (Pharmanex, Inc., Provo, UT) has been marketed as an over-the-counter dietary supplement to 'maintain healthy cholesterol levels'. However, there was a legal dispute between Pharmanex, the FDA and Merck as to whether Cholestin was a drug or a dietary supplement[50]. The most recent court (US District Court, Utah) ruling, in March 2001, was that RYRE or similar products containing lovastatin are unapproved drugs. As a result, Pharmanex removed their RYRE from the market.

Despite the legal controversy, RYRE have been shown to be a potent LDL-lowering agent. One American study[48] and several Chinese studies[51–53] documented the safety and efficacy of RYR and RYRE in healthy hyperlipidemic subjects. Heber and colleagues conducted a double-blind, placebo-controlled, randomized 12-week trial of 83 patients with hypercholesterolemia (LDL > 160 mg/dl)[48]. Subjects had not been previously treated, and were not on other lipid-lowering medications. Subjects consumed a diet similar to the American Heart Association Step 1 Diet and were randomized to either 2.4 g/day of RYRE, delivering 10 mg of total monacolins, or placebo. Compared to placebo, mean total cholesterol and LDL had significantly decreased by 20% at 8 and 12 weeks. Additionally, fasting triglycerides deceased by 11% compared to placebo, while there were no changes in HDL. These impressive reductions in LDL are similar to those obtained by low-dose statins (e.g. 10 mg simvastatin, 20 mg lovastatin). Unlike the statins, however, there are no long-term safety data on RYRE, and their effect on atherosclerotic CVD hard endpoints is unknown.

As far as safety goes, none of the small trials published reported abnormal liver function or muscle enzyme tests. In conclusion, while RYR and RYRE are effective as LDL-lowering agents, their lack of availability in the USA makes this supplement an impractical option for most patients. Using RYR truly as a food or condiment is unlikely to result in clinically meaningful reductions in serum cholesterol, but is probably safe.

Guggul extracts

Gugulipid is an extract of the resin from the mukul myrrh tree (*Commiphora mukul*). This thorny tree has little foliage and is indigenous to Western India. Upon injury, this 4-foot (1.2 m) tree exudes a resin called gum guggul or guggulu, with medicinal uses that date back to 600 BC[54]. The soluble portion of gum guggul is called gugulipid and is extracted using ethyl acetate. Gugulipid has been approved by regulatory bodies in India for the treatment of hypercholesterolemia since 1987. In the USA, gugulipid is available over the counter as a single herb, or more frequently, as part of a multi-herbal preparation marketed for 'maintaining healthy cholesterol levels'. The most active ingredients of gugulipid are the ketones E- and Z-guggulsterones. Like many other lipid-lowering dietary supplements, gugulipid appears to have multiple modes of action, although none are particularly well understood. Animal models indicate that gugulipid works by inhibiting lipogenic enzymes and HMG-CoA reductase in the liver[55]. It is also thought to stimulate lipolytic enzymes, enhance fecal excretion of sterols and act as a bile acid sequestrant[55]. Gugulipid has also been shown to stimulate thyroid function in rats[56]. More recently, scientists have discovered that E- and Z-guggulsterones are potent antagonist ligands for the farnesoid X receptor (FXR)[57]. This nuclear hormone receptor is important in the regulation of bile acid secretion from the liver. These authors found that hepatic, but not serum, cholesterol decreased in cholesterol-fed mice treated with guggulsterones. This latest study establishes a potential biological mechanism for the cholesterol-lowering effect of this natural product.

There are four published human clinical trials evaluating the hyperlipidemic effect of standardized gugulipid, all performed and published in India between 1985 and 1994[58–61]. Two of the four studies were placebo controlled and only one study directly compared gugulipid to another agent (clofibrate). The largest trial was a two-phase multicenter study which included 205 patients[60]. In the first phase of this study, patients were placed on a low-fat diet for 6 weeks before being treated with gugulipid 500 mg three times a day for 12 weeks and then being switched to a matching placebo for an additional 8 weeks. At study entry, this cohort had on average a total cholesterol level of 301 mg/dl and triglycerides of 231 mg/dl. While this was primarily a prevention trial, an unspecified number of patients with stable atherosclerotic CVD were also included. In this first phase of the study, it was noted that gugulipid significantly decreased total cholesterol by 22% and triglycerides by 25% compared to placebo. The most rigorous study to date randomized 60 hyperlipidemic subjects to receive either 50 mg guggulsterones twice a day or placebo for 24 weeks as adjuncts to a high-fiber diet[61]. The gugulipid-treated subjects had a net 22% reduction in LDL and a 23% reduction in fasting triglycerides compared to placebo-treated subjects. Additionally, the authors found an improvement in a marker of lipid oxidation and postprandial glucose measures in the gugulipid-treated group. Overall, gugulipid was well tolerated in clinical trials, with some reports of gastrointestinal distress.

Despite the generally positive results, two anecdotal reports have noted a paradoxical pro-lipidemic effect of gugulipid[62,63]. It is unclear whether this effect represents non-responders (up to 30% of treated patients) or individual variations. Additionally, there is one published report of drug interactions between gugulipid and both diltiazem and propranalol[64]. In this report, a single 1-g dose of gugulipid reduced the bioavailability of these two drugs by 35%. It is unclear at this point whether this pharmacokinetic interaction translates into reduced clinical efficacy. In conclusion, gugulipid appears to have a rational basis for use in modulating cholesterol metabolism. However, the studies performed to date have only been in Asian populations where it appears that up to 70% of patients had a favorable response. More research in Western populations is needed for further definition of the role of guggul extracts in clinical practice.

Policosanols

Policosanols are a group of compounds composed of predominantly five higher primary aliphatic alcohols – tetracosanol, hexacosanol, octacosanol, triacontanol and dotriacontanol[65]. These compounds are derived from sugar cane and beeswax and have been used extensively in South America and the Caribbean to reduce LDL. Most research on policosanols has been carried out in Cuba by one research group at the National Center for Scientific Research. This group has published their findings in over 20 clinical trials involving over 1000 subjects, demonstrating the safety and efficacy of sugar cane-derived policosanols. In fact, policosanols are part of standard pharmacopeias for hyperlipidemia in Cuba and other countries in South America.

While the evidence at the present time is not entirely conclusive, research suggests that policosanols may have multiple mechanisms of action involving suppression of endogenous cholesterol synthesis[65]. Studies suggest that policosanols inhibit cholesterol synthesis at the earliest steps of their biosynthetic pathway in the liver without affecting HMG-CoA reductase (the rate-limiting step in cholesterol biosynthesis)[66,67]. Other possible mechanisms of action include increased LDL uptake by the liver and increased LDL catabolism[65].

Over a dozen double-blind, placebo-controlled clinical trials have been published to date, documenting policosanols' efficacy, safety and tolerability in hyperlipidemic subjects. These clinical studies have included short- and long-term, placebo-controlled and comparative studies versus statins[68–70], fibrates[71] and acipimox[72]. In all of these published studies, policosanol intakes ranging from 2 to 20 mg/day demonstrated statistically and clinically significant improvements in total cholesterol, LDL, HDL and triglycerides[65]. Published studies on policosanols demonstrate that significant results can be obtained within the first 8–12 weeks of use. The results from the placebo-controlled studies produced an average 16% decrease in TC at 10 mg/day, and a 23% decrease in total cholesterol at 20 mg/day after 8-12 weeks. At a daily intake of 10 mg/day of policosanol, LDL-cholesterol levels typically drop by 20–25% within 3 months[65]. These consistent improvements in LDL have been documented in 'special populations' such as diabetics[73], the elderly[74] and patients with established atherosclerotic CVD[75]. When compared to statins, it appears that 10 mg policosanols is equipotent to 10 mg of simvastatin[69] and superior to 20 mg of lovastatin[68,76] and 10 mg of pravastatin[70] with regards to LDL-cholesterol lowering.

Finally, policosanols also appear to have antiplatelet effects which have been documented in animals[77], healthy volunteers[78] and hypercholesterolemic subjects[79]. This effect appears to be equivalent to that of low-dose aspirin, but works via a different mechanism[80]. In all clinical trials conducted so far, policosanols have been well tolerated. There are no reports of abnormal serum biochemical variables. Specifically, no abnormalities of liver or muscle marker enzymes have been reported. Adverse effect frequency was not significantly different between treatment and placebo groups, and the effects were mild and transient[81].

In conclusion, policosanols appear to be a very promising class of natural products, which seem to have potent LDL-lowering effects, similar to those of low-dose statin drugs. More research is needed to establish the long-term safety and efficacy of policosanols in Western populations, and to establish whether policosanols reduce clinical atherosclerotic CVD endpoints. If proved effective, policosanols would be a welcomed addition to our armamentarium of hyperlipidemic agents, especially in patients who cannot tolerate statin drugs. At the time of this writing, however, policosanols are not readily available in the USA.

THERAPIES AIMED AT THE HIGH-DENSITY LIPOPROTEIN–TRIGLYCERIDE AXIS

Although the NCEP has reiterated the primacy of LDL-cholesterol as a primary target of therapy, there is increasing recognition of the relative importance of other lipids in increasing cardiovascular morbidity and mortality[2]. Specifically, the NCEP has recommended that, once LDL has been appropriately addressed, clinicians should focus next on the metabolic syndrome. This is a cluster of metabolic abnormalities including elevated triglycerides, low HDL-cholesterol, elevated blood pressure, central obesity and impaired glucose handling. The NCEP recognized that patients with the metabolic syndrome are at increased risk for developing both diabetes and atherosclerotic CVD[2,82].

One central component of the metabolic syndrome is the disordered HDL–triglyceride axis characterized by a low HDL-cholesterol and elevated fasting triglycerides. There is emerging literature documenting the inverse relationship between atherosclerotic CVD and HDL-cholesterol[83]. Epidemiological studies suggest that for every 1% increase in HDL-cholesterol, the risk of atherosclerotic CVD is reduced by 2–3%[84]. Also, pharmacological therapies to raise HDL-cholesterol in patients with atherosclerotic CVD significantly reduced the incidence of subsequent cardiovascular-related events[85]. Similarly, moderate hypertriglyceridemia has been linked to adverse cardiovascular outcomes, especially in women, the elderly and patients with diabetes and established atherosclerotic CVD[86]. Thus, therapies aimed specifically at the HDL–triglyceride axis might be very important in reducing the risk of atherosclerotic CVD. With this in mind, cheap and well-tolerated CAM therapies that can raise HDL and/or reduce triglycerides might be useful in reducing the burden of atherosclerotic CVD.

Therapies for hypertriglyceridemia

Fish oils are the only CAM therapy to date that have consistently been shown to reduce triglycerides. Concentrated fish oils are a rich source of $n-3$ polyunsaturated fatty acids ($n-3$ PUFA), also known as omega-3 fatty acids. The two major $n-3$ PUFAs are eicosapentaenoic acid (EPA) and docosahexaenoic acid (DHA). Fish oils have been conclusively shown to reduce both fasting and postprandial triglyceride concentrations in a dose-dependent fashion[87]. In a comprehensive review of human studies, Harris concluded that about 4 g of omega-3 fatty acids/day from fish oil decreased serum triglyceride concentrations by 25–30% with accompanying increases in LDL of 5–10% and HDL of 1–3%[88]. The clinical relevance of the modest and inconsistent elevation of LDL is not known at this time[87]. In fact, a large clinical trial of 11 000 patients following myocardial infarction found that low-dose $n-3$ PUFA supplementation (875 mg/day) raised LDL by 2.5% but reduced cardiovascular mortality by 15%[89]. The mechanism of action by which fish oils reduce trigylcerides is believed to be mediated via a reduction in very low-density lipoprotein (VLDL)[87]. Fish oils are now commonly used in patients with severe hypertriglyceridemia (>600 mg/dl) in combination with either fibrates or niacin. Additional benefits of moderate doses of fish oils (approximately 3 g EPA plus DHA/day) that are relevant to patients with the metabolic syndrome include slight reductions in both systolic and diastolic blood pressures[90] as well as reductions in platelet aggregation[91]. Fish oils have also been shown to reduce *in vivo* measures of oxidant stress[92], improving measures of arterial compliance[87] and reducing the risk of cardiac arrthymias[93].

Effective lipid-altering doses of fish oils range from 3 to 5 g EPA plus DHA/day which can only be obtained consistently by supplementation. Because of variability in the concentration of $n-3$ PUFAs in commercially available products, clinicians and patients need to read the label carefully to ensure adequate intake of EPA and DHA. Currently available supplements in the USA contain between 30 and 60% of EPA plus DHA. Therefore, to improve patient adherence with therapy, 50% concentrated capsules (approximately 500 mg EPA plus DHA) should be ingested three times daily with a meal. After a few weeks of acclimation, the dose can be raised to two capsules (1000 mg EPA plus DHA) three times per day for a total of 3 g (six capsules). Side-effects of fish oil therapy can include burping and a fishy aftertaste. Patients taking omega-3 fatty acid supplements should do so only under a physician's care, since the FDA has noted that an intake in excess of 3 g/day could result in excessive bleeding in some individuals[94].

As mentioned above, flaxseed oil, which is rich in ALA, a precursor to EPA and DHA, has also been shown in some studies to lower triglycerides[88]. However, 4 tablespoons (60 ml) of flaxseed oil is needed to accomplish a 20% reduction in fasting triglycerides, making this an impractical and highly caloric solution. Therefore, flaxseed oil is not recommended for specific lowering of triglycerides.

In conclusion, fish oil supplementation is a useful tool in the management of significant hypertriglyceridemia. It can be used safely alone or in combination with traditional pharmacological agents. Its pleotropic effects on other cardiovascular risk factors make this natural product a very attractive option, especially in those patients with metabolic syndrome.

Therapies aimed at raising high-density lipoprotein-cholesterol

Very few CAM therapies seem to have significant HDL effects. Notably, soy protein and flaxseed, which both contain phytoestrogens, do not consistently raise HDL, unlike pure estrogenic agonists such as estradiol. Niacin, a B vitamin, has convincingly been shown to raise HDL at high doses and reduce cardiovascular endpoints. Because niacin is now fully integrated into mainstream clinical practice, I do not consider niacin a CAM therapy and thus do not discuss its use in this review. Some authors advocate the use of inositol hexaniacinate as a 'no flush' alternative to niacin[95,96]. However, there are only scant clinical data to support this, and thus, I do not recommend inositol hexaniacinate for cholesterol reduction at this time.

The only CAM therapies that seem to have some HDL-raising effects are gugulipid and policosanols. As mentioned above, there are scant data to support an HDL-raising effect of guggul extract by 16–36%[97,98], but this effect was seen predominantly in one study using a high dose of unstandardized guggul extract[98]. However, the data supporting the HDL-raising effects of policosanols are much more consistent. In general, policosanols appear to have a clinically important effect on HDL, raising average levels by 2–28%, depending on the study[65]. In the comprehensive review by Drs Berthold, policosanols raised HDL in three out of eight RCTs in general populations and five out of seven studies in special populations[65]. Across all placebo-controlled RCTs, policosanols appeared to raise HDL by 13%. In head-to-head comparisons with statins and fibrates, policosanols were more effective at raising HDL than low-dose statins, and they augmented the effect of the fibrate[65]. Of note, none of these studies were specifically designed to examine the HDL effect of policosanols, so the negative studies are likely to have been underpowered. More research is needed to investigate the HDL-modulating properties of policosanols in populations with low baseline HDL.

Several popular CAM therapies might negatively affect the HDL–triglyceride axis and thus might increase CVD risk. Specifically, there are some data suggesting that over-the-counter androgens such as androstendione, androstenediol and dehydroepiandrosterone may reduce HDL by 5–10%[99–101]. Therefore, caution might be warranted in using such products, especially in patients with HDL levels of < 40 mg/dl. Lastly, a recent report has suggested that the combination of high doses of the antioxidant vitamins (vitamins C and E and selenium) blunted the HDL-raising effect of niacin and simvastatin[102]. This raises for the first time the issue of a potentially negative effect of antioxidant vitamins on any cardiovas-cular risk factors. Clearly, more research is needed to verify these surprising findings.

CONCLUSIONS AND FUTURE DIRECTION

Dyslipidemia continues to be a potent modifiable surrogate marker for increased cardiovascular risk. Even modest improvements in serum cholesterol from a variety of drug and non-drug interventions have been associated with reduced cardiovascular mortality[103]. For every 10% reduction in total cholesterol, cardiac events drop by 15% and total mortality is decreased by 10%[103]. Thus, lifestyle interventions based on a prudent low saturated fat diet, increased physical activity and selected dietary supplements would be extremely useful, especially on a population basis. As far as CAM therapies are concerned, the best data are for plant-based sterols and stanols, and soluble fiber for reductions in LDL-cholesterol. Red yeast rice and policosanols are also potentially useful but need more study before they can be widely recommended. For hypertriglyceridemia, concentrated fish oils are useful adjuncts of therapy.

With the widespread availability and use of many dietary supplements, more research is urgently needed to help clarify which CAM therapies might potentially be safe and effective lipid-lowering agents. The hope is that these agents would then become integrated into common clinical practice like plant sterols and stanols[2]. A rational development plan would be to conduct small phase II human clinical trials on those therapies commonly used by the hypercholesterolemic population. For the majority of CAM therapies however, smaller *in vitro* and animal studies should be performed first, to gain better understanding of their mechanism of action. Those therapies with some mechanistic rationale for a therapeutic effect would then be tested first in uncontrolled pilot studies before moving onto controlled clinical trials.

References

1. Expert Panel on Detection EaToHBC. Third Report of the Expert Panel on Detection, Evaluation, and Treatment of High Blood Cholesterol in Adults (Adult Treatment Panel III) Full Report. NHLBI web site accessed 15 January 2002

2. Expert panel on detection eatohbcia. Executive summary of the third report of the National Cholesterol Education Program (NCEP) expert panel on detection, evaluation, and treatment of high blood cholesterol in adults (Adult Treatment Panel III). *J Am Med Asssoc* 2001;285:2486–97

3. Carter N, Grundy S. Lowering serum cholesterol with plant sterols and stanols, historical perspectives. *Postgrad Med* 1998;Special Report:6–14

4. Ikeda I, Sugano M. Inhibition of cholesterol absorption by plant sterols for mass intervention. *Curr Opin Lipidol* 1998;9:527–31

5. Hallikainen MA, Uusitupa MI. Effects of 2 low-fat stanol ester-containing margarines on serum cholesterol concentrations as part of a low-fat diet in hypercholesterolemic subjects. *Am J Clin Nutr* 1999;69:403–10

6. Miettinen TA, Puska P, Gylling H, Vanhanen H, Vartiainen E. Reduction of serum cholesterol with sitostanol-ester margarine in a mildly hypercholesterolemic population. *N Engl J Med* 1995;333:1308–12

7. Nguyen TT, Dale LC, Von Bergmann K, Croghan IT. Cholesterol-lowering effect of stanol ester in a US population of mildly hypercholesterolemic men and women: a randomized controlled trial. *Mayo Clin Proc* 1999;74:1198–206

8. Gylling H, Puska P, Vartiainen E, Miettinen TA. Retinol, vitamin D, carotenes and alpha-tocopherol in serum of a moderately hypercholesterolemic population consuming sitostanol ester margarine. *Atherosclerosis* 1999;145:279–85

9. Nestel P, Cehun M, Pomeroy S, Abbey M, Weldon G. Cholesterol-lowering effects of plant sterol esters and non-esterified stanols in margarine, butter and low-fat foods. *Eur J Clin Nutr* 2001;55:1084–90

10. Blair SN, Capuzzi DM, Gottlieb SO, Nguyen T, Morgan JM, Cater NB. Incremental reduction of serum total cholesterol and low-density lipoprotein cholesterol with the addition of plant stanol ester-containing spread to statin therapy. *Am J Cardiol* 2000;86:46–52

11. Kritchevsky D. Fiber effects of hyperlipidemia. In Cunnane SC, Thompson LUE, eds. *Flaxseed in Human Nutrition*. Toronto, CA: 1995:174–86

12. Brown L, Rosner B, Willett WW, Sacks FM. Cholesterol-lowering effects of dietary fiber: a meta-analysis. *Am J Clin Nutr* 1999;69:30–42

13. Anderson JW, Davidson MH, Blonde L, et al. Long-term cholesterol-lowering effects of psyllium as an adjunct to diet therapy in the treatment of hypercholesterolemia. *Am J Clin Nutr* 2000;71:1433–8

14. Jenkins DJ, Kendall CW, Vuksan V, et al. Soluble fiber intake at a dose approved by the US Food and Drug Administration for a claim of health benefits: serum lipid risk factors for cardiovascular disease assessed in a randomized controlled crossover trial. *Am J Clin Nutr* 2002;75:834–9

15. Rami B, Zidek T, Schober E. Influence of a beta-glucan-enriched bedtime snack on nocturnal blood glucose levels in diabetic children. *J Pediatr Gastroenterol Nutr* 2001;32:34–6

16. Burke V, Hodgson JM, Beilin LJ, Giangiulioi N, Rogers P, Puddey IB. Dietary protein and soluble fiber reduce ambulatory blood pressure in treated hypertensives. *Hypertension* 2001;38:821–6

17. Lewis JH. Esophageal and small bowel obstruction from guar gum-containing 'diet pills': analysis of 26 cases reported to the Food and Drug Administration. *Am J Gastroenterol* 1992;87:1424–8

18. Opper FH, Isaacs KL, Warshauer DM. Esophageal obstruction with a dietary fiber product designed for weight reduction. *J Clin Gastroenterol* 1990;12:667–9

19. Lichtenstein AH. Soy protein, isoflavones and cardiovascular disease risk. *J Nutr* 1998;128:1589–92

20. Anderson J, Johnstone B, Cook-Newell M. Meta-analysis of the effects of soy protein Intake on serum lipids. *N Engl J Med* 1995;333:276–82

21. Crouse JR3, Morgan T, Terry JG, Ellis J, Vitolins M, Burke GL. A randomized trial comparing the effect of casein with that of soy protein containing varying amounts of isoflavones on plasma concentrations of lipids and lipoproteins. *Arch Intern Med* 1999;159:2070–6

22. Howes JB, Sullivan D, Lai N, et al. The effects of dietary supplementation with isoflavones from red clover on the lipoprotein profiles of post menopausal women with mild to moderate hypercholesterolaemia. *Atherosclerosis* 2000;152:143–7

23. Potter SM, Baum JA, Teng H, Stillman RJ, Shay NF, Erdman JW Jr. Soy protein and isoflavones: their effects on blood lipids and bone density in postmenopausal women. *Am J Clin Nutr* 1998;68(6 Suppl):1375S–9S

24. Wu AH. Soy and risk of hormone-related and other cancers. *Adv Exp Med Biol* 2001;492:19–28

25. Dotzel MM. Food and Drug Administration. *Food Labeling: Health Claims; Soy Protein and Coronary Heart Disease*. Federal Register 64, 57699-57733. 10-26-1999. Electronic citation

26. Thompson LU, Robb P, Serraino M, Cheung F. Mammalian lignan production from various foods. *Nutr Cancer* 1991;16:43–52

27. Hasler CM, Kundrat S, Wool D. Functional foods and cardiovascular disease. *Curr Atheroscler Rep* 2000;2:467–75

28. Nelson GJ, Chamberlain JG. The effect of dietary alpha-linolenic acid on blood lipids and lipoproteins in humans. In Cunnane SC, Thompson LUE, eds. *Flaxseed in Human Nutrition*. Toronto, CA: AOCS Press, 1995:187–206

29. Arjmandi BH, Khan DA, Juma S, et al. Whole flaxseed consumption lowers serum LDL-cholesterol and lipoprotein(a) concentrations in postmenopausal women. *Nutr Res* 1998;18:1203–14

30. Cunnane SC, Hamadeh MJ, Liede AC, Thompson LU, Wolever TM, Jenkins DJ. Nutritional attributes of traditional flaxseed in healthy young adults. *Am J Clin Nutr* 1995;61:62–8

31. Zambon D, Sabate J, Munoz S, et al. Substituting walnuts for monounsaturated fat improves the serum lipid profile of hypercholesterolemic men and women. A randomized crossover trial. *Ann Intern Med* 2000;132:538–46

32. Bock SA, Munoz-Furlong A, Sampson HA. Fatalities due to anaphylactic reactions to foods. *J Allergy Clin Immunol* 2001;107:191–3

33. Stevinson C, Pittler MH, Ernst E. Garlic for treating hypercholesterolemia. A meta-analysis of randomized clinical trials. *Ann Intern Med* 2000;133:420–9

34. Superko HR, Krauss RM. Garlic powder, effect on plasma lipids, postprandial lipemia, low-density lipoprotein particle size, high-density lipoprotein subclass distribution and lipoprotein(a). *J Am Coll Cardiol* 2000;35:321–6

35. Gardner CD, Chatterjee LM, Carlson JJ. The effect of a garlic preparation on plasma lipid levels in moderately hypercholesterolemic adults. *Atherosclerosis* 2001;154:213–20

36. Ackermann RT, Mulrow CD, Ramirez G, Gardner CD, Morbidoni L, Lawrence VA. Garlic shows promise for improving some cardiovascular risk factors. *Arch Intern Med* 2001;161:813–24

37. Berthold HK, Sudhop T. Garlic preparations for prevention of atherosclerosis. *Curr Opin Lipidol* 1998;9:565–9

38. Steiner M, Li W. Aged garlic extract, a modulator of cardiovascular risk factors: a dose-finding study on the effects of age on platelet functions. *J Nutr* 2001;131:980S–4S

39. Ali M, Thomson M. Consumption of a garlic clove a day could be beneficial in preventing thrombosis. *Prostaglandins Leukot Essent Fatty Acids* 1995;53:211–12

40. Srivastava KC, Justesen U. Isolation and effects of some garlic components on platelet aggregation and metabolism of arachidonic acid in human blood platelets. *Wien Klin Wochenschr* 1989;101:293–9

41. Borek C. Antioxidant health effects of aged garlic extract. *J Nutr* 2001;131:1010S–15S

42. Dillon SA, Lowe GM, Billington D, Rahman K. Dietary supplementation with aged garlic extract reduces plasma and urine concentrations of 8-iso-prostaglandin F(2 alpha) in smoking and nonsmoking men and women. *J Nutr* 2002;132:168–71

43. Lau BH. Suppression of LDL oxidation by garlic. *J Nutr* 2001;131:985S–8S

44. Koscielny J, Klussendorf D, Latza R, et al. The antiatherosclerotic effect of *Allium sativum*. *Atherosclerosis* 1999;144:237–49

45. German K, Kumar U, Blackford HN. Garlic and the risk of TURP bleeding. *Br J Urol* 1995;76:518

46. Rose KD, Croissant PD, Parliament CF, Levin MB. Spontaneous spinal epidural hematoma with associated platelet dysfunction from excessive garlic ingestion: a case report. *Neurosurgery* 1990;26:880–2

47. Piscitelli SC, Burstein AH, Welden N, Gallicano KD, Falloon J. The effect of garlic supplements on the pharmacokinetics of saquinavir. *Clin Infect Dis* 2002;34:234–8

48. Heber D, Yip I, Ashley JM, Elashoff DA, Elashoff RM, Go VL. Cholesterol-lowering effects of a proprietary Chinese red-yeast-rice dietary supplement. *Am J Clin Nutr* 1999;69:231–6

49. Heber D, Lembertas A, Lu QY, Bowerman S, Go VL. An analysis of nine proprietary Chinese red yeast rice dietary supplements: implications of variability in chemical profile and contents. *J Altern Complement Med* 2001;7:133–9

50. Havel RJ. Dietary supplement or drug? The case of cholestin. *Am J Clin Nutr* 1999;69:175–6

51. Wang J, Lu Z, Chi J, et al. Multicenter clinical trial of the serum lipid-lowering effects of a *Monascus purpureus* (red yeast) rice preparation from traditional Chinese medicine. *Curr Ther Res* 1997;58:964–78

52. Shen Z, Yu P, Sun M, et al. [A prospective study on Zhitai capsule in the treatment of primary hyperlipidemia] (translation). *Nat Med J China* 1996;76:156–7

53. Wei J, Yang H, Zhang C, et al. A comparative study of xuezhikang and mevalotin in treatment of essential hyperlipidemia. *Chinese J New Drugs* 1997;6:265–8

54. Satyavati GV. Gum guggul (*Commiphora mukul*) – the success story of an ancient insight leading to a modern discovery. *Indian J Med Res* 1988;87:327–35

55. Sheela CG, Augusti KT. Antiperoxide effects of S-allyl cysteine sulphoxide isolated from *Allium sativum* Linn and gugulipid in cholesterol diet fed rats. *Indian J Exp Biol* 1995;33:337–41

56. Tripathi YB, Malhotra OP, Tripathi SN. Thyroid stimulating action of Z-guggulsterone obtained from *Commiphora mukul*. *Planta Med* 1984;1:78–80

57. Urizar NL, Liverman AB, Dodds DT, et al. A natural product that lowers cholesterol as an antagonist ligand for the FXR. *Science* 2002;269:1703–6

58. Agarwal RC, Singh SP, Saran RK, et al. Clinical trial of gugulipid – a new hypolipidemic agent of plant origin in primary hyperlipidemia. *Indian J Med Res* 1986;84:626–34

59. Gopal K, Saran RK, Nityanand S, et al. Clinical trial of ethyl acetate extract of gum gugulu (gugulipid) in primary hyperlipidemia. *J Assoc Physicians India* 1986;34:249–51

60. Nityanand S, Kapoor NK. Hypocholesterolemic effect of *Commiphora mukul* resin (guggal). *Indian J Exp Biol* 1971;9:376–7

61. Singh RB, Niaz MA, Ghosh S. Hypolipidemic and antioxidant effects of *Commiphora mukul* as an adjunct to dietary therapy in patients with hypercholesterolemia. *Cardiovasc Drugs Ther* 1994;8:659–64

62. Das Gupta R. A new hypolipidaemic agent (gugulipid). *J Assoc Physicians India* 1990;38:186

63. Das Gupta RD. Gugulipid: pro-lipaemic effect. *J Assoc Physicians India* 1990;38:598

64. Dalvi SS, Nayak VK, Pohujani SM, Desai NK, Kshirsagar NA, Gupta KC. Effect of gugulipid on bioavailability of diltiazem and propranolol. *J Assoc Physicians India* 1994;42:454–455

65. Gouni-Berthold I, Berthold HK. Policosanol: clinical pharmacology and therapeutic significance of a new lipid-lowering agent. *Am Heart J* 2002;143:356–65

66. Menendez R, Fernandez SI, Del Rio A, et al. Policosanol inhibits cholesterol biosynthesis and enhances low density lipoprotein processing in cultured human fibroblasts. *Biol Res* 1994;27:199–203

67. Menendez R, Amor AM, Gonzalez RM, Fraga V, Mas R. Effect of policosanol on the hepatic cholesterol biosynthesis of normocholesterolemic rats. *Biol Res* 1996;29:253–7

68. Crespo N, Illnait J, Mas R, Fernandez L, Fernandez J, Castano G. Comparative study of the efficacy and tolerability of policosanol and lovastatin in patients with hypercholesterolemia and non-insulin dependent diabetes mellitus. *Int J Clin Pharmacol Res* 1999;19:117–27

69. Ortensi G, Gladstein J, Valli H, Tesone PA. A comparative study of policosanol versus simvastatin in elderly patients with hypercholesterolemia. *Curr Ther Res* 1997;58:390–401

70. Benitez M, Romero C, Mas R, Fernandez L, Fernandez JC. A comparative study of policosanol versus pravastatin in patients with type II hypercholesterolemia. *Curr Ther Res* 1997;58:859–67

71. Marcello S, Gladstein J, Tesone P, Mas R. Effects of bezafibrate plus policosanol or placebo in patients with combined dyslipidemia: a pilot study. *Curr Ther Res* 2000;61:346–57

72. Alcocer L, Fernandez L, Campos E, Mas R. A comparative study of policosanol versus acipimox in patients with type II hypercholesterolemia. *Int J Tiss React* 1999;21:85–92

73. Torres O, Agramonte AJ, Illnait J, Mas FR, Fernandez L, Fernandez JC. Treatment of hypercholesterolemia in NIDDM with policosanol. *Diabetes Care* 1995;18:393–7

74. Castano G, Mas R, Fernandez JC, Illnait J, Fernandez L, Alvarez E. Effects of policosanol in older patients with type II hypercholesterolemia and high coronary risk. *J Gerontol Series A, Biol Sci Med Sci* 2001;56:M186–92

75. Batista J, Stusser R, Saez F, Perez B. Effect of policosanol on hyperlipidemia and coronary heart disease in middle-aged patients. A 14-month pilot study. *Int J Clin Pharm Ther* 1996;34:134–7

76. Castano G, Mas R, Fernandez JC, Fernandez L, Alvarez E, Lezcay M. Efficacy and tolerability of policosanol compared with lovastatin in patients with type II hypercholesterolemia and concomitant coronary risk factors. *Curr Ther Res* 2000;61:137–46

77. Arruzazabala ML, Carbajal D, Mas R, Garcia M, Fraga V. Effects of policosanol on platelet aggregation in rats. *Thromb Res* 1993;69:321–7

78. Valdes S, Arruzazabala ML, Fernandez L, *et al*. Effect of policosanol on platelet aggregation in healthy volunteers. *Int J Clin Pharmacol Res* 1996;16:67–72

79. Arruzazabala ML, Mas R, Molina V, *et al*. Effect of policosanol on platelet aggregation in type II hypercholesterolemic patients. *Int J Tiss React* 1998;20:119–24

80. Arruzazabala ML, Valdes S, Mas R, Carbajal D, Fernandez L. Comparative study of policosanol, aspirin and the combination therapy policosanol–aspirin on platelet aggregation in healthy volunteers. *Pharmacol Res* 1997;36:293–7

81. Pons P, Rodriguez M, Robaina C, *et al*. Effects of successive dose increases of policosanol on the lipid profile of patients with type II hypercholesterolaemia and tolerability to treatment. *Int J Clin Pharmacol Res* 1994;14:27–33

82. Smiley T, Oh P, Shane LG. The relationship of insulin resistance measured by reliable indexes to coronary artery disease risk factors and outcomes – a systematic review. *Can J Cardiol* 2001;17:797–805

83. Assmann G, Schulte H, von Eckardstein A, Huang Y. High-density lipoprotein cholesterol as a predictor of coronary heart disease risk. The PROCAM experience and pathophysiological implications for reverse cholesterol transport. *Atherosclerosis* 1996;124(Suppl):S11–20

84. Boden WE. High-density lipoprotein cholesterol as an independent risk factor in cardiovascular disease: assessing the data from Framingham to the Veterans Affairs High-Density Lipoprotein Intervention Trial. *Am J Cardiol* 2000;86:19L–22L

85. Rubins HB, Robins SJ, Collins D, *et al*. Gemfibrozil for the secondary prevention of coronary heart disease in men with low levels of high-density lipoprotein cholesterol. Veterans Affairs High-Density Lipoprotein Cholesterol Intervention Trial Study Group. *N Engl J Med* 1999;341:410–18

86. Szapary PO, Rader DJ. Pharmacological management of high triglycerides and low high-density lipoprotein cholesterol. *Curr Opin Pharmacol* 2001;1:113–20

87. Nestel PJ. Fish oil and cardiovascular disease: lipids and arterial function. *Am J Clin Nutr* 2000;71(1 Suppl):228S–31S

88. Harris WS. $n-3$ fatty acids and serum lipoproteins: human studies. *Am J Clin Nutr* 1997;65(5 Suppl):1645S–54S

89. Anon. Dietary supplementation with $n-3$ polyunsaturated fatty acids and vitamin E after myocardial infarction: results of the GISSI-Prevenzione trial. Gruppo Italiano per lo Studio della Sopravvivenza nell'Infarto miocardico. *Lancet* 1999;354:447–55

90. Appel LJ, Miller ER III, Seidler AJ, Whelton PK. Does supplementation of diet with 'fish oil' reduce blood pressure? A meta-analysis of controlled clinical trials. *Arch Intern Med* 1993;153:1429–38

91. Mori TA, Beilin LJ, Burke V, Morris J, Ritchie J. Interactions between dietary fat, fish, and fish oils and their effects on platelet function in men at risk of cardiovascular disease. *Arterioscler Thromb Vasc Biol* 1997;17:279–86

92. Mori TA, Dunstan DW, Burke V, *et al*. Effect of dietary fish and exercise training on urinary F2-isoprostane excretion in non-insulin-dependent diabetic patients. *Metabolism* 1999;48:1402–8

93. O'Keefe JH Jr, Harris WS. From Inuit to implementation: omega–3 fatty acids come of age. *Mayo Clin Proc* 2000;75:607–14

94. Lewis C. Letter regarding dietary supplement health claim for omega–3 fatty acids and coronary heart disease. 91N-0103, 1-34. 10-31-2000. Rockville, MD: Office of Nutritional Products, Labeling and Dietary Supplements; Center for Food Safety and Applied Nutrition, Food and Drug Administration, 2000

95. Head KA. Inositol hexaniacinate: a safer alternative to niacin. *Altern Med Rev* 1996;1:176–84

96. Anon. Inositol hexaniacinate. *Altern Med Rev* 1998;3:222–3

97. Nityanand S, Srivastava JS, Asthana OP. Clinical trials with gugulipid. A new hypolipidaemic agent. *J Assoc Physicians India* 1989;37:323–8

98. Verma SK, Bordia A. Effect of *Commiphora mukul* (gum guggulu) in patients of hyperlipidemia with special reference to HDL-cholesterol. *Indian J Med Res* 1988;87:356–60

99. Brown GA, Vukovich MD, Martini ER, *et al*. Endocrine responses to chronic androstenedione intake in 30- to 56-year-old men. *J Clin Endocrinol Metab* 2000;85:4074–80

100. Brown GA, Vukovich MD, Martini ER, *et al*. Endocrine and lipid responses to chronic androstenediol–herbal supplementation in 30 to 58 year old men. *J Am Coll Nutr* 2001;20:520–8

101. Barnhart KT, Freeman E, Grisso JA, *et al*. The effect of dehydroepiandrosterone supplementation to symptomatic perimenopausal women on serum endocrine profiles, lipid parameters, and health-related quality of life. *J Clin Endocrinol Metab* 1999;84:3896–902

102. Cheung MC, Zhao XQ, Chait A, Albers JJ, Brown BG. Antioxidant supplements block the response of HDL to simvastatin–niacin therapy in patients with coronary artery disease and low HDL. *Arterioscler Thromb Vasc Biol* 2001;21:1320–6

103. Gould AL, Rossouw JE, Santanello NC, Heyse JF, Furberg CD. Cholesterol reduction yields clinical benefit: impact of statin trials. *Circulation* 1998;97:946–52

Alternative treatment of insomnia

21

A. S. Attele and C.-S. Yuan

INTRODUCTION

Humans sleep approximately one-third of their lives. Scientists do not fully understand why sleep is needed, and the mechanisms for physical and mental restoration. Sleep disruption creates fatigue and suboptimal performances, causing significant medical, psychological and social disturbances[1,2].

Insomnia (Latin: *in* means 'not', *somnus* means 'sleep') is a widespread health complaint, and the most common of all sleep disorders[3]. In the USA the cost of insomnia, including treatment, lost productivity and insomnia-related accidents, may exceed $100 billion per year[4,5].

Insomnia is or can be defined as the subjective complaint of impairment in the duration, depth, or restful quality of sleep. It is characterized by one or more of the following problems: difficulty falling asleep, difficulty maintaining sleep, early morning wakening and unrefreshing sleep[6]. Approximately 35% of the adult population has insomnia during the course of a year. Up to 17% indicate that the insomnia is chronic, severe, or both[7–9]. In contrast to the occasional sleepless night experienced by most people, insomnia may be a persistent or recurrent problem with serious complications such as anxiety and depression[7,10,11].

SLEEP PHYSIOLOGY

Natural sleep patterns show considerable individual variability. Most adults are comfortable with 6.5–8 h of sleep daily, taken in a single period[12].

Normal sleep consists of four to six behaviorally and electroencephalographically (EEG) defined cycles of two distinct types: non-rapid-eye-movement (NREM) sleep; and rapid-eye-movement (REM) sleep. According to Rechtshaffen and Kales[13], sleep is staged by determining the predominant pattern in 30-s 'epochs' of EEG, muscle and eye movement activity.

Stage 1 NREM sleep represents very light sleep, from which one can easily be aroused. The predominant EEG pattern is a low-voltage, mixed-frequency activity. The majority of a typical night's sleep is spent in stage 2. Stage 2 NREM sleep is defined by the appearance of steep spindles or K-complexes on the EEG. Stages 3 and 4 of NREM sleep are often referred to collectively as delta sleep or slow-wave sleep.

REM sleep consists of relatively low-voltage, mixed-frequency EEG activity, somewhat similar to stage 1 or wakefulness, with the appearance of episodic REMs. One of the prime characteristics of REM sleep is a low level of muscle tone[13].

ETIOLOGY AND CLASSIFICATION

Insomnia is classified as primary or secondary, as well as acute or chronic. It occurs more frequently with aging and in women.

Primary insomnia is sleeplessness that is not attributable to a medical, psychiatric or environmental cause. The etiology of primary insomnia relates in part to psychological conditioning processes. Secondary insomnia is a symptom caused by medical, psychiatric or environmental factors[14]. In secondary insomnia the target of treatment is the underlying disorder.

Acute insomnia is often caused by emotional or physical discomfort, such as stressful life events, or medical problems of recent onset. Various substances (caffeine, nicotine, alcohol, steroids, etc.) can impair both falling asleep and staying asleep[15]. Chronic insomnia can have multiple and varying causes[6]. This may pose a significant therapeutic challenge.

ALTERNATIVE THERAPIES

Over-the-counter sleep aids are becoming popular as an alternative to prescription hypnotics. Surveys of young adults indicate that approximately 10% used non-prescription medications in the past year to improve sleep[9]. Patients report self-medicating with herbs, hormones and amino acids in an effort to improve sleep and avoid the unacceptable side-effects of prescription medications. The most commonly used botanical sleep aids are valerian and hops; physiological substances include melatonin and L-tryptophan. In addition, acupuncture and 'low-energy emission therapy' may be effective.

Medicinal herbs

Valerian (Valeriana officinalis)

In 1996, valerian was one of the 25 best-selling herbs in the USA[16]. The use of the rhizome and roots of *Valeriana officinalis* as an anxiolytic and sleep aid dates back 1000 years[17]. The US Food and Drug Administration (FDA) rates valerian as a GRAS (generally recognized as safe) herb. It is listed in the European Pharmacopea, and is widely used as a hypnotic and daytime sedative[19].

Valerian contains valepotriates, valerenic acid and unidentified aqueous constituents that contribute to its sedative properties[19]. Valepotriates, a 0.5–2% mixture of unstable irridoid compounds, have been identified in valerian. The rhizome and root also contain 0.3–0.7% of a potent-smelling volatile oil containing bornyl acetate and the sesquiterpene derivatives of valerenic acid[20]. The proportion of these constituents can vary greatly between and within species[21]. The primary active ingredient of valerian has not been identified.

Valerian has been shown to have sleep-inducing, anxiolytic and tranquilizing effects in *in vivo* animal studies and clinical trials. An earlier placebo-controlled, cross-over trial of 128 volunteers reported that 400 mg of valerian extract at bedtime led to improved sleep quality and decreased sleep latency, and reduced the number of night awakenings[22]. Two other clinical studies using 400–900 mg of valerian before sleep also improved insomnia[23,24]. In a double-blind, cross-over, placebo-controlled trial, subjective sleep latency and waking time after sleep onset were reduced by more than half after a 900-mg dose, with a smaller effect after 450 mg[25]. One EEG study reported that 135 mg of aqueous, dried extract of valerian, taken three times daily, improved delta sleep and decreased stage-1 sleep[26]. A recent randomized, double-blind, placebo-controlled, cross-over study assessed the subjective and objective effects of sleep efficiency in a 14-day treatment with valerian[27]. Although sleep efficiency increased with both valerian and placebo, valerian showed significant improvement over placebo on parameters for slow-wave sleep. In general, clinical studies with valerian extracts show that the mild hypnotic effects of valerian decrease sleep latency and improve sleep quality.

Valerian extracts cause both central nervous system (CNS) depression and muscle relaxation[28]. Sedation may result from an interaction of valerian constituents with central type A γ-aminobutryric acid (GABA) receptors[29]. Valerenic acid has been shown to inhibit enzyme-induced breakdown of GABA in the brain, resulting in sedation[30]. Aqueous extracts of the root contain appreciable amounts of GABA, which could directly cause sedation, but there is uncertainty about its availability[31]. Although valerian is effective in producing depression of the CNS, neither valepotriates nor valerenic acid has activity alone. It is possible that a combination of volatile oil, valepotriates and other constituents are involved. It is generally recommended to take one or two tablets or capsules (200–1000 mg *V. officinalis* root) 30–60 min before bedtime[19].

While valerian has been shown to be generally safe, there are concerns about its quality and efficacy[30]. Reports on the cytotoxicity of valepotriates warrant further investigation of the possible carcinogenicity of epoxide groups that act as alkylating agents[32]. Patients using large doses over several years can experience serious withdrawal symptoms following abrupt discontinuation[33]. Valerian is generally recommended for the treatment of patients with mild psychophysiological insomnia.

Ginseng

The ginseng root has been used for over 2000 years for its health-promoting properties[34]. In recent years, it has consistently been one of the ten top-selling herbs in the USA[35]. Results of several studies indicate that the effect of ginseng may be, at least in part, related to maintaining normal sleep and wakefulness. Of the several species of ginseng, *Panax ginseng* (Asian ginseng), *Panax quinquefolius* (American ginseng) and *Panax vietnamensis* (Vietnamese ginseng) are reported to have sleep-modulating effects.

Constituents of most ginseng species include ginsenosides, polysaccharides, peptides, polyacetyleinic alcohols and fatty acids[36]. *Panax vietnamensis* contains ocotillol-type saponins, the major one being majonoside-R2 (MR2). Most pharmacological actions of ginseng are attributed to ginsenosides[37]. Except for ginsenoside Ro, the more than 20 ginsenosides that have been isolated belong to a family of steroids named steroidal saponins[38]. There is a wide variation (2–20%) in ginsenoside content of different ginseng species[37]. Furthermore, within a single species cultivated in two different locations, pharmacological differences have been reported[39].

Ginseng has an inhibitory effect on the CNS and may modulate neurotransmission. A mixture of the ginsenosides Rb_1, Rb_2 and Rc from *Panax ginseng* extracts prolonged the duration of hexobarbital-induced 'sleep' in mice[40]. Rhee and colleagues reported that *Panax ginseng* extract decreased the amount of wakefulness during a 12-h light period and increased the amount of slow-wave sleep[41]. Ginseng is known as an 'adaptogen', capable of normalizing physiological disturbances. For example, Lee and associates reported that *Panax ginseng* extract normalized the disturbances caused by food deprivation in sleep–waking states in rats[42]. MR2, a major ocotillol-type saponin,

isolated exclusively from *Panax vietnamensis*, restored the hypnotic activity of pentobarbital that was decreased by two models of psychological stress[43,44]. A recent double-blind study investigating the influence of ginseng on the quality of life of city dwellers revealed that a daily dose of 40 mg of ginseng extract for 12 weeks significantly improved the quality of life, including sleep[45].

There is evidence to suggest that one mechanism for the CNS-depressant action of ginseng extract and ginsenosides is via regulation of GABA-ergic neurotransmission. Ginsenosides have been reported to compete with agonists for binding to $GABA_A$ and $GABA_B$ receptors[46]. Neuronal discharge frequency in the nucleus tractus solitarius was inhibited by *Panax quinquefolius* extract[39] and $GABA_A$ receptor agonist muscimol[47]. The reversal effect of MR2 and diazepam on the psychological stress-induced decrease in pentobarbital sleep was antagonized by flumazenil, a selective benzodiazepine antagonist[44].

There are few reports of severe side-effects of ginseng, despite the fact that over 6 million ingest it regularly in the USA[48]. The most common reported side-effects are nervousness and excitation, but these diminish with continued use or dosage reduction[48]. On the basis of its long-term usage and the relative infrequency of reported significant side-effects, it is safe to conclude that ginseng is usually not associated with serious adverse reactions[49].

The recommended daily dose is 1–2 g of the crude root, or 200–600 mg of extracts[50]. As the possibility of hormone-like or hormone-inducing effects cannot be ruled out, some authors suggest limiting treatment to 3 months of extracts[50].

Kava kava (Piper methysticum)

Kava kava or kava is a large shrub cultivated in the Pacific islands. Therapeutically, the rhizome of this herb is used to treat anxiety, stress and restlessness[51], the underlying causes of insomnia.

The CNS activity of kava is due to a group of resinous compounds known as kavalactones and kavapyrones[20]. Sedative, anticonvulsive, antispasmodic and central muscular relaxant effects are attributed to kava[52]. Studies in animals show that kava extracts and kavalactones induce sleep and muscle relaxation[20]. While the underlying mechanism is not entirely clear, it is possible that kava acts on GABA- and benzodiazepine-binding sites in the brain[53]. A recent meta-analysis of double-blind, randomized, placebo-controlled trials reported that kava extract was superior to placebo as a symptomatic treatment for anxiety[54]. Several relatively short-term clinical studies have also provided favorable evidence that kava is effective in treating anxiety and insomnia[55].

As a sleep aid, 180–210 mg of kavalactones daily are recommended[20]. It is important to note that ethanol and other CNS depressants can potentiate the effects of kava[51].

Passion flower (Passiflora incarnata)

The herb consists of the dried flowering and fruiting top of a perennial climbing vine (family Passifloraceae) (Figure 1). While studies proving its effectiveness are lacking, it is usually used for insomnia[21]. Active components of passion flower may be harmala-type indole alkaloids, maltol and ethyl-maltol and flavonoids[51]. When administered intraperitoneally to rats, passion flower extract significantly prolonged sleeping time[56]. The principal flavonoid, chrysin, was demonstrated to have benzodiazepine-receptor activity[52].

The usual daily dose is 4–8 g taken as a tea[20]. Since harmala compounds are uterine stimulants, passion flower extract is not recommended in pregnant women. Side-effects have not been reported.

Hops (Humulus lupulus)

The dried strobile with its glandular trichomes of *Humulus lupulus* is a popular sleep aid. Hops has been used for centuries in the treatment of intestinal ailments, but more recently as a sedative–hypnotic. Active ingredients in hops include a volatile oil, valerianic acid, estrogenic substances, tannins and flavonoids[51]. The sedative effects of hops have been demonstrated to induce sleep.

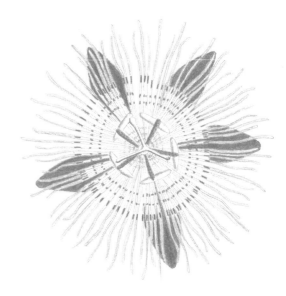

Figure 1 The passion flower, *Passiflora incarnata*

The use of hops for insomnia as an infusion in tea was reported to have a calming effect within 20–40 min of ingestion[57]. The recommended dose is 0.5 g of the dried herb, or its equivalent in extract-based products, taken one to several times daily[50]. Side-effects are uncommon, and large doses have been ingested safely. It is not recommended for pregnant women or women with estrogen-dependent breast cancer[18]. The use of hops is generally regarded to be safe by the FDA[51].

Physiological agents

Melatonin

Melatonin, a hormone secreted by the pineal gland, is considered to be a remedy for insomnia caused by circadian schedule changes, such as jet lag and shift work[58]. Rapid travel across several time zones results in a desynchronization between intrinsic human circadian rhythm and the local environmental photoperiod. The severity and duration of resulting sleep disturbance varies, depending on the number of time zones crossed, direction of travel, departure time and age. A clinical study with flight-crew members who completed a 9-day New Zealand–Los Angeles–England round trip reported that subjects who received melatonin only after arrival had significantly less jet lag overall[59].

Night-shift workers, during their nights off, have problems falling asleep. Folkard and colleagues[60] reported that melatonin increased sleep quality compared with baseline and placebo in night-shift workers. Melatonin has also been shown to have a beneficial effect on the quality of sleep for elderly patients with insomnia[61]. Delayed sleep phase syndrome, a circadian rhythm disorder, is a chronic condition characterized by the persistent inability to fall asleep and rise at conventional times[62]. A recent randomized, double-blind, placebo-controlled, cross-over study showed that a 4-week treatment with melatonin decreased sleep onset latency without altering sleep architecture[63]. Adverse effects of melatonin most commonly reported in the clinical trials include sedation, headache, depression, tachycardia and pruritus[60,64].

Variable melatonin dosages (0.3–5 mg) and drug timing administrations have been studied[58], but the optimal effective dosing is still unclear. The mechanisms of action of melatonin are unknown, but may involve interaction with melatonin receptors in the suprachiasmatic nucleus[6]. A randomized, double-blind, placebo-controlled study that assessed the toxic effects of 10 mg melatonin for 28 days reported that, while there was a significant reduction of stage-1 sleep, there were no toxicological effects that might compromise the use of melatonin[65].

L-Tryptophan and 5-hydroxytryptophan

L-Tryptophan and 5-hydroxytryptophan are precursors of 5-hydroxytryptamine (serotonin). Experimental data and clinical observations have indicated that the serotonergic system plays an important role in sleep regulation. Pharmacological manipulations, in humans and animals, that have affected the serotonergic system, have resulted in profound alterations in sleep[66]. However, the precise role of the serotonergic system in sleep regulation is not fully understood.

L-Tryptophan is an essential amino acid that occurs in plants and animals in concentrations of 1–2%. A dose of 1 g of L-tryptophan has been reported to reduce sleep latency by increasing subjective 'sleepiness' and also decreasing waking time[67]. It functions by increasing serotonin in certain brain cells, thus inducing sleep[68]. Although never approved as a drug, L-tryptophan was widely sold as a sleep aid in health-food stores until 1989[20]. That year, following the deaths of 37 healthy people of eosinophilia–myalgia syndrome after consuming contaminated L-tryptophan, the FDA recalled the product. Until the safety of the marketed product can be assured, the consumption of manufactured L-tryptophan must be avoided[20].

5-Hydroxytryptophan, the immediate precursor of serotonin, is still being used as a sleep aid. A daily dose of 100 mg/day was found to increase slow-wave sleep[68]. Its clinical efficacy has yet to be confirmed by controlled therapeutic studies.

Others

Acupuncture

Acupuncture is best known in the USA as an alternative therapy for chronic pain. However, in traditional Chinese medicine, it is commonly employed for the treatment of insomnia. There are numerous publications in Chinese on the use of acupuncture for insomnia. The literature cited in this review, however, is restricted to articles in English.

Clinical reports on acupuncture therapy verify its efficacy in the treatment of insomnia in psychiatric patients[69,70]. Controlled, clinical trials demonstrating acupuncture's effect on insomnia are rare. A recent study of primary insomniacs treated with acupuncture showed objective as well as subjective improvements in sleep quality[71]. Many previous studies provide only subjective evaluations of sleep. Since acupuncture is an individualized treatment, controlled studies are difficult to execute.

Using scalp, body and ear acupuncture points, positive effects appeared almost immediately after treatment[72]. The mechanisms by which acupuncture treatment modulates insomnia may be understood in terms of the general mechanism by which it produces analgesia[73]. Sites in the CNS where acupuncture signals are integrated also participate in the regulation of sleep–wake cycles in analgesia[73]. Additional clinical studies are necessary to elucidate how acupuncture can reharmonize a disturbed sleep–wake cycle.

Low-energy emission therapy

Low-energy emission therapy (LEET) is a method of delivering low levels of amplitude-modulated radio-frequency electromagnetic fields to humans. The LEET device consists of a signal generator, microprocessor and amplifier. The signal generator is connected to a mouthpiece, which is held between the tongue and palate for the duration of the treatment[74]. Results of some investigations have suggested that LEET may be a potential alternative therapy for chronic insomnia that is refractory to conventional treatment. In healthy volunteers, 15 min of LEET treatment induced EEG changes, and was associated with objective and subjective feelings of relaxation[75]. A double-blind, placebo-controlled study showed that 12 LEET treatments over a 4-week period improved the sleep of chronic insomniacs[76].

The mechanism underlying the effect of LEET is poorly understood. Low levels of electromagnetic field, such as those to which the brain is exposed during LEET, affect *in vitro* and *in vivo* calcium release from neural cells[77], modify the release of GABA[78] and change benzodiazepine receptor concentration in rat brains[79]. In addition, low levels of electromagnetic field modify the release of melatonin in mammals[74]. So far, the administration of LEET treatment is confined to sleep-disorder centers. Unlike conventional therapies, LEET may be administered on an every-other-day basis, and discontinuation does not appear to induce rebound insomnia[76]. LEET therapy-related side-effects have not been reported.

CONCLUSION

Insomnia is the most common sleep disorder. It is often associated with significant medical, psychological and social disturbances. The inability to attain restful sleep in adequate amounts exacts a heavy toll. Conventional treatment for insomnia includes psychological therapy and drugs that exert a depressant effect on the CNS. Most of the drugs prescribed for insomnia involve some risk of overdose, tolerance and addiction. Long-term use of frequently prescribed medications can lead to habituation and problematic withdrawal symptoms. As alternative therapies, herbal products and other agents with sedative–hypnotic effects are increasingly sought after by the general population. The herbs commonly used for their sedative–hypnotic effects are less likely to have the drawbacks of conventional drugs. How alternative therapies compare to conventional therapies warrants further investigation.

References

1. Bixler EO, Kales A, Soldatos CR. Prevalence of sleep disorders in the Los Angeles metropolitan area. *Am J Psychiatry* 1979;1136: 1257–62
2. Lugaresi E, Cirignotta F, Zucconi M, *et al.* Good and poor sleepers: an epidemiological survey of the San Marino population. In Guilleminault C, Lugaresi E, eds. *Sleep/Wake Disorders: Natural History, Epidemiology, and Long Term Evaluation.* New York, NY: Raven, 1983:1–12
3. Morin CM, Mimeault V, Gagne A. Nonpharmacological treatment of late-life insomnia. *J Psychosom Res* 1999;46:103–16
4. Stoller MK. Economic effects of insomnia. *Clin Ther* 1994;16: 873–97
5. Bunney WE Jr, Azarnoff DL, Brown BW Jr, *et al.* Report of the Institute of Medicine Committee on the efficacy and safety of halcion. *Arch Gen Psychiatry* 1999;56:349–352
6. Walsh JK, Benca RM, Bonnet M, *et al.* Insomnia: assessment and management in primary care. *Am Family Physician* 1999;59:3029–38
7. Ford DE, Kamerow DB. Epidemiologic study of sleep disturbances and psychiatric disorders: an opportunity for prevention? *J Am Med Assoc* 1989;262:1479–84

8. Nowell PD, Mazumdar S, Buysse DJ, *et al.* Benzodiazepines and zolpidem for chronic insomnia: a meta-analysis of treatment efficacy. *J Am Med Assoc* 1997;278:2170–7

9. Johnson EO, Roehrs T, Roth T, Breslau N. Epidemiology of alcohol and medication as aids to sleep in early adulthood. *Sleep* 1998;21:178–86

10. Kales JD, Kales A, Bixler EO, *et al.* Biopsychobehavioral correlates of insomnia V: clinical characteristics and behavioral correlates. *Am J Psychiatry* 1984;141:1371–6

11. Mendelson WB. Long-term follow-up of chronic insomnia. *Sleep* 1995;18:698–701

12. Vgontzas AN, Kales A. Sleep and its disorders. *Annu Rev Med* 1999;50:387–400

13. Rechtshaffen A, Kales A. *A Manual of Standardized Terminology, Techniques, and Scoring System for Sleep Stages of Human Subjects.* NIH Report No. 204. Bethesda, MD: National Institute of Health, 1968

14. Eddy M, Walbroehl GS. Insomnia. *Am Fam Physician* 1999;59:1911–15

15. Sharpley AL, Cowen PJ. Effect of pharmacologic treatments on the sleep of depressed patients. *Biol Psychiatry* 1995;37:85–8

16. Grauds CE. Botanical savvy: consultation tips for pharmacists. *Pharma Times* 1996;11:81

17. Foster S, Tyler VE. Valerian. In *Tyler's Honest Herbal.* New York, NY: Haworth Press, 1999:377–78

18. Castleman M. *The Healing Herbs: The Ultimate Guide to the Curative Power of Nature's Medicines.* Emmaus, PA: Rodale Press, 1991

19. Wagner J, Wagner ML, Hening WA. Beyond benzodiazepines: alternative pharmacologic agents for the treatment of insomnia. *Ann Pharmacother* 1998;32:680–91

20. Robbers JE, Tyler VE. Nervous system disorders. In *Tyler's Herbs of Choice.* New York, NY: Haworth Press, 1999:154–7

21. Hobbs C. Valerian. *Herbal Gram* 1989;21:19–34

22. Leathwood PD, Chauffard F, Heck E, Munoz-Box R. Aqueous extract of valerian root (*Valeriana offiinalis* L.) improves sleep quality in man. *Pharmacol Biochem Behav* 1982;17:65–71

23. Leathwood PD, Chauffard F. Aqueous extract of valerian reduces latency to fall asleep in man. *Planta Med* 1985;51:144–8

24. Lindahl O, Lindwall L. Double blind study of a valerian preparation. *Pharmacol Biochem Behav* 1989;32:1065–6

25. Balderer G, Borbely AA. Effect of valerian on human sleep. *Psycho-Pharmacol* 1985;87:406–9

26. Schulz H, Stolz C, Muller J. The effect of valerian extract on sleep polygraphy in poor sleepers: a pilot study. *Pharmacopsychiatry* 1994;27:147–51

27. Donath F, Quispe S, Diefenbach K, Maurer A, Fietze I, Roots I. Critical evaluation of the effects of valerian extract on sleep structure and sleep quality. *Pharmacopsychiatry* 2000;33:47–53

28. Houghton PJ. The biological activity of valerian and related plants. *J Ethnopharmacol* 1988;22:121–42

29. Mennini T, Bernasconi P, Bombardelli E, Morazzoni P. *In vitro* study on the interaction of extracts and pure compounds from *Valeriana officinalis* roots with GABA, benzodiazepine and barbiturate receptors in rat brain. *Fitoterapia* 1993;64:291–300

30. Houghton PJ. The scientific basis for the reputed activity of valerian. *J Pharm Pharmacol* 1999;51:505–12

31. Santos MS, Ferreira F, Faro C, *et al.* The amount of GABA present in aqueous extracts of valerian is sufficient to account for [^{3}H]GABA release in synaptosomes. *Planta Med* 1994;60:2475–6

32. Tortarolo M, Braun R, Hubner GE, Maurer HR. *In vitro* effects of epoxide-bearing valepotriates on mouse early hematopoietic progenitor cells and human T-lymphocytes. *Arch Toxicol* 1982;51:37–42

33. Garges HP, Varia I, Doraiswarmy PM. Cardiac complications and delirium associated with valerian root withdrawal [letter]. *J Am Med Assoc* 1998;280:1566–7

34. Attele AS, Wu JA, Yuan CS. Multiple pharmacological effects of ginseng. *Biochem Pharmacol* 1999;58:1685–93

35. Brevoot P. The US botanical market; an overview. *Herbal Gram* 1996;36:49–57

36. Lee FC. *Facts about Ginseng, the Elixir of Life.* Elizabeth, NJ: Hollyn International, 1992

37. Huang KC. *The Pharmacology of Chinese Herbs.* Boca Raton, FL: CRC Press, 1999

38. Kim YS, Kim DS, Kim SI. Ginsenoside Rh$_2$ and Rh$_3$ induce differentiation of HL-60 cells into granulocytes: modulation of protein kinase C isoforms during differentiation by ginsenoside Rh$_2$. *Int J Biochem Cell Biol* 1998;30:327–38

39. Yuan CS, Wu JA, Lowell T, Gu M. Gut and brain effects of American ginseng root on brainstem neuronal activities in rats. *Am J Chin Med* 1998;26:47–55

40. Takagi K, Saito H, Tsuchiya M. Pharmacological studies of *Panax ginseng* root: pharmacological properties of a crude saponin fraction. *Jpn J Pharmacol* 1972;22:339–46

41. Rhee YH, Lee SP, Honda K, Inoue S. *Panax ginseng* extract modulates sleep in unrestrained rats. *Psychopharmacol* 1990;101:486–8

42. Lee SP, Honda K, Rhee YH, Inoue S. Chronic intake of *Panax ginseng* extract stabilizes sleep and wakefulness in food-deprived rats. *Neurosci Lett* 1990;111:217–21

43. Huong NTT, Matsumoto K, Yamasaki K, Watanabe H. Majonoside-R2 reverses social isolation stress-induced decrease in pentobarbital sleep in mice: possible involvement of neuroactive steroids. *Life Sci* 1997;61:395–402

44. Huong NTT, Matsumoto K, Watanabe H. The antistress effect of majonoside-R2, a major saponin component of Vietnamese ginseng: neuronal mechanism of action. *Meth Find Exp Clin Pharmacol* 1998;20:65–76

45. Marasco AC, Ruiz RV, Villagomex AS, Infante CB. Double-blind study of a multivitamin complex supplemented with ginseng extract. *Drugs Exp Clin Res* 1996;22:323–9

46. Kimura T, Saunders PA, Kim HS, *et al.* Interactions of ginsenosides with ligand-bindings of GABA$_A$ and GABA$_B$ receptors. *Gen Pharm* 1994;25:193–9

47. Yuan CS, Attele AS, Wu JA, Liu D. Modulation of American ginseng on brainstem GABAergic effects in the rat. *J Ethnopharmacol* 1998;63:215–22

48. Punnonen R, Lukola A. Oestrogen-like effect of ginseng. *Br Med J* 1980;281:1110

49. Newall CA, Anderson LA, Phillipson JD. *Herbal Medicines: A Guide for Health-care Professionals.* London: Pharmaceutical Press, 1996:145–50

50. Schulz V, Hansel R, Tyler VE. Rational phytotherapy. In *Agents that Increase Resistance to Diseases.* New York, NY: Springer-Verlag, 1998:269–72

51. Miller LG, Murrey WJ. Herbal medications, nutraceuticals, and anxiety and depression. In: *Herbal Medicine: A Clinician's Guide.* New York, NY: Pharmaceutical Products Press, 1998:211–12

52. Singh YN. Kava: an overview. *J Ethnopharmacol* 1992;37:38

53. Davies LP, Drew CA, Duffield P, *et al*. Kava pyrones and resin: studies on GABA$_A$, and GABA$_B$, and benzodiazepine binding sites in rodent brain. *Pharmacol Toxicol* 1992;71:120

54. Pittler MH, Edzard E. Efficacy of kava extract for treating anxiety: systematic review and meta-analysis. *J Clin Psychopharmacol* 2000;20:84–9

55. Murray MT. *The Healing Power of Herbs*, 2nd edn. Rocklin, CA: Prima Publishing, 1995:210–19

56. Speroni E, Minghetti A. A neuropharmacological activity of extracts from *Passiflora incarnata*. *Planta Med* 1988;54:488–91

57. Mowrey DB. *The Scientific Validation of Herbal Medicine*. New Canaan, CT: Keats Publishing, 1986

58. Chase JE, Gidal BE. Melatonin: therapeutic use in sleep disorders. *Ann Pharmacother* 1997;31:1218–26

59. Petrie K, Dawson AG, Thompson L, Brook R. A double-blind trial of melatonin as a treatment for jet lag in international cabin crew. *Biol Psychiatry* 1993;33:526–30

60. Folkard S, Arendt J, Clark M. Can melatonin improve shift workers' tolerance of the night shift? Some preliminary findings. *Chronobiol Int* 1993;10:315–20

61. Garfunkel D, Laundon M, Nof D, Zisapel N. Improvement of sleep quality in elderly people by controlled release of melatonin. *Lancet* 1990;346:541–3

62. Weitzman ED, Czeisler CA, Coleman RM. Delayed sleep phase syndrome. *Arch Gen Psychiatry* 1981;38:737–46

63. Kayumov L, Brown G, Jindal R, Buttoo K, Shapiro C. A randomized, double-blind, placebo-controlled crossover study of the effect of exogenous melatonin on delayed sleep-phase syndrome. *Psychosom Med* 2001;63:40–8

64. Haimov I, Laudon M, Zisapel N, *et al*. Sleep disorders and melatonin rhythms in elderly people. *Br Med J* 1994;309:167

65. de Lourdes M, Seabra V, Bignotto M, Pinto LR Jr, Tufik S. Randomized, double-blind clinical trial, controlled with placebo, of the toxicology of chronic melatonin treatment. *J Pineal Res* 2000;29:193–200

66. Adriene J. The serotonergic system and sleep–wakefulness regulation. In Kales A, ed. *The Pharmacology of Sleep*. Berlin: Springer Verlag, 1995:91–116

67. Reynolds JEF. *Martindale: The Extra Pharmacopea*, 31st edn. London: Royal Pharmaceutical Society of Great Britain, 1996:336–7

68. Soulairac A, Lambinet H. The effects of 5-hydroxy-tryptophan, a precursor of serotonin, on sleep disorder. *Ann Med Psychol (Paris)* 1977;1:792–7

69. Shi ZX, Tan MZ. An analysis of the therapeutic effect of acupuncture in 500 cases of schizophrenia. *J Trad Chin Med* 1986;6:99

70. Romoli M, Giommi A. Ear acupuncture in psychosomatic medicine: the importance of Sanjiao (triple heater) area. *Acupunct Electrother Res* 1993;18:185–94

71. Montakab H. Acupuncture and insomnia. *Forschende Komplementarmed* 1999;6(Suppl 1):29–31

72. Huang KC. Acupuncture, the past and the present. In *Acupuncture in Internal Medicine*. New York, NY: Vantage Press, 1996:185–6

73. Lin Y. Acupuncture treatment for insomnia and acupuncture analgesia. *Psychiatry Clin Neurosci* 1995;49:119–20

74. Reiter RS. Electromagnetic fields and melatonin production. *Biomed Pharmacother* 1993;51:394–403

75. Higgs L, Reite M, Barbault A. Subjective and objective relaxation effects of low energy emission therapy. *Stress Med* 1994;10:5–14

76. Pasche B, Erman M, Hayduk R, *et al*. Effects of low energy emission therapy in chronic psychophysiological insomnia. *Sleep* 1996;19:327–36

77. Blackman CF. Calcium release from nervous tissue: experimental results and possible mechanisms. In Norden B, Ramel C, eds. *Interaction Mechanisms of Low-level Electromagnetic Fields in Living Systems*. Oxford: Oxford University Press, 1992:107–29

78. Kaczmarek LK, Adey WR. The efflux of $^{45}Ca^{++}$ and gamma-amino butyric acid from cat cerebral cortex. *Brain Res* 1973;63:331–42

79. Lai H, Corino MA, Horita A, Guy AW. Single vs repeated microwave exposure: effects on benzodiazepine receptors in the brain of the rat. *Bioelectromagnetics* 1992;13:57–66

Alternative therapies for type 2 diabetes   22

L. Dey and A. S. Attele

INTRODUCTION

Diabetes mellitus or diabetes is a serious chronic metabolic disorder that has a significant impact on the health, quality of life and life expectancy of patients, as well as on the health-care system. In the USA, diabetes is the sixth leading cause of death[1]. Diabetes is divided into two major categories: type 1 (formerly known as insulin-dependent diabetes mellitus, or IDDM), and type 2 (formerly known as non-insulin-dependent diabetes mellitus, or NIDDM). The overall prevalence of diabetes is approximately 6%, of which 90% is type 2 diabetes[2]. Treatment and care of diabetes represents a substantial portion of the national health-care expenditure. In 1992, for example, diabetes care cost 14.6% of every dollar spent on US health care[3].

Type 2 diabetes represents a syndrome with disordered metabolism of carbohydrate and fat. The most prominent clinical feature is hyperglycemia (fasting plasma glucose level > 126 mg/dl, or glycosylated hemoglobin $A_{1c} > 6.9\%$)[4]. In most patients with type 2 diabetes, the onset occurred in adulthood, and they are over 40 years of age and obese. Hypertension, hyperlipidemia and atherosclerosis are often associated with diabetes.

PATHOPHYSIOLOGY AND COMPLICATIONS

Type 2 diabetes is known to have a strong genetic component with contributing environmental determinants. Although the disease is genetically heterogeneous, there appears to be a fairly consistent phenotype once the disease is fully manifested.

Whatever the pathogenic causes, the early stage of type 2 diabetes is characterized by insulin resistance in insulin-targeting tissues, mainly the liver, skeletal muscle and adipocytes. Insulin resistance in these tissues is associated with excessive glucose production by the liver and impaired glucose utilization by peripheral tissues, especially the muscle. These events undermine metabolic homeostasis but may not directly lead to overt diabetes in the early stage. With increased insulin secretion to compensate for insulin resistance, baseline blood glucose levels can be maintained within normal ranges, but the patients may demonstrate impaired responses to prandial carbohydrate loading and to oral glucose tolerance tests. Thus, this early stage of diabetes features both insulin resistance and a relative insulin deficiency. The chronic overstimulation of insulin secretion gradually diminishes and eventually exhausts the islet β-cell reserve. A state of absolute insulin deficiency ensues and clinical diabetes becomes overt[5–7]. The transition of impaired glucose tolerance to type 2 diabetes can also be influenced by ethnicity, degree of obesity, distribution of body fat, sedentary lifestyle, aging and other concomitant medical conditions[8].

The quality of life of type 2 diabetic patients with chronic and severe hypoglycemia is adversely affected. Characteristic symptoms of tiredness and lethargy can become severe and lead to a decrease in work performance in adults and an increase of falls in the elderly[9]. The most common acute complications are metabolic problems (hyperosmolar hyperglycemic non-ketotic syndrome (HHNS)) and infection. The long-term complications are macrovascular complications (hypertension, dyslipidemia, myocardial infarction, stroke), microvascular complications (retinopathy, nephropathy, diabetic neuropathy, diarrhea, neurogenic bladder, impaired cardiovascular reflexes, sexual dysfunction) and diabetic foot disorders[9].

CONVENTIONAL THERAPIES

The general consensus on treatment of type 2 diabetes is that lifestyle management remains a foremost therapy. In addition to exercise, weight control and medical nutrition therapy, oral glucose-lowering drugs and injection of insulin are the conventional therapies for type 2 diabetes. Since the most important pathological process during the development of diabetes involves three key organs (pancreatic islets, liver and skeletal muscle), almost all anti-diabetic therapies are aimed at these organs. Pharmacological treatment is indicated when fasting glucose level exceeds 140 mg/dl, or the postprandial glucose level exceeds 160 mg/dl, or the level of hemoglobin A_{1c} exceeds 8.0%[10].

Pharmacological treatment and limitations

Oral glucose-lowering drugs

In the USA, five classes of oral agents are approved for the treatment of type 2 diabetes. Oral agent therapy is indicated in any patient with type 2 diabetes in whom diet and exercise fail to achieve acceptable glycemic control[10]. Although the initial responses have been good, oral hypoglycemic drugs may lose their effectiveness in a significant percentage of patients.

Sulfonylureas Both first-generation (e.g. tolbutamide) and second-generation (e.g. glyburide) sulfonylureas enhance insulin secretion from the pancreatic β-cells. A significant side-effect is hypoglycemia. Sulfonylurea therapy is also usually associated with weight gain due to hyperinsulinemia[11,12] which has been implicated as a cause of secondary drug failure[10–12].

Metformin Originally derived from a medicinal plant, *Galega officinalis*, metformin reduces plasma glucose by inhibiting hepatic glucose production and increasing muscle glucose uptake, which reduces

plasma triglyceride and low-density lipoprotein (LDL)-cholesterol levels. The most common side-effects are related to gastrointestinal disturbances.

Acarbose This decreases postprandial glucose levels. It works by interfering with carbohydrate digestion and delaying gastrointestinal absorption of glucose. The major side-effects are related to the gastrointestinal tract.

Thiazolidinediones These are represented by troglitazone, rosiglitazone and pioglitazone. These are relatively expensive oral agents, which work by improving insulin sensitivity in muscle and, to a much lesser extent, in the liver. These drugs decrease plasma triglyceride levels, but this decrease may be associated with weight gain and an increase in LDL-cholesterol levels. Liver toxicity is a concern; therefore, monthly monitoring of liver function is required once therapy with the thiazolidinediones begins. Since troglitazone (Rezulin®) is more toxic to the liver than rosiglitazone and pioglitazone, in March 2000 the Food and Drug Administration (FDA) asked the manufacturer of Resulin to remove the product from the market.

Repaglinide This augments insulin secretion, but weight gain and hypoglycemia are side-effects.

Insulin therapy

Insulin is usually added to an oral agent when glycemic control is suboptimal at maximal doses of oral medications. Some diabetologists prefer to initiate insulin therapy in patients with newly diagnosed type 2 diabetes[10]. Weight gain and hypoglycemia are common side-effects of insulin therapy[13–16]. Vigorous insulin treatment may also carry an increased risk of atherogenesis[14]. Table 1 summarizes some limitations of current drug therapies.

Exercise

Any exercise prescription should be individualized to account for patient interests, physical status, capacity and motivation. Exercising five to six times per week enhances weight reduction. Because many people with diabetes have not been active and are deconditioned, exercise should be started at a low level and gradually increased to avoid adverse effects such as injury, hypoglycemia or cardiac problems[17,18].

Diet therapy

Given the heterogeneous nature of type 2 diabetes, no single dietary approach is appropriate for all patients. Meal plans and diet modifications should be individualized by a registered dietitian to meet a patient's unique needs and lifestyle. In general, diet should be composed of 60–65% carbohydrate, 25–35% fat and 10–20% protein, while alcohol consumption should be limited[19].

ALTERNATIVE THERAPIES

Tremendous effort has been spent in searching for alternative therapies with anti-diabetic activity. Ideal therapies should have a similar degree of efficacy without the troublesome side-effects associated with conventional treatments. Some alternative therapies, which claimed to alleviate or cure diabetes, have become increasingly popular over the past several years[16]. Among them, medicinal herbs, nutritional supplementation, acupuncture and hot-tub therapy may be effective.

Medicinal herbs

Many conventional drugs have been derived from prototypic molecules in medicinal plants. Metformin exemplifies an efficacious oral glucose-lowering agent, and its development was based on the use of *Galega officinalis* to treat diabetes[20]. *Galega officinalis* is rich in guanidine, the hypoglycemic component[21–23]. Because guanidine is too toxic for clinical use, the alkyl diguanides synthalin A and synthalin B were introduced as oral anti-diabetic agents in Europe in the 1920s but were discontinued after insulin became

Table 1 Limitations of some anti-diabetic drugs

Anti-diabetic drugs	Major limitations
Sulfonylureas	hypoglycemia, weight gain
Metformin	gastrointestinal disturbances
Acarbose	gastrointestinal disturbances
Thiazolidinediones	liver toxicity, weight gain, high LDL-cholesterol, high cost
Repaglinide	hypoglycemia, weight gain
Insulin	hypoglycemia, weight gain

LDL, low-density lipoprotein

more widely available. However, experience with guanidine and diguanides prompted the development of metformin[24,25].

To date, over 400 traditional plant treatments for diabetes have been reported[20], although only a small number of these have received scientific and medical evaluation to assess their efficacy. A hypoglycemic effect resulting from the treatment of some herbal extracts has been confirmed in animal models of type 2 diabetes. The World Health Organization Expert Committee on Diabetes has recommended that traditional medicinal herbs be further investigated[20]. The following is a summary of several of the most studied and commonly used medicinal herbs.

Ginseng

The root of ginseng has been used for over 2000 years in the Far East for its health-promoting properties. In recent years, it has consistently been one of the ten top-selling herbs in the USA. Of the several species of ginseng, *Panax ginseng* (Asian ginseng) and *Panax quinquefolius* (American ginseng) are commonly used. Constituents of all ginseng species include ginsenosides, polysaccharides, peptides, polyacetyleinic alcohol and fatty acids[26]. Most pharmacological actions of ginseng are attributed to ginsenosides, a family of steroids named steroidal saponins[27,28]. The chemical composition of ginseng products and their potency may vary with the plant extract derivative, the age of the root, the location where it was grown, the season when it was harvested and the methods of drying[29,30].

Data from animal studies indicate that both Asian ginseng[31,32] and American ginseng[33,34] have significant hypoglycemic action. This blood glucose-lowering effect might be attributed to ginsenoside Rb_2 and, more specifically, to panaxans I, J, K and L in type 1 diabetic models[35–39]. Whether these constituents would have a similar effect on type 2 diabetes is still unknown.

There is some clinical evidence of ginseng's hypoglycemic activity. Sotaniemi and co-workers demonstrated a reduction in the levels of fasting blood glucose and hemoglobin A_{1c} in type 2 diabetics treated with a small dose (100–200 mg) of ginseng relative to placebo[40]. Ginseng also elevated mood, improved psychophysiologial performance and physical activity, and reduced body weight[40]. Recently, Vuksan and associates also demonstrated that 3 g of American ginseng, when given 40 min prior to the test meal, significantly lowered blood glucose in non-diabetic subjects and type 2 diabetic patients[41]. However, when ginseng was given together with meals, this effect did not persist in non-diabetic subjects. Vuksan and colleagues[41] proposed several plausible hypotheses that may work independently or in concert: first, ginseng may slow the digestion of food, decreasing the rate of carbohydrate absorption into the portal hepatic circulation[30,42]; second, ginseng may affect glucose transport, which is mediated by nitric oxide (NO)[32,43–45]; third, ginseng may modulate NO-mediated insulin secretion[46]. It was recently shown that NO stimulated glucose-dependent secretion of insulin in rat islet cells[47].

The most commonly reported side-effects are nervousness and excitation, but these diminish with continued use or dosage reduction[48]. However, there are few reports of noticeable adverse effects of ginseng, despite the fact that over 6 million ingest it regularly in the USA[48]. Ginseng may exert an estrogen-like effect in postmenopausal women, resulting in diffuse mammary nodularity and vaginal bleeding[49,50]. Ginseng may inhibit the effects of warfarin[51], and interact with the monoamine oxidase inhibitor phenelzine[52]. Often, such case reports failed to provide sufficient details concerning the type or quality of ginseng used, or whether the preparation actually contained ginseng or ginsenoside[53,54]. Massive overdose can bring about ginseng abuse syndrome, which is characterized by hypertension, insomnia, hypertonia and edema[48].

The recommended daily ginseng dosage is 1–2 g of the crude root, or 200–600 mg of standardized extracts[55]. As the possibility of hormone-like or hormone-inducing effects cannot be ruled out, some authors suggest limiting treatment to 3 months[55].

Momordica charantia

Momordica charantia (bitter melon), also known as balsam pear or karela, has been referred to as both a vegetable and a fruit and is widely cultivated in Asia, Africa and South America (Figure 1). It has been used extensively in folk medicines as a remedy for diabetes. The blood sugar-lowering action of the fresh juice or unripe fruit has been established in animal experimental models as well as human clinical trials[56,57].

Bitter melon contains several compounds with confirmed anti-diabetic properties. Alcohol-extracted charantin from *Momordica charantia* consists of mixed steroids and is more potent than the oral hypoglycemic agent tolbutamide[58]. Bitter melon also contains an insulin-like polypeptide, polypeptide-P, which decreases blood sugar levels when injected

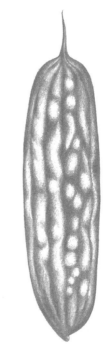

Figure 1 *Momordica charantia*, the bitter melon

subcutaneously into type 1 diabetics, and it appears to have fewer side-effects than insulin. The oral administration of bitter melon preparations has also shown satisfactory results in clinical trials in type 2 diabetic patients. Welihinda and colleagues[56] showed that glucose tolerance was improved in 73% of type 2 diabetics given 57 g of the juice. In another study, 15 g of the aqueous extract of bitter melon produced a 54% decrease in postprandial blood sugar levels and a 17% reduction in glycosylated hemoglobin in six patients[57]. The mechanism of bitter melon's activity in lowering blood glucose is unknown, but in diabetic rabbit models it has been proposed to possess a direct action similar to that of insulin[59]. Karela was also found to be effective in lowering blood glucose in alloxan-treated rabbits[60]. Bailey and Day[20] reported that karela appeared to inhibit the effect of gluconeogenesis.

The recommended bitter melon dosage is 5 ml of tincture two to three times a day, with a total as high as 50 ml/day[61]. However, bitter melon juice is very difficult to make palatable, since it is quite bitter. To avoid the bitter taste, the Indians and Chinese crush karela and form tablets. In Central America, it is prepared as an extract or decoction. Hepatic portal inflammation and testicular lesions in dogs have been reported with excessive administration of cerasee (a component of the wild variety of bitter melon)[62].

Trigonella foenumgraecum

Trigonella foenumgraecum (fenugreek) has been used as a folk remedy for diabetes[63]. The active principle is in the defatted portion of the seed and contains the alkaloid trigonelline, nicotinic acid and coumarin. Administration of the defatted seed (1.5–2.0 g/kg daily) to both normal and diabetic dogs reduced fasting and postprandial blood levels of glucose, glucagon, somatostatin, insulin, total cholesterol and triglycerides, and increased high-density lipoprotein (HDL)-cholesterol levels[64]. Human studies have confirmed these effects[58]. Of the seeds, 50–60% is fiber, and this may constitute another potential mechanism of fenugreek's beneficial effect in diabetic patients[65].

In type 2 diabetics, the ingestion of 15 g of powdered fenugreek seed soaked in water significantly reduced postprandial glucose levels during a glucose tolerance test[65]. The dosage of fenugreek is 625 mg in capsule from two to three times a day[61]. Urine will have a 'maple syrup' smell after fenugreek consumption[66]. No other side-effects have been reported to date.

Gymnema sylvestre

Gymnema sylvestre (gurmar), a plant native to the tropical forests of India, has long been used as a treatment for diabetes. *Gymnema sylvestre* appeared on the US market several years ago, and it was promoted as a 'sugar blocker'[58]. In a study of type 2 diabetes, 22 patients were given *Gymnema sylvestre* extract along with their oral hypoglycemic drugs. All patients demonstrated improved blood sugar control; 21 out of the 22 were able to reduce their oral hypoglycemic drug dosage considerably, and five patients were able to discontinue their oral medication and maintain blood sugar control with the gurmar extract alone[61]. It was postulated that *Gymnema sylvestre* enhances the production of endogenous insulin[67].

The dosage of *Gymnema sylvestre* extract is 400 mg/day. One of its side-effects is that it reduces or abolishes the taste sensation of sweetness and bitterness[61].

Allium cepa and Allium sativum

Allium cepa (onions) and *Allium sativum* (garlic) have demonstrated a blood sugar-lowering action in several studies[68,69]. Volatile oils in raw onion and garlic cloves have been shown to lower fasting glucose concentration in diabetic animals and in human subjects[70]. The active components are believed to be sulfur-containing compounds, allyl propyl disulfide (APDS) and diallyl disulfide (allicin), although other constituents such as flavonoids may play a role as well. Experimental and clinical evidence has suggested that the active components lower glucose levels by competing with insulin for insulin-inactivating sites in the liver[58]. This results in an increase of free insulin.

There is a marked fall in blood glucose levels and an increase in serum insulin level when a dose of 125 mg/kg of APDS is administered to humans. Allicin at doses of 100 mg/kg produces a similar effect[58]. Onion extracts also reduce blood sugar levels in a dose-dependent manner[68]. The dosage of *Allium cepa* is one standardized capsule of 400 mg/day. Excessive amounts can cause liver toxicity[71]. The general daily dosage of garlic is 4 g of fresh garlic or 8 mg of essential oil[72].

Pterocarpus marsupium and other epicatechin-containing plants

Pterocarpus marsupium has a long history of use in India as a treatment for diabetes. The flavanoid, (−)-epicatechin, extracted from the bark of this plant, has been shown to prevent β-cell damage in rats[58]. In addition, both epicatechin and a crude alcohol extract of *Pterocarpus marsupium* have been shown to regenerate functional pancreatic β-cells in diabetic animals[73,74].

Epicatechin and catechin consist of glycosides and esters. They are flavan-3-ols, a group of flavanols, which have anti-diabetic properties[75]. Also, *Camellia sinensis* (green tea polyphenols) and *Acacia catechu* (Burma cutch) are a good source of flavan-3-ols. Since *Pterocarpus* is not very common in the USA, green tea may be the suitable alternative of *Pterocarpus*. The recommended dose of green tea is two 120-ml cups daily or roughly 240 mg of green tea daily. Side-effects of green tea have not been reported.

Vaccinium myrtillus

Vaccinium myrtillus (bilberry or European blueberry) is a shrubby plant that grows in Europe. Leaves of *Vaccinium myrtillus* were widely used as a treatment for diabetes before the availability of insulin[20]. Oral administration of bilberry leaf tea reduced blood sugar level in normal and diabetic dogs, even when glucose was concurrently injected intravenously[76]. Bilberry also has a beneficial effect in microvascular abnormalities of diabetes[77,78]. The anthocyanoside myrtillin is the most active constituent of bilberry.

The standard dose of bilberry extract is based on its anthocyanoside contents and is 80–160 mg three times daily[58]. Animal data suggest that *Vaccinium myrtillus*

administration may be associated with renal and hepatic carcinogenicity[20,79,80].

Atriplex halimu

Atriplex halimu (salt bush) is a branchy woody shrub native to the Mediterranean, North Africa and Southern Europe. Salt bush is rich in fiber, protein and numerous trace minerals including chromium. Human studies with salt bush conducted in Israel demonstrated improved blood glucose regulation and glucose tolerance in type 2 diabetic patients[58]. The dose used in the trial was 3 g/day.

Nutritional supplements

The treatment of diabetes requires nutritional supplementation, as these patients have a greatly increased need for many nutrients. Supplying the diabetic with additional key nutrients has been shown to improve blood sugar control as well as helping to prevent or ameliorate many major complications of diabetes.

Chromium

Chromium is an essential micronutrient for humans. Considerable experimental and epidemiological evidence now indicates that chromium levels are the major determinant of insulin sensitivity, and that chromium functions as a cofactor in all insulin-regulating activities[81]. Chromium works closely with insulin in facilitating the uptake of glucose into cells. Supplemental chromium has been shown to decrease fasting glucose levels, improve glucose tolerance, lower insulin levels and decrease total cholesterol and triglyceride levels while increasing HDL-cholesterol levels in normal, elderly and type 2 diabetic patients[82,83]. Without chromium, insulin's action is blocked, and glucose levels are elevated[82].

Chromium picolinate, a trivalent chromium (Cr^{3+}), is the only form of chromium that exhibits biological activity[84], and is an integral component of the so-called 'glucose tolerance factor' (GTF) when combined with two molecules of nicotinic acid. Chromium deficiency may be an underlying contributing factor in a large number of Americans suffering from diabetes, hypoglycemia and obesity, and marginal chromium deficiency is common in the USA[58].

A large clinical study in 180 diabetics clearly documented the benefit of chromium for type 2 diabetics. In the study, while patients continued their normal medication, they were placed in one of three groups: placebo group, group receiving 100 µg chromium picolinate twice a day, and group reveiving 500 µg chromium picolinate twice a day. There were significant dose- and time-dependent decreases in glycosylated hemoglobin, fasting glucose, 2-h postprandial glucose levels, fasting and 2-h postprandial insulin values and total cholesterol[85]. Supplementing the diet with chromium also lowers body weight while increasing lean body mass, and these chromium effects appear to be due to an increased insulin sensitivity. However, not all studies on chromium have yielded positive results. In a controlled 6-month study to determine the effect of chromium picolinate on individuals with type 2 diabetes, Lee and Reasner[86] reported an improvement in triglyceride level but no statistical difference between control and chromium-treated subjects with respect to measured parameters of glucose control. Joseph and colleagues[87] also found no added benefit of chromium supplementation when it was provided in addition to resistance training.

Although no recommended daily allowance (RDA) has been established for chromium, over 200 µg/day appears to be necessary for optimal blood sugar regulation[53]. A good supply of chromium is assured by adequate daily intake of about 50–200 µg[88], and the best dietary sources are brewer's yeast[63] and barley flour[89]. Interestingly, some aromatic plants, which are utilized by diabetics as medicinal plants, contain a high level of chromium[89]. Refined sugars, white-flour products and lack of exercise can deplete chromium levels. In addition to the regular consumption of chromium-rich foods, diabetics and hypoglycemics should supplement their diet with chromium polynicotinate, chromium picolinate and chromium-enriched yeast[89].

Trivalent chromium has long been considered to be a safe nutritional supplement[90]. Although the hexavalent form of chromium is a known human respiratory tract carcinogen in high-exposure industrial use, there is no evidence of any carcinogenesis in humans from the trivalent form of chromium found in chromium picolinate[91,92]. However, concerns about possible chromosomal damage from long-term, high-dose chromium picolinate have recently been raised[93,94]. Further evaluation of the safety and efficacy of trivalent chromium in diabetes treatment is warranted.

Magnesium

Magnesium is involved in several areas of glucose metabolism and there is considerable evidence that diabetics need supplemental magnesium. It has been reported that magnesium deficiency is common in diabetics and magnesium may prevent some of the complications of diabetes, such as retinopathy and heart disease[95]. Because most Americans consume a diet high in refined foods, meat and dairy products, low magnesium levels are common. The best dietary sources of magnesium are tofu, legumes, seeds, nuts, whole grains and green leafy vegetables. In addition to a diet high in magnesium, supplementation with 300–500 mg of magnesium as aspartate or citrate is recommended for non-diabetic adults, and diabetics may need twice this amount. Diabetics should also take at least 50 mg/day of vitamin B_6, as intracellular vitamin B_6 appears to be intricately linked to the magnesium of the cell[58].

Zinc

Zinc is involved in synthesis, secretion and utilization of insulin metabolism. Zinc also has a protective effect against β-cell destruction and has an antiviral effect[58]. Diabetics typically excrete excessive amounts of zinc in the urine and thus require supplementation[96]. It has been shown that zinc can improve insulin levels in both type 1 and type 2 diabetes[97]. In addition, zinc helps to improve wound healing in diabetics[98]. Zinc is found in good amounts in whole grains, legumes, nuts and seeds. The recommended level of zinc supplementation for diabetics should be over 30 mg/day[58].

Besides chromium, magnesium and zinc, there a number of other minerals such as calcium, potassium and vanadium that appear to improve insulin sensitivity. Some amino acids, such as L-carnitine, taurine and L-arginine may also play a role in the reversal of insulin resistance. Vitamins E, C and B$_6$ and biotin are also effective in diabetic patients. Other nutrients, such as glutathione, fish oils (omega−3 essential fatty acids), coenzyme Q$_{10}$ and lipoic acid may also have therapeutic potential for diabetics[99]. Nutrients used in type 2 diabetes are summarized in Table 2.

Fiber

Supplementation with plant fibers (e.g. guar gum at a dosage of 5 g/meal and pectin 10 g/meal) has demonstrated a positive impact on diabetes control[58]. Guar gum or cluster bean is the powder extracted by milling

Table 2 Supplemental nutrients used in type 2 diabetes

Nutrients	Effect
Chromium picolinate	improves glucose tolerance
Magnesium	improves glucose metabolism
Zinc	improves glucose metabolism
Calcium	improves insulin sensitivity
Potassium	may improve insulin sensitivity
Vanadyl sulfate	improves insulin sensitivity
L-Carnitine	improves insulin sensitivity after intravenous infusion
Taurine	may improve insulin sensitivity
L-Arginine	improves insulin sensitivity after intravenous infusion
Vitamin E	reduces glycosylation and antioxidant activity
Vitamin C	reduces glycosylation and antioxidant activity
Vitamin B$_6$	improves glucose metabolism and nerve function
Biotin	improves glucose metabolism and nerve function
Glutathione	improves insulin sensitivity after intravenous infusion
Omega−3 essential fatty acids	improves insulin sensitivity
Coenzyme Q$_{10}$	improves insulin sensitivity
Lipoic acid	improves insulin sensitivity
Inositol	improves glucose metabolism

Cyamopsis tetragonoloba[72]. It has been reported to decrease fasting blood glucose and postprandial glucose, and improve insulin sensitivity[100–102]. Many experts in diabetes are now using these fiber supplements, along with the standard American Diabetic Association diet[103]. When diabetic patients ate between 14 and 26 g/day of guar, they required less insulin and had less glycosuria[104,105]. However, fiber-supplemented diets are not as effective as the high-carbohydrate, high-plant-fiber diet and they are reserved for the type 2 diabetics who are unwilling to implement the more difficult dietary change[58].

Acupuncture

Acupuncture is best known in the USA as an alternative therapy for chronic pain. However, considerable progress has been made in the treatment of diabetes by acupuncture since 1970[106]. There are numerous publications in Chinese on the use of acupuncture for diabetes, but only those published in English are cited here. It is believed that acupuncture is effective not only in treating diabetes, but also in preventing and managing complications of the disease[106].

The effects of acupuncture on diabetes have been observed experimentally and clinically[107]. Animal experiments have shown that acupuncture can activate glucose-6-phosphatase, an important enzyme in carbohydrate metabolism, and affect the hypothalamus to a certain extent[108]. Acupuncture can act on the pancreas to enhance insulin synthesis, increase the number of receptors on target cells, accelerate the utilization of glucose and, thus, help to lower the blood sugar[107]. Data from another study showed the beneficial anti-obesity effect of acupuncture[109], which is the most modifiable risk factor for type 2 diabetes. It appears that the therapeutic effect of acupuncture on diabetes was not the result of its action on a single organ, but on multiple systems.

The four commonly used points are:

(1) *Zusanli* point, located 3 in (8 cm) below the lateral knee depression, one finger width from the lateral side of the anterior crest of the tibia;

(2) *Sanyinjiao* point, located 3 in above the tip of the inner ankle, on the posterior margin of the metatarsal bone;

(3) *Feishu* point, located 1.5 in (4 cm) lateral and inferior to the spinous process of the third thoracic vertebra in a prone position;

(4) *Shenshu* point, located 1.5 in lateral to the posterior midline, lateral and inferior to the spinous process of the second lumbar vertebra in a prone position.

The selection of acupuncture points was based on traditional Chinese medicine theory. During the treatment, other points can be added according to symptoms and signs[106]. Other methods have also been employed such as point injection with normal saline, a small dose of insulin or Chinese herbal medicine extracts. Treatment is generally given once a day or once every other day as a course of 14–21 treatments. It is believed that the longer the course of treatment, the more marked the effect. Effects of acupuncture usually appear after 25 treatments and the therapy generally lasts 2–5 months[106].

Acupuncture is more effective when the course is mild or moderate, and less effective in severe cases with a prolonged course. It is often very effective in treating diabetic complications, usually with marked improvement in clinical symptoms. However, in patients with ketoacidosis, the therapeutic results are poor[106]. Patients with a strong needling sensation often show a better therapeutic effect than those with a weak needling sensation. Usually obese patients have better therapeutic results. Results of treatment are often unsatisfactory in depressed or emotionally unstable individuals. Better therapeutic results are obtained in patients with dietary control than in those without it. Proper physical exercises, breathing exercises and massage can help improve the therapeutic effect.

Although acupuncture shows some effectiveness in treating diabetes, its mechanisms of action are still obscure. Integration of scientific advances and research methods would further develop acupuncture treatment for diabetes.

Hot-tub therapy

Since hot-tub therapy can increase blood flow to skeletal muscles, it has been recommended for patients with type 2 diabetes who are unable to exercise[110]. A study reported that eight patients were asked to sit in a hot tub for 30 min daily for 3 weeks. During the study period, the patients' weight, mean plasma glucose level and mean glycosylated hemoglobin decreased[111]. Proper water sanitation and appropriate guidance should be considered when prescribing hot-tub therapy for diabetic patients.

CONCLUSIONS

Type 2 diabetes is a chronic metabolic disease that has a significant impact on the health, quality of life and life expectancy of patients, as well as on the healthcare system. Exercise, diet and weight control continue to be essential and effective means of improving glucose homeostasis. However, these lifestyle management measures may be insufficient, and conventional drug therapies (oral glucose-lowering agents and insulin injection) are indicated in most of the patients. In addition to adverse effects, drug treatments are not always satisfactory in maintaining euglycemia and avoiding late-stage diabetic complications. Alternative therapies have often been used in chronic conditions that may be only partially alleviated by conventional treatment. Herbal medication is the most commonly used alternative therapy, but its safety and hypoglycemic effects need to be further evaluated via carefully planned animal research, and well-designed controlled clinical studies. Although herbs used for diabetes are less likely to have the drawbacks of conventional drugs, potential adverse herb–drug interactions should be kept in mind for patients also receiving conventional anti-diabetic medications.

References

1. National Institutes of Diabetes and Digestive and Kidney Diseases. *Diabetes Statistics*. NIH publication no. 96-3926. Bethesda, MD: NIDDK, 1995
2. American Diabetes Association. *Diabetes 1996 Vital Statistics*. Alexandria, VA: American Diabetes Association, 1996
3. Rubin RJ, Altman WM, Mendelson DN. Health care expenditures for people with diabetes mellitus, 1992. *J Clin Endocrinol Metab* 1994;78:809A–F
4. Report of the Expert Committee on the Diagnosis and Classification of Diabetes Mellitus. *Diabetes Care* 1997;20:1183-91
5. DeFronzo RA. The triumvirate: B-cell, muscle, liver. A collusion responsible for NIDDM. *Diabetes* 1988;37:667–87
6. Seely BL, Olefsky JM. Potential cellular and genetic mechanisms for insulin resistance in common disorders of obesity and diabetes. In Moller D, ed. *Insulin Resistance and its Clinical Disorders*. London: John Wiley & Sons, 1993:187–252
7. Olefsky JM. Insulin resistance and pathogenesis of non insulin dependent diabetes mellitus: cellular and molecular mechanisms. In Efendic S, Ostenson CG, Vranic M, eds. *New Concepts in the Pathogenesis of NIDDM*. New York, NY: Plenum Publishing, 1999
8. Clark CM Jr. The burden of chronic hyperglycemia. *Diabetes Care* 1998;21(Suppl. 3):C32–4
9. Davidson MB. *Diabetes Mellitus: Diagnosis and Treatment*, 3rd edn. New York, NY: Churchill Livingstone, 1991
10. DeFronzo RA. Pharmacologic therapy for type 2 diabetes mellitus. *Ann Intern Med* 1999;131:281–303
11. Parving HH, Gall MA, Skott MA, *et al.* Prevalence and causes of albuminuria in non-insulin dependent diabetic patients. *Kidney Int* 1992;41:758–62
12. Kelley DE. Effects of weight loss on glucose homeostasis in NIDDM. *Diabetes Rev* 1995;3:366-77
13. United Kingdom Prospective Diabetes Study 24 (UKPDS 24). A 6-year, randomized, controlled trial comparing sulfonylurea, insulin, and metformin therapy in patients with newly diagnosed type 2 diabetes that could not be controlled with diet therapy. United Kingdom Prospective Diabetes Study Group. *Ann Intern Med* 1998;128:165–75
14. United Kingdom Prospective Diabetes Study 33 (UKPDS 33). Intensive blood-glucose control with sulphonylureas or insulin compared with conventional treatment and risk of complications in patients with type 2 diabetes. United Kingdom Prospective Diabetes Study Group. *Lancet* 1998;352:837-53
15. United Kingdom Prospective Diabetes Study 34 (UKPDS 34). Effect of intensive blood-glucose control with metformin on complications in overweight patients with type 2 diabetes. UK Prospective Diabetes Study Group. *Lancet* 1998;352:854-65
16. Sinha A, Formica C, Tsalamandris C, *et al.* Effect of insulin on body composition in patients with insulin-dependent and non-insulin-dependent diabetes. *Diabetes Med* 1996;13:40–6
17. American Diabetes Association. *Medical Management of Non-insulin-dependent (Type ll) Diabetes*, 3rd edn. Alexandria, VA: American Diabetes Association, 1994:22–39
18. American Diabetes Association. Clinical practice recommendations 1995. Position statement: diabetes mellitus and exercise. *Diabetes Care* 1995;18(Suppl 1):28
19. Schlichtmann J, Graber MA. Hematologic, electrolyte, and metabolic disorders. In: Graber MA, Toth PP, Herting RL, eds. *The Family Practice Hand Book*. 3rd edn. St Louis, MO: Mosby-Year Book, 1997:192–251
20. Bailey CJ, Day C. Traditional plant medicines as treatments for diabetes. *Diabetes Care* 1989; 12:553–65
21. British Herbal Medicine Association. *British Herbal Pharmacopoeia*. Keighley, UK: British Herbal Medicine Association, 197
22. Hermann M. *Herbs and Medicinal Flowers*. New York, NY: Galahad, 1973
23. Petricic J, Kalogjera Z. Bestimmung des Galegins und die Antidiabetische Wirkung der Droge Herba Galegae. *Planta Med* 1982;45:140
24. Sterne J. Pharmacology and mode of action of the hypoglycemic agents. In Campbell GD, ed. *Oral Hypoglycemic Agents: Pharmacology and Therapeutics*. New York, NY: Academic, 1969: 193–245
25. Bailey CJ. Metformin revisited: its action and indications for use. *Diabetic Med* 1988;5:315–20
26. Lee FC. *Facts about Ginseng, the Elixir of Life*. Elizabeth, NJ: Hollyn International, 1992
27. Huang KC. *The Pharmacology of Chinese Herbs*. Boca Raton, FL: CRC Press, 1999
28. Attele AS, Wu JA, Yuan CS. Ginseng pharmacology, multiple constituents and multiple actions. *Biochem Pharm* 1999;58:1685–93
29. Reis CA, Sahud MA. Agranulocytosis caused by Chinese herbal medicine: dangers of medications containing aminopyrine and phenylbutazone. *J Am Med Assoc* 1975;231:352
30. Yuan CS, Wu JA, Lowell T, Gu M. Gut and brain effects of American ginseng root on brainstem neuronal activities in rats. *Am J Chin Med* 1998;26:47–55
31. Liu CX, Xiao PG. Recent advances on ginseng research in China. *J Ethnopharmacol* 1992;36:27–38
32. Ohnishi Y, Takagi S, Miura T, *et al.* Effect of ginseng radix on GLUT2 protein content in mouse liver in normal and epinephrine-induced hyperglycemic mice. *Biol Pharm Bull* 1996;19:1238–40
33. Oshima Y, Sato K, Hikino H. Isolation and hypoglycemic activity of quinquefolans A, B, and C, glycans of *Panax quinquefolium* roots. *J Nat Prod* 1987;50:188–90
34. Martinez B, Staa EJ. The physiological effects of Aralia, Panax and Eleutherococcus on exercised rats. *Jpn J Pharmacol* 1984;35: 79–85
35. Tomoda M, Shimada K, Konno C, Sugiyama K, Hikino H. Partial structure of Panaxan A: a hypoglycemic glycan of *Panax ginseng* roots. *Planta Med* 1984;50:436–8
36. Konno C, Sugiyama K, Kano M, Takahashi M, Hikino H. Isolation and hypoglycemic activity of panaxans A, B, C, D, and E: glycans of *Panax ginseng* roots. *Planta Med* 1984;50:436–8
37. Konno C, Murakani M, Oshima Y, Hikino H. Isolation and hypoglycemic activity of panaxans Q, R, S, R, and U: glycans of *Panax ginseng* roots. *J Ethnopharmacol* 1985;14:69-74
38. Yokozawa T, Kobayashi T, Oura H, Kawashima Y. Studies on the mechanism of the hypoglycemic activity of ginsenoside-Rb2 in streptozotocin-diabetic rats. *Chem Pharm Bull* 1985;33:869–72
39. Oshima Y, Kkonno C, Hikino H. Isolation and hypoglycemic activity of panaxans I, J, K and L, glycans of *Panax ginseng* roots. *J Ethnopharmacol* 1985;14:255–9

40. Sotaniemi EA, Happakoski E, Rautio A. Ginseng therapy in non-insulin dependent diabetic patients. *Diabetes Care* 1995;18:1373–5

41. Vuksan V, Sievenpiper JL, Koo VY, *et al.* American ginseng (*Panax quinquefolius* L) reduces postprandial glycemia in nondiabetic subjects and subjects with type 2 diabetes mellitus. *Arch Intern Med* 2000;60:1009–13

42. Suzuki Y, Ito Y, Konno C, Furuya T. Effects of tissue culture of ginseng on gastric secretion and pepsin activity [in Japanese]. *Yakugaku Zasshi* 1991;111:770–4

43. Hasegawa H, Matsumiya S, Murakami C, *et al.* Interaction of ginseng extract, ginseng seperated fractions, and some triterpenoid saponins with glucose transporters in sheep erythrocytes. *Planta Med* 1994;60:153–7

44. Gills CN. *Panax ginseng* pharmacology: a nitric oxide link? *Biochem Pharmacol* 1997;54:1–8

45. Roy D, Perrault M, Marette A. Insulin stimulation of glucose uptake in skeletal muscle and adipose tissue *in vivo* is NO dependent. *Am J Physiol.* 1998;274:E692–9

46. Kimura M, Waki I, Chujo T, *et al.* Effects of hypoglycemic components in ginseng radix on blood insulin level in alloxan diabetic mice and on insulin release from perfused rat pancreas. *J Pharmacobiodyn* 1981;4:410–17

47. Spinas GA, Laffranchi R, Francoys I, David I, Richter C, Reinecke M. The early phase of glucose-stimulated insulin secretion requires nitric oxide. *Diabetologia* 1998;41:292–9

48. Punnonen R, Lukola A. Oestrogen-like effect of ginseng. *Br Med J* 1980;281:1110

49. Palmer BV, Montgomery ACV, Monteiro JCMP. Ginseng and mastalgia. *Br Med J* 1978;1:1284

50. Hammond TG, Whitworth JA. Adverse reactions to ginseng. *Med J Aust* 1981;1:492

51. Janetzky K, Morreale AP. Probable interaction between warfarin and ginseng. *Am J Health Syst Pharm* 1997;54:692–3

52. Jones BD, Runkis AM. Interaction of ginseng with phenelzine. *J Clin Psychopharmacol* 1987;7:201–2

53. Cui J, Garle M, Eneroth P, Bjorkhem I. What do commercial ginseng preparations contain? *Lancet* 1994;344:134

54. Awang DVC. Maternal use of ginseng and neonatal androgenization. *J Am Med Assoc* 1991;266:363

55. Schulz V, Hansel R, Tyler VE. Rational phytotherapy. In *Agents that Increase Resistance to Diseases.* New York, NY: Springer-Verlag, 1998:269–72

56. Welihinda J, Karunanaya EH, Sherrif MHR, Jayasinghe KSA. Effect of *Momordica charantia* on the glucose tolerance in maturity onset diabetes. *J Ethnopharmacol* 1986;17:277–82

57. Srivastava Y, Venkatakrishna-Bhatt H, Verma Y, *et al.* Antidiabetic and adaptogenic properties of *Momordica charantia* extract. An experimental and clinical evaluation. *Phytother Res* 1993;7:285–9

58. Murray MT, Pizzorno JE Jr. Diabetes mellitus. In Pizzorno JE Jr, Murray MT, eds. *Textbook of Natural Medicine,* 2nd edn. Edinburgh: Churchill Livingstone, 1999:1193–218

59. Akhtar MS, Athar MA, Yaqub M. Effect of *Momordica charantia* on blood glucose level of normal and alloxan diabetic rabbits. *Planta Med* 1981;42:205–12

60. Larner J, Haynes C. Insulin and hypoglycemia drugs, glycogen. In Gilman GG, Goodman LS, Rall TW, Murad F, eds. *The Pharmacological Basis of Therapeutics,* 5th edn. New York, NY: Macmillan Publishing, 1975:1507–28

61. Mozersky RP. Herbal products and supplemental nutrients used in the management of diabetes. *J Am Osteopath Assoc* 1999;99:S4–9

62. Dixit VP, Khanna P, Bhargava SK. Effects of *Momordica charantia* L fruit extract on the testicular function of dog. *Planta Med* 1978;34:280–6

63. Miller LG. Herbal medications, nutraceuticals, and diabetes. In Miller LG, Murray WJ, eds. *Herbal Medicinals, A Clinician's Guide.* Binghamton, NY: Pharmaceutical Products Press, Imprint of the Haworth Press, 1998:115–33

64. Ribes G, Sauvaire Y, Baccou JC, *et al.* Effects of fenugreek seeds on endocrine pancreatic secretions in dogs. *Ann Nutr Metab* 1984;28:37–43

65. Madar Z, Abel R, Samish S, Arad J. Glucose-lowering effect of fenugreek in non-insulin dependent diabetes. *Eur J Clin Nutr* 1988;42:51–4

66. Bartley GB, Hymd H, Andreson BD, Clairmont AC, Maschke SP. 'Maple syrup' urine odor due to fenugreek ingestion. *N Engl J Med* 1981;305:467

67. Shanmugasundaram ERB, Rajeswara G, Baskaran K, Kumar BRJ, Shanmugasundaram KR, Arhmath BK. Use of *Gymnema sylvestre* leaf extract in the control of blood glucose in insulin-dependent diabetes mellitus. *J Ethnopharmacol* 1990; 30:281–94

68. Sharma KK, Gupta S, Samuel KC. Antihyperglycemic effect of onion: effect on fasting blood sugar and induced hyperglycemia in man. *Ind J Med Res* 1977;65:422–9

69. Sheela CG, Augusti KT. Antidiabetic effects of S-allyl cysteine sulphoxide isolated from garlic (*Allium sativum*, Linn.). *Ind J Exp Biol* 1992;30:523–6

70. Jain RC, Vyas CR, Mahatama OP. Hypoglycemic action of onion and garlic [letter]. *Lancet* 1973;2:1491

71. Augusti KT, Benaim ME. Effect of essential oil of onion (allyl propyl disulphide) on blood glucose, free fatty acid and insulin levels of normal subjects. *Clin Chim Acta* 1975;60:121–3

72. Herbal monographics. In Gruenwald J, Brendler T, Jaenicke C, eds. *PDR for Herbal Medicines,* 2nd edn. Montvale, NJ: Medical Economics Company, 2000:376–8

73. Chakravarthy BK, Gupa S, Gambhir SS, Gode KD. Pancreatic beta-cell regeneration in rats by (−)-epicatechin. *Lancet* 1981;2:759–60

74. Chakravarthy BK, Gupa S, Gode KD. Functional beta cell regeneration in the islets of pancreas in alloxan induced diabetic rats by (−)-epicatechin. *Life Sci* 1982;31:2693–7

75. Subramanian SS. (−)Epicatechin as an antidiabetic drug. *Ind Drugs* 1981;18:259

76. Allen FM. Blueberry leaf extract. Physiological and clinical properties in relation in carbohydrate metabolism. *J Am Med Assoc* 1927;89:1577–81

77. Scharrer A, Ober M. Anthocyanosides in the treatment of retinopathies. *Klin Monatsbl Augenheikd* 1981;178:386–9

78. Caselli L. Clinical and electroretinographic study on activity of anthocyanosides. *Arch Med Int* 1985;37:29–35

79. Devillers J, Boule P, Vasseur P, *et al.,* Enviromental and health risks of hydroquinone. *Ecotoxicol Environ Safety* 1990;19:327–54

80. Shibata MA, Hirose M, Tanaka H, Asakawa E, Shirai T, Ito N. Induction of renal cell tumors in rats and mice, and enhancement of hepatocellular tumor development in mice after long-term hydroquinone treatment. *Jpn J Cancer Res* 1991;82:1211–19

81. Offenbacher E, Stunyer F. Beneficial effect of chromium-riched yeast on glucose tolerance and blood lipids in elderly patients. *Diabetes* 1980;29:919–25

82. Mooradian AD, Failla M, Hoogwerf B. Selected vitamin and mineral in diabetes. *Diabetes Care* 1994;17:464–79

83. Baker B. Chromium supplements tied to glucose control. *Fam Practice News* 1996;15:5

84. Mertz M. Chromium occurrence and function in biologic systems. *Physiol Rev* 1969;49:163–237

85. Anderson R, *et al*. Beneficial effect of chromium for people with type 2 diabetes. *Diabetes* 1996;45:124A/454

86. Lee NA, Reasner CA. Beneficial effect of chromium supplementation on serum triglyceride levels in NIDDM. *Diabetes Care* 1994;17:1449–52

87. Joseph LJ, Farrell PA, Davey SL, *et al*. Effect of resistance training with or without chromium picolinate supplementation on glucose metabolism in older men and women. *Metabolism* 1999;48:546–53

88. Anderson RA, Bryden NA, Polansky M. Dietary chromium intake. Freely chosen diets, institutional diet, and individual foods. *Biol Trace Element Res* 1992;32:117

89. Castro VR. Chromium in a series of Portuguese plants used in the herbal treatment of diabetes. *Biol Trace Element Res* 1998;62:101–6

90. Nielsen FH. Chromium. In Shils ME, Olson JA, Shike M, eds. *Modern Nutrition in Health and Disease*, 8th edn. Philadelphia, PA: Lea & Febiger, 1994:264–8

91. Reading SA, Wecker L. Chromium picolinate. *J Fla Med Assoc* 1996;83:29–31

92. Stearns DM, Wetterhahn KE. Chromium (III) picolinate [letter, author's reply]. *FASEB J* 1996;10:367–9

93. Stearns DM, Belbruno JJ, Wetterhahn KE. A prediction of chromium (III) accumulation in humans from chromium dietary supplements. *FASEB J* 1995;9:1650–7

94. Stearns DM, Wise JP Sr, Patierno SR, Wetterhahn KE. Chromium (III) picolinate produces chromosome damage in Chinese hamster ovary cells. *FASEB J* 1995;9:1643–8

95. White JR, Campbell RK. Magnesium and diabetes. A review. *Ann Pharmacother* 1993;27:775–80

96. Mooradian AD, Morley JE. Micronutrient status in diabetes mellitus. *Am J Clin Nutr* 1987;45:877–95

97. Hegazi SM. Effect of zinc supplementation on serum glucose, insulin, glucose-6-phosphatase, and mineral levels in diabetics. *J Clin Biochem Nutr* 1992;12:209–15

98. Engel ED, Erlich NE, Davis RH. Diabetes mellitus. Impaired wound healing from zinc deficiency. *J Am Pediatr Assoc* 1981;71:536–44

99. Kelly GS. Insulin resistance: lifestyle and nutritional interventions. *Altern Med Rev* 2000;5:109–32

100. Tagliaferro V, Cassader M, Bozzo C, *et al*. Moderate guar-gum addition to usual diet improves peripheral sensitivity to insulin and lipaemic profile in NIDDM. *Diabetes Metab* 1985;11:380–5

101. Landin K, Holm G, Tengborn L, Smith U. Guar gum improves insulin sensitivity, blood lipids, blood pressure, and fibrinolysis in healthy men. *Am J Clin Nutr* 1992;56:1061–5

102. Fairchild RM, Ellis PR, Byrne AJ, *et al*. A new breakfast cereal containing guar gum reduces postprandial plasma glucose and insulin concentrations in normal-weight human subjects. *Br J Nutr* 1996;76:63–73

103. Vahouny G, Kritchevsky D. *Dietary Fiber in Health and Disease*. New York, NY: Plenum Press, 1982

104. Jenkins DJA, Wolever TMS, Bacon S, *et al*. Diabetic diets: high carbohydrate combined with high fiber. *Am J Clin Nutr* 1980;33:1729–33

105. Jenkins DJA, Wolever TMS, Taylor RH, *et al*. Glycemic index of foods: a physiological basis for carbohydrate exchange. *Am J Clin Nutr* 1981;24:362–6

106. Hui H. A review of treatment of diabetes by acupuncture during the past forty years. *J Trad Chin Med* 1995;15:145–54

107. Chen JF, Wei J. Changes of plasma insulin level in diabetics treated with acupuncture. *J Trad Chin Med* 1985;5:79–84

108. Wateri N. Reviews of presentation of the *7th World Congress of Acupuncture*, 1982:74

109. Lei ZP. Treatment of 42 cases of obesity with acupuncture. *J Trad Chin Med* 1988;8:125–6

110. Hooper PL. Hot-tub therapy for type 2 diabetes mellitus. *N Engl J Med* 1999;341:924–5

111. Hooper PL. Hot-tub therapy for type 2 diabetes mellitus. *N Engl J Med* 2000;342:218–19

Are there any remedies for obesity?

23

L. Dey and C.-S. Yuan

INTRODUCTION

Obesity is defined as body weight 30% over the ideal body weight. The body mass index (BMI) has emerged as an indicator of obesity[1,2]. BMI is defined as weight in kilograms divided by height in meters squared (i.e. $BMI = kg/m^2$, or $BMI = lb/in^2 \times 705$). The American Heart Association (AHA) has adopted the BMI as an indicator of adiposity. A person who has a BMI of > 25 kg/m^2 is considered overweight, and > 27 kg/m^2 is considered obese.

Obesity is a chronic condition that affects approximately one-third of the US population[3,4]. Obesity is the second leading cause of preventable death in the USA[4,5] and it causes or exacerbates many health problems, both independently and in association with other diseases. For example, it is associated with the development of coronary heart disease, type 2 diabetes, an increased incidence of several forms of cancer, respiratory complications (obstructive sleep apnea) and osteoarthritis of large and small joints[6].

The economic burden of the condition is substantial. The weight-loss industry accrues about $33 billion each year. The estimated medical costs of treating obesity are about $238 billion per year, of which approximately $100 billion covers the cost of treating co-morbid conditions[2].

FACTORS INFLUENCING OBESITY

Obesity is not a single disorder but a heterogeneous group of conditions with multiple causes. Body weight is determined by an interaction between genetic, environmental and psychological factors acting through the physiological mediators of energy intake and expenditure[6].

According to the first law of thermodynamics, obesity results from an imbalance between energy intake and energy expenditure. Energy expenditure can be divided into three major components: thermic effect of food; resting energy expenditure; and physical activity. The sympathetic nervous system controls part of the energy expenditure process[7].

Elements of the system that control obesity are also presented as a feedback model[8,9]: a controlled system that ingests, metabolizes and stores food; afferent signals (e.g. cholecystokinin and leptin) that tell the brain about the internal and external environment; the central controller in the brain (e.g. serotonin, adrenergic and noradrenergic receptors in the hypothalamus) that transduces messages from the periphery into action; and the efferent or action system (e.g. endocrine and autonomic nervous system).

ALTERNATIVE THERAPIES

Medicinal herbs

Ma huang (Ephedra)

Ma huang (Chinese name), also known as desert herb, contains ephedra, a compound that is similar to ephidrine. Dietary supplements that contain ephedra alkaloids (ma huang) are widely promoted and used in the

USA as a means of losing weight and increasing energy. Ephedra has been shown to increase heart rate, affect blood pressure variably and increase 24-h energy expenditure in humans[10]. These effects are probably associated with the thermogenic effect of direct β_1 and β_2 agonism[11].

Cardiovascular symptoms, such as hypertension, followed by palpitation, tachycardia, or both, and central nervous system side-effects, such as stroke and seizures, have been reported. Death and permanent disability have also been noted. The Food and Drug Administration (FDA) has proposed establishing limits on the dose and duration of the use of ephedra, owing to the recently reported adverse effects. The FDA also requested an independent review of reports of adverse events related to the use of supplements that contained ephedra alkaloids to assess causation and to estimate the level of risk posed by the use of these supplements to consumers[12]. Haller and Benowitz[12] reviewed 140 reports of adverse events related to the use of dietary supplements. Their report indicated that the use of dietary supplements that contain ephedra alkaloids may pose a health risk to some persons. These findings indicate the need for a better understanding of individual susceptibility to the adverse effects of such dietary supplements.

Ma huang is usually available in dried branchlets and tablet form, in combination with guarana (see below). Some commercial weight-reduction products (e.g. Metabolife®) contain a combination of ma huang and guarana. The usual dose for ma huang is 20 mg ephedrine equivalent, and for guarana is 200 mg caffeine equivalent, three times daily[13].

Guarana

Guarana is derived from the seeds of *Paullinia cupana*, and is also known as brazilian cocoa. It contains the chief alkaloid caffeine, in addition to small amounts of theophylline and theobromine. Guarana is used by Brazilian Indians in a stimulating beverage similar to coffee or tea. Several studies have shown that guarana may be effective in treating obesity when it is used with ma huang.

A controlled study of 180 obese patients showed significantly greater weight loss using guarana in combination with ma huang, over a 24-week period[14]. However, Breum and colleagues[15] reported that 54% of patients treated with the guarana and ma huang combination experienced central nervous system side-effects, especially agitation, but noted that these side-effects declined markedly after the first month of treatment. In another study, the hemodynamic side-effects, such as increased systolic, but not diastolic, blood pressure and increased heart rate, were transient, while the thermogenic effects on energy expenditure were persistent[16]. As mentioned above, the usual dose for guarana is 200 mg caffeine equivalent three times daily.

Garcinia cambogia and Garcinia indica

Garcinia cambogia and *Garcinia indica*, which is also known as brindleberry, is isolated from the fruit of the Malabar tamarind. It is native to southern India, where it is dried and used extensively in curries.

Garcinia cambogia and *Garcinia indica* are now incorporated into many commercial weight-loss products. Hydroxycitric acid is the active ingredient; it competitively inhibits the extramitochondrial enzyme adenosine triphosphate-citrate (pro-3S)-lyase. In many *in vitro* and *in vivo* studies, investigators have demonstrated that hydroxycitric acid not only inhibited the actions of the citrate cleavage enzyme and suppressed fatty acid synthesis[17], but also increased rates of hepatic glycogen synthesis[18], suppressed food intake[19] and decreased body weight gain[20].

Six published human studies have examined hydroxycitric acid in weight loss. Of these studies, five reported positive results, but all had experimental inadequacies[21]. A randomized controlled study over a 12-week period found no differences in weight loss between a group of obese individuals given 3000 mg of *Garcinia cambogia* (50% hydroxycitric acid) daily and a control group given placebo[21]. However, this study did not measure either the appetite-suppressant effect or the plasma concentration of hydroxycitric acid. Opponents of this study have postulated that the high-fiber diet used in the study may have limited the bioavailability, thus rendering the study ineffective and leading to the disappointing results[22]. It appears that hydroxycitrate may offer a safe, natural aid for weight loss when taken at a dose of 500 mg three times daily[23].

Green tea

Green tea has been widely consumed in China and Japan for many centuries. Using an *in vitro* intercapsular brown adipose tissue system, Dulloo and colleagues[24] showed that the effect of green tea on thermogenesis and fat oxidation may be attributed to an interaction between the high content of catechin polyphenols and caffeine[24]. In *in vivo* animal experiments, Kao and associates[25] demonstrated that green tea epigallocatechin gallate reduced food intake. Human studies by Dulloo and co-workers[26] observed that administration of capsules containing the green tea extract resulted in a significant increase in 24-h energy expenditure, thermogenesis, fat oxidation and urinary noradrenalin relative to placebo. These findings could be of value in assisting the management of obesity. The dosage used in the clinical study was green tea extract (50 mg caffeine and 90 mg epigallocatechin gallate). No adverse effects have been reported.

Gymnema sylvestre (gurmar)

The leaves of *Gymnema sylvestre* have been highly valued as folk medicine for diabetes in India for more than 2000 years[27]. Gymnemic acid, a mixture of triterpene glycosides extracted from the leaves of *Gymnema sylvestre*, can improve glucose tolerance and decrease the blood glucose level in diabetic patients[28,29]. On the basis of this effect, gymnemic acid has been suggested as a useful agent in therapy for obesity[30], since overingestion of carbohydrates is a well-documented cause of obesity. Wang and associates[31] observed that gymnemic acid also potently inhibited oleic acid absorption in the rat intestine, dose-dependently and reversibly. To date, no controlled studies have been conducted to evaluate the efficacy of *Gymnema* extract on obesity.

The recommended dose of *Gymnema* extract is 400 mg/day. An undesirable effect of this agent is that it reduces or abolishes the taste sensation of sweetness and bitterness[32].

Ginseng

There are over a dozen articles reporting the effects of ginseng on animal body-weight changes. However, in most cases, the reports on ginseng's body-weight effects were based on one of the measurements in the study, rather than being the primary goal of the project. Interestingly, these results are highly variable: six articles showed an increase in body-weight effect, three showed a decreased effect and another four showed no effect.

Several studies reported an increase in body weight after treatment with *Panax ginseng* root. Rats fed a diet containing purified ginseng saponin extract[33,34] and ginseng root extract[35,36] showed an increase in body weight. In addition, some studies reported that treatment with *Panax ginseng* extract or ginsenosides prevented stress-associated weight loss[37,38]. Other studies reported that *Panax ginseng* root had a body-weight-reducing effect. Park and co-workers[39] observed that red ginseng total saponins caused a significant drop in the body weight of rats. A single high dose of red ginseng total saponins significantly reduced the weight of rats and mice[40]. Administration of panaxatriol (isolated from *Panax ginseng* root) to healthy mice suppressed their maturity-associated increase in body weight[41]. Results of other studies failed to show an association between ginseng and body weight[42–45]. It is important to point out that these studies used different ginseng preparations and components in different animal species and models.

A clinical trial[46] that investigated anti-diabetic effects of ginseng root reported that, in addition to an improvement in fasting blood glucose levels, the subjects experienced a reduction in body weight. In this study of patients with type 2 diabetes, patients in both the control and the ginseng-treated group were encouraged to reduce body weight by exercise and food intake control. Thus, patients in the ginseng-treated group as well as the placebo group lost weight. It appears that the anti-obesity effect of ginseng is inconclusive.

The recommended daily ginseng dose is 1–2 g of the crude root, or 200–600 mg of standardized extracts[47]. As the possibility of hormone-like or hormone-inducing effects cannot be ruled out, some authors suggest limiting treatment to 3 months[47].

Kelp

Kelp generically refers to seaweed species including *Laminaria*, *Macrocystis*, *Nereocystis* and *Fucus*. It has been used as an anti-obesity agent presumably by supplying iodine, hence increasing thyroid hormone production with consequent increased metabolism and removal of fat. Iodine content is different in kelp products. Hyperthyroidism has been reported after the use of a kelp product[48]. Potassium iodide content may result in hypersensitivity reactions in sensitive patients. Concomitant use of kelp with levothyroxine could result in excessive replacement, producing typical symptoms of hyperthyroidism[49]. Since kelp and related seaweed products contain sodium, they should consequently be avoided by those who must restrict their salt intake. In addition, using any thyroid hormone-related product to control body weight is inadvisable and should be discouraged.

Capsaicin

Capsaicin is the major pungent principle in various species of capsaicin fruits, such as hot chilli peppers, and has long been globally used as an ingredient of spices, preservatives and medicines (Figure 1)[50].

Dietary supplementation of capsaicin in high-fat diets lowered the peripheral adipose tissue weight and serum triglyceride concentration in rats, owing to enhancement of energy metabolism[51,52]. Watanabe and co-workers[53,54] have investigated the neurophysiolgical functions of capsaicin and have demonstrated that capsaicin increases energy metabolism by catecholamine secretion from the adrenal medulla through sympathetic activation via the central nervous system. In a human study, Yoshioka and associates[55] observed

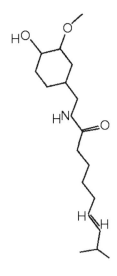

Figure 1 Chemical structure of capsaicin

that energy expenditure increased immediately after a meal containing red pepper, whereas this enhancement of energy metabolism by a red pepper diet was inhibited after the administration of the β-adrenergic blocker propranolol. In a recent human study, Matsumoto and co-workers[56] investigated the effect of capsaicin on sympathetic nervous system activity and energy metabolism in 16 lean and obese young women, matched for age and height. Their observation supported previous investigations and reinforced the finding that the altered specific sympathetic function related to thermogenic capacity may be a significant sign reflecting the autonomic state in human obesity. However, data from their study also indicated that the reduced sympathetic responsiveness to thermogenic perturbation such as that found in a diet including capsaicin, which may cause impaired diet-induced thermogenesis and further weight gain, could be an important etiological factor leading to obesity in young women. The dose in the study was 3 mg of capsaicin in spicy yellow curry sauce.

Guggul gum (gugulipid)

This resin from the myrrh species, in addition to being used as a cholesterol-lowering agent, is found in some over-the-counter diet products. Gugulipid has been shown to stimulate the release of endogenous thyroid hormone in rats[57], although there are no additional animal or human studies supporting this claim. Gugulipid is available in the extract form, powdered resin and concentrated tablets.

Nutritional supplements

Chromium

Chromium has lately gained a great deal of public attention as an aid to weight loss. One of the key goals for enhancing weight loss is to increase insulin sensitivity of cells throughout the body, on the basis that chromium plays an important role in cellular sensitivity to insulin[58].

Preliminary studies with chromium demonstrated that chromium picolinate promoted an increase in percentage of lean body weight and a decrease in percentage of body fat, which may lead to weight loss[58,59]. Greater muscle mass has greater fat-burning potential. Chromium supplementation also improves blood sugar control and lowers cholesterol and triglyceride levels[60].

Several forms of chromium are available, such as chromium picolinate, chromium polynicotinate, chromium chloride and chromium-enriched yeast. The recommended chromium dose is 200–400 μg daily[23]. There have been reports of possible tissue accumulation and damage to DNA and renal damage following long-term ingestion of large doses of chromium[61,62].

5-Hydroxytryptamine (serotonin)

There are three clinical studies with 5-hydroxytryptamine (5-HT) in overweight women[63–65] and these studies showed that 5-HT appeared to promote weight loss by promoting satiety, leading to fewer calories being consumed at meals. Besides mild nausea, no other side-effects were reported.

The recommended starting dose of 5-HT is 50–100 mg 20 min before meals for 2 weeks, and then double the dosage to a maximum of 300 mg if weight loss is less than 1 lb (0.45 kg) per week. Higher doses of 5-HT are associated with nausea, but this symptom disappears after 6 weeks of use[23].

L-Carnitine

L-Carnitine is an amino acid found in meat and dairy products; it is formed from the amino acids lysine and methionine, in the liver and kidney. Its proposed action is an increase in fat metabolism. Two studies have shown no changes in the rate of fat oxidation following L-carnitine supplementation[66,67]. Control studies examining the effects of L-carnitine on weight loss have not been published. Oral supplementation may cause diarrhea, but no other major adverse effects have been noted.

Medium-chain triglycerides

Medium-chain triglycerides are saturated fats (which can be extracted from coconut oil) whose chains range in length from six to 12 carbon atoms. Unlike regular fats and long-chain triglycerides, medium-chain triglycerides appear to promote weight loss rather than weight gain. They may promote weight loss by increasing thermogenesis[68]. A study demonstrated that oil of medium-chain triglycerides given over a 6-day period could increase diet-induced thermogenesis by 50%[69]. In order to gain the benefit from medium-chain triglycerides, a diet must remain low in long-chain triglycerides. Medium-chain triglycerides can be used as an oil for salad dressing or a bread spread, or simply be taken as a supplement. Dosage recommendation is 1–2 tablespoons per day. Diabetics and individuals with liver disease should be monitored very closely when using medium-chain triglycerides, as they may develop ketoacidosis.

Coenzyme Q10

Coenzyme Q_{10} is an essential compound required in the transport and breakdown of fatty acids into energy. In one study, coenzyme Q_{10} levels were found to be low in 52% of overweight subjects tested. In the study, nine subjects (five with low coenzyme Q_{10} levels and four with normal levels) were given 100 mg/day of coenzyme Q_{10} along with a low-calorie diet. After 9 weeks, mean weight loss in the coenzyme Q_{10}-deficient group was 29.7 lb (13.4 kg), compared with 12.8 lb (5.8 kg) in those with initially normal levels of coenzyme Q_{10}[70]. The recommended dose is 100–300 mg/day.

Chitosan

Chitosan is an amino polysaccharide derived from the powdered shells of marine crustaceans such as prawns and crabs. Some clinical studies have shown lipid-lowering effects[71], as well as weight loss[72–74]. The proposed action of chitosan is binding to dietary fat, preventing digestion and storage. However, in a recent controlled trial in 17 individuals, the weight-reduction effect of chitosan was not confirmed[75]. Risks such as steatorrhea and malabsorption of essential nutrients are possible.

Fiber

Increasing the amount of dietary fiber promotes weight loss. The best fiber sources for weight loss are psyllium, chitin, guar gum, glucumannan, gum karaya and pectin, which are rich in water-soluble fibers. When taken with water before meals, these fiber sources bind to water in the stomach to form a gelatinous mass, which induces a sense of satiety[23]. Fiber supplements have been shown to enhance blood sugar control, decrease insulin levels and reduce the number of calories absorbed by the body[76]. The most impressive results in studies of weight loss have been achieved with guar gum, a water-soluble fiber obtained from the Indian cluster bean (*Cyamopsis tetragonoloba*).

The starting dose should be between 1 and 2 g before meals and at bedtime, with gradual increase of the dose to 5 g[23]. Water-soluble fibers are fermented by intestinal bacteria; therefore, a great deal of gas can be produced, leading to increased flatulence and abdominal discomfort.

Acupuncture

One indication for acupuncture is obesity[77]. Ernst[78] reviewed the results of sham/placebo-controlled clinical trials of acupuncture/acupressure for obesity. His goal was to determine whether these therapies have specific effects on appetite and reduction of body weight. Two studies suggested a positive effect of acupuncture on appetite and body weight[79,80], whereas two other trials showed no effect of acupuncture or acupressure[81,82].

Richards and Marley[83] studied the effectiveness of transcutaneous electrical nerve stimulation of specific auricular acupuncture points on appetite suppression. They observed that frequent stimulation of a specific auricular acupuncture point was an effective method of appetite suppression, leading to weight loss. It has been postulated that acupuncture stimulation of certain parts of the ear can reduce appetite by activating the satiety center within the hypothalamus[84], or control stress and depression via endorphin and dopamine production[83].

CONCLUSIONS

In the USA, weight loss is a national obsession. Over one-third of all Americans are obese, and they spend over $30 billion annually to lose weight. Clinically, obesity is a serious medical disorder, because it can cause a myriad of health problems, such as heart disease, hypertension and adult-onset diabetes. Alternative therapies, especially herbal medicines, are increasingly used by obese people and some non-obese people who want to lose weight. Ephedra (ma huang) and ephedra-containing products are often effective, especially at high doses of ephedra alkaloids. However, ephedra may cause significant cardiovascular and central nervous system adverse effects, particularly in individuals with increased susceptibility to these effects. Most herbs and nutritional supplements are used in conjunction with prescription anti-obesity drugs. Potential adverse herb–drug interactions should also be kept in mind for patients who are receiving conventional pharmacological agents. In addition, since a single herb (e.g. ephedra) may be used in different commercial anti-obesity dietary preparations, consumers should not take more than one product simultaneously, to avoid any undesirable additive effects.

References

1. Hollander P. Strategies for reducing weight to increase insulin sensitivity. In *Drug Benefit Trends*. Darien, CT: Cliggott Publishing Co., Division of SCP/ Cliggott Communications, Inc. 2000; 12(Suppl A):57–65

2. Negro AD. *It's Time to Treat Obesity*. American Heart Association Scientific Sessions, 2000

3. Kuczmarski RJ, Carroll MD, Flegal KM, Troiano RP. Varying body mass index cutoff points to describe overweight prevalence among U.S. adults: NHANES III (1988–1994). *Obes Res* 1997;5:542–8

4. Flegal KM, Carroll MD, Kuczmarski RJ, Johnson CL. Overweight and obesity in the United States: prevalence and trends, 1960–1994. *Int J Obes* 1998;22:39–47

5. McGinnis JM, Forge WH. Actual causes of death in the United States. *J Am Med Assoc* 1993;270:2207–12

6. Kopelman PG. Obesity as a medical problem. *Nature (London)* 2000;404:635–51

7. de Jonge L, Bray GA. The thermic effect of food and obesity: a critical review. *Obes Res* 1997;5:622–31

8. Bray GA. Drug treatment of obesity: don't throw the baby out with the bath water. *Am J Clin Nutr* 1998;67:1–4

9. Bray GA. *Diabetes and Endocrinology Clinical Management*, vol 3. *Physiology and Consequences of Obesity*. New York, NY: Medscape, 2000

10. White LM, Gardner SF, Gurley BJ, Marx MA, Wang Pl. Pharmaco-kinetics and cardiovascular effects of ma-huang (*Ephedra sinica*) in normotensive adults. *J Clin Pharmacol* 1997;37:116–22

11. Shannon JR, Gottesdiener K, Jordan J, *et al.* Acute effect of ephidrine on 24-h energy balance. *Clin Sci (Colch)* 1999;96:483–91

12. Haller CA, Benowitz NL. Adverse cardiovascular and central ner-vous system events associated with dietary supplements containing ephedra alkaloids. *N Engl J Med* 2000;343:1833–8

13. Morelli V, Zoorob RJ. Alternative therapies: Part 1. Depression, diabetes, obesity. *Am Fam Physician* 2000;62:1051–60

14. Astrup A, Breum L, Toubro S, Hein P, Quadde F. The effect and safety of an ephedrine/caffeine compound compared to ephidrine, caffeine and placebo in obese subjects on an energy restricted diet. A double blind trial. *Int J Obes Relat Metab Disord* 1992;16:269–77

15. Breum L, Pedersen JK, Ahlstrom F, Frimodt-Moller J. Comparison of an ephedrinc/caffeine combination and dexfluramine in the treat-ment of obesity. A double-blind multi-center trial in general practice. *Int J Obes Relat Metab Disord* 1994;18:99–103

16. Astrup A, Toubro S. Thermogenic, metabolic and cardiovascular responses to ephedrine and caffeine in man. *Int J Obes Relat Metab Disord* 1993;17(Suppl 1):S41–3

17. Lowenstein JM. Effect of (−)-hydroxycitrate on fatty acid synthesis by rat liver *in vivo*. *J Biol Chem* 1971;246:629–32

18. Sullivan AC, Triscari J, Neal Miller O. The influence of (−)-hydroxy-citrate on *in vivo* rates of hepatic glycogenesis: lipogenesis and cholesterol genesis. *Fed Proc* 1974;33:656

19. Sullivan AC, Triscari J, Hamilton JG, Neal Miller O. Effect of (−)-hydroxycitrate upon the accumulation of lipid in the rat: appetite. *Lipids* 1973;9:129–34

20. Nageswara Rao R, Sakeriak KK. Lipid-lowering and antiobesity effect of (−) hydroxycitric acid. *Nutr Res* 1988;8:209–12

21. Heymsfield SB, Allison DB, Vasselli JR, Pietrobelli A, Greenfield D, Nunez C. *Garcinia cambogia* (hydroxycitric acid) as a potential antiobesity agent: a randomized controlled trial. *J Am Med Assoc* 1998;280:1596–600

22. Firenzuoli F, Gori L. *Garcinia cambogia* for weight loss. *J Am Med Assoc* 1999;282:234

23. Murray MT, Pizzorno JE Jr. Obesity. In Pizzorno JE Jr, Murray MT, eds. *Textbook of Natural Medicine*, 2nd edn. Churchill Living-stone, 1999;429–39

24. Dulloo AG, Seydoux J, Girardier L, Chantre P, Vandermander J. Green tea and thermogenesis: interactions between catechin-poly-phenols, caffeine and sympathetic activity. *Int J Obes* 2000;24:252–8

25. Kao YH, Hiipakka RA, Liao S. Modulation of endocrine systems and food intake by green tea epigallocatechin gallate. *Endocrinology* 2000;141:980–7

26. Dulloo AG, Duret C, Rohrer D, *et al.* Efficacy of a green tea extract rich in catechin polyphenols and caffeine in increasing 24-h energy expenditure and fat oxidation in humans. *Am J Clin Nutr* 1999;70:1040–5

27. Nadkarni KM. *Gymnema sylvestre*, R.Br. or *Asclepias geminata*. In Nadkarni KM, ed. *Indian Materia Medica*. Bombay: Popular Praka-shan, 1982;1:596–9

28. Baskaran, K, Kizar AB, Radha SK, Shanmugasundaram ER. Anti-diabetic effect of a leaf extract from *Gymnema sylvestre* in non-insulin dependent diabetes mellitus patients. *J Ethnopharmacol* 1990;30:295–300

29. Shanmugasundaram ER, Rajeswari G, Baskaran, K, Rajesh KBR, Radha SK, Kizar AB. Use of *Gymnema sylvestre* leaf extract in the control of blood glucose in insulin dependent diabetes mellitus. *J Ethnopharmacol* 1990;30:281–94

30. Terasawa H, Miyoshi M, Imoto T. Effects of long term administra-tion of *Gymnema sylvestre* watery-extract on variations of body weight, plasma glucose, serum triglyceride, total cholesterol and insulin in Wistar fatty rats. *Yonago Acta Med* 1994;37:117–27

31. Wang LF, Luo H, Imoto T, Hiji Y, Sasaki T. Inhibitory effect of gymnemic acid on intestinal absorption of oleic acid in rats. *Can J Physiol Pharmacol* 1998;76:1017–23

32. Mozersky RP. Herbal products and supplemental nutrients used in the management of diabetes. *J Am Osteopath Assoc* 1999;99:54–9

33. Rhee DK, Lim CJ, Kim DH, Hong SK, Park EH, Han YN. Studies on the acute and subacute toxicity of ginseng saponin. *Yakhak Hoe Chi* 1982;26:209–14

34. Rim KT, Choi JS, Lee SM, Cho KS. Effect of ginsenosides from red ginseng on the enzymes of cellular signal transduction system (Korean). *Koryo Insam Hakhoechi* 1997;21:19–27

35. Hong SA. Effects of *Panax ginseng* on the general behavioral activity and survival time of food deprivation in rats. *Ch'oesin Uihak* 1972;15:81–91

36. Eui S, Kim BY, Paik TH, Joo CN. The effect of ginseng on alcohol metabolism. *Hanguk Saenghwa Hakhoe Chi* 1978;11:1–15

37. Fujimoto K, Sakata T, Ishimaru T, et al. Attenuation of anorexia induced by heat or surgery during sustained administration of ginsenoside Rg$_1$ into rat third ventricle. *Psychopharmacology* 1989;99:257–60

38. Zierer R. Prolonged infusion of *Panax ginseng* saponins into the rat does not alter the chemical and kinetic profile of hormones from the posterior pituitary. *J Ethnopharmacol* 1991;34:269–74

39. Park CW, Kim JG, Lee YS, Kim GJ, Kim KS, Cho DH. Subacute toxicity study of red ginseng total saponin in rats. *J Toxicol Publ Health* 1998;14:77–82

40. Kim JG, Park CW, Lee YS, Kim JG, Kim KS, Cho DH. Acute toxicity study of red ginseng total saponin in rats and mice. *J Toxicol Publ Health* 1998;14:69–75

41. Kim YS, Kang KS, Kim S II. Effects of a cytotoxic substance, panaxytriol from *Panax ginseng* C.A. Meyer on the immune responses in normal mice. *Korean J Toxicol* 1990; 6:13–19

42. Hong BJ, Kim CI, Kim UH, Rhee YC. Effect of feeding ginseng crude saponin on body weight gain and reproductive function in chicken. *Hanguk Ch'uksan Hakhoe Chi* 1976;18:355–61

43. Hess FG Jr, Parent RA, Cox GE, Stevens KR, Beci PJ. Reproduction study in rats of ginseng extract G115. *Food Chem Toxicol* 1982;20:189–92

44. Hess FG Jr, Parent RA, Stevens KR, Cox GE, Becci PJ. Effects of subchronic feeding of ginseng extract G115 in beagle dogs. *Food Chem Toxicol* 1983;21:95–7

45. Murphy LL, Cadena RS, Chavez D, Ferraro JS. Effect of American ginseng (*Panax quinquefolium*) on male copulatory behavior in the rat. *Physiol Behav* 1998;64:445–50

46. Sotaniemi EA, Haapakoski E, Rautio A. Ginseng therapy in non-insulin-dependent diabetic patients. *Diabetes Care* 1995;18:1373–75

47. Schulz V, Hansel R, Tyler VE. Rational phytotherapy. In *Agents that Increase Resistance to Diseases*. New York, NY: Springer-Verlag, 1998:269–72

48. Foster S, Tyler VE, eds. *Tyler's Honest Herbal. A Sensible Guide to the Use of Herbs and Related Remedies*, 4th edn. Binghamton, NY: Haworth Press, 1999:233–9

49. Miller LG. Herbal medications, nutraceuticals, and diabetes. In Miller LG, Murray WJ, eds. *Herbal Medicinals, A Clinician's Guide*. Binghamton, NY: Pharmaceutical Products Press, Imprint of Haworth Press, 1998:115–33

50. Suzuki T, Iwai K. Constituents of red pepper spices: chemistry, pharmacology and food science of the pungent principle of *Capsicum* species. In Bross A, ed. *The Alkaloids*. New York, NY: Academic Press, 1984;23:227–9

51. Kawada T, Hagiharaa K, Iwai K. Effects of capsaicin on lipid metabolism in rats fed a high fat diet. *J Nutr* 1986;116:1272–8

52. Kawada T, Watanabe T, Takaishi T, Tanaka T, Iwai K. Capsaicin-induced β-adrenergic action on energy metabolism in rats: influence of capsaicin on oxygen consumption, the respiratory quotient, and substrate utilization. *Proc Soc Exp Biol Med* 1986;183:250–6

53. Watanabe T, Kawada T, Iwai K. Enhancement by capsaicin of energy metabolism in rats through secretion of catecholamine from adrenal medulla. *Agric Biol Chem* 1987;51:75–9.

54. Watanabe T, Kawada T, Kurosawa M, Sato A, Iwai K. Adrenal sympathetic efferent nerve and catecholamine secretion excitation caused by capsaicin in rats. *Am J Physiol* 1988;255:E23–7

55. Yoshioka M, Lim K, Kikuzato S, et al. Effects of red-pepper diet on the energy metabolism in men. *J Nutr Sci Vitaminol* 1995;41:647–56

56. Matsumoto T, Miyawaki C, Ue H, Yuasa T, Miyasuji A, Moritani T. Effects of capsaicin-containing yellow curry sauce on sympathetic nervous system activity and diet-induced thermogenesis in lean and obese young women. *J Nutr Sci Vitaminol* 2000;46:309–15

57. Tripathi YB, Malhotra OP, Tripathi SN. Thyroid stimulation action of Z-guggulsterone obtained from *Commiphora mukul*. *Planta Med* 1984;1:78–80

58. Anderson RA. Effects of chromium on body composition and weight loss. *Nutr Rev* 1998;56:266–70

59. Evans GW. Chromium picolinate is an efficacious and safe supplement. *Int J Sport Nutr* 1993;3:117–22

60. Press RI, Gellaer J, Evans GW. The effect of chromium picolinate on serum cholesterol and apolipoprotein fractions in human subjects. *West J Med* 1993;152:41–5

61. Stearns DM, Belbruno JJ, Wetterhahn KE. A prediction of chromium (III) accumulation in humans from chromium dietary supplements. *FASEB J* 1995;9:1650–7

62. Cerulli J, Grabe DW, Gauthier l, Malone M, McGoldrick MD. Chromium picolinate toxicity. *Ann Pharmacother* 1998;32:428–31

63. Ceci F, Cangiano C, Cairella M, et al. The effects of oral 5-hydroxytryptophan administration on feeding behavior in obese adult female subjects. *J Neural Transm* 1989;76:109–17

64. Cangiano C, Ceci F, Cairella M, et al. Effects of 5-hydroxytryptophan on eating behavior and adherence to dietary prescriptions in obese adult subjects. *Adv Exp Med Biol* 1991;294:591–3

65. Cangiano C, Ceci F, Cascino A, et al. Eating behavior and adherence to dietary prescriptions in obese adult subjects treated with 5-hydroxytryptophan. *Am J Clin Nutr* 1992;56:863–7

66. Sulkers EJ, Lafeber HN, Degenhart HJ, Przyrembel H, Schlotzer E, Sauer PJ. Effects of high carnitine supplementation on substrate utilization in low-birth-weight infants receiving total parenteral nutrition. *Am J Clin Nutr* 1990;52:889–94

67. Vukovich MD, Costill DL, Fink WJ. Carnitine supplementation: effect on muscle carnitine and glycogen content during exercise. *Med Sci Sports Exerc* 1994;26:1122–9

68. Baba N, Bracco EF, Hashim SA. Enhanced thermogenesis and diminished deposition of fat in response to overfeeding with diet containing medium chain triglyceride. *Am J Clin Nutr* 1982;35:678–82

69. Hill JO, Peters JC, Yang D, et al. Thermogenesis in humans during over feeding with medium-chain triglycerides in man. *Am J Clin Nutr* 1986;44:630–34

70. Van Gaal L. Exploratory study of coenzyme Q$_{10}$ in obesity. In Folkers K, Yamamura Y, eds. *Biomedical and Clinical Aspects of Coenzyme Q$_{10}$*. Amsterdam: Elsevier Science, 1984;4:369–73

71. Ventura P. Lipid lowering activity of chitosan, a new dietary integrator. In Muzzarelli RAA, ed. *Chitin Enzymology*. Ancona, Italy: Atec Edizioni, 1996;2:55–62

72. Maezaki Y, Tsuji K. Hypochlosterolaemic effect of chitosan in adult males. *Biosc Biochem Biotech* 1993;57:1439–44

73. Abelin J, Lassus AL. *112 Bipolymar- Fat [Binder] as a Weight Reducer in Patients with Moderate Obesity*. Medical research report. A study performed at Ars Medicinar, Heisinki, August–October, 1994

74. Veneroni G, Veneroni F, Contos S. Effect of a new chitoson on hyperlipidaemia and overweight in obese patients. In Muzzarelli RAA, ed. *Chitin Enzymology*. Ancona, Italy: Atec Edizioni, 1996;2:63–7

75. Pittler MH, Abbot NC, Harkness EF, Ernst E. Randomized, double-blind trial of chitosan for body weight reduction. *Eur J Clin Nutr* 1999;53:379–81

76. Spiller GA. *Dietary Fiber in Health and Nutrition*. Boca Raton, FL: CRC Press, 1994

77. Cassell DK, Larocca FE. *The Encyclopedia of Obesity and Eating Disorders*. New York, NY: Fact on File, 1994

78. Ernst E. Acupuncture/acupressure for weight reduction? A systemic review. *Wien Klin Wochenschr* 1997;109:60–2

79. Giller RM. Auricular acupuncture and weight reduction. A controlled study. *Am J Acupuncture* 1975;3:151–3

80. Shafshak TS. Electroacupuncture and exercise in body weight reduction and their application in rehabilitating patients with knee osteoarthritis. *Am J Clin Med* 1995;13:15–25

81. Mok MS, Parker LN, Voina S, Bray GA. Treatment of obesity by acupuncture. *Am J Clin Nutr* 1976;29:832–5

82. Allison DB, Krie K, Heshka S, Heymsfield SB. A randomised placebo-controlled clinical trial of an acupressure device for weight loss. *Int J Obes* 1995;19:653–8

83. Richards D, Marley J. Stimulation of auricular acupuncture points in weight loss. *Aust Fam Physician* 1998;27(Suppl 2):73–7

84. Huang MH, Yang RC, Hu SH. Preliminary results of triple therapy for obesity. *Int J Obes* 1996;20:830–6

Warning: adverse effects of ephedra-containing dietary supplements

24

H. H. Aung, L. Dey and C.-S. Yuan

ADVERSE EFFECTS OF EPHEDRA-CONTAINING SUPPLEMENTS

In the USA, weight loss is a national obsession. Over 60% of American adults are either overweight or obese[1]. It is estimated that one-half of women and one-third of men are trying to lose weight at any given time, and spend over $33 billion annually to lose weight[2,3]. Successful weight loss and healthy weight management depend on long-term lifestyle changes, such as reducing calorie consumption and increasing physical activity. However, because these changes are difficult to achieve and current pharmacological treatment has limitations, easily obtainable, non-prescription weight-loss herbal products become an alternative to consumers. Since herbal product exposure has increased through television, magazines and the Internet, it is not surprising that weight-loss dietary supplements are popular among obese people.

In the past several years, ephedra has gained popularity as a weight-loss aid. In 1998, 2% of obese Americans and 1% of the general population took over-the-counter weight-loss products containing ephedra[4]. In 2000, ephedra was one of the most commonly used herbs in the USA, with over 3 billion servings of ephedra products consumed[5]. These figures are likely to increase in the future, particularly in light of the recent withdrawal of phenylpropanolamine, another popular over-the-counter drug for weight loss, from the market. Ephedra-containing products are targeted not only toward the obese, but also

toward the non-obese, for boosting energy level and enhancing athletic performance.

EFFECTS OF EPHEDRA

Ephedra, known as ma huang in Chinese, is a traditional Chinese medicine used to treat respiratory conditions, such as asthma and bronchitis. Most ephedra used in the USA is imported from China. Ephedra contains alkaloids including ephedrine, pseudoephedrine, norephedrine, methylephedrine and norpseudoephedrine[6].

Ephedrine, the predominant active compound, is a non-catecholamine sympathomimetic agent. It exhibits α_1, β_1 and β_2 activities by acting directly at adrenergic receptors and indirectly by releasing endogenous norepinephrine (noradrenaline) from sympathetic neurons. Ephedrine has caused dose-dependent increases in blood pressure and heart rate[7], with an elimination halflife of approximately 5–6 h[8]. However, ephedra alkaloids inconsistently increased heart rate and blood pressure in healthy, normotensive volunteers after a single dose[9].

Ephedra products have stimulant properties and are purported to decrease weight when used in combination with other herbs, through thermogenesis and reduced appetite. It is believed that, at the appropriate dose (limited to 24 mg/day), ephedra, in combination with caffeine, is effective and may be used in physician-monitored programs for patients who are not at high risk for certain cardiovascular and cerebrovascular disorders[10,11]. In a randomized controlled trial, an ephedra–caffeine preparation produced significant weight loss in obese subjects[12]. In that study, however, 23% of the actively treated subjects withdrew because of side-effects.

Ephedra has also gained popularity as an ergogenic (physical performance enhancing) aid. Individual ephedrine alkaloids did not affect physical performance[13], but the combination of ephedrine and caffeine improved physical performance as determined by exercise time to exhaustion[14]. This combination of ephedrine and caffeine may be unsafe, because it also causes greater tachycardia than either placebo or ephedrine alone. Moreover, ephedrine is a banned substance in amateur sporting events and is likely to disqualify athletes in drug-tested events[13].

ADVERSE EFFECTS OF EPHEDRA

The use of ephedra has raised serious safety concerns. Haller and Benowitz reviewed 140 adverse event reports submitted to the US Food and Drug Administration (FDA) related to the use of dietary supplements containing ephedra alkaloids[15]. They observed that 31% of cases were considered to be related to the use of these supplements and another 31% were deemed to be possibly related. Among the adverse events, 47% involved cardiovascular symptoms and 18% involved the central nervous system[15]. Most of these adverse events have occurred in healthy young or middle-aged adults who used ephedra for losing weight and increasing energy[16]. In at least one case, ephedra was also associated with eosinophilic myocarditis[17].

Recently, an updated review of the FDA's Center for Food Safety and Applied Nutrition's Special Nutritionals Adverse Event Monitoring System (SN/AEMS) reported that there were 3308 adverse events for all dietary supplements between 1993 and 2001, of which 42% were associated with ephedra alkaloid dietary supplements[18]. Adverse events associated with dietary supplements containing ephedra alkaloids coincide with known effects of sympathomimetic agents on various organ systems[19,20]. It is essential that the adverse event data for ephedrine should be considered along with the growing body of evidence indicating that ephedra-containing dietary supplements may not be safe. Potential adverse effects associated with ephedra-containing dietary supplements are listed in Table 1.

Long-term use of sympathomimetic agents such as ephedrine alkaloids, even at very low levels, could cause serious adverse events, including cardiomyopathy and myocardial necrosis, which can result in death[21–23]. Thus, ephedrine use may lead to the cardiomyopathy typically seen with catecholamine excess[24]. In addition, use of ephedrine alkaloids during periods of intense physical activity resulted in enhanced or synergestic actions on the sympathetic nervous system[23]. It has also been shown that ephedrine alkaloids down-regulate the β-adrenergic receptor, which may cause refractory hypotension after anesthesia[25–27]. Extended use also results in tachyphylaxis from depletion of endogenous catecholamine stores and may contribute to perioperative hemodynamic instability[28].

Table 1 Potential adverse effects associated with ephedra-containing dietary supplements. From references 18, 19, 48–51

Organ systems	Potential adverse effects
General manifestations	numbness, tingling, dizziness, fatigue, lethargy, weakness, myopathy
Cardiovascular effects	mild to severe hypertension, palpitation, tachycardia, arrhythmias, angina, myocardial infarct, cardiac arrest, myocarditis, sudden death
Central nervous system effects	stroke (secondary to intracranial and subarachnoid hemorrhage, vasculitis and ischemia), seizures, transient ischemic attack
Neuropsychiatric effects	anxiety, nervousness, tremor, hyperactivity, insomnia, altered behavior, memory changes, altered or loss of consciousness, mania, psychosis, suicide
Gastrointestinal effects	nausea, vomiting, diarrhea, constipation, altered liver enzymes, hepatitis, ischemic colitis
Renal effects	urinary retention, renal stones, rhabdomyolysis, leading to acute renal failure
Dermatological reactions	rashes, exfoliative dermatitis

Cytotoxicity data showed that ephedra extract had a higher neurocytotoxic potential than a standardized dose of synthetic ephedrine hydrochloride alone[29]. These authors suggested that this increased toxic effect might be attributable to the combination of different ephedrine alkaloids or to other unknown compounds present in the ephedra extract, but not present in pure synthetic ephedrine. Adverse events may also occur from various herbal products found in combination with ephedra. More research is required on the effects of the combined herbal products.

Ephedra-containing dietary supplements are widely used worldwide, and the reported number of adverse events are relatively small. However, adverse events could be underreported, as there is no central mechanism for mandatory reporting, as there is for conventional medications[28]. Other contributing factors to underreporting are the possibilities that physicians do not recognize adverse events[30] and that patients are reluctant to report and seek treatment for adverse reactions associated with dietary supplements[31].

In 1997, the FDA proposed restrictions on dietary supplements containing ephedrine alkaloids with a labelling statement that instructs ephedra users to seek the advice of a health-care provider[32]. In particular, the agency proposed:

(1) To restrict the amount of ephedrine alkaloids in dietary supplements to 8 mg or less;

(2) To limit the intake of ephedra alkaloids to 8 mg in a 6-h period and 24 mg in a day;

(3) To require a warning against use for more than 7 days;

(4) To require the label statement 'Taking more than the recommended serving may result in heart attack, stroke, seizure, or death';

(5) To prohibit the combination of ephedrine alkaloids with other stimulants[16].

These proposals were subsequently withdrawn, owing to criticisms by the General Accounting Office that additional evidence was needed to support these restrictions[33]. However, the FDA continues to monitor adverse events associated with the use of products containing ephedra[4,34]. In addition, a Canadian government agent has issued a public advisory statement, warning consumers not to use products containing ephedra[35]. Some US states have individually adopted regulations similar to those proposed by the FDA. Recently, a public citizen's health research group petitioned the FDA to ban the production and sale of ephedra-containing dietary supplements[18].

INDIVIDUAL RISK FACTORS

Although the reported number of ephedra-induced adverse events is relatively low, the severity of the events, such as permanent disability or death in young, otherwise healthy individuals, signals a high risk. Cardiovascular adverse effects associated with ephedra are not limited to massive doses[36]; ephedra-induced serious adverse effects can occur in susceptible people even at low doses.

It has been shown that genes that control metabolic functions, receptor numbers and types may influence individual susceptibility to sympathomimetic agents[32]. Table 2 shows that ephedrine alkaloids may pose a significant health risk to a selected population. For example, use of ephedra in diabetic patients could result in adverse effects, especially in the presence of uncontrolled hypertension[4]. Other factors that may influence sensitivity to ephedra, similar to sympathomimetic agents, are also shown in Table 2. These findings indicate the need for a better understanding of individual susceptibility to ephedra-containing dietary supplements.

POTENTIAL EPHEDRA–DRUG AND EPHEDRA–HERB INTERACTIONS

The adverse effects of ephedra may be considerably greater in combination with other medications. Patients on many hypertensive drugs may be more sensitive to vasoconstrictors, such as ephedra, and loss of blood pressure control may result[19]. Some herbs

Table 2 Patients' medical conditions and factors that may increase susceptibility to ephedra alkaloids or other sympathomimetic agents

Patients' conditions	Possible adverse effects
Pre-existing coronary occlusive disease*	myocardial infarction due to constriction of coronary arteries, coronary vasospasm and positive inotropic and chronopic effects on the heart[52,53]; cardiac arrhythmias due to adrenergic effects of ephedrine, shortening cardiac refractory periods
Hypertension	further increase in blood pressure due to peripheral vasoconstriction and cardiac stimulation[31]
Cerebrovascular disease and seizure disorders	enhanced ephedra susceptibility[32]
Neuropsychiatric disease	depression, anxiety and schizophrenia, enhancing susceptibility[32]
Diabetes	promotion of hyperglycemia due to enhancing gluconeogenesis and glycogenolysis, and inhibiting insulin and glycogen synthase[54]
Hyperthyroidism	increased susceptibility[55]
Autonomic insufficiency	augmenting of pressure response to stimulants; damage to nerves controlling blood vessels, resulting in increased sensitivity to sympathomimetics' constricting effects[56]
Renal disease	reduction of rate of drug elimination[55]
Prostate disease	acute urinary retention due to prostatic hypertrophy[57]
Narrow-angle glaucoma	enhanced susceptibility[32,58]
Genetics	increased susceptibility, particularly in those with genes controlling metabolic function, receptor numbers and types[32]
Elderly	increased cariovascular sensitivity; urinary retention[19]
Children	central stimulant or sedative[19]
Pregnancy	ephedra crossing the placenta and increasing fetal heart rate and beat-to-beat variability[59]; increased rate of congenital malformations[59]
Lactation	infant toxicity via breast milk[60,61]
Hyperdynamic or exercise	augmenting cardiovascular stress; sympathetic nervous system activation, leading to increased blood pressure and heart rate[62,63]
Long-term use	cardiomyopathy even at low doses, possibly due to catecholamine-mediated cytotoxicity, and myocardial necrosis that can result in death[53,64,65]

*However, underlying cardiovascular disease is not a prerequisite for ephedra-related adverse events[36]

can also increase the likelihood, frequency and severity of the adverse effects of ephedra. Potential ephedra–drug and ephedra–herb interactions are summarized in Tables 3 and 4, respectively.

VARIABILITY IN EPHEDRA-CONTAINING DIETARY SUPPLEMENTS

Safety concerns are greatly heightened when herbal preparations with unknown concentrations of the active ingredients are consumed. Variations in composition are very common in dietary supplements. The active ingredients are not identified unequivocally and their presence or amount is not consistent from batch to batch. In addition, because of a lack of good agricultural practice standards, herbal products in one geographic location may differ from a similar product in another location with respect to active dose, ingredients and bioactivity. For example, 11 of

20 ephedra supplements tested failed to list the ephedrine alkaloid content on the label, or there was more than 20% difference between the actual amount and the amount listed on the label[6]. The dose of ephedrine alkaloids found in prescription or over-the-counter medications is constant and known, but such consistency is not found in ephedra-containing dietary supplements. Variability of ephedrine content per dosage unit in different ephedra products was highly significant (Figure 1).

Pharmacological activities of herbal medications have been observed in both animal studies and human clinical trials. However, the increasing variety of marketed dietary supplement products and the use of multiple herbs with variable phytochemical contents in a given product make conducting well-controlled clinical trials difficult and make comparison between data from different trials undependable. Providing a consistent dose of the active ingredients is a challenge to the herbal industry.

Table 3 Potential ephedra/ephedrine–drug interactions

Drugs	Potential interactions
Caffeine	synergistic adverse effects to enhance cardiovascular and central nervous system effects, by competitively antagonizing the receptors for adenosine, leading to blood vessel constriction and increase of catecholamine release[66]; increase in an individual's susceptibility to adverse events, such as stroke[67]
Theophylline	increase in adverse effects of theophylline without enhancing therapeutic response[68]
Phenelzine, tranylcypromine and other monoamine oxidase inhibitors	acute hypertensive crisis (marked headache, severe hypertension and stroke), vasculitis, necrotizing angiitis and ischemia[69]; marked increase in risk of sympathomimetic activities[70]
Amphetamine	necrotizing angiitis and ischemic strokes[22,67]
Fluoxetine, paroxetine and other selective serotonin reuptake inhibitors	excessive serotonergic activity and serotonin syndrome (changes in mental status, hypertension, restlessness, myoclonus, hyper-reflexia, diaphoresis, shivering and tremor)[71]
Cold remedies containing pseudoephedrine	increased susceptibility to adverse events, such as stroke[32]; serotonin syndrome[71]
Phenylpropanolamine*	increased susceptibility to adverse events, such as stroke[72,73]
Sibutramine	enhanced adverse effects due to stimulation of norepinephrine and dopamine release at nerve terminals[70]
Phentermine	development of serotonin syndrome and enhanced adverse effects due to noradrenergic and serotonergic actions[70]
Thiazides, furosemide	increased risk of arrhythmias due to depletion of body potassium[32]
Propranolol, timolol, and other non-selective β-receptor blocking agents	development of severe hypertensive reaction and/or marked bradycardia due to unopposed α-vasoconstriction and increased reflex vagal tone[19]
Halothane	development of intraoperative ventricular arrhythmias due to halothane, sensitizing the myocardium to ventricular arrhythmias caused by exogenous catecholamines[74]
Sodium bicarbonate, aluminum hydroxide and other urinary alkanizers	prolonged ephedra effect by reducing elimination rate, owing to alkalination of urine[75]
Guanethidine	decreased effect of guanethidine[58]; antagonism of the hypotensive action of guanethidine by interfering with its uptake into adrenergic neurons[76]

* Phenylpropanolamine, a sympathomimetic agent, is an ingredient used in prescription and over-the-counter (OTC) drug products. Since the compound could have an independent risk factor for hemorrhagic stroke in women[77], the Food and Drug Administration ordered that phenylpropanolamine-containing OTC medications be removed from the market[78]

ABUSE POTENTIAL OF EPHEDRA-CONTAINING DIETARY SUPPLEMENTS

Marketers of ephedra say it will produce euphoria, enhance energy levels, aid in weight loss, heighten awareness, or increase sexual sensations[37]. Herbal 'ecstasy' (the street name for 4-methyl-2-dimethoxy-amphetamine) is an alternative drug of abuse usually containing both ephedrine and caffeine. Many products containing ephedra combined with guarana or kola nut (caffeine sources) are available on the market with different street names[35]. Such products are shrewdly marketed on the Internet and in magazines targeting those leading alternative lifestyles. They can be easily obtained in unrestricted quantities via mail order. It has been reported that more than 150 million pills of 'herbal ecstasy' have been sold in 4 years[38]. In particular, a stimulant overdose syndrome has been reported in children and teenagers who have used these products[20].

Ephedra-containing dietary supplements often contain a combination of different ephedrine alkaloids, including norpseudoephedrine, a schedule IV controlled substance. These dietary supplements have the ability to mimic the effects of amphetamines[39]. In a study of the physiological and behavioral effects of ephedrine, data showed that ephedrine was able to produce subjective effects similar to those of amphetamines and, therefore, the authors proposed that they had comparable abuse potential[40]. Although it is a single alkaloid, ephedrine has a less addictive profile than amphetamines[41]; its effects are potentiated by the concomitant use of caffeine. In fact, the combination of ephedrine and caffeine at individually subthreshold quantities is synergistically able to produce an effect that is similar to that of amphetamines[42]. This is especially significant, because many ephedra-containing dietary supplements often contain caffeine or other stimulants. Illicit use of ephedrine as a cheap alternative to amphetamines has been shown to induce

Table 4 Potential ephedra/ephedrine–herb interactions

Herbs	Potential interactions
Guarana, green tea, verbamate, kola nut, and other caffeine-containing herbs[79,80]	same as caffeine in Table 3
Senna, aloe, buckthorn and other laxative herbs	increased risk of arrhythmias due to depletion of body potassium[32,81]
Uva ursi, and other diuretic herbs	increased risk of arrhythmias due to depletion of body potassium[32,82]
St John's wort	increased risk of adverse effects by inhibition of monoamine oxidase activity, and augmented effects of catecholamines released by ephedra[83,84]
Synephrine and octopamine, citrus aurantium and other natural sources of adrenergic agonists	elevated mean arterial blood pressure and augmented cardiovascular effects[85]
Ginseng	increased hypertension and central nervous system (CNS) stimulation[86]
Willow bark	increased risk of adverse effects due to salicin, reducing renal clearance and rate of ephedrine elimination[52]
Yohimbine and other α-selective adrenoreceptor blocking agents	enhanced elevating blood pressure, heart rate, tremor and anxiety due to stimulation of CNS[87,88]

myocardial infarction in an individual with a history of substance abuse[43].

The SN/AEMS data include reports of addiction, withdrawal and dependence. Some women reported continued use of ephedra-containing products despite adverse effects of withdrawal symptoms such as fatigue and weight gain[18]. Furthermore, seven of 36 users described ephedrine dependence[44]. In April 1996, the FDA issued a public health warning to consumers not to purchase or consume compounds portrayed as alternatives to illegal street drugs such as 'ecstasy'[37]. Interestingly, while ephedra-containing dietary supplements are readily available in the USA without prescription, ephedra's potential for abuse is much more emphasized in China, owing to the fact that chemical structure modification can turn ephedra into an illicit substance (Dr J.J. Yin of the FDA, personal communication).

COMMENTS

The continuing increase in the rate of obesity in the USA and the attractiveness and ease of obtaining weight loss herbals will probably increase the use of herbal products. Consumers often assume that dietary supplements are from natural sources and, thus, have no adverse effects even at high doses. Many patients may not inform their physicians about the use of herbal products, including the use of ephedra-containing

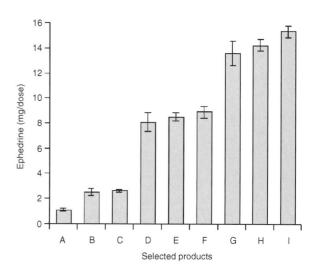

Figure 1 Variability of ephedrine content in selected ephedra products. Data adapted from reference 6

dietary supplements. Although the beneficial effects of herbal medications are documented[45], of primary importance to physicians are issues of herbal safety, potential herb–drug interactions and herb–herb interactions[28,46]. Therefore, there is a great need for health-care professionals to take an active role in educating themselves to enable them to help their patients make appropriate choices. Questioning patients about consumption of herbal products should be part of routine medical visits.

In anti-obesity combat, the main goal of the patients and their health-care providers should be to improve health by reducing co-morbid risk factors rather than to achieve dramatic weight loss. The risks of not managing obesity should be compared with the potential risks of ephedra. When considering using ephedra, the patient's age and lifestyle, concomitant disease states and medications should be taken into consideration. For example, the correlation between body mass index and mortality may weaken with increasing age, and it is unknown whether weight loss in patients over 65 years will prolong life.[47] It seems that the benefits should also be weighed carefully against the potential adverse effects of ephedra.

Unlike vitamins and minerals, ephedra alkaloid supplements are not essential for proper nutrition[15]. Therefore, it seems inappropriate to call products containing ephedra alkaloids a dietary supplement. Data from the SN/AEMS, the American Association of Poison Control Centers and the medical literature indicate that ephedra-containing dietary supplements present an unreasonable risk of illness and injury to American consumers. Because herbal products are not currently subject to the same rigorous FDA regulations required for prescription and over-the-counter products, and because there is no central mechanism for mandatory reporting of herbal adverse effects as there is for conventional medications, there is a potential unknown risk when taking ephedra-containing products. Based on reported risks and adverse effects and potential drug interactions, ephedra-containing weight-loss products should not be used indiscriminately.

References

1. National Institutes of Health. *Clinical Guidelines on the Identification, Evaluation, and Treatment of Overweight and Obesity in Adults*. Bethesda, MD: Department of Health and Human Services; National Institutes of Health; National Heart, Lung, and Blood Institute, 1998

2. Wolf AM, Colditz GA. The cost of obesity: the US perspective. *Pharmacoeconomics* 1994;5(Suppl 1):34–7

3. Serdula MK, Mokdad AH, Williamson DF, Galuska DA, Mendlein JM, Heath GW. Prevalence of attempting weight loss and strategies for controlling weight. *J Am Med Assoc* 1999;282:1353–8

4. Blanck HM, Khan LK, Serdula MK. Use of nonprescription weight loss products: results from a multistate survey. *J Am Med Assoc* 2001;286:930–5

5. Ephedra Education Council website. Available at: http://www.ephedrafacts.com. (Accessed 3 December 2001)

6. Gurley BJ, Gardner SF, Hubbard MA. Content versus label claims in ephedra-containing dietary supplements. *Am J Health Syst Pharm* 2000;57:963–9

7. Hoffman BB, Lefkowitz RJ. Catecholamines, sympathomimetic drugs, and adrenergic receptor antagonists. In Hardman JG, Gilman AG, Limbird LE, eds. *Goodman and Gilman's The Pharmacological Basis of Therapeutics*, 9th edn. New York, NY: McGraw-Hill, 1996: 199–248

8. Gurley BJ, Gardner SF, White LM, Wang PL. Ephedrine pharmacokinetics after the ingestion of nutritional supplements containing *Ephedra sinica* (ma huang). *Ther Drug Monit* 1998;20:439–45

9. White LM, Gardner SF, Gurley BJ, Marx MA, Wang PL, Estes M. Pharmacokinetics and cardiovascular effects of ma-huang (*Ephedra sinica*) in normotensive adults. *J Clin Pharmacol* 1997;37:116–22

10. Astrup A, Breum L, Toubro S, Hein P, Quaade F. The effect and safety of an ephedrine/caffeine compound compared to ephedrine, caffeine, and placebo in obese subjects on an energy restricted diet: a double blind trial. *Int J Obes Relat Metab Disord* 1992;16:269–77

11. Astrup A, Toubro S, Cannon S, Hein P, Madsen J. Thermogenic synergism between ephedrine and caffeine in healthy volunteers: a double-blind, placebo controlled study. *Metabolism* 1997;40:323–9

12. Boozer CN, Nasser JA, Heymsfield SB, Wang V, Chen G, Solomon JL. An herbal supplement containing ma huang-guarana for weight loss: a randomized, double-blind trial. *Int J Obes* 2001;25:316–24

13. Bucci LR. Selected herbals and human exercise performance. *Am J Clin Nutr* 2000;72:624s–36s

14. Bell DG, Jacobs I, Zamecnik J. Effects of caffeine, ephedrine and their combination on time to exhaustion during high-intensity exercise. *Eur J Appl Physiol* 1998;77:427–33

15. Haller CA, Benowitz NL. Adverse cardiovascular and central nervous system events associated with dietary supplements containing ephedra alkaloids. *N Engl J Med* 2000;343:1833–8

16. Nightingale SL. From the Food and Drug Administration. *J Am Med Assoc* 1997;278:15

17. Zaacks SM, Klein L, Tan CD, Rodriguez ER, Leikin JB. Hypersensitivity myocarditis associated with ephedra use. *J Toxicol Clin Toxicol* 1999;37:485–9

18. Wolfe SM, Ardati AK, Woosley R. Petition to the Food and Drug Administration (FDA) requesting the ban of production and sale of dietary supplements containing ephedrine alkaloids. HRG Publication no. 1590. (Accessed 30 January 2002)

19. Dollery C, ed. Ephedrine (hydrochloride). In *Therapeutic Drugs*, vol. 1. New York, NY: Churchill Livingstone, 1991:E26–9

20. Food and Drug Administration. Adverse events with ephedra and other botanical dietary supplements. *FDA Med Bull* 1994;24:3

21. Lynch J, House MA. Cardiovascular effects of methamphetamine. *J Cadiovasc Nurs* 1992; 6:12–19

22. Karch SB. Other naturally occurring stimulants. In Karch SB, ed. *The Pathology of Drug Abuse*. Boca Raton, FL: CRC Press, 1996: 177–98

23. Karch SB. Synthetic stimulants. In Karch SB, ed. *The Pathology of Drug Abuse*. Boca Raton, FL: CRC Press, 1996:199–240

24. Van Mieghem W, Stevens E, Cosemans J. Ephedrine induced cardiopathy [letter]. *Br Med J* 1978;1:816–42

25. Perkins JP, Hausdorff WP, Lefkowitz RJ. Mechanisms of ligand-induced desensitization of beta-adrenergic receptors. In Perkins JP, ed. *The Beta-Adrenergic Receptor*. Clifton: Humana Press, 1991:73–124

26. Williams BR, Barber R, Clark RB. Kinetic analysis of agonist-induced down-regulation of the beta(2)-adrenergic receptor in BEAS-2B cells reveals high- and low-affinity components. *Mol Pharmacol* 2000;58:421–30

27. Hanzawa S, Nemoto M, Etoh S, Onoda N, Sakio H. A case of amphetamine-induced down-regulation of beta-adrenoceptor [In Japanese]. *Masui* 2001;50:1242–5

28. Ang-Lee MK, Moss J, Yuan CS. Herbal medicines and perioperative care. *J Am Med Assoc* 2001;286:208–16

29. Lee MK, Cheng BW, Che CT, Hsieh DP. Cytotoxicity assessment of ma-huang (ephedra) under different conditions of preparation. *Toxicol Sci* 2000;56:424–30

30. Perharic L, Shaw D, Murray V. Toxic effects of herbal medications and food supplements. *Lancet* 1993;342:180–1

31. Barnes J, Mills SY, Abbot NC, Willoughby M, Ernst E. Different standards for reporting ADRs to herbal remedies and conventional OTC medicines: face-to-face interviews with 515 users of herbal remedies. *Br J Clin Pharmacol* 1998;45:496–500

32. Food and Drug Administration. Dietary supplements containing ephedrine alkaloids. *Federal Register* 1997;62:30677–7024

33. Anon. FDA backs away from elements of plan to regulate ephedrine supplements. *Am J Health-Syst Pharm* 2000;57:922

34. Food and Drug Administration. Dietary supplements containing ephedrine alkaloids *Federal Register* 2000;65:17477

35. Health Canada 2001, June 14. Advisory: not to use products containing ephedra or ephedrine. Available at: http://www.hc-sc.gc.ca/english/archives/warnings/2001/2001. (Accessed 30 January 2002)

36. Samenuk D, Link MS, Homoud MK, *et al.* Adverse cardiovascular events temporally associated with ma huang, an herbal source of ephedrine. *Mayo Clin Proc* 2002;77:12–16

37. Nightingale SL. From the Food and Drug Administration. *J Am Med Assoc* 1996;275:1534 (abstr)

38. Hamilton K, Murr A. We're squeaky clean. *Newsweek* 1996;May 6:64

39. Glennon RA, Young R. (+)Amphetamine-stimulus generalization to an herbal ephedrine product. *Pharmacol Biochem Behav* 2000; 65:655–8

40. Martin W, Sloan J, Sapira J, Jasinski D. Physiologic, subjective, and behavioral effects of amphetamine, methamphetamine, ephedrine, phenmetrazine, and methylphenidate in man. *Clin Pharmacol Ther* 1971;12:245–58

41. Chait L. Factors influencing the reinforcing and subjective effects of ephedrine in humans. *Psychopharmacology* 1994;13:381–7

42. Young R, Gabryszuk M, Glennon RA. (−)Ephedrine and caffeine mutually potentiate one another's amphetamine-like stimulus effects. *Pharmacol Biochem Behav* 1998;61:169–73

43. Cockings J, Brown M. Ephedrine abuse causing acute myocardial infarction. *Med J Aust* 1997;167:199–200

44. Gruber A, Pope HGJ. Ephedrine abuse among 36 female weight-lifters. *Am J Addict* 1998;7: 256–61

45. Ernst E. The risk–benefit profile of commonly used herbal therapies: ginkgo, St. John's wort, ginseng, echinacea, saw palmetto, and kava. *Ann Intern Med* 2002;136:42–53

46. Miller LG. Herbal medicinals: selected clinical considerations focusing on known or potential drug–herb interactions. *Arch Intern Med* 1998;158:2200–11

47. National Heart, Lung, and Blood Institute. *Clinical Guidelines on the Identification, Evaluation, and Treatment of Overweight and Obesity in Adults. The Evidence Report*. NIH publication no. 98. Washington, DC: US Department of Health and Human Services, 1998:4083

48. Pentel P. Toxicity of over the counter stimulants. *J Am Med Assoc* 1984;252:1898–903

49. Tang DH. Ephedra (ma huang). *Clin Toxicol Rev* 1996;18:1–2

50. Anon. Sympathomimetics. In Reynolds JEF, ed. *Martindale: The Extra Pharmacopoeia*, 31st edn. London: Royal Pharmaceutical Society of Great Britain, 1996:1563–76

51. Powell T, Hsu FF, Turk J, Hruska K. Mahuang strikes again: ephedrine nephrolithiasis. *Am J Kidney Dis* 1998;32:153–9

52. Wiener I, Tilkian AG, Palazzolo M. Coronary artery spasm and myocardial infarction in a patient with normal coronary arteries: temporal relationship to pseudoephedrine ingestion. *Cathet Cardiovasc Diagn* 1990;20:51–3

53. To LB, Sangster F, Rampling D. Ephedrine induced cardiomyopathy. *Med J Aust* 1980;2:35–6

54. Bravo EL. Metabolic factors and the sympathetic nervous system. *Am J Hypertens* 1989;2:339S–44S

55. Weiner N. Norephedrine, epinephrine and the sympathomimetic amines. In Goodman LS, Gilman AG, eds. *The Pharmacological Basis of Therapeutics*, 7th edn. New York, NY: Macmillan, 1985:145–80

56. White LM, Gardner SF, Gurley BJ, Marx MA, Wang PL, Estes M. Pharmacokinetics and cardiovascular effects of ma-huang (*Ephedra sinica*) in normotensive adults. *J Clin Pharmacol* 1997;37:6–22

57. Hoffman BB. Catecholamines, sympathomimetic drugs, and adrenergic receptor antagonists. In Hardman JG, Limbird LE, Gilman AG, eds. *Goodman and Gilman's The Pharmacological Basis of Therapeutics*, 10th edn. New York, NY: McGraw-Hill, 2001:215–45

58. Roth LS. Ephedra. In Como D, Myers T, Barbarick K, eds. *Mosby's Handbook of Herbs and Natural Supplements*. St Louis, MO: Mosby, 2001:318–22

59. Anastasio GD, Harston P. Fetal tachycardia associated with maternal use of pseudoephedrine and over the counter oral decongestant. *J Am Board Fam Pract* 1992;5:527–8

60. Chung KF, Barnes PJ. Treatment of asthma. *Br Med J (Clin Res Ed)* 1987;294:103–5

61. Mortimer EA. Drug toxicity from breast milk? *Pediatrics* 1977;60:780–1

62. Christensen NJ, Galbo H. Sympathetic nervous activity during exercise. *Annu Rev Physiol* 1983;45:139–53

63. Eisenhofer G, Rundqvist B, Friberg P. Determinants of cardiac tyrosine hydroxylase activity during exercise-induced sympathetic activation in humans. *Am J Physiol* 1998;274:R626–34

64. Karch SB. Cocaine: cardiovascular system. In Karch SB, ed. *The Pathology of Drug Abuse*. Boca Raton, FL: CRC Press, 1996:83–124

65. Gaultieri J, Harris C. Dilated cardiomyopathy in a heavy ephedrine abuser. *J Toxicol Clin Toxicol* 1996;34:581–2 (abstr)

66. Benowitz NL. Clinical pharmacology of caffeine. *Annu Rev Med* 1990;41:277–88

67. Stoessl AJ, Young GB, Feasby TE. Intracerebral hemorrhage and angiographic beading following ingestion of catecholaminergics. *Stroke* 1985;16:734–6.

68. Weinberger M, Bronsky T, Bensch GW, Bock GN, Yecres JJ. Interaction of ephedrine and theophylline. *Clin Pharmacol Ther* 1975;17:585–92

69. Hirsch MS, Walter RM, Hasterlik RJ. Subarachnoid hemorrhage following ephedrine and MAO inhibitor. *J Am Med Assoc* 1965;194:1259

70. ASHP. Therapeutic position statement on the safe use of pharmacotherapy for obesity management in adults. Developed by the ASHP Commission on Therapeutics and approved by the ASHP Board of Directors on April 23, 2001. *Am J Health-Syst Pharm* 2001;58:1645–55

71. Skop BP, Finkelstein JA, Mareth TR, Magoon MR, Brown TM. The serotonin syndrome associated with paroxetine, an over the counter cold remedy and vascular disease. *Am J Emerg Med* 1994;12:642–4

72. Fallis RJ, Fisher M. Cerebral vasculitis and hemorrhage associate with phenylpropanolamine. *Neurology* 1985;35:405–7

73. Lake CRS, Gallant EM, Miller P. Adverse drug effects attributed to phenylpropanolamine: a review of 142 case reports. *Am J Med* 1990;89:195–208

74. Roizen MF. Anesthetic implications of concurrent diseases. In Miller RD, ed. *Anesthesia*, 4th edn. New York, NY: Churchill Livingstone, 1994:903–1014

75. Stockley IH. Sympathmimetic drug interactions. In Stockley IH, ed. *Drug Interactions*, 3rd edn. Cambridge: Blackwell Scientific Publications, 1994:727–36

76. Griffin JP. Interactions with drug used to treat hypertension. In Griffin JP, D'Arcy PF, eds. *A Manual of Adverse Drug Interactions*, 5th edn. Amsterdam: Elsevier Science, 1997:147–77

77. Yale University Study on Phenylpropanolamine (PPA). Available at: http://www.ppaaction.com/yalestudy.doc. (Accessed 30 January 2002)

78. US Food and Drug Administration Center for Drug Evaluation and Research. Phenylpropanolamine (PPA) information page. Available at: http://www.fda.gov/cder/drug/infopage/ppa/default.htm. (Accessed 30 January 2002)

79. Liberti L. Guarana (monograph). In *The Lawrence Review of Natural Products, Facts and Comparisons*. St Louis, MO: Wolters Kluwer Company, 1991; May:1–2

80. Liberti L. Mate (monograph). In *The Lawrence Review of Natural Products, Facts and Comparisons*. St Louis, MO: Wolters Kluwer Company, 1988; April:1–2

81. Liberti L. Senna (monograph). In *The Lawrence Review of Natural Products, Facts and Comparisons*. St Louis, MO: Wolters Kluwer Company, 1991; January:1–3

82. Liberti L. Herbal diuretics (monograph). In *The Lawrence Review of Natural Products, Facts and Comparisons*. St Louis, MO: Wolters Kluwer Company, 1989; May: 1–2

83. Bennet DA Jr, Phun L, Polk JF, *et al.* Neuropharmacology of St. John's wort (*Hypericum*). *Ann Pharmacother* 1998;32:1201–8

84. Nathan P. The experimental and clinical pharmacology of St. Johns wort. *Mol Psychiatry* 1999;4:333–8

85. Huang Y, Wang G, Chen C, *et al.* Fructus aurantii reduced portal pressure in portal hypertensive rats. *Life Sci* 1995;57:2011–20

86. Roth LS. Ginseng. In Como D, Myers T, Barbarick K, eds. *Mosby's Handbook of Herbs and Natural Supplements*. St Louis, MO: Mosby, 2001:1380–5

87. Wilkerson RD. Cardiovascular effects of coccaine enhancement by yohimbine and atropine. *J Pharmacol Exp Ther* 1989;248:57–61

88. Liberti L. Yohimbine (monograph). In *The Lawrence Review of Natural Products, Facts and Comparisons*. St Louis, MO: Wolters Kluwer Company, 1993:1–2

Natural products and cancer 25

W. Sampson

DEFINITIONAL AND HISTORICAL PROBLEMS OF HERBAL THERAPIES IN CANCER

Some questions of definition arise when considering the roles of herbs and other natural substances in cancer. First, natural products may be sources for specific chemical compounds, which may be extracted and used in purified form. Other natural substances may be consumed as a tea, the rough equivalent of an aqueous extract. Others are consumed whole, as foods, in the normal diet. Some whole foods are wild species, but most modern food varieties have been cultivated, selected and bred over centuries for qualities of taste and appearance. Cultivated varieties may or may not be considered 'natural'. For purposes here, all plant foods and herbs are considered, but only those of considerable interest are described in detail.

Many differentiate herbs from other natural products. According to the *Random House College Dictionary*, an herb is 'a flowering plant whose stem above ground does not become woody' and 'such a plant valued for its medicinal properties, flavor, scent...'. Some authors include the property of being an annual plant. It is implied that the herb plant is not a common food source, and is not commonly known to be particularly toxic – at least in its folklore. Taste and trial and error over millennia probably eliminated many toxic plants from medicinal use.

Most would consider an herb to be taken in small quantities for either medicinal purpose or to impart flavor. This chapter considers relations of cancer to herbs, whole foods and specific products derived from them.

NATURAL PRODUCT HISTORICAL PERSPECTIVE

Most traditional uses as recorded in standard references were for conditions no longer common, or for which the definitions have been changed, for instance, the disorders quinsy, erysipelas and inflammatory rheumatism. Some disorders, such as smallpox and polio, have been practically eliminated, and the frequency of rheumatic fever has been markedly diminished. Some conditions, such as systemic lupus and other autoimmune disorders, were not recognized or accurately defined a century ago. Pernicious (megaloblastic) anemia was found to have three or four different causes, and those not due to vitamin B_{12} deficiency have been renamed and have different specific treatments.

Until one and a half centuries ago, cancer was identifiable in life only through changes visible on the body surface. Internal cancers were unknown before formal body dissections were carried out in the 16th century, and leukemias were not classified until the 20th century. Diagnoses were made on gross appearance only – the microscope and tissue slides not being in common use until the 1800s. Radiographs appeared in the 20th century. Traditional diagnoses were frequently erroneous or lacked relevance to modern classification, and some were based mainly on symptoms. Therefore, traditional observations of herb and natural product effects were also erroneous or are irrelevant to modern disease concepts.

In addition, older uses were based on almost uniformly faulty observations. Spontaneous recovery from self-limited illness was often misinterpreted as caused by whichever herb or other remedy was applied at the time. This mistaken attribution is a common source of error made by unsystematic observation.

Finally, controlled clinical trials were not routinely performed until after World War II, and many refinements have been made only in the past two decades. All of these considerations have rendered traditional uses close to meaningless. The historical conclusion, then, is that there is little to no rational historical foundation on which to base any human study, which in turn makes it unlikely for new controlled trials to uncover significant effects of traditional herbs and plants. Endpoints for controlled trials on traditional natural products are essentially equal to randomly chosen ones. Most meaningful studies will have been devised from modern understanding of herb and plant components, or on recently discovered properties such as antioxidant, enzyme-inhibiting or enzyme-inducing properties, or neutralizing of pathways of cell differentiation, growth and apoptosis.

PRINCIPLES OF CANCER

General principles regarding the nature of cancer also set limits on the possibilities for treatment with natural substances. First, cancer cells closely resemble normal cells from the tissue from which they are derived. This fact makes it unlikely that any particular substance would have an effect on cancer cells markedly different from that on normal cells. In fact, most anticancer agents have a narrow therapeutic ratio, meaning that the dosage difference between desired anticancer effect and undesirable or toxic effects is quite small. Doses have to be carefully drawn, and unwanted effects monitored (hence the poor reputation of anticancer chemotherapy even with purified, standardized materials). The use of raw, impure and combined materials, with variable and uncontrollable contents, has potential for producing more harm than good. Natural substances do not contain any beneficent or other property that confers special qualities of effectiveness in cancer.

Since cancer cell metabolism differs only slightly and in special circumstances from normal cell metabolism, substances necessary for normal cell growth are also necessary for cancer cell growth. This principle

makes it possible for any natural herb or food substance even to stimulate cancer cell growth.

The complexities of natural substances magnify the problems. Some natural substances interfere with pharmaceuticals by several different mechanisms. Some, such as St John's wort, induce enzymes (e.g. cytochrome P450) that metabolize drugs, causing the drugs to be removed more rapidly from circulation. This mechanism is responsible for the diminished effect of cyclosporin, an immune suppressant used in organ transplants and in autoimmune diseases, and of protease inhibitors in HIV disease.

Other substances reduce the effectiveness of those enzymes, thus increasing the amount of circulating drug, as in the interaction between grapefruit and statin drugs for cholesterol lowering. Other substances displace drugs from circulating binding proteins, releasing free drug, thus increasing the activity. Many substances displace warfarin, increasing the concentration of free drug, causing that anticoagulant's dosage to be difficult to control. On the other hand, vitamin K in the diet counters the effects of warfarin. Not much is known about botanical interactions with anticancer medications.

Herbal contents vary depending on several factors. All plant contents vary according to season or time of year of planting; time of harvest; soil, moisture, heat and sun conditions; conditions of manufacture; conditions of storage; length of storage; and degree of insect, mold and bacterial infestation. One method attempting to create more consistency is being developed at the University of Guelph, through cloning of plant cells and using constant growing conditions[1].

Because of lax oversight, contamination and adulteration are a source of morbidity, as illustrated by the epidemic of renal failure in hundreds of Belgian women who took a Chinese herbal tea for weight loss. The herbal mixture contained the wrong herb, mistakenly substituted for another because of similar sounding names. Many of the women later developed renal pelvis cancers[2]. Another type of contamination, adulteration, probably occurred in the herbal mixture PC-SPES, in which added pharmaceuticals were found to be responsible for its anticancer actions (described below.) Often, the particular active materials are unknown, further complicating evaluation.

In regard to increasing resistance or anticancer immunity, no such activity has been described as being due to a natural product, despite references to such properties in some of the literature on natural products. In fact, no material, natural or synthetic, has properties of increasing any form of host resistance to cancer. This is an important principle to keep in mind, as several herbs such as echinacea and ginseng (*Panax*) as well as other substances have been used for presumed stimulation of the immune system or other unspecified form of resistance.

Nevertheless, a number of whole herbal and whole plant materials have been proposed as treatments for cancer. None of them has succeeded in clinical trials, or has been shown to have enough activity in experimental animal or tissue culture systems to warrant further investigation in human trials.

Some products proposed as active cancer-fighting agents are echinacea, evening primrose oil, St John's wort and turmeric[3]. Another reference lists 32 botanicals that have been proposed or have been studied for their effect on cancer[4].

Whole herbal and other natural plant materials have been proposed as cancer preventives based largely on antioxidant qualities (Table 1).

Others have been proposed as having anticancer, antiproliferative activity. The evidence for antioxidant activity is adequate for some, but antioxidant activity is limited to a preventive role (Table 2).

As mentioned, the products were selected mainly because of known or presumed antioxidant properties. However, there is no known activity of antioxidants on established cancers, and there is no plausible mechanism for such action. Therefore, it is not surprising that researchers have not found herbs to have activity against established human cancer. One should note that antioxidant natural products can neutralize effects of anticancer agents such as bleomycin and alkylating agents, actions of which depend partially on their oxidant properties.

DIETARY APPROACHES

Soy-based diets

Soy is the focus of study because of the lower incidence of breast and other cancers (prostate, colon) in Asian countries, where soy is a major component of many diets. Observational studies of diets in different cultures

Table 1 Herbal remedies with antioxidant qualities

Adrographis (*Andrographis panniculus*)
Arnica (*Arnica montana*)
Bilberry fruit (*Chelidonium majus*)
Ginseng (*Panax ginseng*)
Licorice (*Glycyrrhiza*)
Melilotus (*Melilotus officinalis*)
Pau d'arco

Table 2 Evidence for effects of herbal remedies

Botanical	Claimed action	Evidence (quality)
Aloe	marrow stimulation	none
	anticancer	none
Astragalus	anticancer	none
Barberry	marrow stimulation	none
	anticancer	none
Beet root	anticancer	none
	'detoxification'	none
Bromelain	anticancer	none
Burdock	anticancer	none
Chapparal	anticancer	none
Chlorella	anticancer	none
Cottonseed	anticancer	none
Essiac	anticancer	none
Garlic	anticancer	none
	antioxidant	some (adequate)
Goldenseal	marrow stimulation	none
	anticancer	none
Green tea	antioxidant (prevention)	conflicting
	anticancer	none
Hoxsey formula	anticancer	none
Milk thistle	anti-liver toxicity	poor
	anticancer	none
Mistletoe	anticancer	none
Noni juice	marrow stimulation	none
	anticancer	none
Pau d'arco	anticancer	none
PC-SPES	anticancer (prostate)	none
Soy	anticancer (breast, prevention)	some (adequate)
Red clover	anticancer	none
Saw palmetto	anticancer (prostate)	poor
Siberian ginseng	anticancer	none
Turmeric	antioxidant	some
	anticancer	none
Wheatgrass	'detoxification'	none
	anticancer	none

show a negative correlation between soy-containing diets and breast cancer incidence. Studies on soy-based diets show that soy may have an inhibitory effect on breast cancer generation if the diet is consumed from an early age. There is no good evidence that a soy diet affects an established cancer.

Isoflavones, genistein

Isoflavones and lignans are subtypes of phytoestrogens. Genistein, one of the isoflavones, is abundant in many legumes, especially soybeans.

Studies on phytoestrogens range from comparative observational studies on the diets of whole populations, analyses of the proportions of isoflavones and soy, to studies of isoflavones and specific compounds such as genistein in animals and cells. Phytoestrogens may, like other hormone analogs and response modifiers such as tamoxifen and raloxifene, demonstrate either mild estrogenic activity or inhibitory activity, depending on the conditions of the experiment, the clinical situation, the target tissue and perhaps the types and amounts of other isoflavonoids in the diet. Activity is difficult to predict, and must be determined by observation and experiment.

Studies on genistein in animal breast cancers and on breast cancer cells show a complex of actions. Some studies show a negative influence of cancer incidence, but a few show stimulation of established breast cancer cells[5]. The genistein-precursor genistin also shows stimulation of breast cancer cell growth[6].

In males, phytoestrogens have an antitestosterone action, as might be anticipated from the mild estrogenic activity of these compounds. Substrates of lignans and isoflavonoid phytoestrogens inhibit the conversion of testosterone to dihydrotestosterone, and inhibit 5α-reductase activity[7].

Overall, the anticarcinogenic mechanisms of dietary genistein and soy products seem to predominate, favoring some degree of breast cancer prevention, possibly if the diet is begun before maturity. It is uncertain whether effects are due directly to soy or to reduced intake of other carcinogen-containing foods. Evidence is incomplete for prevention of other cancers. Evidence warrants caution in the presence of established breast cancer, especially estrogen- and progesterone receptor-positive tumor[8].

A few studies have tried to assess the value of vegetable- and fruit-based diets in established cancer. One such study used a vegetable mixture plus herbs, and claimed to have shown increased survival in lung cancer. However, these claims were based on a non-randomized, small number of subjects, with the treatment group affected by one long-term survivor[9].

At the same time, researchers in nutrition and biochemistry are discovering specific food component compounds and their mechanisms of cancer prevention. At this point in time, most authorities agree that a few simple actions can optimize the reduction in likelihood of cancer development. They involve a diet predominantly of grains, leafy and pigmented vegetables and fruits, especially tomato products and cruciferous vegetables, moderate fish and meat intake, and minimizing intake of charcoal-broiled meats. No known supplement adds to the effects of this simple dietary approach.

NATURAL SUBSTANCES IDENTIFIED WITH ANTICARCINOGENIC ACTIONS

Carotenes

Carotenoids are pigment compounds that have antioxidant and other chemical properties, and are found mainly in vegetables and fruits. β-Carotene is a precursor of vitamin A. Because of its antioxidant property and because foods containing it were associated negatively with cancer incidence, β-carotene supplements were tested prospectively. Several studies found paradoxically that cancer incidence increased with carotene supplementation, especially in smokers[10]. The mechanisms for these results are not known, although some antioxidants act as pro-oxidants under some circumstances (see ascorbate, below).

In addition, in ferrets, whose cellular processes closely resemble those of humans, there is evidence of changes in other intracellular processes. Daily pharmacological doses of β-carotene reduced (beneficial) levels of retinoic acid, and the retinoic acid receptor-β declined in lung tissues. Indicators of cell proliferation (gene products) increased. Lung tissues showed precancerous squamous metaplasia that increased with added daily exposure to cigarette smoke[11]. These changes might help explain the increase in cancer incidence in the human β-carotene trials.

Lycopenes

Lycopenes are carotenoids also found in red and yellow vegetables, especially in tomatoes. The amount of available lycopene is increased by cooking and the richest sources are in tomato paste. In a prospective controlled trial, prostate cancer patients preparing for surgery received 3 weeks of lycopene supplement and at surgery showed reduced cancer markers and microscopic evidence of cell regression and apoptosis when compared to controls[12]. This treatment period seems short for the surprising amount of changes found.

Lycopene blood levels were inversely correlated with breast cancer as well[13]. As with other findings on botanical approaches, such intriguing results have to be verified. Other carotenes, such as lutein, have not been tested extensively.

Cruciferous plants and sulforaphane

Other classes of fruits and vegetables have become objects of study. Population studies seem to point to the genus *Brassica* of the Crucifera family (broccoli and cauliflower) as cancer inhibitors. The search began for agents that neutralize highly reactive oxygen free radicals, natural carcinogens and chemicals resulting from oxidant processes, and resulted in finding large amounts of isothiocyanates, especially sulforaphane.

Instead of directly neutralizing oxygen and other free radicals, the isothiocyanate compounds were found in a variety of animal models to work indirectly. Two mechanisms are involved. First, they inhibit phase 1 enzymes involved in carcinogen activation. Second, they induce enzymes that accelerate the inactivation or metabolism of carcinogens (phase 2 enzymes).

These isothiocyanates have variable potencies as enzyme inducers, depending partly on their intracellular concentrations and area under the curve (integral of concentration and duration of presence)[14].

The matter is further complicated because of natural compounds in brassica vegetables that themselves act as inducers or promoters of carcinogenesis. Indole glucosinolates, which predominate in the mature vegetable, may give rise to degradation products (e.g. indole-3-carbinol) that can enhance tumorigenesis[15].

Small quantities of cruciferous sprouts may protect against the risk of cancer as effectively as much larger quantities of mature vegetables of the same variety. In a series of experiments on plants of various ages, Talalay and his group found that 3-day-old sprouts of cultivars of broccoli and cauliflower contained 10–100 times higher levels of glucoraphanin (the glucosinolate of sulforaphane) than did the corresponding mature plants[16]. This finding has launched a search for methods to prolong high quantities of sulforaphane in mature plants.

Curcumin

These are a lesser known series of naturally occurring compounds, derived from plants of the ginger family. They are also inducers of phase 2 enzymes. A number of natural and synthetic structural analogs of the dietary constituent also capably induce phase 2 detoxification enzymes[17].

Green tea

In 1992, Japanese researchers reported on epidemiological findings of a reduced incidence of esophageal and gastric cancer in one Western Japanese prefecture. They found the most marked reduction in areas where green tea was habitually produced and drunk, with frequent refreshing of the tea leaves. Residents had decreased incidence of death from other cancers also. Subsequent animal experiments showed that both initiation and promotion and growth were slowed by administration of a tannin component of the tea, catechin[18–20].

However, subsequent studies failed to find similar relationships. 'In a population-based, prospective cohort study in Japan, we found no association between green-tea consumption and the risk of gastric cancer'[21]. Because of conflicting reports, the effects of green tea remain unknown.

PC-SPES

The history of PC-SPES serves as a warning example of how difficult it is to evaluate a material's true nature by following strictly defined evidence-based guidelines. PC-SPES enjoyed a period of scientific legitimacy before it was found to be inactive or misrepresented.

Clinicians' interest in the herbal supplement PC-SPES flared after a 1998 report in the *New England Journal of Medicine* showed the herb's therapeutic effect on prostate cancer[22]. The popularity was unusual, given the product's known existence of only 10 years. PC-SPES is a mixture of seven Asian herbs and one North American herb, including chrysanthemum, isatis, licorice, *Ganoderma lucidum*, *Panax pseudoginseng*, *Rabdosia rubescens*, saw palmetto (*Serenoa repens*) and skullcap. The herbs contain a range of plant chemicals including flavonoids, alkanoids, polysaccharides, amino acids and trace minerals.

PC-SPES was developed in the early 1990s by Chen, who claimed to have created the formula by integrating modern science and ancient Chinese herbal wisdom. However, there is not much rationale given for why the specific herbs were selected. By the mid-1990s, the formula became widely promoted in the USA and was named PC-SPES[23]. PC stands for prostate cancer and SPES comes from the Latin root for hope.

Chinese herbs are used for conditions defined in traditional Chinese medicine (TCM), which do not relate or conform to modern scientific or tissue diagnoses. Therefore, PC-SPES had no historic use in prostate cancer. Before systematic identification of the contents began, clinical trials studied the herbal mixture. Most clinical trials use identified and purified compounds. The PC-SPES materials were produced in Taiwan, from sources in mainland China without effective regulation. Nevertheless, earlier studies demonstrated anticancer activity in

animals and in *in vitro* experiments on human tissue. Early and later clinical trials showed activity against both hormone-sensitive and hormone-resistant prostate cancer[24].

By 2001 researchers had identified a number of cellular mechanisms through which the herbal combination apparently worked[25]. None of the individual herbs had the same magnitude or variety of effects as did the mixture. Taken singly, three herbs inhibited cell activity, and five of the eight stimulated cancer cell activity *in vitro*. 'Our results show that the cytotoxic and cytostatic properties of PC SPES are not entirely dependent on the presence of AR [androgen receptor]. The antitumor mechanism of PC SPES is complex. It involves multiple metabolic pathways, such that the whole extract acts on redundant mechanisms, which otherwise will permit cell survival if a single-target agent is used.' Three herbs lowered intracellular and secreted prostate-specific antigen (PSA), while the remaining herbs actually increased PSA expression[26]. It is 'unlikely that the activity of a single herb can account for the overall effects of PC-SPES.' The authors implied that the whole mixture was required for full effect and that the contents interacted in a yet undetermined way.

In October 2001, researchers reported bleeding in a patient on PC-SPES. Warfarin was found in the blood, as well as in the PC-SPES mixture. On 9 February 2002, the Food and Drug Administration (FDA) issued a recall of PC-SPES and recommended that all people cease taking it. California authorities also found the companion supplement, SPES, to be contaminated with the sedative alprazolam (Xanax®).

In 2002 independent research oncologist Nagourney, who followed the PC-SPES reports from 1996, reported finding varying amounts of diethylstilbestrol in samples which decreased over 4 years, during which warfarin levels increased[27]. He also identified the anti-inflammatory drug indomethacin in the herb mixture. Anti-inflammatory, cyclo-oxygenase-2 inhibitors are a class of drugs effective against colon and prostate cancer[27]. PC-SPES activity against prostate cancer was apparently found to be due to adulteration with pharmaceuticals.

UNPROVED AND DISPROVED SUBSTANCES

The following are a number of diet- and plant-based cancer treatments that are promoted by a few individuals and have large followings from time to time. Advocates synthesize claims without experimental or epidemiological evidence. The claims lack plausibility, have not been evaluated or have been disproved by surveys or clinical trials. Nevertheless, many non-research-based dietary approaches to cancer have been claimed by their advocates to prevent, slow the growth of, or cure cancer. Most involve strict adherence to food and supplement plans and other lifestyle methods.

Laetrile

Laetrile is the commercial name given to an extract of fruit pits: amygdalin from apricots, prunasin, linamarin and other cyanogenic glycosides from other fruits and cassava root. Laetrile marketed in the 1970s was mainly amygdalin. Its structure is a benzene molecule with a side arm of two sequential glycosides and a CN moiety on the adjacent carbon. It contains 6% cyanide by weight[28]. The proposed theory of action was an invention of E.T. Krebs Jr, a one-time medical student, who tried to find an explanation for his father's claim to have found a cancer cure in these compounds. He theorized that amygdalin's cyanide, released by the enzyme β-glucosidase in cancer tissue, would kill the cancer cell. He claimed that the neutralizing enzyme rhodanese would protect normal cells by converting cyanide to thiocyanate. The major error was that human tissue, including cancer, does not contain significant amounts of β-glucosidase. Glucosidase occurs naturally in the amygdalin-containing food and intestinal bacteria. The glucosidase in the gut cleaves the sugar from the benzene moiety, and hydrolysis releases cyanide on further digestion. Cyanide released by ingested food in the gut is absorbed, and both cancer cells and normal cells are affected equally.

The theory was invented to give plausibility to a fraudulent stock investment scheme on Canadian stock exchanges and in the USA. The promoters were convicted of fraud in Canadian and US courts in the 1970s. Two FDA-sponsored studies showed insignificant Laetrile activity in human cancer[29,30].

Iscador (*Viscum album*, mistletoe)

Iscador is an extract of the common parasitic vine, mistletoe. An early 20th century spiritual philosopher, Rudolph Steiner, theorized that mistletoe would be effective against cancer by using the doctrine of signatures (like cures like – a principle of homeopathy). He conceived mistletoe to share qualities of parasitism similar to the role of a cancer to its host. Mistletoe became part of his methods called anthroposophical medicine. Mistletoe is popular in Germany, where many citizens believe in natural and philosophical approaches to treatment, although most regular physicians do not prescribe it. Certain extracts have been shown to have some effect on cancer cells *in vitro*[31]. However, no convincing evidence of effect in humans has been forthcoming[32]. The effectiveness of adjuvant mistletoe treatment was shown in a controlled trial in resesected head and neck cancer patients[33,34]. Some components of Iscador have been shown to function as oxidants[35].

Ascorbate (vitamin C)

Ascorbate was proposed and popularized as having anticancer activity by biochemist Linus Pauling, based on the theory that it strengthened connective tissue, which would prevent cancer from spreading. The strength of connective tissue has not been shown to affect cancer growth or spread.

Ascorbate is a powerful antioxidant and may have some role, along with other food constituents, in reducing cancer development by neutralizing DNA damage by oxygen free radicals. However, in some circumstances ascorbate is a pro-oxidant, and acts to augment oxidation, resulting in DNA damage[36]. Ascorbate's most beneficial effects are found through intake of foods high in ascorbate rather than in supplement form. Pauling's anticancer theory lacked plausibility and the action was disproved in two clinical trials at the Mayo Clinic[30,37].

Essiac

Essiac (Caisse backwards) is an herbal mixture introduced by nurse R. Caisse, who obtained the formula from a patient who attributed it to a Canadian Chippewa medicine man. The tea is made from the following contents: burdock root, sheep sorrel, Turkish rhubarb, slippery elm bark; blessed thistle, red clover and kelp, added to later formulations. It has been tested in humans with no effect found[38].

Hoxsey formula

Hoxsey formula is a water extract of a mixture of pokeweed, burdock root, licorice, barberry, buckthorn, stillingia, red clover, prickly ash and sometimes other materials. The promoter, Harry Hoxsey, claimed that a poultice of the herbs cured a cancer on his grandfather's horse's leg. (A microscopic diagnosis of cancer was not possible at the time.) Lacking any plausibility, it has not been studied seriously. It was declared fraudulent by the US FDA, although it is marketed through clinics in Mexico and somewhat clandestinely in the USA.

Gerson therapy

Gerson therapy is a mix of strict vegetarian and juice diet, supplements and coffee enemas. Available in Mexico, it has no demonstrable effect.

Other nutrition-based methods include the Kelley (grape) and Gonzales methods, wheatgrass, Di Bella (Italy) and other varieties of dieting.

COMPLEMENTARY METHODS

True complementary methods are not treatments or therapies[39]. They are a variety of unrelated methods that satisfy esthetic or 'spiritual' needs of people or help to integrate a philosophy, ideology or other set of ideas into a psychological heuristic system that either makes sense for or adds meaning to the person whose humanity and existence are threatened. The methods may be as simple as exercise and relaxation or as complex as a religion. The practical help these methods supply includes reduction of symptoms, increase in life quality, aid in traversing difficult treatments and aid in adjustment to illness and death.

No measurement of effectiveness is necessary for these methods. Claims of effectiveness are few, and would be difficult to prove, because they are not used alone, but in conjunction with measurable and proved treatments. There is little to prove, as each person may find one or a combination of methods attractive and useful, and the intent is to offer qualitative support. They include the following.

Knowledge

This is often forgotten as a means of psychological support, but knowledge of the disease process and of one's clinical status reduces uncertainty, and thus decreases anxiety.

Arts

These include drawing and painting, music, dance and poetry (reading and composition). These have the benefit of being practiced without the aid of others. Groups and instructors can also be used, of course.

Self-help groups

Psychological support groups are increasingly popular. Some meet in person, others such as Internet discussion groups may serve the same purpose for those who are unable, or do not desire, to travel to meeting places. A drawback of unsupervised groups is the dissemination of false and sometimes harmful suggestions. Initial studies showing increased survival by participating in groups failed in subsequent trials and were shown to have been incorrectly devised[40].

Massage

Massage requires a helper or a professional, but even lay helpers or relatives can learn basic techniques quickly and be of help. Massage may provide relaxation, relief of tension and anxiety, and even an opportunity to open discussion of concerns that might otherwise be kept private.

Occupational and physical therapies

These services are supplied at most hospitals and in many medical groups, using trained and sometimes specialty-educated and licensed personnel. They are important during recovery from surgery and other debilitating procedures.

Stress reduction, relaxation and meditation techniques

These are relatively recently developed techniques intended, as named, to reduce stress and induce a more relaxed state in order to reduce perception of pain and other uncomfortable symptoms, and provide a sense of control. They were developed in recent decades, and are associated with some New Age and other philosophies, and Eastern (Asian) religious practices. They may not appeal to everyone. Some techniques are accompanied by music or recorded voice tapes.

Hospice

The hospice movement developed in the 1970s and includes home care, and attention to relief of pain and other symptoms. The concept was not new, as home symptom care for dying patients had been in use before and had simply not been given a name.

Humanistic, patient-centered approaches

The idea that the patient could be in charge of his own care and that one might choose among treatment options and supportive measures was also not new, or a manifestation of complementary medicine. The concept became more formalized and was given a name in the late 20th century.

CONCLUSION

Regional and cultural differences in cancer incidence suggest strongly that environmental factors are important determinants of carcinogenesis. The diet is the most common vehicle for carcinogen transport into the body – the other routes being inhalation and skin absorption (including radiation.) Along with other environmental differences, nutritional factors may account for as much as 30% or more of cancer incidence. Despite the difficulties in determining the roles of individual compounds and specific conditions, research on natural products will remain a fertile field for decades, and will have potential for making a significant contribution to human health. Nutrition will also lead into unavoidable, unproductive cul-de-sacs and will be a fertile field for unfounded claims.

References

1. Murch SJ, KrishnaRaj, S, Saxena P. Phytopharmaceuticals: mass production, standardization, and conservation. *Sci Rev Altern Med* 2000;4:39–43
2. Betz W. Herbal crisis in Europe: a review of the epidemic of reno-toxicity from Chinese herbal remedies. *Sci Rev Altern Med* 2000;4:23–8
3. Mills S, Bone K. *Principles and Practice of Phytotherapy*. London: Churchill Livingstone, 2000:614
4. Labriola D. *Complementary Cancer Therapies*. Roseville, CA: Prima Publishing, 2000:173–4
5. Allred CD, Allred KF, Ju YH, Virant SM, Helfrich WG. Soy diets containing varying amounts of genistein stimulate growth of

estrogen-dependent (MCF-7) tumors in a dose dependent manner. *Cancer Res* 2001;61:5045–50

6. Allred CD, Ju YH, Allred KF, Chang J, Helferich WG. Dietary genistin stimulates growth of estrogen-dependent breast cancer tumors similar to that observed with genistein. *Carcinogenesis* 2001;10:1667–73

7. Evans BF, Griffith K, Morton MS. Inhibition of 5α-reductase in genital skin fibroblasts and prostate tissue by dietary lignans and isoflavonoids. *J Endocrinol* 1995;147:295–302

8. Tham DM, Gardner CD, Haskell,WL. Potential health benefits of dietary phytoestrogens: a review of the clinical, epidemiological, and mechanistic evidence. *J Clin Endocrinol Metab* 1999;83:2223–35

9. Sun AS, Yeh HC, Wang LH, *et al*. Pilot study of a specific dietary supplement in tumor-bearing mice and in stage IIIB and IV non-small cell lung cancer patients. *Nutr Cancer* 2001;39:85–95

10. Omenn G, Goodman GE, Thornquist MD, *et al*. Effects of a combination of beta carotene and vitamin A on lung cancer and cardiovascular disease. *N Engl J Med* 1996;334:1150–5

11. Wolf G. The effect of low and high doses of beta-carotene and exposure to cigarette smoke on the lungs of ferrets. *Nutr Rev* 2002;60:88–90

12. Kucuk O, Sarkar FH, Sakr W, *et al*. Phase II randomized clinical trial of lycopene supplementation before radical prostatectomy. *Cancer Epidemiol Biomarkers Prev* 2001;10:861–8

13. Hulten K, Van Kappel AL, Winkvist A, *et al*. Carotenoids, alpha-tocopherols, and retinol in plasma and breast cancer risk in northern Sweden. *Cancer Causes Control* 2001;12:529–37

14. Zhang Y, Talalay P. Mechanism of differential potencies of isothiocyanates as inducers of anticarcinogenic Phase 2 enzymes. *Cancer Res* 1998;58:4632–9

15. Bjeldanes L, Kim J, Grose KR, Bartholemew JC, Bradfield CA. Receptor agonists generated from indole-3-carbinol *in vitro* and *in vivo*. *Proc Natl Acad Sci* 1991;88:9534–47

16. Fahey J, Zhang Y, Talalay P. Broccoli sprouts: an exceptionally rich source of inducers of enzymes that protect against chemical carcinogens. *Proc Natl Acad Sci USA* 1997;94:10367–72

17. Dinkova-Kostova AT, Talalay P. Relation of structure of curcumin analogs to their potencies as inducers of Phase 2 detoxification enzymes. *Carcinogenesis* 1999;20:911–14

18. Sano M, Ozeki K, Taguchi M, Oguni I. Effects of green tea and tea catechins on the development of mammary gland. *Biosci Biotechnol Biochem* 1996;60:169–70

19. Yamane T, Nakatani H, Kikuoka N, *et al*. Inhibitory effects and toxicity of green tea polyphenols for gastrointestinal carcinogenesis. *Cancer* 1996;77(Suppl 8):1662–7

20. Mabe K, Yamada M, Oguni I, Takahashi T. *In vitro* and *in vivo* activities of tea catechins against *Helicobacter pylori*. *Antimicrob Agents Chemother* 1999;43:1788–91

21. Tsubono Y, Nishino Y, Komatsu S, *et al*. Green tea and the risk of gastric cancer in Japan. *N Engl J Med* 2001;344:632–6

22. DiPaola RS, Zhang H, Lambert GH, *et al*. Clinical and biologic activity of an estrogenic herbal combination (PC-SPES) in prostate cancer. *N Engl J Med* 1998;339:785–91

23. Anon. *Complementary and Alternative Cancer Methods*. Atlanta, GA: American Cancer Society, 2000:251–2

24. Small EJ, Frohglich MW, Bok R, *et al*. Prospective trial of the herbal PC-SPES in progressive cancer of the prostate. *J Clin Oncol* 2000;18:3595–603

25. De La Taille A, Hayek OR, Buttyan R, Bagiella E, Burchardt M, Katz AE. Effects of phytotherapeutic agent, PC-SPES, on prostate cancer: a preliminary investigation on human cell lines and patients. *Br J Urol Int* 1999;84:845–50

26. Hsieh TC, Wu JM. Mechanism of action of herbal supplement PC-SPES: elucidation of effects of individual herbs of PC-SPES on proliferation and prostate specific gene expression in androgen-dependent LNCaP cells. *Int J Oncol* 2002;3:583–8

27. Sovak M, Seligson AL, Konas M, *et al*. PC-SPES in prostate cancer: an herbal mixture currently containing warfarin and previously diethylstilbestrol and indomethacin. *Trans Am Assoc Cancer Res* 2002;LB152 [http://aacr02.agora.com/planner/displayabstract.asp?presentationid=10056]

28. Herbert V, Barrett S. *Vitamins and Health Foods*. Amherst, NY: Prometheus Books, 1980:12–15

29. Ellison NM, Byar DP, Newell GR. Special report on Laetrile: the NCI Laetrile review. *N Engl J Med* 1978;299:549–52

30. Moertel CG, Fleming TR, Rubin J, *et al*. A clinical trial of amygdalin (Laetrile) in the treatment of human cancer. *N Engl J Med* 1982;306:201–6

31. Kutton G, Menon LG, Antony S, Kuttan R. Anticarcinogenic and antimetastatic activity of Iscador. *Anticancer Drugs* 1997;1:S15–16

32. Steuer-Vogt MK, Bonkowsky V, Ambrosch P, *et al*. The effect of an adjuvant mistletoe treatment programme in resected head and neck cancer patients: a randomized controlled clinical trial. *Eur J Cancer* 2001;37:23–31

33. Kaegi E. Unconventional therapies for cancer: 3. Iscador. *CMAJ* 1998;158:1157–9

34. Maier G, Fiebig HH. Absence of tumor growth stimulation in a panel of 16 human tumor cell lines by mistletoe extracts *in vitro*. *Anticancer Drugs* 2002;13:373–9

35. Bussing A, Schaller G, Pfuller U. Generation of reactive oxygen intermediates (ROI) by the thionins from *Viscum album* L. *Anticancer Res* 1998;18:4291–6

36. Saltman P. Oxidative stress; a radical view. *Semin Hematol* 1989;26:249–56

37. Moertel CG, Fleming TR, Creagan ET, Rubin J, O'Connell MJ, Ames MM. High-dose vitamin C versus placebo in the treatment of patients with advanced cancer who have had no prior chemotherapy. A randomized double-blind comparison. *N Engl J Med* 1985;312:137–41

38. Kaegi E. Unconventional therapies for cancer. 1. Essiac. The task force on alternative therapies of the Canadian Breast Cancer Research Initiative. *CMAJ* 1998;158:897–902

39. Bruss K, ed. *American Cancer Society Guide to Complementary and Alternative Cancer Methods*. Atlanta, GA: American Cancer Society, 2000

40. Sampson W. Mind and cancer: explaining decades of erroneous positive results. *Semin Oncol* 2002;29:in press

Complementary and alternative medicine and cancer: facts, fiction and challenges

26

B. A. Bauer

INTRODUCTION

The explosion in interest in complementary and alternative medicine (CAM), especially among cancer patients, is a potentially overwhelming phenomenon for both the patient and the physician. 'Cures' seem to populate websites as fast as new websites can be created. Faced with an overwhelming flood of information (and misinformation), a busy physician might be justified in longing for a time when there was not so much interest in 'alternative' or 'natural' therapies. In truth, the concept that a cure for cancer should come from nature has been present perhaps for as long as the notion of cancer itself. Hippocrates (460–377 BC) advanced the concept of *vis medicatrix naturae* (the healing force of nature). Paracelsus (1493–1541) stated 'The art of healing comes from nature, not from the physician', and in the Jacksonian America of the 19th century, people rebelled against the harsh 'heroic' conventional medicine of the age, turning instead to homeopathy, herbs and self-treatment. So profound was this rebellion against the prevailing conventional medicine of the day that, by 1840, most states had repealed their medical licensing laws. Thus, it seems clear that the quest for an alternative to conventional medicine is not a new phenomenon. Especially when the disease is incurable or the conventional treatment particularly harsh or dangerous, people have sought and continue to seek treatments that promise help without the attendant costs in side-effects or discomfort.

What has perhaps changed in recent years is the ready availability of information regarding alternative treatments. In this regard, the World Wide Web (WWW) has played no small role. In fact, it seems to be the confluence of these two powerful social phenomena (CAM and the Internet) that has yielded an almost insatiable interest in CAM cancer treatments.

This creates tremendous challenges for both the cancer patient and the physician caring for the patient with cancer. Twenty or thirty years ago, a patient wishing to find information about other sources of treatment for a particular cancer might have searched laboriously in a local library and found only a few articles or mentions of 'alternative' treatments. Today, that patient may go to the WWW, use a robust search engine such as Google™, enter the terms 'alternative', 'medicine', and 'cancer' and find over 500 000 sites, purveying information of amazing breadth. Trying to sort through the barrage of sites to find information that is true and useful is a daunting task even when one feels well and is not distracted by the demands of a severe illness such as cancer. The quiet desperation that often accompanies a cancer diagnosis makes it significantly more difficult for such a patient to separate the 'good from the bad'.

This proliferation of information (and misinformation) poses challenges to the physician as well. As a patient advocate, the physician must be able to win-now the 'wheat from the chaff' and provide reliable and accurate information to the patient. At the same time, the patient expects to be heard and have their questions addressed in a comprehensive and non-judgemental fashion. The physician must be even-handed and provide sufficient education and interpretation of available information to allow the patient to make a well-informed decision.

It is therefore important for physicians and other health-care providers to have an understanding of the scope of the issue and a framework that allows some understanding of the potential positives and negatives associated with the cancer patient's exploration of CAM modalities. This chapter first considers general usage trends, then reviews a few popular non-herbal therapies used by cancer patients (herbal and botanical therapies are addressed in Chapter 25). This brief review will be used to help formulate a strategy for communicating with cancer patients. Done well, such communication and education will allow patients with cancer the ability to make informed choices in regards to their care.

USAGE IN GENERAL

Eisenberg's studies[1,2] have become well known and are frequently cited when considering the general use of CAM in the USA. These studies showed that the use of CAM rose from 34% in 1993 to 42% in 1998. More recently, Gray and co-workers[3] performed a survey of 4400 health-plan members who were stratified by number of chronic diseases. Forty-two per cent reported use of at least one CAM therapy, with the most common being relaxation techniques (18%), massage (12%), herbal medicine (10%) and mega-vitamin therapy (9%). Those who used a CAM therapy generally perceived that it was efficacious (from a low of 76% for hypnosis to a high of 98% for energy healing). Demographic information revealed typical findings with users more likely to be female, young, better educated and employed. Briefly, these and other studies indicate a continued interest in, and usage of, CAM by the general population.

USAGE BY CANCER PATIENTS

Many surveys have been performed to assess the use of CAM therapies by patients with cancer. Because of the variability in the definitions of CAM used by various investigators, results are often variable. In 1998, Ernst and Cassileth[4] published a summary of 26 international surveys that investigated the prevalence of CAM usage in patients with cancer. Thirteen countries were represented in the surveys that showed a usage of CAM therapies ranging from a low of 7% to a high of 64%. The average prevalence of usage across the studies was 31.4%.

In Norway, Risberg and colleagues[5] found that 20% of hospitalized cancer patients had used a CAM therapy. Only 10% expected their CAM therapy to contribute to a cure for their cancer. Most sought relief of symptoms or increased strength. Interestingly, users of CAM therapies reported that they received less hope of a cure (30%) from their physician, compared to non-users (50%).

A study in Australia[6] found that, among 156 cancer patients attending an oncology clinic at a teaching hospital, 81 (52%) had used at least one CAM therapy subsequent to their diagnosis. Meditation and relaxation techniques were employed by nearly 30% of patients, with a similar number employing dietary changes. Multivitamins, antioxidants, high-dose vitamin C and herbs were also popular. Most patients felt that the therapy would aid their conventional treatment and also provide them with a sense of control of their health care. Most patients did not expect a cure from the therapy they chose.

More recently, Kappauf and co-workers[7] surveyed 128 patients, of whom 65% were suffering from malignancies. Fifty per cent of the patients with a malignancy used an unconventional medicine, compared with 10% of those patients without a malignancy. Only 18% of the patients with a malignancy who used a CAM therapy expected the therapy to increase the chance of a cure. Among this same group, 60% felt that they experienced a distinct or mild improvement in their physical well-being and 62% felt that they had an improvement in psychological well-being.

Another study[8] evaluated 104 consecutive patients with advanced cancer patients in the community and

50 consecutive patients with advanced cancer in a tertiary palliative care unit. A face-to-face survey regarding CAM use was employed. Many patients were excluded (96), largely owing to cognitive impairment. Of the 58 remaining patients, 28% were found to be using CAM therapies. The most common therapies included herbs (57%), shark cartilage (21%) and vitamins (9%). The mean cost was $156 (Canadian)/month. A majority (81%) of those using CAM therapies felt that they had received some benefit from the treatments.

Patients with breast cancer deserve special mention, as they have generally been found to be aggressive users of CAM therapies. A 2000 study[9] compared 288 breast cancer patients with 329 patients with other primary site diagnoses and found that CAM therapies were used consistently by 84% of the breast cancer patients versus 66% of patients with other cancers.

A comprehensive evaluation of breast cancer patients and their interest in and usage of CAM therapies was conducted at the University of Texas MD Anderson Cancer Center[10] between December 1997 and June 1998. Richardson and colleagues studied 453 breast cancer patients. They found that 83% had used at least one CAM approach following their diagnosis.

An important issue to consider is how the fascination with CAM might translate into problems with conventional cancer research trials. For instance, Neuhouser and associates[11] studied dietary supplement use among participants in the Prostate Cancer Prevention Trial. Over 15 000 men completed food frequency questionnaires and dietary supplement questionnaires. Of the men enrolled in the trial, 44% used a multivitamin, 35% used single supplements of vitamin C or E, and 10–15% used antioxidant mixtures or single supplements of vitamins A or D, zinc or β-carotene. Overall, 60% of the men reported regular use of at least one supplement during the previous year. The authors pointed out that 'because supplements, especially antioxidants, may confer independent cancer-preventive effects, analytic models of study findings should include exposure measurements of dietary supplements with appropriate tests for interaction'[11].

For example, the α-tocopherol and β-carotene study[12], which was targeted at primary prevention of lung cancer, actually noted a 32% reduction in prostate cancer. Similarly, a study of selenium as a treatment to reduce skin cancer[13] also found an unexpected 60% decrease in prostate cancer incidence. Thus, both the clinician and the cancer researcher must be aware of the high likelihood that a significant number of their patients are using some form of CAM. CAM therapies might be beneficial, harmful or neutral in and of themselves, but their combination with chemotherapy may result in unexpected side-effects. Research may be confounded if careful inquiry is not carried out with each patient. The first step in helping patients make wise health-care decisions regarding CAM and cancer is a simple, nonjudgemental inquiry into their current use and/or interest in such therapies.

SURVIVAL AND QUALITY OF LIFE

CAM therapies have the potential to impact both survival and quality of life. Both effects are important and need to be addressed for the cancer patient trying to make a decision regarding usage of a particular therapy. In regards to survival, there is not much literature to suggest a significant benefit when considering general CAM usage in cancer patients. Risberg and colleagues[14] followed 252 cancer patients from 1990 to 1996. Only 110 patients were alive at the 5-year follow-up. The authors calculated that 45% of the patients used a non-proven therapy, with women (50%) being more likely to be users compared to men (31%). There was no difference in the 5-year observed survival rate between users of non-proven therapies and non-users. This lack of effect on survival of CAM usage has also been observed in other studies[15,16]. However, many specific therapies have yet to be subjected to rigorous trials, so it is premature to make any broad generalization regarding CAM and survival.

What is safe to say is that quality of life has become increasingly recognized as an important consideration, one worthy of rigorous investigation. A pilot study[17] from Australia compared 29 cancer patients being treated by conventional therapy with 29 being treated by both complementary and conventional therapy. The authors found a benefit in psychological distress using the Brief Symptom Inventory scale.

Researchers are continuing to refine the ability to measure disparate markers of quality of life. The question of how the patient feels is becoming increasingly recognized to be nearly as important as how the patient is doing clinically.

Besides basic compassion and the physician's core value to relieve suffering, there may be additional reasons to focus on quality of life in cancer patients. There are studies that seem to support the notion that quality of life is an independent prognostic factor for survival in various types of cancer[18,19]. Specifically in breast cancer patients, Fraser and co-workers[20] found that quality of life at trial entry predicted both response to chemotherapy and survival.

What has been debated is whether or not 'psychological interventions designed to improve quality of life can enhance response to adjuvant or neoadjuvant chemotherapy for breast cancer'[21]. Fortunately, there is a burgeoning interest in studying and improving quality of life in patients with cancer.

TYPES OF THERAPY

With the above overview as background, it is appropriate to focus on the therapies that cancer patients are likely to encounter. Therapies can be broadly considered as falling into one of three main categories: supplemental, complementary and alternative.

Supplemental

Many cancer patients are turning to CAM modalities, not in an effort directly to attack the disease, but in an effort to sustain quality of life while undergoing chemotherapy, surgery or radiation. Hence, many are turning to massage therapy, music therapy or healing touch to help them weather the often significant ravages of conventional treatment. Such treatments are intended to supplement, not replace, conventional therapies. They are generally non-invasive and unlikely to interfere with the efficacy of the treatment being offered. In fact, as mentioned above, there are a growing number of studies that seem to indicate real benefit from measures aimed at improving quality of

life. Such therapies pose little risk, may be helpful and can generally be incorporated into the conventional regimen in a manner that is supportive of the patient's interest in such approaches.

Complementary

Another approach is the introduction of therapies that are geared towards 'boosting the immune system' or otherwise 'helping the body to fight'. This includes the use of herbs, vitamins and other dietary supplements. The theory generally expounded is that cancer is the result of a breakdown in the body's natural defense system. Helping 'rejuvenate' or 'strengthen' the immune system is viewed as contributing to the body's own ability to fight cancer. Claims to this effect are made for antioxidants, cat's claw (*Uncaria tomentosa*), mega-vitamin therapy and a host of other therapies.

Here the realm becomes much murkier. For example, antioxidants are generally viewed as positive in their effects on the body, acting as scavengers of free radicals, and thus limiting the damage these reactive oxygen species can cause. Epidemiological studies suggest that populations with high intake of certain vitamins have reduced rates of cancer. Such findings bolster the current public fascination with mega-dose vitamin therapy as a means of preventing and/or treating cancer. At the worst, most physicians have felt that such treatments were generating little risk, except the financial cost of purchasing the vitamins. However, the CARET trial[22] unexpectedly showed that high intake of β-carotene actually increased the risk of lung cancer in a population at high risk for the disease. This was a wake-up call in many respects for physicians and patients alike that simply ingesting mega-doses of any agent might potentially have unintended consequences.

Also, cancer patients, aware of the role of oxidants in some cancers, and bombarded with the message that antioxidants are beneficial, have begun adding mega-dose vitamin therapy to their conventional treatment regimens, frequently without notifying their care-givers. However, many chemotherapeutic agents rely in some part for their effectiveness on the generation of free radicals. It is potentially feasible that taking high-dose antioxidant therapy at the time of chemotherapy or radiation therapy could potentially blunt the effectiveness of the treatment. Debate is ongoing and the available literature is inconclusive.

Alternative

Finally, there are those treatments that are advertised and promoted as replacements for conventional therapies. Here lie some of the greatest risks and dangers to a cancer patient sifting the volumes of information from lay journals, well-meaning friends and family members, and the websites. The promotion of a CAM modality as being 'natural', 'gentle' or 'non-toxic' can be a siren song to the patient who only knows vague rumors of the challenges of conventional therapy. Fearing hair loss, nausea and vomiting, and depleted immune function as inevitable outcomes of conventional therapy, many patients are quick to latch onto the hope provided by a professional-appearing website, promoting a cure that is free of side-effects.

There are literally thousands of alternative 'cures' being promoted today. Because the greatest risks to patients are posed by therapies that are specifically intended to replace conventional therapy, five of these (Cancell, cellular therapy, Coley's toxins, shark cartilage and 714X) will be reviewed. This review will serve to frame the discussion of how a physician can work collaboratively with the patient facing cancer and a murky sea of claims and promises.

Cancell

Background   Cancell (also called Entelev, Sheridan's Formula, Jim's Juice, Crocinic Acid and Cantron) was developed by James V. Sheridan, a former researcher at Michigan Cancer Center, in the 1930s. He claimed to have received the formula in a dream inspired by God and consequently offered the treatment to patients free of charge. The exact formula has varied according to the manufacturer, but generally contains

inositol, nitric acid, sodium sulfate, potassium hydroxide, sulfuric acid and catechol. Sheridan believed that the formula lowers the voltage of the cancer cell, allowing the body to recognize it as foreign. This then allows the body to 'digest' the cancer cells.

Evidence/clinical trials   Animal studies done at the National Cancer Institute in the late 1970s and 1980 failed to detect any substantial anticancer activity. Further investigations in the early 1990s were also negative. No clinical trials have been published to date.

Toxicity   There are no published reports of serious toxicity related to treatment with Cancell. Some of the manufacturers' Websites suggest that mild nausea can occur.

Cellular treatment

Background   Cellular therapy is known by a variety of names (e.g. live cell therapy, cellular suspensions, glandular therapy, embryonic cell therapy and organotherapy). Popularized in the 1930s by a Swiss physician (Paul Niehans MD, 1882–1971), the treatment consists of injections of processed tissues from animal embryos, fetuses or organs. Cells are harvested from the animal organ that corresponds to the diseased organ of the patient. For example, a lung cancer patient might receive embryonic lung cells from an animal 'donor'. Usually, sheep and cows are the primary 'donor' animals. In 1970, Wolfram Kuhnau MD, one of Dr Niehans' associates, began providing cellular therapy to cancer patients in Tijuana, Mexico. Similarly to homeopathic reasoning, 'like cells help like cells' is the underpinning to this therapy. Injected cells are theorized to travel to the diseased organ and there revitalize it.

Evidence/clinical trials   There are no clinical trials reporting results of cancer patients treated with cellular therapy.

Toxicity   Most conventional researchers view such treatment as dangerous, since the consequences of injecting foreign animal material into the human body is rife with potential complications.

Coley's toxins

Background   William B. Coley, a surgeon at what is now Memorial Sloan Kettering Cancer Center, observed in the early 1900s that sarcoma patients who developed bacterial infections after surgery had a better survival rate than those who did not. He hypothesized that toxins associated with the bacteria stimulated the immune system and enhanced the antitumor effect against the sarcoma. He formulated a mixture of bacterial toxins that came to be known as Coley's toxins. Proponents suggest that the toxins could boost the production of interferon, interleukin-2 and/or tumor necrosis factor.

Evidence/clinical trials   The University of Texas MD Anderson Cancer Center[23] summarized all available research regarding Coley's toxins to December 2000. This review identified 30 human studies, with only three being randomized controlled trials. Methodological concerns and possible bias limit the interpretability of the studies but, in essence, little clinical benefit could be identified.

Shark cartilage

History   In the early 1950s, Dr John F. Prudden, at the Columbia Presbyterian Medical Center, used bovine cartilage to promote wound healing in surgical patients. He also used cartilage powder to treat a woman with an ulcerated breast cancer. She was reported to have done well until she died of unrelated causes 12 years later. Interest in this therapy was revitalized in the early 1990s when Dr I. William Lane published a book entitled *Sharks Don't Get Cancer*. Subsequent research demonstrated that sharks do in fact develop cancers, but the public fascination with shark cartilage as a possible cancer cure was already established.

Although a modest antiangiogenic effect has been observed in laboratory experiments, it has not been demonstrated that feeding shark cartilage to humans significantly inhibits angiogenesis in patients with cancer. Others have postulated an immune-enhancing effect to be the mechanism of benefit.

Evidence/clinical trials   A comprehensive summary of the literature to 2001 has been published on the MD Anderson Cancer Center site[23]. Of 17 human studies, seven were incomplete or preliminary phase I/II studies. Of the remaining ten studies, nine were prospective cohort trials without controls and one was a 'best case' series. Prudden's early studies were encouraging, but most of the more recent trials have failed to demonstrate a significant benefit.

A large trial sponsored by the National Cancer Institute (NCI) and the National Center for Complementary and Alternative Medicine (NCCAM) is underway, hopefully to provide definitive information on the utility of shark cartilage in the treatment of cancer.

Toxicity   There have been few reports of toxicity associated with shark cartilage. Five patients withdrew from one cartilage study because of gastrointestinal symptoms[24], and one possible case of hepatitis has been reported[25].

714X

History   714X is an aqueous solution containing camphor, nitrogen, ammonium salts and ethanol. Gaston Naessens, a scientist from Quebec, developed the formula. He theorized that within the human body there are living organisms called 'somatids'. He was able to view these creatures using a special microscope of his own design, called a 'somatoscope'. Based on his observations on the life cycles of these somatids, he determined that cancer cells produce co-cancerogenic factor (CKF), which prevents the immune system from recognizing cancer cells. 714X provides extra nitrogen that causes the cancer cells to cease production of CKF. This allows the immune system to recognize and eliminate cancer cells.

Evidence/clinical trials   A comprehensive review conducted by staff of the MD Anderson Cancer Center found only four published human trials of 714X to August 2001[23]. Each of these are case reports, published primarily in lay publications.

Toxicity According to the review by the Task Force on Alternative Therapies of the Canadian Breast Cancer Research Initiative, no published reports were found on infection associated with the use of 714X, although localized redness, tenderness and swelling at the injection site was common[26].

The above five treatments, and thousands more like them, are appealing to patients for a number of reasons. Foremost, they have at least a scientific veneer that makes the claims seem plausible. Many have been discovered and or promoted by individuals with impressive credentials. Almost all of them, on superficial review, seem to a desperate and scientifically naive patient, to be novel, effective and largely non-toxic.

The issues become even more complex when one moves deeper into promotional sites on the Web. Several themes emerge when the websites that promote these and similar 'cures' are examined closely. First, most purveyors of a 'cure' generally claim to have unique knowledge or insight into cancer. This may be in the form of a novel concept of how cancer is caused (e.g. somatids) or on the method needed to attack cancer cells (e.g. nitrogen). Usually, there is a disclaimer that physicians, pharmaceutical companies or both are suppressing this unique knowledge. The implication, veiled (or sometimes not), is that the 'cure' is being suppressed to allow physicians and companies to profit from the treatment of cancer. The claims will usually include promises that the treatment being promoted is 'natural', 'safe' and devoid of side-effects.

HOW A PHYSICIAN HELPS A PATIENT THROUGH THE MAZE OF CLAIMS, PROMISES AND OUTRIGHT FALSEHOODS IS CRITICAL

The realm of CAM and cancer is one in a state of flux. Both patients and, increasingly, physicians are showing interest in the importance of quality of life for the cancer patient. This has led to some cancer treatment centers incorporating music and massage therapy into their usual treatment regimens. Studies are increasingly being undertaken to look at these therapies, not so much to determine whether they increase survival but whether they increase the quality of life. Simply being able to ask the question 'Does this make a patient feel better?' as opposed to focusing only on 'Does this make a patient live longer?' is an important step in the ongoing development of the medical profession.

At the same time, CAM therapies are being studied to see whether they can work in a truly complementary, or even synergistic, fashion with conventional treatments. The study of ginkgo biloba as a potential preventive for the development of chemotherapy-related cognitive decline is one such example. The known protective effects of ginkgo on the brain (e.g. cerebral vasodilatation, antioxidant function, platelet inhibition) suggest that it might indeed decrease the long-term sequelae of chemotherapy commonly referred to as 'chemo brain'. The previously discussed concerns regarding the administration of antioxidants at the time of chemotherapy should sound a cautionary note. The fact that patients have already begun using ginkgo and other antioxidants at the time of chemotherapy highlights the need for definitive, rigorous scientific studies.

Finally, into this generally positive milieu of changing attitudes and re-prioritization of values, comes the specter of the 'cure'. Whether peddled by a well-intentioned friend or more commonly by a profit-oriented huckster, there is a proliferation of companies and individuals each claiming unique truth in the battle against cancer. The huckster of the 1800s, peddling generally worthless cures, can be forgiven as he generally provided some entertainment and his nostrums generally were less harmful than the mercury and bloodletting a patient might expect at the hands of a conventional physician. That scenario has changed dramatically now, with many cancers being curable and a significant proportion controllable through the use of chemotherapy, radiation therapy and/or surgery. Rapidly improving detection tools continue to advance the point in the continuum of disease when many tumors can be detected. As a result, a person with a small breast tumor has a real chance to be cured when the full forces of modern medicine are brought to bear. That same patient, however, if fearful of conventional treatment and desirous of a natural alternative, could well end up expending her initial efforts on such treatments. Time spent on these treatments potentially allows the tumor to progress to the point that a previously curable cancer is so no longer, by the time she returns to seek conventional care.

Thus, the physician or other health-care provider, who truly wishes to benefit the cancer patient with treatment, must be open-minded and uncritical in their thinking. Listening carefully to what the patient is asking is a basic step, but one that frequently is pushed aside in the modern age of cost-containment and brief encounters. Once the patient's question is understood, resources can be assembled and both physician and patient can learn together. Websites maintained by the American Cancer Society[27] and the NCI[28] have sections devoted to CAM and some of the most commonly encountered therapies. The MD Anderson Cancer Center[23] site has recently been updated and includes excellent in-depth summaries of many CAM therapies used by patients. For excellent, referenced information on herbs and dietary supplements, the Natural Medicine Comprehensive Database[29] is an excellent resource. It is a proprietary site but the content is updated frequently and is linked to references (and frequently directly to the full article).

Using such resources, a physician can bring back important information to the patient. Potential risks and benefits can be discussed in a rational manner. Then, if the patient decides to incorporate some aspect of CAM into their treatment regimen, the physician will know of the decision. Patient and physician can be partners to watch for side-effects and also monitor whether the treatment is achieving the agreed-upon outcomes. Thus, a CAM therapy that is not beneficial to the patient's health or quality of life can be stopped. If the patient finds some benefit, the physician–patient team can monitor the results together. The physician who takes the extra time to learn about CAM therapies and then shares that information with their patient is fulfilling one of the most ancient and important aspects of being a doctor – teaching. Together, armed with a rapidly growing body of reliable research, physicians and patients can be partners in choosing and safely combining the best that conventional medicine and CAM have to offer.

References

1. Eisenberg DM, Kessler RC, Foster C. Unconventional medicine in the United States: prevalence, costs, and patterns of use. *N Engl J Med* 1993;328:246–52

2. Eisenberg DM, Davis RB, Ettner SL, *et al.* Trends in alternative medicine use in the United States, 1990–1997: results of a follow-up national survey. *J Am Med Assoc* 1998;280:1569–75

3. Gray CM, Tan AWH, Pronk NP, O'Connor PJ. Complementary and alternative medicine use among health plan members: a cross-sectional survey. *Eff Clin Pract* 2002;5;17–22

4. Ernst E, Cassileth BR. The prevalence of complementary/alternative medicine in cancer. *Cancer* 1998;83:777–82

5. Risberg T, Kaasa S, Wist E, Melsom H. Why are cancer patients using non-proven complementary therapies? A cross-sectional mulitcentre study in Norway. *Eur J Cancer* 1997;33:575–80

6. Miller M, Boyer M, Butow P, Gattellaria M, Dunn S, Childs A. The use of unproven methods of treatment by cancer patients: frequency, expectations and cost. *Support Care Cancer* 1998;6:337–47

7. Kappauf H, Leykauf-Ammon D, Bruntsch U, *et al.* Use of and attitudes held towards unconventional medicine by patients in a department of internal medicine/oncology and haematology. *Support Care Cancer* 2000;8:314–22

8. Oneschuck D, Hanson J, Bruera E. Complementary therapy use: a survey of community- and hospital-based patients with advanced cancer. *Palliat Med* 2000;14:432–4

9. Morris KT, Johnson N, Homer L, Walts D. A comparison of complementary therapy use between breast cancer patients and patients with other primary tumor sites. *Am J Surg* 2000;179:407–11

10. Richardson M, Sanders T, Palmer J, Greisinger A, Singletary S. Complementary/alternative medicine use in a comprehensive cancer center and the implications for oncology. *J Clin Oncol* 2000; 18:2505–14

11. Neuhouser ML, Kristal AR, Patterson RE, Goodman PJ, Thompson IM. Dietary supplement use in the prostate cancer prevention trial: implications for prevention trials. *Nutr Cancer* 2001;39:12–18

12. Heinonen OP, Albanes D, Virtamo J, *et al.* Prostate cancer and supplementation with alpha-tocopherol and beta-carotene: incidence and mortality in a controlled trial. *J Natl Cancer Inst* 1998;90:440–6

13. Clark LC, Combs GF, Turnbull BW, *et al.* Effects of selenium supplementation for cancer prevention in patients with carcinoma of the skin. A randomized controlled trial. Nutritional Prevention of Cancer Study Group. *J Am Med Assoc* 1996;276:1957–63

14. Risberg T, Lund E, Wist E, Kaasa S, Wilsgaard T. Cancer patients use of nonproven therapy: a 5-year follow-up study. *J Clin Oncol* 1998;16:6–12

15. Bagenal FS, Easton DF, Harris E, *et al.* Survival of patients with breast cancer attending Bristol Cancer Help Centre. *Lancet* 1990;336:606–10

16. Cassileth BR, Lusk EJ, Guerry D, *et al.* Survival and quality of life among patients receiving an unproven as compared with conventional therapy. *N Engl J Med* 1991;324:1180–5

17. Gilbar O, Iron G, Goren A. Adjustment of illness of cancer patients treated by complementary therapy along with conventional therapy. *Patient Educ Counsel* 2001;44:243–9

18. Weeks J. Quality of life assessment: performance status upstaged? *J Clin Oncol* 1992;10:1827–9

19. Coates A, Porzsolt F, Osoba D. Quality of life in oncology practice: prognostic value of EORTC QLQ-C30 scores in patients with advanced malignancy. *Eur J Cancer* 1997;33:1025–30

20. Fraser SCA, Ramirez AJ, Ebbs SR, *et al.* A daily diary for quality of life measurement in advanced breast cancer trials. *Br J Cancer* 1993;67:341–6

21. Walker LG, Walker MB, Ogston K, *et al.* Psychological, clinical and pathological effects of relaxation training and guided imagery during primary chemotherapy. *Br J Cancer* 1999;80:262–8

22. Omenn GS, Goodman GE, Thornquist MD, *et al.* Effects of a combination of beta carotene and vitamin A on lung cancer and cardiovascular disease. *N Engl J Med* 1996;334:1150–5

23. http://www.mdanderson.org/departments/cimer/

24. Miller DR, Granick JL, Stark JJ, Anderson GT. Phase I/II trial of the safety and efficacy of shark cartilage in the treatment of advanced cancers. *J Clin Oncol* 1998;16:3649–55

25. Ashar B, Vargo E. Shark cartilage-induced hepatitis [letter]. *Ann Intern Med* 1996;125:780–1

26. Kaegi E. Unconventional therapies for cancer: 6. 714X. *Can Med Assoc J* 1998;158:1621–4

27. www.cancer.org/

28. www.nci.nih.gov/

29. www.naturaldatabase.com/

Complementary and alternative medicine in the perimenopause and menopause

27

E. J. Bieber and J. S. Gell

INTRODUCTION

This text has focused on many of the alternative and integrative methodologies for treatment of both normally occurring physiological processes (such as the menopause) versus pathological states. The areas of menopause and perimenopause treatment have been very active in the last few years with exciting medical studies being completed and with new, and in some cases, very unexpected data (such as the Heart and Estrogen/progestin Replacement Study (HERS) and the Women's Health Initiative (WHI) trials) being published. There are multiple cross references throughout this text to the agents discussed within this chapter. Patients have significant interest in the available options for menopausal treatment and there is a tremendous need for valid clinical information. We have tried to include recent, relevant trials and information to guide you and your patients in making important health-care decisions.

The extent of alternative therapy use during the menopausal transition is probably much greater than previously appreciated. In a recent survey of Washington State HMO patient's aged 45–65, 23% of patients reported past or present soy product usage[1]. Not surprisingly, patients not taking exogenous estrogen were twice as likely to use alternative treatments to manage symptoms.

As the population of the USA continues to age, more women than ever before are reaching menopause. While the average age of menopause remains at 51 years, many women begin to experience symptoms classically associated with menopause well before their menses cease. The World Health Organization defines the perimenopause as the age of onset of menopausal symptoms until 1 year after the final menstrual period with menopause being defined as the permanent cessation of menstruation resulting from the loss of ovarian follicular activity. The clinical features of the menopause transition include menstrual irregularities, vasomotor symptoms and urogenital atrophy. While traditional hormonal therapies are an option, many women look to complementary and alternative medicine to alleviate their symptoms.

PERIMENOPAUSE: THE BIOLOGY

The ovarian follicular apparatus is laid down during embryonic development. Oocyte mitosis occurs early in gestational life with the maximum number of oocytes being present in the ovary at about 20 weeks of gestational age. Primary oocytes begin meiosis but the process is arrested in the diplotene stage of the first meiotic division. At this point, the primary oocyte is surrounded by a layer of primitive granulosa cells and becomes a primordial follicle. Oocytes that are not incorporated into follicles undergo degeneration and account for the majority of oocytes that disappear by birth. The oocytes remain arrested until puberty, and with the onset of ovulation, the first meiotic division is completed. The second meiotic division begins after ovulation and is completed after fertilization. This process continues throughout reproductive life. The perimenopausal transition coincides with a marked decrease in the number of primordial follicles within the ovary. With the decrease in follicle number, fewer granulosa cells are present resulting in diminished inhibin secretion leading to increased follicle stimulating hormone (FSH) secretion[2]. Estradiol levels are initially maintained; however, greater fluctuations in secretion occur. Finally, estradiol levels begin to decline substantially within the year or two preceding the final menses.

Recently, a prospective study categorized the symptoms and their prevalence in a large cohort of women throughout the menopausal transition[3]. The symptoms most specifically linked to the hormonal changes of menopausal transition are vasomotor complaints, vaginal dryness and breast tenderness.

PHYTOESTROGENS

Phytoestrogens are one of the main alternatives women turn to as an alternative to estrogen replacement therapy. Phytoestrogens are diphenolic compounds found in grains, legumes and grasses. Because they possess a phenolic ring, they are able to bind to estrogen receptors[4]. Most phytoestrogens, however, have a greater affinity for the estrogen receptor-β than the estrogen receptor-α. The clinical consequences of these relationships remain to be elucidated. An important point is that even though these compounds can bind to the estrogen receptor, they are much weaker than human estrogens[5]. While many classes of phytoestrogens exist, ones pertinent to treating menopausal symptoms are isoflavones, ligans and coumestans (Figures 1–3). Lignans are found in grains and cereals such as linseed oil, coumestans are found in sprouts such as alfalfa[6] and isoflavones are found primarily in legumes such as soybeans and soy products.

Soybeans, which contain 1–2 mg of isoflavone per gram of soy protein, are the richest food source of isoflavones. The amount of phytoestrogen found in a soy product depends on how it is processed (Table 1). Soymilk and flour contain less phytoestrogen than soybeans and some soy powders and capsules have no remaining isoflavone after being processed with an

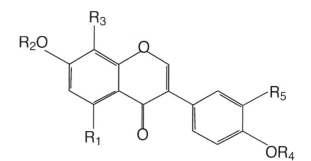

Figure 1 Chemical structure of isoflavone

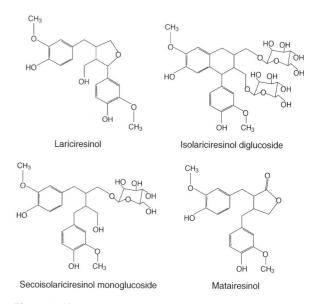

Lariciresinol

Isolariciresinol diglucoside

Secoisolariciresinol monoglucoside

Matairesinol

Figure 2 Chemical structures of the lignans, lariciresinol, isolariciresinol diglucoside, secoisolariciresinol monoglucoside and matairesinol

alcohol extract[5]. Soybeans contain three different types of isoflavones: genistein, daidzein and glyciten (Figure 4). Red clover is another source of isoflavone. Similar to soy products, red clover extracts contain genistein and daidzein in addition to formononetin and biochanin[7].

Genistein has 1/400–1/1000 the potency of 17β-estradiol and binds much more readily to the estrogen β-receptor than the α-receptor. Depending on the tissue type and the amount of endogenous circulating estrogens, genistein may exhibit either estrogenic or antiestrogenic effects. Due to these properties, isoflavones are used by women to treat various perimenopausal symptoms and complaints.

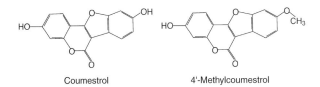

Coumestrol   4'-Methylcoumestrol

Figure 3 Chemical structures of the coumestans, coumestrol and 4'-methylcoumestrol

Table 1 Isoflavone content of soy products

	Amount (cup)	Isoflavone (mg)	Calories (kcal)	Fat (g)
Low-fat tofu	Half	35	60	2
Regular tofu	Half	35	110	6
Soy milk	One	30	130–150	4
Low-fat soy milk	One	20	105	2
Soy nuts	Quarter	60	195	9

THERAPEUTIC USE OF PHYTOESTROGENS

The hot flash is the classic and clearly the most bothersome symptom of the perimenopause. Accordingly, many recent studies have investigated the efficacy of phytoestrogens for treating hot flashes. Given that only 10–14% of Asian women, who have a much higher dietary intake of soy products, experience hot flashes as compared to 70–80% of women in the USA, Brzezinski and colleagues looked at the effects of a short-term, phytoestrogen-rich diet on menopausal symptoms[8]. Women were randomized to either a diet rich in phytoestrogens or to a regular diet with instructions to avoid specific soy products and flax seed. The phytoestrogen-rich diet included 80 g of tofu (containing approximately 75 mg/g daidzein and 200 mg/g genistein), 400 ml of soy drink (7 mg/g daidzein and 20 mg/g genistein), one teaspoon of miso (40 mg/g daidzein and 35 mg/g genistein) and two teaspoons of ground flax seed (4 mg/g lignans). Throughout the study period, the women recorded the severity of their menopausal symptoms and also had assays performed for gonadotropins, estradiol, sex hormone binding globulin (SHBG) and phytoestrogens. Menopause symptoms

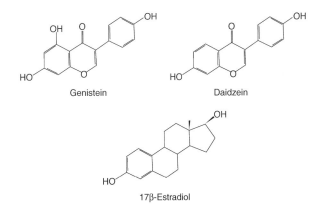

Genistein   Daidzein

17β-Estradiol

Figure 4 Chemical structures of genistein, daidzein and 17β–estradiol

improved overall in both groups; however, hot flashes and vaginal dryness were more significantly reduced in the phytoestrogen group as compared to the control group. SHBG also increased in the women eating a phytoestrogen-rich diet but there was no significant difference in estradiol levels.

St Germain and colleagues compared the differences of an isoflavone-rich soy protein (80.4 mg/day), an isoflavone-poor soy protein (4.4 mg/day) and a control (whey protein) for the treatment of hot flashes and night sweats[9]. In this study, women were randomized to one of the three groups and filled out a weekly menopausal diary at baseline, 12 weeks and 24 weeks of the study. Frequency of hot flashes decreased in all groups, as did night-sweat frequency. However, no difference existed between the treatment groups and placebo.

Other investigators have looked at the effects of soy supplementation on menopausal symptoms. Albertazzi and co-workers performed a double-blind, placebo-controlled trial in which 104 women were randomized to either 60 g of casein as a placebo or 60 g of isolated soy protein daily consisting of 76 mg of isoflavones[10]. All women were asked to record the number and severity of hot flashes and night sweats for a 12-week period. At the completion of the study, women in the isoflavone group experienced a 45% decrease in hot flashes as compared to a 30% decrease in the casein group (Figure 5). In a follow-up study, Albertazzi and colleagues evaluated the change in serum levels of isoflavones after the 60-g/day soy supplementation. Marked increases were seen in

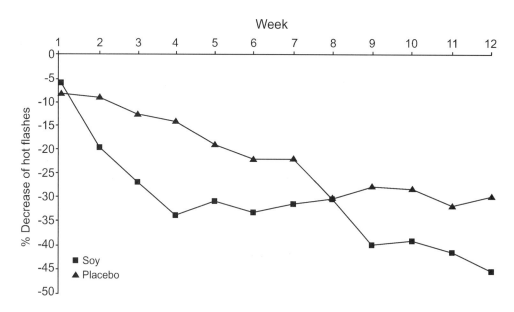

Figure 5 Weekly decrease (%) in the number of hot flashes experienced by women taking either soy protein or a placebo. The difference was significant after week 2, with the exception of week 8. Reproduced from reference 10 with permission

genistein, daidzin and equol[11] (Figure 6). Interestingly, these marked increases did not correlate with decreases in vasomotor symptoms. They also noted large inter- and intra-individual variation in levels of isoflavones.

Washburn investigated soy supplementation and menopausal symptoms in perimenopausal women supplementing their diet with either placebo or once-daily administration of phytoestrogens or twice-daily administration of phytoestrogens[12]. Women recorded both the frequency and severity of hot flashes and night sweats. Hot flash severity declined in the twice-daily group and night-sweat severity improved slightly but did not reach statistical significance.

Scambia assessed a standardized soy extract containing 50 mg/day isoflavone as compared to placebo or in combination with conjugated equine estrogens[13]. Initially, women received either placebo or the soy supplement alone; after 6 weeks, 0.625 mg of conjugated equine estrogens were given to each group. Women taking soy alone had a significant reduction in hot flash frequency and severity. An even greater decrease was seen when conjugated equine estrogens were added. Consistent with these studies is an interesting prospective cohort study, which evaluated premenopausal females in Takayama, Japan[14]. In patients

who began to have vasomotor symptoms during the 6 years of follow-up, hot flashes were inversely correlated with low levels of soy (total consumption) or isoflavone intake.

In evaluating the best clinical trials to date regarding soy supplementation there seems to be some data to suggest that soy does have an effect which may be greater than placebo if high enough doses are ingested. There are other reasons to have a diet high in isoflavones and these areas are intentionally not covered in this chapter. An interesting issue is the present use of tablets containing isolated isoflavones. Unfortunately, ingestion of isoflavones in this manner may not offer the same value as a lifetime of exposure to naturally derived high isoflavone foodstuffs. An additional concern is the variability in conversion of soy isoflavones in the gastrointestinal system to the more potent equol. As Albertazzi demonstrated, even measurements in the same patient, ingesting the same daily amount, demonstrated wide fluctuations in levels. Albertazzi recently made an accurate observation about the continued need for well-done clinical trials in this important area. He noted, 'Above all, when using isolated nutrients such as isoflavones in tablet form, it is important to assess their bioavailability first, before attempting to assess clinical efficacy.

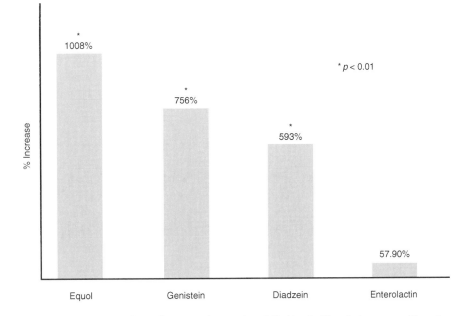

Figure 6 Change in serum levels of isoflavones after isoflavone supplementation of 60 g/day for 12 weeks in women with moderate to severe hot flashes. Reproduced from reference 11 with permission

A lot of these phytoestrogen preparations may, in fact, just be very expensive pellets that once ingested are, literally speaking, going down the drain! This lack of rigor will, if allowed to persist, ultimately undermine the credibility of the whole field of phytoestrogens among both scientists and consumers alike, thus dooming compounds that could potentially have extremely attractive health-giving properties.'[15]

Another source of isoflavones is red clover. Red clover is a medicinal herb traditionally used by Native Americans for a multitude of conditions. Red clover contains four primary isoflavones: genistein, daidzein and their methylated precursors biochanin and formonometin[16]. Unlike soy products, which in some cultures are dietary staples, red clover, if eaten at all by humans, is consumed in small quantities as flavoring. Recently, standardized extracts of red clover have been developed to treat menopausal symptoms. Baber and colleagues investigated the use of Promensil™, a standardized red clover extract containing 40 mg per tablet of total isoflavones for hot flashes[17]. Women with at least three hot flash episodes per day were randomized to either Promensil or placebo for 3 months then crossed over to the alternate treatment. Hot flash

severity and frequency decreased in both groups but was not different in the red clover group. There was no change in endometrial thickness in the red clover group suggesting lack of endometrial stimulation. Unfortunately, the short study interval limits this interpretation. Urine isoflavone analysis demonstrated high urinary isoflavone excretion in both Promensil and placebo groups suggesting that women in the placebo group also ingested isoflavones in their regular diets. Decreased flashing frequency was, however, correlated to increased urinary isoflavone excretion.

Another group looked at the effects of increasing doses of Promensil on hot flash severity and frequency[18]. Study participants had at least three hot flashes per day. Women were randomized to placebo, 40 mg daily of Promensil or 160 mg daily of Promensil. Each active tablet contained 4.0 mg of genistein, 3.5 mg of daidzein, 24.5 mg of biochanin and 8.0 mg of formononetin. Flashing frequency decreased in all groups over the 12-week trial with no significant difference between the groups. Urinary isoflavone levels demonstrated a dose-dependent increase between women receiving the isoflavone tablets. However, a small increase was also observed for women receiving placebo suggesting that these women also increased dietary consumption of isoflavones.

ISOFLAVONES AND NEOPLASIA

Since isoflavones have estrogenic effects, a concern is that they are able to stimulate the endometrium which could theoretically lead to the development of endometrial hyperplasia or endometrial adenocarcinoma. In fact, a case report describes a 39-year-old woman with a body mass index of 19 who developed a grade 1 adenocarcinoma of the endometrium with her only identifiable risk factor being significant consumption of soy and isoflavone containing supplements[19].

Several studies have looked at the effect of isoflavone treatment on both endometrial thickness and vaginal maturation. Wilcox found an increase in maturation index in women supplementing their diet with soya flour, red clover sprouts and linseed[20]. However, other studies have not demonstrated an increase in vaginal maturation with increasing isoflavone content in the diet or supplementation[21]. Scambia and co-workers evaluated endometrial thickness after treatment with either placebo or soy supplementation and did not find any difference between the groups[14]. Finally, Duncan and colleagues evaluated endometrial histology obtained by endometrial biopsy performed at baseline and after treatment phases[21]. There was no difference between baseline and after consumption of isoflavone-enriched diets. Histological findings included inactive endometrium and proliferative endometrium, which was found in both groups at baseline and after treatment.

Another area of interest and potential concern is in soy or phytoestrogen ingestion in patients who have previously been diagnosed with breast cancer. There are 175 000–185 000 new cases of breast cancer per year in the USA with many of these patients being symptomatic in the peri- or newly menopausal stage. Often these patients have been dissuaded by their clinicians or are afraid of estrogen ingestion based on lay media reports, and turn to soy products as an alternative for their vasomotor symptomology. In addition, patients

who are beginning tamoxifen treatment may experience significant exacerbation of vasomotor symptoms. In a well-done clinical trial, 177 breast cancer survivors with vasomotor symptoms were enrolled in a randomized, double-blind, crossover trial in which the patients consumed 150 mg/day of soy (equivalent to approximately three glasses of soy milk)[22]. Soy was not more effective than placebo at reducing vasomotor instability and patients actually preferred the placebo.

In addition to the lack of efficacy data, little clinical safety information exists to allow us to reassure these patients. Indeed, several studies have suggested that, in mice, genistein and soy at typical levels may be stimulatory to breast cancer cells[23].

In another recent trial, Ju and colleagues evaluated the impact of genistein on the efficacy of tamoxifen, again in a mouse model. Of concern, was that ingestion of dietary genistein negated the effect of tamoxifen, and actually increased the expression of genes known to be modulated by estrogen[24]. No human data are currently available regarding this issue, although in populations with high soy diets such as those seen in Japan, breast cancer survival appears unaffected.

BLACK COHOSH

Cimicifugae racemosae rhizoma (Black cohosh) is a herb native to Eastern North America and has been traditionally used by Native Americans to treat gynecological conditions including menopause[25]. Black cohosh was commercially marketed in the 19th century as Lydia Pinkham's Vegetable Compound (Figure 7), in the 20th century as Huntington's 11 and most recently in the 21st century as Remifemin®. The primary active constituents in black cohosh are triterpenes and flavonoids[26]. In a recent study evaluating estrogenic activity *in vitro*, black cohosh did not appear to induce the growth of a human breast cancer cell line or activate either the estrogen receptor-β or estrogen receptor-α in cells transfected with an estrogen-dependent reporter plasmid[27]. Clinically, black cohosh has been used to treat hot flashes in breast cancer patients. One placebo-controlled, randomized trial did not demonstrate a difference between placebo or black cohosh[28]. Both groups experienced a decrease in frequency and severity of hot flashes.

Given that black cohosh's effects may be dose-dependent, a recently reported 6-month trial compared the standard 40 mg/day of black cohosh to a higher dose (127.3 mg/day)[29]. Both groups reported improvement in hot flashes; however, a placebo was not included in this study. In addition, there was no effect on vaginal maturation index in either group.

No long-term studies on black cohosh exist and, thus, treatment has been recommended to last no longer than 6 months. Side-effects are limited but include gastrointestinal upset, bradycardia, headaches and nausea.

VITAMIN E

Vitamin E has also been suggested as an alternative to estrogen and progestin for reducing vasomotor symptoms (Figure 8) . Limited case reports had previously suggested efficacy. However, a randomized, placebo-controlled, crossover study performed by Barton and colleagues in breast cancer survivors failed to demonstrate improvement greater than placebo[30]. Patients received 400 IU of vitamin E succinate b.i.d. for 4 weeks in a crossover design.

DONG QUAI AND CHINESE HERBS

Dong quai is a Chinese herbal commonly used for a number of gynecological conditions. Often extracted from the root of *Angelica senesis* it has been used through the centuries to treat menstrual disorders and menopausal symptoms as well as nervousness, dizziness and insomnia. There are multiple chemicals that can be found in Dong quai but the primary active compounds are believed to be coumarin derivatives including psoralen, osthol and oxypeucedanin.

In a randomized, double-blind clinical trial performed in the Kaiser system, Dong quai 4.5 g/day in a standardized extract was compared to placebo in postmenopausal patients with a FSH level > 30 mIU/ml[31]. Patients were evaluated at baseline

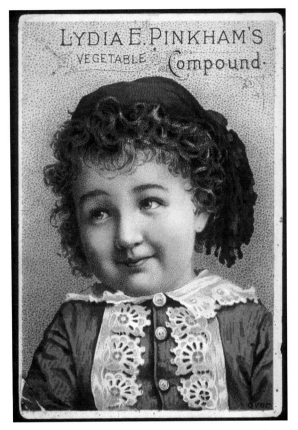

Figure 7 A label from Lydia Pinkham's Vegetable Compound. Courtesy of the National Library of Medicine

and at 6, 12 and 24 weeks. Both placebo and treatment groups had equivalent reductions in hot flashes with no difference noted in endometrial thickness, vaginal maturation index or Kupperman index. The Kupperman index is an index based on 11 menopausal symptoms including vasomotor, nervousness, insomnia, melancholia, paresthesia, formication, fatigue, headache, palpitation, arthralgia and vertigo. While some herbalists have suggested Dong quai exerts an estrogenic effect, this study would not support that claim. Critics of this trial have suggested that Dong quai is not used alone in traditional Chinese medicine. However, in the USA, Dong quai is often purchased in this fashion at health food stores. Another concern was that the dose used in this trial was lower than often prescribed.

Side-effects of Dong quai are infrequent but can include phototoxicity from external application.

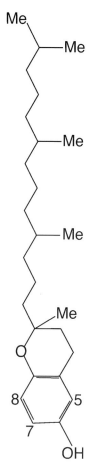

Figure 8 Chemical structure of vitamin E

Since coumarin derivatives are present there is a theoretical concern regarding bleeding; however, there are no clinical reports to date. Herbal pharmacopeias suggest Dong quai is an abortifacient and should thus not be used in pregnancy. Most recently, Amato and colleagues at Baylor College of Medicine, Texas, evaluated Dong quai for evidence of estrogenicity as well as ability to stimulate breast cancer cells *in vitro*[27]. While Dong quai did not demonstrate evidence of an estrogen-like effect on either cells or tissue, there was a significant stimulatory effect on the human breast cancer cell line MCF-7. This would suggest caution in using this agent in patients with known breast cancer.

Davis and colleagues from Australia are one of the few groups to attempt to study prospectively a defined combination of Chinese medicinal herbs[32]. Of interest is the fact that their combination did not

include Dong quai as one of the constituents. They did use a menopause-specific quality-of-life questionnaire (MENQOL) as part of their double-blind, randomized, placebo-controlled trial. Chinese herbs were found to reduce vasomotor events by 15%; however, placebo had a 31% decrease and this almost reached statistical significance in favor of placebo, $p = 0.09$. Both groups had score reductions on the MENQOL questionnaire that were equivalent. Several important points come out of this trial. It is very important to have control groups; in this trial the authors even attempted to flavor the placebo to match the treatment. This trial looked at a specific grouping of 12 Chinese herbs at specific doses. A different combination at varying doses could well have produced dissimilar results.

PROGESTERONE CREAMS

A highly popular movement in the USA is for the use of topical progesterone creams for treatment of vasomotor symptoms, premenstrual syndrome (PMS) and osteoporosis. Some practitioners have also used topical progesterones in place of oral progestins in patients on combined hormone replacement therapy (HRT). In light of the WHI trial, one wonders if this practice will increase. The Mexican wild yam (*Dioscorea villosa*) has been used as a means to derive progestins and other steroids synthetically and has found favor as an extract for the treatment of a multitude of menopausal symptoms (Figure 9). Because of the widespread use of these treatments, it is important to be familiar with some interesting recent studies.

While extracts of wild yam cream are popular, human beings are not capable of converting the plant sterol dioscorea to progesterone. Thus, one would expect no clinical progestational effect. Whether other constituents of *Dioscorea* are active remains to be elucidated. It has been suggested that diosgenin, another sterol in the Mexican yam has estrogenic effects[33]. It should be noted that all yams are not the same and this discussion applies only to *Dioscorea villosa*. A small (23 patients) double-blind, placebo-controlled, crossover trial with 3 months' treatment per arm found that wild yam cream was ineffective[34].

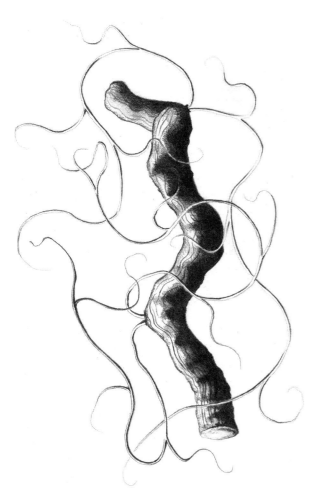

Figure 9 The Mexican wild yam (*Dioscorea villosa*)

No significant differences between placebo and wild yam cream were found in levels of FSH, cholesterols, estradiol, serum or salivary progesterone. Similarly, there were no differences in the number of flashing events or their severity.

It is possible that actual progesterone may exert effects when used in cream form. One of the larger trials compared application of a quarter teaspoon of 20 mg of progesterone cream to placebo for 1 year[35]. They noted improvement or resolution of hot flashes in 25 of 30 (83%) patients receiving the progesterone cream versus five of 26 (19%) receiving placebo, $p < 0.001$. Bone density was unchanged after the first year.

There has been confusion regarding the best means of accessing progesterone levels: serum, free or salivary versus progesterone metabolites. Lewis and colleagues evaluated progesterone pharmacokinetics in a three-arm randomized, double-blind, placebo-controlled trial of menopausal patients not on HRT[36]. Their three arms included placebo and 20 mg or 40 mg of compounded progesterone cream b.i.d. Interestingly, salivary progesterone levels have been suggested to be more predictive of serum levels and effect, and were variable, ranging from 0.25 to 82.11 nmol/l and correlated poorly with serum levels. Actual plasma progesterone increased in both the 20 and 40 mg groups but only slightly. Erythrocytes have been suggested as the means by which progesterone is transported; however, in this trial, erythrocyte progesterone levels were even lower than the low plasma levels[36].

A study by Wren and colleagues has raised concern for patients who are using progesterone cream to oppose oral or transdermal estrogen[37]. They treated postmenopausal patients aged 50–65 for 12 weeks with a weekly estrogen patch (0.1 mg of 17β-estradiol) and randomized patients to one of three doses of micronized progesterone cream, 16 mg, 32 mg or 64 mg, which was applied topically for the last 2 weeks of each 4-week cycle. Serum progesterone levels were performed after 2 weeks of estrogen alone and at the end of month 3 (after the three treatments of progesterone for 14 days). There was a small increase in progesterone levels between the two samples but of greatest concern was the lack of transformation to a secretory endometrium, a finding that would be expected in the face of an adequate amount of progesterone. Given the high incidence of endometrial hyperplasia after treatment with unopposed estrogen (20–50%) the lack of response is worrying. Based on these data, we would recommend that patients on oral or transdermal estrogen using clinically unsubstantiated doses of progesterone should undergo intermittent endometrial sampling.

ALTERNATIVE PHARMACEUTICALS FOR VASOMOTOR SYMPTOMS

It is worthwhile to consider the additional alternatives that exist for women who are significantly symptomatic with vasomotor complaints. As has been detailed in this chapter, increasing isoflavone intake substantially, and possibly use of black cohosh, may impact on vasomotor instability. Several additional non-traditional pharmacological options exist to enhance further our treatment strategies and opportunities to optimize patient satisfaction

Progestins such as norethindrone acetate or medroxyprogesterone acetate (MPA) have been evaluated and found to be successful in ameliorating hot flashes. In early work, Schiff found that oral MPA at a dose of 20 mg/day effectively decreased vasomotor flashes by 73.9%[38]. Lobo noted that depo-MPA compared favorably to 0.625 mg of conjugated equine estrogens in a short-term study[39]. Not surprisingly, megesterol acetate at doses of 40–80 mg/day also markedly decreased hot flashes[40]. More recently, Hornstein and associates evaluated norethindrone acetate 5 mg/day compared to estrogen and progesterone as add-back in patients on gonadotropin releasing hormone agonist and found equivalent efficacy in vasomotor relief (Table 2)[41].

Bellergal, a combination of phenobarbital (40 mg), belladonna alkaloids (0.2 mg) and ergotamine tartrate (0.6 mg), has been successfully used for short-term management of vasomotor symptoms. The exact method of action or key component in this mixture is unknown. The PDR suggests that the combination in some way impacts on the autonomic nervous system; however, data are lacking in this regard. Several trials have demonstrated efficacy although no recent studies have been identified. In one double-blind trial, hot flashes were noted to decrease by 50%[42]. In a second trial published in the mid-1980s, investigators in

The Netherlands found a short-term benefit 2 and 4 weeks after starting the agent but noted a loss of efficacy by 8 weeks[43].

Bellergal has multiple contraindications including coronary artery disease, peripheral vascular disease, hypertension, impaired renal or hepatic function, glaucoma, porphyria, asthma and obstructive uropathy. Bellergal should only be used for short-term use, as phenobarbital is addictive. Patients should also be counseled regarding the sedative effect.

α-Adrenergic agents such as clonidine and methyldopa can also be used as agents for decreasing vasomotor flashing. It has been suggested that norepinephrine is involved in hot flashes and thus these agents may impact on autonomic neurons in the central nervous system. Methyldopa seems to be the least effective of the agents. Several studies in the 1980s failed to provide consistent and convincing evidence for an effect. One trial from 1981, which was a double-blind, crossover design, suggested that Aldomet® was more effective than placebo (65% versus 38% reduction)[44]. However, in a subsequent study by Hammond and colleagues using 250 mg t.i.d. the authors noted some minor degree of improvement but felt the incidence of side-effects limited practical usage[45].

More recently, clonidine has become increasingly utilized as an alternative to sex steroids. Initial trials used higher doses than are currently employed and found good efficacy but noted significant patient intolerance and drop out[46]. In an interesting trial by Freedman and Dinsay, postmenopausal patients with and without hot flashes were injected with intravenous clonidine[47]. Interestingly, clonidine increased the sweating threshold in symptomatic women while

Table 2 Vasomotor symtoms in women treated for 12 months with leuprolide acetate depot (3.75 mg every 4 weeks) alone and in combination with three hormonal add-back regimens. Reproduced from reference 41 with permission

	Group A Placebo	Group B Norethindrone acetate (5 mg)	Group C Norethindrone acetate (5 mg) + CEE (0.625 mg)	Group D Norethindrone acetate (5 mg) + CEE (1.25 mg)
Percent with hot flashes	88	47★	58†	40‡
Median days of hot flashes	28	0‡	2‡	0‡
Median maximum number of hot flashes in 24 h	6	0‡	1★	0‡

CEE, conjugated equine estrogens; ★$p \leqslant 0.01$; †$p \leqslant 0.05$; ‡$p \leqslant 0.001$ compared with Group A

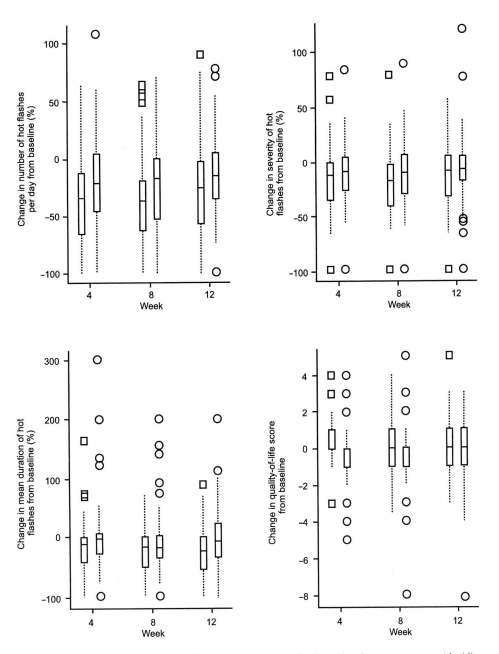

Figure 10 Changes in hot flash symptoms and quality-of-life score compared with baseline values, by treatment group (clonidine or placebo) and study week. For each week, the left-hand box-plot with squares represents the clonidine group and the right-hand box-plot with circles represents the placebo. Reproduced with permission from reference 48

decreasing the threshold in asymptomatic patients. More recent trials have used lower doses such as 0.1 mg/day in an effort to decrease the risk of intolerance. One such trial evaluated this dose in 194 postmenopausal women with a prior history of breast cancer who were being treated with tamoxifen and

were symptomatic with hot flashes[48]. In this 8-week placebo-controlled trial there were significant differences found with clonidine use with a 37% versus 20% decrease at 4 weeks and 38% versus 24% at 8 weeks (Figure 10). Noteworthy was the fact that the clonidine patients had a statistically greater incidence of difficulty sleeping, the opposite of what one might believe in patients who have amelioration of their hot flashes. Transdermal clonidine has also been used with limited success. Goldberg and colleagues found that transdermal clonidine statistically decreased vaso-motor symptoms[49]. However, there was only a 20% decrease in frequency and only a 10% decrease in severity from baseline. Patients experienced side-effects such as mouth dryness, constipation, itchiness from the patch and drowsiness.

The most recent advance in the treatment of vaso-motor symptoms has been the finding that reuptake inhibitors, such as venlafaxine, which affect serotonin and norepinephrine reuptake and slightly impact on dopamine uptake, and selective serotonin reuptake inhibitors (SSRIs), such as paroxetine and fluoxetine, significantly decrease vasomotor symptoms. Loprinzi and colleagues investigated the use of venlafaxine (Effexor®) in three doses (37.5 mg, 75 mg, and 150 mg) versus placebo in the treatment of 191 breast cancer survivors with significant hot flashes[50]. Hot flashes were reduced in all four groups with both the 75 and 150 mg doses decreasing the number from base-line by 61%. The lower dose of 37.5 mg only decreased the number by 37%, which was only slightly better than placebo at 27%. Side-effects included nausea, dry mouth, decreased appetite and constipation, which were more frequent at the higher doses. The same authors reported the intermediate follow-up in this same cohort who were allowed, if desired, to con-tinue use of venlafaxine in a non-randomized fashion. Efficacy was maintained and side-effects did not increase in this intermediate term study[51]. Similarly, a small pilot trial of 20 mg paroxetine in 30 patients demonstrated a 67% decrease in hot flash frequency and a 75% reduction in severity[52]. The most com-mon side-effect was somnolence. At the conclusion of the trial, 83% of patients chose to continue being treated. Most recently fluoxetine (Prozac®) 20 mg was also investigated. Loprinzi and co-workers found

a 50% reduction in hot flash scores, which they defined as frequency times severity, after 4 weeks of treatment which was slightly better than placebo at 36%[53]. Further trials are needed to elucidate optimal dose and long-term compliance and success. How-ever, SSRIs may offer the most effective alternative to patients who are significantly symptomatic or who are not relieved by soy or black cohosh. They are also potentially the safest options for breast cancer survi-vors given the questions regarding even natural alter-natives. It is important in discussing SSRIs as an option for patients that they understand that they are being prescribed the medication for vasomotor relief and not as antidepressants, as there continues to be stigma attached to use of these agents.

CONCLUSION

This chapter has reviewed a number of agents that may be used for the various symptoms that might be encountered in the perimenopause and menopause. There are many areas open to research and investiga-tion given the short nature of many of the studies as well as the lack of appropriate control groups and ran-domization. The National Institute of Health (NIH) and many other investigators are currently conduct-ing such trials. Since the publication of the initial results from the estrogen and progestin arm of the WHI many patients have chosen to stop hormone replacement therapy. Millions of others who will enter the menopausal transition in the next several decades may choose never to start the use of estrogen. Hopefully, the NIH and other trials underway will provide data that will shed further light on which therapies are most appropriate in what situations and for which patients. This will allow clinicians and care providers the greatest opportunity to improve patients' quality of life.

References

1. Newton KM, Buist DS, Keenan NL, Anderson LA, LaCrois AZ. Use of alternative therapies for menopause symptoms: results of a population-based survey. *Obstet Gynecol* 2002;100:18–25

2. Burger HG, Dudley EC, Hopper JL, *et al.* The endocrinology of the menopausal transition: a cross-sectional study of a population-based sample. *J Clin Endocrinol Metab* 1995;80:3537–45

3. Dennerstein L, Dudley EC, Hopper JL, *et al.* A prospective population-based study of menopausal symptoms. *Obstet Gynecol* 2000;96:351–8

4. Mackey R, Eden J. Phytoestrogens and the menopause. *Climacteric* 1998;1:302–8

5. Glazier MG, Bowman MA. A review of the evidence for the use of phytoestrogens as a replacement for traditional estrogen replacement therapy. *Arch Intern Med* 2001;161:1161–72

6. Hudson T. Soy and women's health. *The Female Patient* 2001;26:26–37

7. Clifton-Bligh PB, Baber RJ, Fulcher GR, *et al.* The effect of isoflavones extracted from red clover (rimostil) on lipid and bone metabolism. *Menopause* 2001;8:259–65

8. Brzezinski A, Adlercreutz H, Shaoul R, *et al.* Short-term effects of phytoestrogen-rich diet on postmenopausal women. *Menopause* 1997;2:89–94

9. St Germaine A, Peterson CT, Robinson JG, *et al.* Isoflavone-rich or isoflavone-poor soy protein does not reduce menopausal symptoms during 24 weeks of treatment. *Menopause* 2001;8:17–26

10. Albertazzi P, Pansini F, Bonaccorsi G, *et al.* The effect of dietary soy supplementation on hot flashes. *Obstet Gynecol* 1998;91:6–11

11. Albertazzi P, Pansini F, Bottazzi M, *et al.* Dietary soy supplementation and phytoestrogen levels. *Obstet Gynecol* 1999;94:229–31

12. Washburn S, Burke GL, Morgan T, Anthony M. Effect of soy protein supplementation on serum lipoproteins, blood pressure and menopausal symptoms in perimenopausal women. *Menopause* 1999;6:7–13

13. Scambia G, Mango D, Signorile PG, *et al.* Clinical effects of a standardized soy extract in postmenopausal women: a pilot study. *Menopause* 2000;7:105–11

14. Nagata C, Takatsuka N, Kawakami, Shimizu H. Soy product intake and hot flashes in Japanese women: results from a community-based prospective study. *Am J Epidemiol* 2001;153:790–3

15. Albertazzi P. Soy supplement. Why is the effect so elusive. *J Clin Endocrinol Metab* 2002;87:3508

16. Fugh-Berman A, Kronenberg F. Red clover (*Trifolium pratense*) for menopausal women: current state of knowledge. *Menopause* 2001;8:333–7

17. Baber RJ, Templeman C, Morton T, *et al.* Randomized placebo-controlled trial of an isoflavone supplement and menopausal symptoms in women. *Climacteric* 1999;2:85–92

18. Knight DC, Howes JB, Eden JA. The effect of promensil, an isoflavone extract, on menopausal symptoms. *Climacteric* 1999;2:79–84

19. Johnson EB, Muto MG, Yanushpolsky EH, Mutter GL. Phytoestrogen supplementation and endometrial cancer. *Obstet Gynecol* 2001;98:947–50

20. Wilcox G, Wahlquist ML, Burger HG, Medley G. Oestrogenic effects of plant foods in postmenopausal women. *Br Med J* 1990;301:905–6

21. Duncan AM, Underhill KEW, Xu X, *et al.* Modest hormonal effects of soy isoflavones in postmenopausal women. *J Clin Endocrinol Metab* 1999;84:3479–84

22. Quella SK, Loprinzi CL, Barton DL, *et al.* Evaluation of soy phytoestrogens for the treatment of hot flashes in breast cancer survivors: a North Central Cancer Treatment Group trial. *J Clin Oncol* 2000;18:1068–74

23. Allred CD, Allred KF, Ju YH, Virant SM, Helferich WG. Soy diets containing varying amounts of genistein stimulate growth of estrogen-dependent (MCF-7) tumors in a dose-dependent manner. *Cancer Res* 2001;61:5045–50

24. Ju YH, Doerge DR, Allred KF, Allred CD, Helferich WG. Dietary genistein negates the inhibitory effect of tamoxifen on growth of estrogen-dependent human breast cancer (MCF-7) cells implanted in athymic mice. *Cancer Res* 2002;62:2474–7

25. McKenna DJ, Jones K, Humphrey S, Hughes K. Black cohosh: efficacy, safety and use in clinical and preclinical applications. *Alter Ther Health Med* 2001;7:93–100

26. Tyler VE. Honest herbalist; the bright side of black cohosh. *Prevention* 1997;49:76–9

27. Amato P, Christophe S, Mellon PL. Estrogenic activity of herbs commonly used as remedies for menopausal symptoms. *Menopause* 2002;9:145–50

28. Jacobson JS, Troxel AB, Klaus EJ, *et al.* Randomized trial of black cohosh for the treatment of hot flashes among women with a history of breast cancer. *J Clin Oncol* 2001;19:2739–45

29. Liske E, Hanggi W, Henneicke-von Zepelin HH, *et al.* Physiological investigation of a unique extract of black cohosh (*Cimicifugae racemosae* rhizoma): a 6-month clinical study demonstrates no systemic estrogenic effect. *J Womens Health Gend Based Med* 2002;11:163–74

30. Barton DL, Loprinzi CL, Quella SK, *et al.* Prospective evaluation of vitamin E for hot flashes in breast cancer survivors. *J Clin Oncol* 1998;16:495–500

31. Hirata JD, Swierz LM, Zell B, Small R, Ettinger B. Does Dong quai have estrogenic effects in postmenopausal women? A double-blind placebo-controlled trial. *Fertil Steril* 1997;68:981–6

32. Davis SR, Briganti EM, Chen RQ, *et al.* The effects of Chinese medicinal herbs on postmenopausal vasomotor symptoms of Australian women. A randomized contolled trial. *Med J Aust* 2001;174:68–71

33. Mirkin G. Estrogen in yams. *J Am Med Assoc* 1991;265:912

34. Komesaroff PA, Black CV, Cable V, Sudhir KE. Effects of wild yam extract on menopausal symptoms, lipids and sex hormones in healthy menopausal women. *Climacteric* 2001;4:144–50

35. Leonetti HB, Longo S, Anasti JN. Transdermal progesterone cream for vasomotor symptoms and postmenopausal bone loss. *Obstet Gynecol* 1999;94:225–8

36. Lewis JG, McHill H, Patton VM, Elder PA. Caution on the use of saliva measurements to monitor absorption of progesterone from transdermal creams in postmenopausal women. *Maturitas* 2002;41:1–6

37. Wren BG, McFarland K, Edwards L. Micronized transdermal progesterone and endometrial response. *Lancet* 1999;354:1447–8

38. Schiff I, Tulchinsky D, Cramer D, Ryan KJ. Oral medroxy-progesterone in the treatment of postmenopausal symptoms. *J Am Med Assoc* 1980;244:1443–5

39. Lobo RA, McCormick W, Singer F, Roy S. Depo-medroxy-progesterone acetate compared with conjugated estrogens for the treatment of postmenopausal women. *Obstet Gynecol* 1984;63:1–5

40. Erlik Y, Meldrum DR, Lagasse LD, Judd HL. Effect of megesterol acetate on flushing and bone metabolism in post-menopausal women. *Maturitas* 1981;3:167–72

41. Hornstein MD, Surrey ES, Weisberg GW, *et al*. Leuprolide acetate depot and hormonal add-back in endometriosis: a 12 month study. *Obstet Gynecol* 1998;91:16–24

42. Lebherz TB, French LT. Nonhormonal treatment of the menopause syndrome: a double-blind evaluation of an autonomic system stabilizer. *Obstet Gynecol* 1969;33:795–9

43. Bergmans MG, Merkus JM, Corbey RS, *et al*. Effect of Bellergal retard on climacteric complaints: a double-blind, placebo controlled study. *Maturitas* 1987;9:227–34

44. Nesheim BI, Saete T. Reduction of menopausal hot flushes by methyldopa. A double-blind crossover trial. *Eur J Clin Pharmacol* 1981;20:413–16

45. Hammond MG, Hatley L, Talbert LM. A double-blind study to evaluate the effect of methyldopa on menopausal vasomotor flushes. *J Clin Endocrinol Metab* 1984;58:1158–60

46. Laufer LR, Erlik Y, Meldrum DR, *et al*. Effect of clonidine on hot flashes in postmenopausal women. *Obstet Gynecol* 1982;60:583–6

47. Freedman RR, Dinsay R. Clonidine raises the sweating threshold in symptomatic but not in asymptomatic postmenopausal women. *Fertil Steril* 2000;74:20–3

48. Pandya KJ, Raubertas RF, Flynn PJ, *et al*. Oral clonidine in post-menopausal patients with breast cancer experiencing tamoxifen-induced hot flashes. *Ann Intern Med* 2000;132:788–93

49. Goldberg RM, Loprinzi CL, O'Fallon JR, Veeder MH. Transdermal clonidine for ameliorating tamoxifen induces hot flashes. *Clin Oncol* 1994;12:155–8

50. Loprinzi CL, Kugler JW, Sloan JA, *et al*. Venlafaxine in management of hot flashes in survivors of breast cancer: a randomized controlled trial. *Lancet* 2000;356:2025–6

51. Barton D, La VB, Loprinzi C, *et al*. Venlafaxine for the control of hot flashes: results of a longitudinal continuation study. *Oncol Nursing Forum* 2002;29:33–40

52. Stearns V, Issacs C, Rowland J, Crawford J. A pilot trial assessing the efficacy of paroxetine hydrochloride (Paxil) in controlling hot flashes in breast cancer survivors. *Ann Oncol* 2000;11:17–22

53. Loprinzi CL, Sloan JA, Perez EA, *et al*. Phase III evaluation of fluoxetine for treatment of hot flashes. *J Clin Oncol* 2002;20:1578–83

Complementary and alternative options for mood disorders, premenstrual syndrome and mastalgia

28

E. J. Bieber and J. S. Gell

MOOD DISORDERS

Population-based studies of the menopause transition have evaluated the incidence of mood complaints. Dennerstein and colleagues reported increased symptoms such as nervous tension and sadness in the late perimenopause although the increase was not statistically significant[1]. Still, many women look to alternative therapies to improve mood.

St John's wort

St John's wort, or *Hypericum perforatum*, is commonly used for treatment of depression especially in patients who fear either adverse effects or the perceived stigma associated with prescription antidepressants. In Germany, St John's wort is prescribed more often than any pharmaceutical in the treatment of depression. St John's wort may act similarly to selective serotonin reuptake inhibitors in that it decreases the rate of reuptake of monoamine neurotransmitters such as serotonin[2,3]. However, this has not been consistently demonstrated[4]. St John's wort is most often made from the flower and based in an ethanolic extract standardized to 0.3% hypericin, one of the proposed active constituents of the plant. There may well be multiple other active components including pseudohypericin

and flavonoids. Indeed, more recently, hypericin has been called into question as the main active component since it does not cross the blood–brain barrier. Hyperforin, another potential active constituent has been suggested as the key component. Importantly, significant differences in concentrations of these substances exist depending on when, what and how harvesting of St John's wort is performed. This may account for some of the variability seen in results of clinical trials.

Multiple studies have been performed evaluating hypericum extracts for treatment of depression. A German group looked at an extract of hypericum as compared to placebo for treatment of mild to moderate depression[5]. The treatment group showed an improvement in depression scores as compared to the placebo group with no adverse effects in either group. Other groups have evaluated hypericum as compared to selective serotonin reuptake inhibitors in the treatment of mild to moderate depression. In an evaluation of extract LI 160 as compared to sertraline, clinical response was noted in 47% of the patients receiving hypericum and 40% of the patients receiving sertraline[6]. Another study investigated the use of hypericum extract as compared to fluoxetine[7]. Both treatment groups demonstrated improvement in multiple depression scoring systems. Several meta-analyses have similarly suggested that in patients with mild to moderate depression, St John's wort has similar efficacy to low-dose tricyclic antidepressants but may be better tolerated[8,9].

Two recent studies from the USA have evaluated St John's wort in patients with moderate to severe depression. In the first multicenter trial, St John's wort was found to be no better than placebo, with similar decreases in the Hamilton Depression Scale score (HDS) in both groups after 8 weeks (Figure 1)[10]. In subgroup analysis, it was noted that patients in the St John's wort group did have higher remission rates of 14.3% versus 4.9% for placebo. The second trial was a randomized, placebo-controlled study evaluating the use of LI 160 extract of hypericum as compared to sertraline and placebo for the treatment of moderate to severe depression[11]. These investigators did not detect any significant difference between either treatment group or placebo. A concern with this trial was that over one-third of patients had been depressed for over 2 years. Another concern for both trials is that these patients had higher levels of depression (moderate to severe) as evaluated by the HDS than most of the patients who are commonly treated with St John's wort.

While these studies did not specifically evaluate mood disorders in perimenopausal or menopausal women, they do suggest a potential therapeutic benefit for mild depression. St John's wort extracts are generally well tolerated and the adverse effects such as gastrointestinal symptoms, sedation and photosensitivity are relatively uncommon[12]. However, several recently communicated adverse effects are noteworthy. St John's wort has been reported to decrease cyclosporine levels resulting in organ transplantation rejection[13]. Also, recent reports have suggested St John's wort may decrease oral contraceptive efficacy with resultant increased breakthrough bleeding and risk of pregnancy[14]. Warfarin, theophylline, digoxin, indinavir and amitriptyline may all also interact with hypericum causing reductions in therapeutic efficacy[15]. Consistent with this, cessation of hypericum while on one of these agents may cause higher than desired levels. A recent report also associated a hypertensive crisis with initiation of St John's wort use[16].

Ginseng

Ginseng, which is covered in Chapter 16, has also been widely used by women. An interesting study of young adults (mean age 25–27 years), evaluating ginseng for psychological enhancement, including changes in mood and affect found no effect[17]. This randomized, double-blind, controlled trial used both 200 and 400 mg for an interval of 8 weeks. Fewer data exist regarding treatment of menopausal patients, although ginseng remains widely used for this purpose. In one of the few trials published, Norwegian investigators evaluated 384 patients randomly assigned to a standardized ginseng extract or placebo[18]. No treatment effect was noted after 16 weeks on vasomotor symptoms, follicle stimulating hormone (FSH), estradiol levels, endometrial thickness or vaginal maturity index. However, evaluation of the Psychological General Well Being Index (a validated questionnaire) found improvement in the depression, well-being and health subscales in the ginseng group.

Side-effects reported with ginseng include tachycardia, palpitations, hypertension and insomnia. In addition, mastalgia, postmenopausal bleeding and estrogen-like effects have been suggested[19]. However, in Amato's study, ginseng demonstrated little estrogenic activity[20]. Of concern, as with Don quai, was

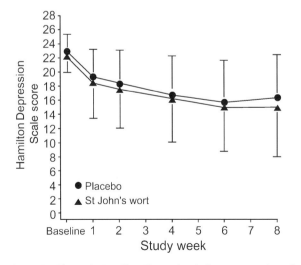

Figure 1 Change in Hamilton Depression Scale scores over 8-week trial comparing St John's wort with placebo in treatment of severe depression. Reproduced from reference 10 with permission

the stimulatory effect of ginseng on the breast cancer cell line MCF-7.

PREMENSTRUAL SYNDROME

Premenstrual syndrome (PMS) is a common complaint of women, with surveys suggesting as many as 50–80% of all women have some or all of the common symptoms of bloating, breast tenderness (see previous section), sleep abnormalities, dysphoria, poor concentration, etc. A much smaller percentage, approximately 2–5% of patients have severe symptoms. Often, complaints which are referred to as 'PMS', are more consistent with normal cyclical changes or menstrual symptomatology. It is thus important to have patients evaluate symptoms prospectively over several menstrual cycles to determine the relationship of symptoms to the luteal phase as well as their severity. Multiple questionnaires have been developed for this purpose. Since PMS is such a common complaint, a multitude of treatments have been used in an effort to improve symptoms. Only some of these treatments seem to have efficacy. As discussed in the previous section, it is also important to differentiate PMS dysphoria from significant depression, which may require a very different treatment.

Several vitamins and minerals have been investigated either alone or in combinations. Few of these seem to have value; however, vitamin B$_6$ (pyridoxine), magnesium and calcium are worthy of consideration based on data published to date. In an interesting older study, Abraham noted that PMS patients had significantly different dietary patterns compared to a group of non-PMS patients[21]. PMS patients were noted to have less zinc, manganese and iron in their diets while ingesting a much higher amount of refined sugar and carbohydrates. Vitamin B$_6$ may impact on the neurotransmitters dopamine and serotonin and has been used as a treatment in several trials. Kleijnen and colleagues have thoughtfully reviewed data on this subject[22]. Some of the reports did demonstrate efficacy while others were negative. Another review of the subject found that in evaluating nine randomized double-blind, placebo-controlled trials the overall odds ratio was 2.32 in favor of

pyridoxine[23]. Unfortunately, the dataset was poor and thus limits the validity of the conclusions. The usual dose in clinical trials ranged from 50 to 500 mg/day. No data to date demonstrate a dose–response relationship. It is important for patients to be aware of the potential for neurotoxicity from ingestion of excessive doses of pyridoxine.

Magnesium has also been used alone and in combination with other agents for PMS symptomatology. In one trial, 360 mg of magnesium pyrrolidone carboxylic acid was administered t.i.d. in the luteal phase[24]. In this small trial of 32 patients of short duration, magnesium was noted to decrease negative affect. In another trial, magnesium oxide 200 mg/day was noted to decrease fluid retention in patients after two cycles[25]. The same group later published on the successful use of magnesium and pyridoxine together to decrease anxiety symptoms[26].

Calcium supplementation may be the most exciting area of nutritional support in PMS patients. Several studies have suggested that patients with PMS may have aberrations in calcium homeostasis and metabolism[27,28]. Indeed, several trials have demonstrated increased rates of osteoporosis in PMS patients. In a small initial trial, Thys-Jacobs and colleagues evaluated the use of calcium carbonate at a dose of 1000 mg/day in the treatment of PMS[29]. This small randomized, double-blind, placebo-controlled, cross-over study demonstrated reductions in negative affect, water retention and pain in the luteal phase and decreased pain during menses. A subsequent smaller study using both manganese and calcium (1336 mg/day) also demonstrated improvement in pain, water retention and mood scores[30]. These studies led to development of a large well-designed follow-up trial in which Thys-Jacobs and co-workers administered 1200 mg/day of elemental calcium in the form of 2-TUMS E-X (1500 mg of calcium carbonate) tablets b.i.d. to 497 women with moderate to severe PMS[31]. The trial, was a 3-month prospective, randomized, double-blind, placebo-controlled design. Consistent with the earlier pilot trial, significant improvement was noted after the 2nd and 3rd month compared to placebo (48% reduction in total symptom scores from baseline; Figure 2). All four of the major symptom complexes were also noted to be

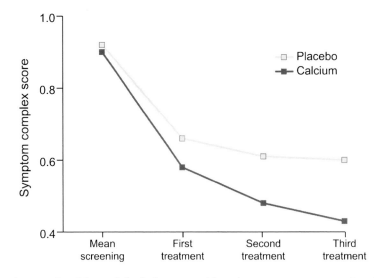

Figure 2 Mean symptom complex scores for calcium and placebo in women with moderate to severe premenstrual syndrome during treatment with calcium 1200 mg/day for 3 months. Adapted from reference 31 with permission

reduced including pain, water retention and negative mood affect and food cravings (Figure 3).

The chaste tree, *Vitex agnus castus*, has been commonly used in alternative medicine for the treatment of PMS symptoms. Both the berries, which may contain flavonoids, and the leaves have been used for these purposes.

A recent large German trial evaluated 1634 patients with PMS[32]. Unfortunately, this was an open-label trial with no control arm. The authors report that 93% of patients experienced improvement in one of the four symptom complexes after 3 months. A total of 81% of the patients subjectively reported being very much better at the trial conclusion.

A more recent and better-designed trial from Huttenberg, Germany evaluated 170 PMS patients in a prospective randomized, placebo-controlled trial of 3 months' duration[33]. Patients were administered agnus castus fruit (ZE440), the berry, which was standardized for casticin, 20 mg/day, or a placebo that was matched for taste, smell, etc. The authors found significant improvement with treatment for mood alteration, anger, headache, irritability and breast fullness. Bloating was not affected by treatment. Responder rates, which the authors defined as a 50% or greater reduction in symptoms from baseline, were

markedly higher in the treatment group – 52% versus 24%. No significant adverse events were noted and the treatment was well tolerated.

Another commonly used treatment for PMS is the use of progesterone in a multitude of forms. It was certainly conceptually appealing to believe that PMS might emanate from a deficiency of the key luteal hormone progesterone, and that supplementation might alleviate a number of the symptoms. A key proponent of this concept was Professor K. Dalton from the UK whom I still remember delivering an eloquent and compelling lecture on this topic in the 1980s. Unfortunately, as science has done in so many areas, concepts that might seem correct are just not born out in truth when well-designed trials are performed. Such is the case with progesterone and PMS. As early as 1979, small studies began to discredit the commonly held belief that progesterone vaginal suppositories impacted PMS symptoms[34]. However, the best data to date come from Freeman and colleagues who studied 168 PMS patients in a randomized, placebo-controlled, double-blind, crossover study[35]. Progesterone suppositories were administered at doses of 400 and 800 mg/day silencing some critics who had believed that inadequate doses had been used in prior trials. Consistent with other trials none of the

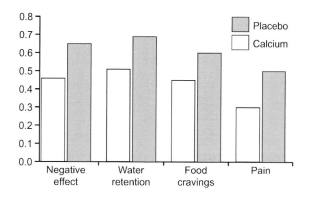

Figure 3 Effects of calcium treatment on four symptom factor scores. Adapted from reference 30 with permission

multitude of symptom clusters or individual symptoms showed any improvement with progesterone suppository treatment. Some continued proponents of progesterone therapy have suggested that route may be important to efficacy. In a smaller trial than Freeman's, Dennerstein and co-workers studied the use of 300 mg/day of oral micronized progesterone in PMS patients[36]. They noted improvement in several symptom areas including vasomotor reactivity, fluid retention, anxiety, swelling and depression. Still, the most common method of administering exogenous progesterone remains the use of progesterone creams that may be commonly obtained over the counter. The use of these creams was discussed for vasomotor relief in Chapter 27. Unfortunately, there are few reasonable data to support the effectiveness of the common practice of administering 200–400 mg of progesterone cream in the luteal phase. Given the large number of women currently using these treatment options, it is an area worth further investigation.

Other treatment options for PMS include use of reflexology, yoga, acupuncture, massage and multiple additional dietary and supplement regimens. While some limited case reports and poor trials have been published, little reliable information exists from which to make recommendations. Thus, these areas are neither accepted nor refuted based on this lack of data. Certainly, the majority of these options are either low risk or risk free and may be tried alone or in combination with more traditional treatments.

BREAST TENDERNESS AND DYSMENORRHEA

Women of reproductive age, and often during the early perimenopausal years, complain of significant breast tenderness. Although this symptom decreases as women enter menopause (Figures 4 and 5), in some cases, it is severe enough for women to look for some sort of intervention[1]. A wide range of therapeutic options have been used in the treatment of mastalgia ranging from well-fitted bras to gonadotropin releasing hormone analogs and surgery[37].

The etiology of cyclic mastalgia is unclear but may be less related to circulating hormone levels than previously believed. Instead, some investigators have suggested that women with cyclic mastalgia have an altered proportion of fatty acid esters as compared to non-affected women[38]. Therefore, one therapeutic option is supplemental fatty acid intake. Evening primrose oil contains two essential fatty acids, linoleic acid and gamma linoleic acid[39]. Australian data suggest evening primrose oil at a dose of 1000 mg three times daily improves cyclic mastalgia[40]. In addition, a cohort of 66 Asian women treated with gamolenic acid demonstrated a marked reduction in cyclic mastaglia after 6 months of treatment[41]. Side-effects such as occasional nausea, indigestion and headache occurred in 12% of the women but were easily tolerated and not a cause for discontinuation of therapy. In contrast, an analysis of the literature to 1996 by Budeiri and colleagues failed to find

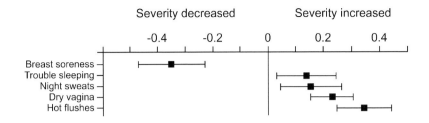

Figure 4 Mean changes in symptom severity scores (± 95% confidence intervals) comparing premenopausal and early perimenopausal scores with late perimenopausal and postmenopausal scores. Adapted from reference 1 with permission

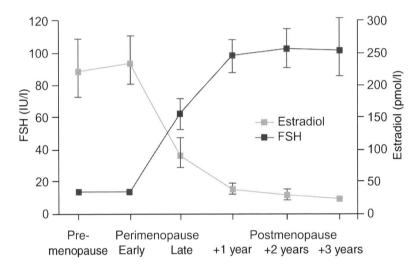

Figure 5 Geometric means (± 95% confidence interval) of hormone levels by menopausal status (*n* = 172). FSH, follicle stimulating hormone. Reproduced with permission from reference 1

compelling evidence that evening primrose oil altered symptoms in PMS patients[42]. The authors do state that no large trials were available for analysis and thus some treatment effect could not be completely ruled out.

An interesting review of dietary interventions in patients with fibrocystic breast disease failed to identify any of the commonly used modalities as truly being supported by evidence-based medicine[43]. These included vitamin E, evening primrose oil, caffeine restriction or pyridoxine. It should also be noted that these interventions are low risk (as many CAM treatments are) and although further investigation is warranted, such treatments may be starting points for non-medical intervention.

A recent randomized prospective trial of 500 units of vitamin E was performed in 100 16–18-year-old female students who noted primary dysmenorrhea[44]. Patients were given the vitamin E or placebo tablets 2 days prior to menses until 3 days into menses. While the trial only lasted 2 months, vitamin E had a greater effect on pain reduction than placebo.

CONCLUSIONS

Alterations in mood, PMS symptomatology and mastalgia are all reasonably common complaints for premenopausal, perimenopausal and menopausal transition patients. Multiple therapeutic alternatives exist for the savvy clinician. Acuity and severity of patient symptoms will dictate appropriate treatment alternatives as well as the possible need for intervention by other trained professionals such as counselors, dieticians, psychologists or psychiatrists. However, for many patients non-traditional alternatives offer a starting point for treatment, especially for the many women who have only limited symptoms. The interesting data regarding use of calcium supplementation should serve as a starting point for treating many patients. Additional options such as chaste berries may be additionally added or tried independently. While the current data are conflicting regarding St John's wort, the widespread use of this agent as an initial treatment option for patients with mild depression is intriguing. Additional options such as diet modification while not presently evidence-based, or alternatives such as yoga or other positive lifestyle alterations are to be encouraged, if for nothing more than the promotion of a healthy low-stress lifestyle. There is no question that many clinical trials need to be performed in this area and will likely give further credence to some treatments while demonstrating that others are less than helpful. The reader is encouraged to continue to read the literature actively since many of these trials are presently underway. To this end, most of us would not have believed that calcium would have any impact on PMS symptoms; unfortunately, the converse is not true. Lack of supporting trials should not cause us to accept treatments complacently as being efficacious. That is what makes watching this exciting area so interesting.

References

1. Dennerstein L, Dudley EC, Hopper JL, *et al*. A prospective population-based study of menopausal symptoms. *Obstet Gynecol* 2000;96:351–8
2. Perovic S, Muller WEG. Pharmacological profile of hypericum extract. Effect of serotonin uptake by postsynaptic receptors. *Arzneimittel forschung* 1995;45:1145–8
3. http://nccam.nih.gov/
4. Bennett DA Jr, Phun L, Polk JF, *et al*. Neuropharmacology of St. John's Wort. *Ann Pharmacother* 1998;32:1201–8
5. Kalb R, Trautmann-Sponsel RD, Kieser M. Efficacy and tolerability of hypericum extract WS 5572 versus placebo in mildly to moderately depressed patients. A randomized double-blind multicenter clinical trail. *Pharmacopsychiatry* 2001;34:96–103
6. Brenner R, Azbel V, Madhusoodanan S, Pawlowska M. Comparison of an extract of hypericum (LI 160) and sertraline in the treatment of depression; a double-blind, randomized pilot study. *Clin Ther* 2000;22:411–19
7. Behnke K, Jensen GS, Graubaum HG, Gruenwald J. *Hypericum perforatum* versus fluoxetine in the treatment of mild to moderate depression. *Adv Ther* 2002;19:43–52
8. Linde K, Ramirez G, Mulrow CD, *et al*. St. John's Wort for depression. *Br Med J* 1996;313:253–8
9. Gaster B, Holroyd J. St. John's Wort for depression: a systematic review. *Arch Intern Med* 2000;160:152–6
10. Shelton RC, Keller MB, Gelenberg A, *et al*. Effectiveness of St John's wort in major depression. A randomized controlled trial. *J Am Med Assoc* 2001;285:1978–86
11. Hypericum Depression Trial Study Group. Effect of *Hypericum perforatum* (St. John's Wort) in major depressive disorder. A randomized controlled trial. *J Am Med Assoc* 2002;287:1807–14
12. Ernest E, Rand JI, Barnes J, Stevinson C. Adverse effects profile of herbal antidepressant St. John's Wort. *Eur J Clin Pharmacol* 1998;54:589–94
13. Ernst E. St. John's Wort supplements endanger the success of organ transplantation. *Arch Surg* 2002;137:316–19
14. Ratz AE, von Moos M, Drewe J. St. John's Wort: a pharmaceutical with potentially dangerous interaction. *Schweiz Rundsch Med Prax* 2001;90:843–9
15. Baede-van Dijk PA, van Galen E, Lekkerkerker JF. Drug interaction of *Hypericum perforatum* are potentially hazardous. *Ned Tijdschr Geneesk* 2000;144:811–12
16. Patel S, Robinson R, Burk M. Hypertensive crisis associated with St. John's Wort. *Am J Med* 2002;112:507–8
17. Cardinal BJ, Engels HJ. Ginseng does not enhance psychological well-being in healthy, young adults. Results of a double-blind placebo-controlled randomized clinical trial. *J Am Diet Assoc* 2001;101:655–60
18. Wiklund IK, Mattsson LA, Lindgren R, Limoni C. Effects of a standardized ginseng extract on quality of life and physiological parameters in symptomatic postmenopausal women: a double blind, placebo controlled trial. *Int J Clin Pharmacol Res* 1999;19:89–99
19. Greenspan EM. Ginseng and vaginal bleeding. *J Am Med Assoc* 1983;249:2018
20. Amato P, Christophe S, Mellon PL. Estrogenic activity of herbs commonly used as remedies for menopausal symptoms. *Menopause* 2002;9:145–50
21. Abraham GE. Nutritional factors in the etiology of the premenstrual tension syndrome. *J Reprod Med* 1983;28:446–64
22. Kleijnen J, Ter Riet G, Knipschild P. Vitamin B$_6$ in the treatment of the premenstrual syndrome – a review. *Br J Obstet Gynaecol* 1991;97:847–52
23. Wyatt KM, Dimmock PW, Jones PW, *et al*. Efficacy of vitamin B-6 in the treatment of premenstrual syndrome: systematic review. *Br Med J* 1999;318:1375–81
24. Facchinetti F, Borella P, Sances G, *et al*. Oral magnesium successfully relieves premenstrual mood changes. *Obstet Gynecol* 1991;78:177–81
25. Walker AF, DeSouza MC, Vickers MF, *et al*. Magnesium supplementation alleviates premenstrual symptoms of fluid retention. *J Womens Health* 1998;7:1157–65

26. DeSouza MC, Walker AF, Robinson PA, Bolland K. A synergistic effect of a daily supplement for 1 month of 200 mg magnesium plus 50 mg vitamin B6 for the relief of anxiety-related premenstrual symptoms: a randomized, double-blind, crossover study. *J Womens Health Gend Based Med* 2000;9:131–9

27. Thys-Jacobs S. Micronutrients and the premenstrual syndrome: the case for calcium. *J Am Coll Nutr* 2000;19:220–7

28. Thys-Jacobs S, Ceccarelli S, Bierman A, *et al*. Calcium supplementation in premenstrual syndrome. *J Gen Intern Med* 1989;4:183–9

29. Thys-Jacobs S, Silverton M, Alvir J, *et al*. Reduced bone mass in women with premenstrual syndrome. *J Womens Health* 1995;4:161–8

30. Penland JG, Johnson PE. Dietary calcium and manganese effects on menstrual cycle symptoms. *Am J Obstet Gynecol* 1993;168:1417–23

31. Thys-Jacobs, Starkey P, Bernstein D, *et al*. Calcium carbonate and the premenstrual syndrome: effects on premenstrual and menstrual symptoms. *Am J Obstet Gynecol* 1998;179:444–52

32. Loch EG, Selle H, Boblitz N. Treatment of premenstrual syndrome with a phytopharmaceutical formulation containing *Vitex agnus castus*. *J Womens Health Gend Based Med* 2000;9:315–20

33. Schellenberg R. Treatment for the premenstrual syndrome with agnus castus fruit extract: prospective, randomized, placebo controlled study. *Br Med J* 2001;322:134–7

34. Sampson GA. Premenstrual syndrome: a double blind controlled trial of progesterone and placebo. *Br J Psychiatry* 1979;135:209–15

35. Freeman E, Rickels K, Sondheimer SJ, Polansky M. Ineffectiveness of progesterone suppository treatment for premenstrual syndrome. *J Am Med Assoc* 1990;264:349–53

36. Dennerstein L, Spencer-Gardner C, Gotts G, *et al*. Progesterone and the premenstrual syndrome: a double blind crossover trial. *Br Med J* 1985;290:1617–21

37. BeLieu RM. Mastodynia. *Obstet Gynecol Clin N Am* 1994;21:461–78

38. Gately CA, Maddox PR, Pritchard GA, *et al*. Plasma fatty acid profiles in benign breast disorders. *Br J Surg* 1992;79:407–9

39. Strid J, Jepson R, Moore V, *et al*. Evening primrose oil or other essential fatty acids for the treatment of pre-menstrual syndrome (PMS). (Protocol for a Cochrane Review). *Cochrane Library*, 2002;issue 2

40. Wetzig NR. Mastalgia; a 3 year Australian study. *Aust NZ J Surg* 1994;64:329–31

41. Cheung KL. Management of cyclical mastalgia in oriental women: pioneer experiment of using gamolenic acid (Efamast) in Asia. *Aust NZ J Surg* 1999;69:492–4

42. Budeiri D, Li Wan Po A, Doran JC. Is evening primrose oil of value in the treatment of premenstrual syndrome? *Cont Clin Trials* 1996;17:60–8

43. Horner NK, Lampe JW. Potential mechanisms of diet therapy for fibrocystic breast conditions show inadequate evidence of effectiveness. *J Am Diet Assoc* 2000;1000:1368–80

44. Ziaei S, Faghihzadeh S, Sohrabvand F, Lamyian M, Emamgholy T. A randomized placebo-controlled trial to determine the effect of vitamin E in treatment of primary dysmenorrhoea. *BJOG* 2001;108:1181–3

Alternative therapies for sexual dysfunction

29

H. H. Aung and V. Rand

INTRODUCTION

Sexual dysfunction is characterized by disturbances in sexual desire and in the psychophysiological changes associated with the sexual response cycle[1]. Sexual dysfunction is highly prevalent in both genders, ranging from 10% to 52% of men and 25% to 63% of women, according to several studies[2–4]. Laumann and co-workers reported that the incidence of sexual dysfunction in the USA was higher in women (43%) than in men (31%)[5].

Advances have occurred in the understanding of the neurovascular mechanisms of sexual response in men and women[6–8]. Several new classes of drugs have been identified that offer significant therapeutic potential for the treatment of male erectile disorder[9–11] while other agents have been indicated for disorders of sexual desire and orgasm disorders[10,12,13]. In addition to conventional therapies, however, people with sexual dysfunction also seek alternative therapies. This Chapter reviews alternative therapies for erectile and ejaculation disorders in men and sexual dysfuntion in women.

SEXUAL DYSFUNCTION IN MEN

Penile erection is mediated by the parasympathetic nervous system, which, when stimulated, can cause arterial dilatation and relaxation of the cavernosal smooth muscle. The increased blood flow into the corpora cavernosa in association with reduced venous outflow results in penile rigidity. Nitric oxide (NO) is a chemical mediator of erection. It is released from nerve endings and vascular endothelium, causing smooth muscle relaxation, resulting in venous engorgement and penile tumescence.

Erectile dysfunction is defined as the inability to achieve and maintain an erection sufficient to permit satisfactory sexual intercourse[14]. It has been estimated to affect 20 million to 30 million men in the USA[15,16]. Erectile dysfunction can be classified as psychogenic, organic (neurogenic, hormonal, arterial, cavernosal, or drug-induced), or mixed psychogenic and organic[17]. Treatment options have progressed from psychosexual therapy and penile prostheses (1970s), through revascularization, vacuum constriction devices and intracavernous injection therapy (1980s), to transurethral and oral drug therapy (1990s). The NO–cyclic GMP pathway for erectile function and the development of sildenafil citrate (Viagra®) are recent advances[17].

Herbal medicines

Yohimbine

Yohimbine is an alkaloid derived from the bark of the central African tree *Corynanthe yohimbe* (Figure 1). It may cause penile vasodilatation via α_2-receptor antagonism. The results from a meta-analysis suggest that yohimbine is effective for erectile disorder. No trial has yet been conducted to compare yohimbine with sildenafil citrate, but indirect comparison of placebo-controlled trials suggests that yohimbine is less effective but relatively safer[18]. Combination of yohimbine and L-arginine (see below) is in early phase III development[19]. In addition, yohimbine is also effective in the treatment of antidepressent-induced sexual dysfunction in patients with depression, including those receiving selective serotonin reuptake inhibitors and tricyclic antidepressants[20,21].

Patients generally receive oral yohimbine doses between 5 and 10 mg three times a day, which are well tolerated, and without side-effects. The side-effects of yohimbine are clearly dose dependent[22]. Doses over 30 mg occasionally cause small increases in blood pressure and doses over 50 mg or higher (100 mg) sometimes increase heart rate in normotensive subjects.

Tribulus terrestris and protodioscin

Protodioscin is a phytochemical agent derived from the plant *Tribulus terrestris* L, which has been clinically proven to improve sexual desire and enhance erection via the conversion of protodioscin to dehydroepiandrosterone (DHEA)[23]. Protodioscin-containing components have also been proved to be effective in increasing fertility in subfertile men and improve erectile dysfunction in both diabetic and non-diabetic men[23].

Ginkgo biloba

Ginkgo biloba, or ginkgo, facilitates the microvascular circulation that may physiologically lead to improvement in sexual function[24]. There is evidence that ginkgo extract may directly produce smooth muscle relaxation, probably via effects on the NO pathway[25,26]. An uncontrolled pilot study assessed the effects of ginkgo extract in antidepressant-induced sexual dysfunction, and it appears to be efficacious[27].

Ginseng

Ginseng is widely believed to have aphrodisiac effects for patients with sexual dysfunction[28]. One placebo-controlled study assessed 90 patients, who were treated with either ginseng or trazodone. Although no intergroup differences were reported for frequency of intercourse, the results suggested superiority of

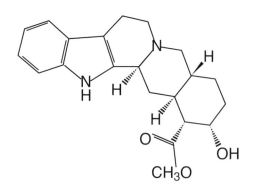

Figure 1 Chemical structure of yohimbine

ginseng for penile rigidity, girth, libido and satisfaction[29]. Ginsenosides, the primary active component of ginseng, have been shown to increase NO production in endothelial cells[30,31], which may be due to upregulation of NO synthase activity by the compounds[30]. Therefore, the effects of ginsenosides on NO production have implications for improved sexual function. In addition, ginseng was demonstrated to increase spermatozoon count and motility in infertility patients[32].

Mucuna pruriens and Withania somnifera

A non-uncontrolled study assessed the potential of mustong, an oriental herbal preparation from *Mucuna pruriens* and *Withania somnifera*, as an option for treating male sexual dysfunction[33]. The report suggested improvement of sexual function in 16 of 25 diabetics with impotence. Mustong was given in two tablets twice daily for 7–8 weeks. Each tablet contained 155 mg from *Mucuna pruriens* and 100 mg from *Withania somnifera*. No adverse effects were observed.

Damiana

Damiana (*Turnera diffusa, Turnera aphrodisiaca*) has been traditionally used as a tonic for the central nervous and hormonal systems in Latin America[34]. It has been shown that damiana has receptor activity as a phytoprogestin[35]. Sexually impaired rats treated with damiana increased their rates of copulatory performance[36].

Others

Eurycoma longifolia, *Pimpinella pruacen*, *Muara puama*, homy goat weed, ashwangandha, ginger, faba beans, nettle, oats, pumpkin, pygeum, saw palmetto and maca root are also believed to enhance sexual function. More research studies are needed to evaluate their efficacy.

Vitamins and minerals

There is evidence that vitamins and minerals enhance sexual function. B-complex vitamins are important for the activity of many enzymes and for energy metabolism. Low levels of circulating folate and vitamin B_6 increase the risk of peripheral vascular disease, leading to potential reduction of sexual function[37]. Vitamin B_{12} injections have increased sperm counts in men[38,39]. Vitamin E supplementation has been shown to increase fertility in men[40].

Zinc is a fundamental mineral in the maintenance of human reproductive function. Low zinc levels have been shown to cause sexual dysfunction, and are associated with infertility in males[41].

L-Arginine

L-Arginine is an amino acid that functions as a precursor to the formation of NO, which mediates the relaxation of smooth muscle. Preliminary studies in men appear promising. Attempts have been made using a combination of L-arginine and yohimbine for both men and women with sexual dysfunction[42].

Acupuncture

One randomized controlled trial evaluated acupuncture as a treatment for patients with non-organic erectile dysfunction[43]. Nine patients were treated with acupuncture points and six received placebo acupuncture twice weekly for 6 weeks. Improvements in sexual function were reported in the treatment group that were not significantly different from those in the control group. Data from non-controlled studies have indicated some positive effects on the quality of erection and sexual activity in erectile dysfunction due to non-organic[44] and mixed[45] etiologies.

Biofeedback

A controlled trial of biofeedback training assessed patients with psychogenic erectile dysfunction. The first group received feedback plus the viewing of segments of erotic film. The second group received film without feedback and the third group received no feedback and no film. There were no intergroup differences in erectile functioning during a 1-month follow-up period[46]. It was concluded that the therapeutic value of biofeedback in erectile dysfunction remains undemonstrated.

Hypnotherapy

Two randomized controlled trials assessed the effects of hypnotic suggestions on sexual function[47]. Both studies originated from the same research group and included patients with no detectable organic cause. These studies found some improvements in sexual function and reported that hypnotic suggestion was significantly more effective than the administration of oral placebo.

Pelvic floor exercise

Pelvic floor exercises apply pressure on the glans penis to trigger reflex contractions of the ischiocavernosus muscles and the perineal muscles. The exercise may reinforce the strength of perineal muscles and facilitate penile rigidity during erection[48]. One controlled trial compared a pelvic floor exercise program with surgery[49]. A total of 150 patients with erectile dysfunction and proven vascular leakage were included; 78 were randomized to the training program. Prior to the study, pelvic floor exercises were demonstrated to the patients, who also underwent general muscle consciousness training to help them differentiate between abdominal, gluteal, femoral adductor and pelvic floor muscles. Patients were also instructed in a home exercise program in the prone, sitting and standing positions. This was given five times in weekly sessions and supervised by a trained physiotherapist. The study data suggested that, in mild to moderate venous leakage, pelvic floor exercise is an alternative to surgery. However, surgery intervention is recommended for severe cases.

SEXUAL DYSFUNCTION IN WOMEN

Female sexual response consists of a three-phase model: desire, arousal and orgasm[50]. In female sexual function, neurotransmitter-mediated vascular smooth muscle relaxation results in increased vaginal lubrication, vaginal wall engorgement and vaginal luminal diameter expansion, as well as increased clitoral length and diameter[51]. Female sexual dysfunction is characterized by decreased libido, vaginal dryness, pain and discomfort with intercourse, decreased genital sensation, decreased arousal and difficulty in achieving orgasm. These dysfunctions are due to vasculogenic, neurogenic, hormonal or psychogenic etiologies[42]. For example, atherosclerotic vascular disease can result in conditions such as insufficient vaginal engorgement and clitoral erectile syndromes.

During menopause, there is vaginal atrophy and declination of sexual function. It is believed that NO is involved in both of these conditions[52]. Estrogen withdrawal appears to play a role in the regulation of vaginal NO synthase expression and apoptosis in nerves, smooth muscle, vascular endothelium and epithelium of the vagina, implying an NO-related mechanism in female sexual function. As an NO precursor, L-arginine has been shown to be essential to sexual maturation in the female rat[53].

Female sexual dysfunction is a complex result of psychological and physiological factors, and no efficacious pharmaceutical therapies are currently available.

Administration of sildenafil citrate in 30 postmenopausal women did not significantly improve sexual function, although there was some increase in vaginal lubrication and clitoral sensitivity[54].

Some herbal medicines have been tested in treating sexual dysfunction in women. In a study of women with hypoactive sexual desire, yohimbine had no significant effect on improving sexual desire, although it increased methoxy-4-hydroxyphenylglycol, the major central nervous system metabolite of norepinephrine (noradrenaline), to a plasma level similar to that seen in men[55]. In a pilot study, ginkgo seemed efficacious in the treatment of antidepressant-induced sexual dysfunction, particularly in women[27]. In addition, vitamin E supplementation has also been shown to increase fertility in women[40]. In a Hungarian randomized, double-blind, controlled trial, multivitamin supplementation has been shown to enhance fertility by 5% in women[56].

In a controlled study using a nutritional supplement for enhancement of female sexual function, notable improvements were observed in sexual desire, reduction in vaginal dryness, frequency of sexual intercourse and orgasm, and clitoral sensation, without significant side-effects[57]. The nutritional supplement has a combination of the following ingredients: ginseng (containing 30% ginsenosides), ginkgo (24% flavone glycosides, 6% terpene lactones), damiana leaf, L-arginine, along with vitamins A, B_6, B_{12}, biotin, folate, niacin, pantothenic acid, riboflavin, thiamin, antioxidant vitamins (C and E), calcium, iron and zinc. Although the exact mechanism of action of this supplement is not known, the proposed action is believed to occur via enhancement of the NO pathway. As discussed above, NO derived from L-arginine is a main contributor to smooth muscle relaxation, vascular dilatation and regulation of circulation.

SUMMARY

There is convincing evidence for the effectiveness of yohimbine for male erectile dysfunction from organic or non-organic causes. Comparative studies with conventional oral medication, such as sildenafil citrate, are not available at present, but it has been suggested that yohimbine is less effective but probably safer. However, whether yohimbine is safe for long-term use remains to be tested in future controlled studies. There are some data supporting gingko's use for impotence due to arterial insufficiency and selective serotonin reuptake inhibitors. However, patients on blood thinners, such as warfarin and aspirin, should be cautious in using gingko. Despite the huge popularity of ginseng for centuries, there is a lack of solid data to support its use for sexual concerns. Since L-arginine is a precursor to the formation of NO, it may play a role in treating male and female sexual dysfunction. Other approaches, such as hypnotherapy, although the evidence is not compelling, may be beneficial for some patients, owing to the possibility of a large placebo response.

References

1. American Psychiatric Association. *Diagnostic and Statistical Manual of Mental Disorders*, 4th edn. Washington, DC: American Psychiatric Association, 1994:493–522

2. Frank E, Anderson C, Rubinstein D. Frequency of sexual dysfunction in 'normal' couples. *N Engl J Med* 1978;299:111–15

3. Spector IP, Carey MP. Incidence and prevalence of the sexual dysfunctions: a critical review of the empirical literature. *Arch Sex Behav* 1990;19:389–408

4. Rosen RC, Taylor JF, Leiblum SR, Bachmann GA. Prevalence of sexual dysfunction in women: results of a survey study of 329 women in an outpatient gynecological clinic. *J Sex Marital Ther* 1993;19:171–88

5. Laumann EO, Paik A, Raymond C. Sexual dysfunction in the United States: prevalence and predictors. *J Am Med Assoc* 1999;281:537–44

6. Rajfer J, Aronson WJ, Bush PA, Dorey FJ, Ignarro LJ. Nitric oxide as a mediator of relaxation of the corpus cavernosum in response to nonadrenergic, noncholinergic neurotransmission. *N Engl J Med* 1992;326:90–4

7. Burnett AL. The role of nitric oxide in the physiology of erection. *Biol Reprod* 1995;52:485–9

8. Park K, Goldstein I, Andry C, Siroky MB, Krane RJ, Azadzoi KM. Vasculogenic female sexual dysfunction: the hemodynamic basis for vaginal engorgement insufficiency and clitoral erectile insufficiency. *Int J Impot Res* 1997;9:27–37

9. Heaton JP, Morales A, Adams MA, Johnston B, el-Rashidy R. Recovery of erectile function by the oral administration of apomorphine. *Urology* 1995;45:200–6

10. Morales A, Heaton JP, Johnston B, Adams M. Oral and topical treatment of erectile dysfunction: present and future. *Urol Clin N Am* 1995;22:879–86

11. Boolell M, Gepi-Attee S, Gingell JC, Allen MJ. Sildenafil: a novel effective oral therapy for male erectile dysfunction. *Br J Urol* 1996;78:257–61

12. Rosen RC, Ashton AK. Prosexual drugs: empirical status of the 'new aphrodisiacs'. *Arch Sex Behav* 1993;22:521–43

13. Segraves RT, Saran A, Segraves K, Maguire E. Clomipramine versus placebo in the treatment of premature ejaculation: a pilot study. *J Sex Marital Ther* 1993;19:198–200

14. NIH Consensus Development Panel on Impotence. NIH Consensus Conference: impotence. *J Am Med Assoc* 1993;270:83–90

15. Feldman HA, Goldstein I, Hatzichristou DG, Krane RJ, McKinlay JB. Impotence and its medical and psychosocial correlates: results of the Massachusetts Male Aging Study. *J Urol* 1994;151:54–61

16. Benet AE, Melman A. The epidemiology of erectile dysfunction. *Urol Clin N Am* 1995;22:699–709

17. Lue TF. Erectile dysfunction. *N Engl J Med* 2000;342:1802–13

18. O'Leary M. Erectile dysfunction. In Godlee F, ed. *Clinical Evidence*. London: BMJ Books, 1999

19. Padma-Nathan H, Giuliano F. Oral drug therapy for erectile dysfunction. *Urol Clin N Am* 2001;28:321–34

20. Segraves RT. Treatment emergent sexual dysfunction in affective disorder. *J Clin Psychiatry* 1993;11:1–4

21. Price J, Grunhaus LJ. Treatment of clomipramine-induced anorgasmia with yohimbine: a case report. *J Clin Psychiatry* 1990;51:32–3

22. Tam SW, Worcel M, Wyllie M. Yohimbine: a clinical review. *Pharmacol Ther* 2001;91:215–43

23. Adimoelja A. Phytochemicals and the breakthrough of traditional herbs in the management of sexual dysfunctions. *Int J Androl* 2000;23 (Suppl 2):82–4

24. Welt K, Weiss J, Koch S, Fitzl G. Protective effects of *Ginkgo biloba* extract EGb 761 on the myocardium of experimentally diabetic rats. II. Ultrastructural and immunohistochemical investigation on microvessels and interstitium. *Exp Toxicol Pathol* 1999;51:213–22

25. Paick JS, Lee JH. An experimental study of the effect of *Ginkgo biloba* extract on the human and rabbit corpus cavernosum tissue. *J Urol* 1996;156:1876–80

26. Chen X, Salwinski S, Lee TJ. Extracts of *Ginkgo biloba* and ginsenosides exert cerebral vasorelaxation via a nitric oxide pathway. *Clin Exp Pharmacol Physiol* 1997;24:958–9

27. Cohen AJ, Bartlik B. *Ginkgo biloba* for antidepressant-induced sexual dysfunction. *J Sex Marital Ther* 1998;24:139–43

28. Vogler BK, Pittler MH, Ernst E. The efficacy of ginseng. A systematic review of randomized clinical trials. *Eur J Clin Pharmacol* 1999;55:567–75

29. Choi HK, Seong DH, Rha KH. Clinical efficacy of Korean red ginseng for erectile dysfunction. *Int J Impot Res* 1995;7:181–6

30. Chen X, Lee TJ. Ginsenosides-induced nitric oxide-mediated relaxation of the rabbit corpus cavernosum. *Br J Pharmacol* 1995;115:15–18

31. Han SW, Kim H. Ginsenosides stimulate endogenous production of nitric oxide in rat kidney. *Int J Biochem Cell Biol* 1996;28:573–80

32. Salvati G, Genovesi G, Marcellini L, Paolini P, De Nuccio I, Pepe M, Re M. Effects of *Panax ginseng* C.A. Meyer saponins on male fertility. *Panminerva Med* 1996;38:249–54

33. Ojha JK, Roy CK, Bajpai HS. Clinical trial of mustong on secondary sexual impotence in male married diabetics. *J Med Assoc Thailand* 1987;70:228–30

34. Foster S. Herbs and sex: seperating fact from fantasy. *Health Food Business* 1991;74:573–80

35. Zava DT, Dollbaum CM, Blen M. Estrogen and progestin bioactivity of foods, herbs, and spices. *Proc Soc Exp Biol Med* 1998; 217:369–78

36. Arletti R, Benelli A, Cavazzuti E, Scarpetta G, Bertolini A. Stimulating property of *Turnera diffusa* and *Pfaffia paniculata* extracts on the sexual-behavior of male rats. *Psychopharmacology (Berl)* 1999;143: 15–19

37. Robinson K, Arheart K, Refsum H, *et al*. Low circulating folate and vitamin B6 concentrations: risk factors for stroke, peripheral vascular disease, and coronary artery disease. European COMAC Group. *Circulation* 1998;97:437–43

38. Sandler B, Faragher B. Treatment of oligospermia with vitamin B12. *Infertility* 1984;7:133–8

39. Kumamoto Y, Maruta H, Ishigami J, *et al*. [Clinical efficacy of mecobalamin in the treatment of oligozoospermia – results of double-blind comparative clinical study.] In Japanese. *Hinyokika Kiyo* 1988;34:1109–32

40. Bayer JR. Treatment of infertility with vitamin E. *Intern J Fertil* 1960;5:70–8

41. Mohan H, Verma J, Singh I, Mohan P, Marwah S, Singh P. Interrelationship of zinc levels in serum and semen in oligospermic infertile patients and fertile males. *Indian J Pathol Microbiol* 1997; 40:451–5

42. Berman JR, Berman LA, Werbin TJ, Goldstein I. Female sexual dysfunction: anatomy, physiology, evaluation and treatment options. *Curr Opin Urol* 1999;9:563–8

43. Aydin S, Ercan M, Çaskurlu T, *et al*. Acupuncture and hypnotic suggestions in the treatment of non-organic male dysfunction. *Scand J Urol Nephrol* 1997;31:271–4

44. Kho HG, Sweep CG, Chen X, Rabsztyn PR, Meuleman EJ. The use of acupuncture in the treatment of erectile dysfunction. *Int J Impot Res* 1999;11:41–6

45. Yaman LS, Kilic S, Sarica K, Bayar M, Saygin B. The place of acupuncture in the management of psychogenic impotence. *Eur Urol* 1994;26:52–5

46. Reynolds BS. Biofeedback and facilitation of erection in men with erectile dysfunction. *Arch Sex Behav* 1980;9:101–13

47. Aydin S, Odabas O, Ercan M, Kara H, Agargun MY. Efficacy of testosterone, trazodone, and hypnotic suggestion in the treatment of non-organic male sexual dysfunction. *Br J Urol* 1996;77:256–60

48. Lavoisier P, Proulx J, Courtois F, De Carufel F, Durand LG. Relationship between perineal muscle contraction, penile tumescence and penile rigidity during nocturnal erections. *J Urol* 1988;139:176–9

49. Claes H, Baert L. Pelvic floor exercise versus surgery in the treatment of impotence. *Br J Urol* 1993;71:52–7

50. Kaplan HS. *The New Sex Therapy*. London: Baillière Tindall, 1974

51. Goldstein I, Berman JR. Vasculogenic female sexual dysfunction: vaginal engorgement and clitoral erectile insufficiency syndromes. *Int J Impot Res* 1998;10 (Suppl 2):S84–90; discussion S98–101

52. Berman JR, McCarthy MM, Kyprianou N. Effect of estrogen withdrawal on nitric oxide synthase expression and apoptosis in the rat vagina. *Urology* 1998;51:650–6

53. Pau MY, Milner JA. Dietary arginine and sexual maturation of the female rat. *J Nutr* 1982;112:1834–42

54. Kaplan SA, Reis RB, Kohn IJ, *et al*. Safety and efficacy of sildenafil in postmenopausal women with sexual dysfunction. *Urology* 1999;53:481–6

55. Piletz JE, Segraves KB, Feng YZ, Maguire E, Dunger B, Halaris A. Plasma MHPG response to yohimbine treatment in women with hypoactive sexual desire. *J Sex Marital Ther* 1998;24:43–54

56. Czeizel AE, Metneki J, Dudas I. The effect of preconceptional multivitamin supplementation on fertility. *Int J Vitam Nutr Res* 1996;66:55–8

57. Ito TY, Trant AS, Polan ML. A double-blind placebo-controlled study of ArginMax, a nutritional supplement for enhancement of female sexual function. *J Sex Marital Ther* 2001;27:541–9

Availability of medicinal herbs to boost HIV patients' immune systems

30

J. A. Wu and C.-S. Yuan

INTRODUCTION

The acquired immunodeficiency syndrome (AIDS) is a result of human immunodeficiency virus (HIV) infection which subsequently leads to significant suppression of immune functions. AIDS is an unprecedented threat to nations as well as to global health[1,2]. It is estimated that each year HIV infects at least 2 million people in the USA and more than 10 million people worldwide. Therefore, the search for effective therapies to treat AIDS is urgently needed. In order to combat HIV, a colossal amount of money and manpower has been dedicated to searching for compounds that can be developed as therapeutic agents. In the past two decades, several chemical anti-HIV agents have been developed. However, besides the high cost, there are adverse effects and limitations associated with using chemotherapy for the treatment of HIV infection. Herbal medicines have frequently been used as an alternative medical therapy by HIV-positive individuals and AIDS patients. The aim of this chapter is to summarize research findings for herbal medicines that are endowed with the ability to inhibit HIV. In this chapter, we emphasize a Chinese herbal medicine, *Scutellaria baicalensis* Georgi and its identified components (i.e. baicalein and baicalin), which have been shown to inhibit infectivity and replication of HIV.

CONVENTIONAL CHEMOTHERAPY FOR HIV INFECTION

According to De Clercq, the replicative cycle of HIV is composed of ten steps that may be adequate targets for chemotherapeutic intervention[3,4]. Most of the substances that have been identified as anti-HIV agents can be assigned to one of these ten classes of HIV inhibitors based on the stage at which they interfere with the HIV replicative cycle. These ten steps are:

(1) Viral adsorption to the cell membrane;

(2) Fusion between the viral envelope and the cell membrane;

(3) Uncoating of the viral nucleocapsid;

(4) Reverse transcription of the viral RNA to proviral DNA;

(5) Integration of the proviral DNA to the cellular genome;

(6) DNA replication;

(7) Transcription of the proviral DNA to RNA;

(8) Translation of the viral precursor mRNA to mature mRNA;

(9) Maturation of the viral precursor proteins by proteolysis, myristoylation and glycosylation;

(10) Budding, virion assembly and release.

Step 4, a key step in the replicative cycle of retroviruses, which makes it distinct from the replicative cycle of other viruses, is the reverse transcription catalyzed by reverse transcriptase. Another target for therapeutic intervention is step 9, particularly the proteolysis of precursor proteins by HIV protease. The majority of chemotherapeutic strategies have, therefore, focused on the development of retroviral enzyme inhibitors.

The US Food and Drug Administration (FDA) has approved a number of anti-HIV drugs for clinical use[5]. However, these medications have limitations such as high cost, peripheral neuropathy and decreased sensitivity due to the rapid emergence of drug-resistant mutant virus strains, and adverse effects such as bone marrow suppression and anemia[6,7]. Therefore, more effective and less toxic anti-HIV agents are still needed. In addition, alternative approaches, including herbal therapies, long-term screening of plant extracts, particularly anti-infective or immunomodulating medicinal herbs, and the structural modification of leading compounds, have been attempted.

STUDIES OF MEDICINAL HERBS ON HIV INFECTION

Use of herbs in Asia and North America

Herbal medicine has been used in China for centuries. Even after opening its doors to Western medicine two centuries ago, China still relies heavily on traditional medicine and herbal therapies because of their efficacy. Indeed, the recent focus of the Chinese government has been to propel research at its institutes and universities towards developing efficacious herbal drugs, particularly as anticancer, anticardiovascular disease and immunomodulating agents[8].

In China, medicinal herbs are being used in the treatment of HIV-positive subjects and AIDS patients. One example is the traditional Chinese medicinal herb Tian-Hua-Fen (*Trichosanthes kirilowii*), which appears in the classical Chinese medical reference work *Compendium of Materia Medica* from the late 14th century. Tian-Hua-Fen has been used in China for hundreds of years to reset menstruation and expel retained placentas. Trichosanthin, an active protein component isolated from Tian-Hua-Fen, has been shown to inhibit HIV infection and has been used in the clinical treatment of AIDS[9].

In addition to the study of Tian-Hua-Fen, two multiple screening approaches have been applied to aqueous extracts of 19 herbs in Hong Kong[10] and 35 herbs in Beijing[11] in order to detect antiviral agents. Also, an oriental remedy called *Xiao-Chai-Hu-Tang* (Chinese name) or *Sho-saiko-to* (SST or TJ9, Japanese name), which consists of a mixture of aqueous extracts from seven commonly used herbs, has been used in AIDS patients in China and Japan[12–14].

Scientists from both Thailand and Japan have worked together to screen the anti-HIV activity of 413 plants grown in Thailand. Significant inhibitory activity has been found in 81 of these plants[15].

In the USA, the use of herbs as an alternative medical treatment for many illnesses has increased steadily over the past decade. Because herbs are categorized as natural food products or dietary supplements, they are not currently subject to strict control by the FDA[8]. However, many patients with AIDS are using herbal medical therapies in addition to conventional treatment. One study reported that, in 1991, 22% of AIDS patients had used one or more herbs for medicinal purposes in the previous 3 months[16]. Recently, this percentage has increased[17]. Our group evaluated a new Chinese herbal medicine formulation, Qian-Qun-Ning, which consists of a mixture of aqueous extracts from 14 different herbs, and showed efficacy in a pilot clinical trial of HIV-positive subjects[18].

Since 1987, the US National Cancer Institute has worked with the Chinese Academy of Sciences to study Chinese medicinal herbs for anti-AIDS application. Over 1000 Chinese traditional medicines were screened using different solvent extraction forms and more than 140 different herbs were found to have HIV inhibition activity. Among them, more than 20 herbs have exhibited significant HIV inhibitory activity[19].

In the USA experimental studies are in progress to isolate anti-HIV agents from medicinal plants and their natural products. In one such study, conducted by the National Cancer Institute, approximately 4500 plant samples are currently screened per year for *in vitro* anti-HIV activity, based on a random selection of plants[20].

At the University of Illinois at Chicago[21], a simple *in vitro* method has been developed for screening the HIV type 1 (HIV-1) reverse transcriptase inhibitory potential of natural products. More than 100 plant extracts have been evaluated, and 15 of these extracts show significant inhibitory activity. A total of 156 natural products have been examined in this system[22].

Bioactive components from the herbs

A number of articles that discuss the HIV inhibitory activity of herbs and their natural products[19,20,23–27] suggest that a variety of chemically disparate molecules, produced by species distributed across the plant kingdom, such as algae, pine trees and flowering plants, are effective at inhibiting the activity of HIV. These compounds are composed of: aliphatic ketones and aldehydes; terpenoids; alkaloids; coumarin derivatives; flavonoids; xanthone; flavone-xanthone C-glucoside; hyperlein; tannins; gossypol acetic acid; polysaccharides; and proteins.

Because of their potential systemic effects and prophylactic action against HIV infection, plant-derived antiviral agents are prime study candidates. They may also be useful as topical agents to inactivate newly formed viruses, or as adjuvants with other antiviral drugs.

In the isolation of natural products, it is essential to adhere to the following steps. First, the plant kingdom as a source of new antiviral leading compounds should continue to be explored. Second, leading compounds that have been shown to inhibit HIV activity should be developed through modern pharmacological methods to increase activity and decrease toxicity. Finally, herbal medicines or natural products as part of drug combination regimens for the treatment of HIV infections should be encouraged and continued[26].

Anti-HIV activity of flavonoids and *Scutellaria baicalensis* Georgi

Various flavonoids have been shown, *in vitro*, to inhibit the reverse transcriptase of certain retroviruses, including HIV (step 4 of the replicative cycle), as well as cellular DNA polymerases. These products exhibited selective anti-HIV-1 activity[28,29], whereas baicalein (5,6,7-trihydroxyflavone), a constituent isolated from *Scutellaria baicalensis* Georgi (*Huang Qin* in Chinese, *Worgon* in Japanese), specifically inhibited HIV reverse transcriptase[8,30].

In AIDS treatment, the inhibition of HIV reverse transcriptase is currently considered a useful approach, therefore natural products that show inhibitory activity have been extensively explored[24].

Effects of baicalein and baicalin

Oho and colleagues showed the effects of baicalein on the activity of various reverse transcriptases. They demonstrated that 1 μg/ml baicalein inhibited 90% of the activity of murine leukemia virus reverse transcriptase, and that 2 μg/ml baicalein inhibited 90% of the activity of HIV reverse transcriptases[31].

Tang and colleagues[11] found that baicalin, which is isolated from *Scutellaria baicalensis* Georgi, inhibited HIV reverse transcriptase, with an IC_{50} value of 22 μmol/l. Some pharmacological test results have demonstrated non-competitive inhibition of retroviral reverse transcriptase activity in HIV-1-infected H9 cells[32], HIV-1 specific core antigen p24 expression and quantitative focal syncytium formation on CEM-SS monolayer cells[33]. Baicalin and its derivative 7-glucuronic acid 5,6-dihydroxyflavone were also efficacious in inhibiting reverse transcriptase of other retroviruses[34]. The difference in HIV-1 reverse transcriptase inhibitory activity between baicalein and baicalin has been examined[35]. The results show that the HIV-1 reverse transcriptase inhibitory activity of baicalein was four times higher than that of baicalin. The inhibition of HIV-1 integration (step 5 of the replicative cycle) by baicalein was investigated biochemically and by means of structure–activity relationships. It was reported that the IC_{50} for HIV integrase inhibition by baicalein was 4.3 µmol/l[36].

An investigation into the metabolism of baicalin has been published[37]. The results indicated that baicalin was first metabolized into baicalein (Figure 1), and the final metabolite was identified as baicalein 6-O-sulfate by comparing its retention time in high-performance liquid chromatography (HPLC) and electrospray ionization mass spectra (ESI-MS)/MS methods with that of an authentic sample.

Mechanisms of action

As for the mechanism of the anti-HIV-1 effect of baicalin, it was found that baicalin and baicalein have an inhibitory effect on various cellular DNA and RNA polymerases[30,38]. In the case of baicalein, the mode of inhibition was of the competitive type (murine leukemia virus reverse transcriptase and HIV-1 reverse transcriptase) with respect to the template primer ((rA)n·(dT)12-18), or mixed type, suggesting that baicalein also inhibits HIV-1 reverse transcriptase activity by interfering with the binding of viral RNA to the reverse transcriptase molecule near the active site of the enzyme. Baicalin does not inhibit the activity of HIV-2 reverse transcriptase, or murine leukemia virus reverse transcriptase. Futhermore, baicalin neither inhibited the binding of OKT4A monoclonal antibody to the gp120 binding site of CD4, nor interfered with the gp 120–CD4 binding. This rules out the possibility that baicalin interferes with the virus adsorption step (step 1 of the replicative cycle). Flavonoids such as gardennin, myricetin and baicalein were found to inhibit HIV-1 protease. However, the IC_{50} value of baicalein was 480 µmol/l, almost 44 times that of gardennin (IC_{50}=11 µmol/l)[39].

Efficacy of the herbal formulation

As mentioned above, Xiao-Chai-Hu-Tang or Sho-saiko-to consists of a mixture of aqueous extracts from seven different plants. Of this, 7.5 g contains 4.5 g of dried extract, which is prepared from boiled water extracts of seven herbs: 7.0 g of *Bupleurum* root, 5.0 g of *Pinellia* tuber, 3.0 g of *Scutellaria* root, 3.0 g of *Jujube* fruit, 3.0 g of *Ginseng* root, 2.0 g of *Glycyrrhiza* root and 1.0 g of ginger rhizome[40,41]. Some research groups have demonstrated that, among the active components of Sho-saiko-to, baicalein and baicalin were found to be mainly responsible for antioxidative[40,42], antitumor[28,43–47], antiproliferative[48–50] and anti-HIV[12,37] activity.

It is interesting to note that data on antioxidative activity between Sho-saiko-to and *Scutellaria* root using MeOH extracts were very similar[40]. Our group and other researchers have shown that the water extracts of *Scutellaria* root also have significant antioxidant activity[51]. In the four major constituents, the order of antioxidant activity is baicalein > baicalin >> worgonin > wogonoside[52]. Antioxidant and other mechanisms may also play a role in the anti-HIV effects of baicalin and baicalein[30].

An oral dose toxicity study of Sho-saiko-to in rats has been reported[53]. Two oral doses (2 and 6.4 g/kg) of Sho-saiko-to were administered to the animal after overnight fasting, and no death was observed.

Combination of herbal medicine and chemotherapy

Combination therapy for AIDS patients has been applied, discussed and standardized[7]. Synergistic anti-HIV-1 effects of baicalin with 3'-azido-2',3'-dideoxythymidine (AZT) have been reported[54], suggesting

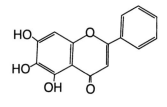

Figure 1 Chemical structures of baicalin and baicalein

that baicalin might be potentially useful as part of a drug combination regimen for the treatment of HIV-1 infections. The use of Sho-saiko-to as an adjuvant with other antiviral drugs such as 3TC has been published[14]. A patent for anti-AIDS-virus effect-enhancing agents containing Sho-saiko-to or baicalein has been approved in Japan[55].

Discovery and development of plant-derived natural products and their analogs as anti-HIV agents

Although the history of Chinese herbal medicines dates back thousands of years, herb–drug interactions should not be overlooked[56]. With any anti-AIDS drug, attention must be paid to adverse effects, long-term sustainable effects and increased toxicity due to drug–drug interaction in a person receiving multiple drug therapies. The search for effective and less toxic anti-AIDS agents of single structure still continues. One approach is to modify novel, leading compounds derived from plants. Some promising research developments from different groups have been reported[6,19,57,58].

A successful example is the study by Lee and Morris-Natschke[6]. Through a bioactivity-directed search for plant-derived, naturally occurring compounds, the leading compound sukudorfin was isolated from the fruit of *Lomatium suksorfii* and its structure was identified. Sukudorfin inhibited HIV-1 replication in H9 lymphocytes with an *in vitro* IC_{50} value of 1.3 μmol/l and a therapeutic index ($TI = LD_{50}/IC_{50}$) value of over 40. The discovery of sukudorfin led to the synthesis of 42 khellactone derivatives by structure modification. Among these synthetic compounds, the most promising leading compound was 3′,4′-di-O-(S)-(−)-camphanoyl-(3′R,4′R)-(+)-*cis*-khellactone (DCK), which showed extremely potent activity ($IC_{50} = 0.00041$ μmol/l) against HIV-1 replication in the H9 cell line, and had a remarkable TI value of 136 719. In comparison, the values of AZT in the same assays were 0.15 μmol/l and 12 500, respectively. As an anti-HIV chemotherapeutic agent, DCK is a candidate for an anti-AIDS clinical trial[6,57,58].

When baicalein was first found to be a strong inhibitor of reverse transcriptase activity, the question arose as to the necessary structural requirements of the flavonoid for such activity. It is believed that number, position of the putative functional groups (hydroxyl groups) and flavone or flavonoid structure[59] are important. Research on structural modification and structure–activity relationship of baicalin and baicalein has been reported. The results indicated that the flavonoids with hydroxyl groups at C-5 and C-7 in the A-ring, and with a C-2–C-3 double bond were the most potent inhibitors of HIV growth. In general, the presence of substituents (hydroxyl and halogen) in the B-ring increased toxicity and/or decreased activity[28,60,61].

According to the above information on structure–activity relationships, structure modification methods can also be used for flavonoid leading compounds, which are derived from plants with possible anti-HIV activity. As a potential target, the heteroatom in position 1 of the C-ring of the flavonoid compounds has been considered. Therefore, similar or even new biological activities could be anticipated when the oxygen of bioactive flavonoids is replaced by another atom such as nitrogen or sulfur, which is closely aligned with oxygen in the periodic table. Thus, a series of 5,6,7,8-substituted 2-phenylthio-chromen-4-ones have been synthesized and evaluated for anti-HIV activity[28]. Among them, one new compound was the most active (IC_{50} value of 0.65 μmol/l) against HIV in acutely infected H9 lymphocytes, and had a TI of approximately 5.

SUMMARY

Medicinal herbs may have practical value as an alternative medical therapy in the inhibition of HIV activity. There is considerable evidence that sukudorfin, baicalin and baicalein are important leading compounds for the development of antiviral and/or virucidal drugs against HIV. Baicalin and baicalein might be useful as topical agents to deactivate a newly formed virus, or act as an adjuvant with other antiviral drugs. However, it is essential that the plant kingdom, as a source of new anti-HIV herbal medicines, should be explored further.

References

1. Fauci AS, Masur H, Gelmann EP, Markham PD, Hahn BH, Lane HC. NIH Conference. The acquired immunodeficiency syndrome: an update. *Ann Intern Med* 1985;102:800–13

2. Fauci AS, Artlett JG. Guideline for the use of antiretroviral agents in HIV-infected adults and adolescents. *Ann Intern Med* 1998;128:1079–100

3. De Clercq E. Antiviral therapy for human immunodeficiency virus infections. *Clin Microbiol Rev* 1995;8:200–39

4. De Clercq E. Toward improved anti-HIV chemotherapy: therapeutic strategies for intervention with HIV infections. *J Med Chem* 1995;38:2491–517

5. De Clercq E. Perspectives of non-nucleoside reverse transcriptase inhibitors (NNRTIs) in the therapy of HIV-1 infection. *II Farmaco* 1999;54:26–45

6. Lee KH, Morris-Natschke SL. Recent advances in the discovery and development of plant-derived natural products and their analogs as anti-HIV agents. *Pure Appl Chem* 1999;71:1045–51

7. Vandamme AM, Van Vaerenbergh K, D'Clercq E. Anti-human immunodeficiency virus drug combination strategies. *Antivir Chem Chemother* 1998;9:187–203

8. Huang KC. *The Pharmacology of Chinese Herbs.* Boca Raton, FL: CRC Press, 1999

9. Zhao J, Ben LH, Wu YL et al. Anti-HIV agent trichosanthin enhances the capabilities of chemokines to stimulate chemotaxis and G protein activation, and this is mediated through interaction of trichosanthin and chemokine receptors. *J Exp Med* 1999;190:101–11

10. Collins RA, Ng TB, Fong WP, Wan CC, Yeung HW. A comparison of human immunodeficiency virus type 1 inhibition by partially purified aqueous extracts of Chinese medicinal herbs. *Life Sci* 1997;60:345–51

11. Tang XS, Chen HS, Zhang XQ. Inhibition of human immunodeficiency virus reverse transcriptase by Chinese medicines *in vitro*. *Proc CAMS PUMC* 1990;5:140–4

12. Buimovici-Klein E, Mohan V, Lange M, Fenamore E, Inada Y, Copper LZ. Inhibition of HIV replication in lymphocyte cultures of virus-positive subjects in the presence of Sho-saiko-to, an oriental plant extract. *Antivir Res* 1990;14:279–86

13. Wu XS, Akatsu H, Okada H. Apoptosis of HIV-infected cells following treatment with Sho-saiko-to and its components. *Jpn J Med Sci Biol* 1995;48:79–87

14. Piras G, Makino M, Baba M. Sho-saiko-to, a traditional kampo medicine, enhances the anti-HIV-1 activity of Lamivudine (3TC) *in vitro*. *Microbiol Immunol* 1997;41:835–9

15. Yamamoto T, Takahashi H, Sakai K, Kowithayakorn T, Koyano T. Screening of Thai plants for anti-HIV-1 activity. *Nature Med* 1997;51:541–6

16. Kassler WJ, Blanc P, Greenlatt R. The use of medicinal herbs by human immunodeficiency virus-infected patients. *Arch Intern Med* 1991;151:2281–8

17. Phillips LG, Nichols MH, King WD. Herbs and HIV: the health food industry's answer. *South Med J* 1995;88:911–13

18. Xue YX, Liu CH, Zhang L, Yuan CS. Traditional Chinese medicine and AIDS. *Am J Compreh Med* 1999;1:542–4

19. Luo SD, Chen JJ, Wang HY. Natural compounds with anti-HIV activity. *Chin Tradit Herb Drug (Suppl)* 1999;30:40–3

20. Vlietinck AJ, De Bruyne T, Vanden Berghe DA. Plant substances as antiviral agents. *Curr Org Chem* 1997;1:307–44

21. Tan GT, Pezzuto JM, Kinghorn AD. Evaluation of natural products as inhibitors of human immunodeficiency virus type 1 (HIV-1) reverse transcriptase. *J Nat Prod* 1991;54:143–54

22. Tan GT, Miller JF, Kinghorn AD, Hughes SH, Pezzuto JM. HIV-1 and HIV-2 reverse transcriptases: a comparative study of sensitivity to inhibition by selected natural products. *Biochem Biophys Res Commun* 1992;185:370–8

23. Chu CK, Cutler HG. *Natural Products as Antiviral Agents.* New York, NY: Plenum Press, 1992

24. Ng TB, Huang B, Fong WP, Yeung HW. Anti-human immunodeficiency virus (anti-HIV) natural products with special emphasis on HIV reverse transcriptase inhibitors. *Life Sci* 1997;61:933–49

25. Cragg GM, Boyd MR, Christini MA, et al. Screening of natural products of plant, microbial and marine origin: the NCI experience. *Spec Publ R Soc Chem* 1997;200:1-29

26. Vlietinck AJ, Bruyne TD, Apers S, Pieters LA. Plant-derived leading compounds for chemotherapy of human immunodeficiency virus (HIV) infection. *Planta Med* 1998;64:97–109

27. Lee KH. Antitumor agents.188. Highlights of research on plant-derived natural products and their analogs with antitumor, anti-HIV, and antifungal activity. In Cutler SJ, Cutler HG, eds. *Biologically Active Natural Products: Agrochemicals and Pharmaceuticals.* Symposium Series. Washington, DC: American Chemical Society, 2000:73–94

28. Wang HK, Xie Y, Yang ZY, Morris-Natschke SL, Lee KH. Recent advances in the development of flavonoids and their analogues as antitomor and anti-HIV agents. In Manthey JA, Buslig BS, eds. *Flavonoids in the Living System.* New York, NY: Plenum Press, 1998:191–225

29. Mahmood N, Pizza C, Aquino R, et al. Inhibition of HIV by flavonoids. *Antivir Res* 1993;22:189–99

30. Kitamura K, Honda M, Yoshizaki H, et al. Baicalin, an inhibitor of HIV-1 production *in vitro*. *Antivir Res* 1998;37:131–40

31. Oho K, Nakane H, Fukushima M, Chermann JC, Barre-Sinoussi F. Inhibition of reverse transcriptase activity by a flavonoid compound, 5,6,7,-trihydroxyflavone. *Biochem Biophy Res Commun* 1989; 160:982–7

32. Zhang XQ, Tang XS, Chen HS. Inhibition of HIV replication by baicalin and *S. baicalensis* extract in H9 cell culture. *Chin Med Sci J* 1991;6:230–2

33. Li BQ, Fu T, Yan YD, Baylor NW, Ruscetti FW, Kung HF. Inhibition of HIV infection by baicalin – a flavonoid compound purified from Chinese herbal medicine. *Cell Mol Biol Res* 1993;39:119–24

34. Baylor NW, Fu T, Yan YD, Ruscetti FW. Inhibition of human T cell leukemia virus by the plant flavonoid baicalin (7-glucuronic acid, 5,6-dihydroxyflavone). *J Infect Dis* 1992;165:433–7

35. Zhao J, Zhang ZP, Chen HS, Zhang XQ, Chen XH. Synthesis of baicalin derivatives and evaluation of their anti-human immunodeficiency virus (HIV-1) activity. *Acta Pharmaceut Sin* 1998; 33:22–7

36. Raghavan K, Buolamwini JK, Fesen MR, Pommier Y, Kohn KW, Weinstein JN. Three-dimensional quantitative structure–activity relationship (QSAR) of HIV integrase inhibitors: a comparative molecular field analysis (CoMFA). *J Med Chem* 1995;38:890–7

37. Muto R, Motozuka T, Nakano M, Tatsumi Y, Sakamoto F, Kosaka N. The chemical structure of new substance as the metabolite of baicalin and time profiles for the plasma concentration after oral administration of Sho-saiko-to in human. *Yakugaku Zasshi* 1998;118:79–87

38. Ono K, Nakane H. Mechanisms of inhibition of various cellular DNA and RNA polymerases by several flavonoids. *J Biochem* 1990;108:609–13

39. Brinkworth RI, Stoermer MJ, Fairlie DP. Flavones are inhibitors of HIV-1 proteinase. *Biochem Biophys Res Commun* 1992;188:631–7

40. Shimizu I, Ma YR, Mizobuchi Y, *et al*. Effects of Sho-saiko-to, a Japanese herbal medicine, on hepatic fibrosis in rats. *Hepatology (Philadelphia)* 1999;29:149–60

41. Geerts A, Rogiers V. Sho-saiko-to: the right blend of traditional oriental medicine and liver cell biology. *Hepatology (Philadelphia)* 1999;29:282–4

42. Yoshino M, Ito M, Okajima H, Haneda M, Murakam K. Role of baicalein compounds as antioxidant in the traditional herbal medicine. *Biomed Res* 1997;18:349–52

43. Tsutsumi M, Kitada H, Shiraiwa K, *et al*. Inhibitory effects of combined administration of antibiotics and anti-inflammatory drugs on lung tumor development initiated by N-nitrosobis(2-hydroxypropyl)amine in rats. *Carcinogenesis* 2000;21:251–6

44. Liu W, Kato M, Akhand AA, *et al*. The herbal medicine Sho-saiko-to inhibits the growth of malignant melanoma cells by upregulating Fas-mediated apoptosis and arresting cell cycle through downregulation of cyclein-depedent kinases. *Int J Oncol* 1998;12:1321–6

45. Kato M, Liu W, Yı H, *et al*. The herbal medicine Sho-saiko-to inhibits growth and metastasis of malignant melanoma primarily developed in *ret*-transgenic mice. *J Invest Deramatol* 1998;111:640–4

46. Mizushima Y, Kashii T, Tokimitsu Y, Kobayashi M. Cytotoxic effect of herbal medicine Sho-saiko-to on human lung cancer cell lines *in vitro*. *Oncol Rep* 1995;2:91–4

47. Motoo Y, Sawabu N. Antitumor effects of saikosaponins, baicalin and baicalein on human hepatoma cell lines. *Cancer Lett* 1994;86:91–5

48. Inoue T, Jackson EK. Strong antiproliferative effects of baicalein in cultured rat hepatic stellate cells. *Eur J Pharm* 1999;378:129–35

49. Ono M, Miyamura M, Kyotani S, Saibara T, Ohnishi S, Nishioka Y. Effects of Sho-saiko-to extract on liver fibrosis in relation to the changes in hydroxyproline and retinoid levels of the liver in rats. *J Pharm Pharmacol* 1999;51:1079–84

50. Yagura M, Murai S, Kojima H, Tokita H, Kamitsukasa H, Harada H. Changes of liver fibrosis in chronic hepatitis C patients with no response to interferon-α therapy: including quantitative assessment by a morphometric method. *J Gastroenterol* 2000;35:105–11

51. Shao ZH, Li CQ, Vanden Hock TL, *et al*. Extract from *Scutellaria baicalensis* Georgi attenuates oxidant stress in cadiomyocytes. *J Mol Cardiol* 1999;31:1885–95

52. Gao Z, Huang K, Yang, X, Xu H. Free radical scavenging and antioxidant activities of flavonoids extracted from the radix of *Scutellaria baicalensis* Georgi. *BBA-Biomembranes* 1999;1472:643–50

53. Minematsu S, Takei H, Sudo K, Honda K, Fujii Y, Oyama T. A single oral dose toxicity study of TSUMURA Sho-saiko-to (TJ-9) in rats. *Jpn Pharmacol Ther* 1995;23:29–32

54. Inada Y, Watanabe K, Miyamoto K, Maitra U, Klein EB, Lange M. Regulatory activities of Sho-saiko-to in immune responses, eicosanoid pathway and HIV production. In *Proceedings of the Tenth International Conference on AIDS Satellite Symposium*. Yokohama, Japan: 1994

55. Maikeru R, Erena BK, Utopare M, *et al*. Anti-AIDS virus effect-enhancing agents containing Shosaikoto. [Japanese Patent.] *Jpn Koka Tokkyo Koho* 1996:5

56. Fugh-Berman A. Herb–drug interactions. *Lancet* 2000;355:134–8

57. Xie L, Takeuchi Y, Cosentino LM, Lee K-H. Anti-AIDS agents. 37. Synthesis and structure–activity relationships of $(3'R,4'R)$-(+)-*cis*-khellactone derivatives as novel potent anti-HIV agents. *J Med Chem* 1999;42:2662–72

58. Kashiwada Y. Studies on bioactive natural products: plant-derived natural products and analogues as anti-HIV agents. *Nature Med* 1999;53:153–8

59. Oho K, Nakane H, Fukushima M, Chermann JC, Barre-Sinoussi F. Differential inhibitory effects of various flavonoids on the activities of reverse transcriptase and cellular DNA and RNA polymerases. *Eur J Biochem* 1990;190:469–76

60. Zhao J, Zhang ZP, Chen HS, Chen XH, Zhang XQ. Preparation and anti-HIV activity study of baicalein and its benzylated derivatives. *Acta Pharmaceut Sin* 1997;32:140–3

61. Hu CQ, Chen K, Shi Q, Kilkuskie RE, Cheng YC, Lee KH. Anti-AIDS agents 10. Acacetin-7-O-β-D-galactopyranoside, an anti-HIV principle from *Chrysanthemum morifolium* and a structure–activity correlation with some related flavonoids. *J Nat Prod* 1994;57:42–51

Complementary and alternative therapies for other disorders

31

L. Dey, J. L. Gnerlich and C.-S. Yuan

ANXIETY

Anxiety disorders, the most prevalent psychiatric illnesses in the general community, are present in 15–20% of medical clinic patients. The US National Comorbidity Survey suggests a 1-year prevalence of anxiety disorders of 17% and a lifetime prevalence of almost 25%[1].

Anxiety, defined as a subjective sense of unease, dread, or foreboding, can indicate a primary psychiatric condition or can be a component of, or reaction to, a primary medical disease. The primary anxiety disorders are classified according to their duration and course and the existence and nature of precipitants. Panic disorder with or without agoraphobia, generalized anxiety disorder, phobic disorders, stress disorder and obsessive–compulsive disorder are the common anxiety disorders. Benzodiazepines are the most commonly used conventional therapy, but they are associated with serious adverse effects such as dependence, sedation and memory impairment[2,3].

Forty-three per cent of people who suffer from anxiety attacks have used complementary and alternative medicine in the previous 12 months, and approximately a quarter of them have visited a practitioner of complementary and alternative medicine (CAM) for treatment[4]. The most commonly used CAM therapies include relaxation, exercise, herbs, massage, aromatherapy, meditation, spiritual healing and biofeedback.

Relaxation

In a randomized controlled trial, relaxation was shown to be less effective than cognitive therapy for panic disorder, but both were superior to minimal contact control[5]. For management of agoraphobia, relaxation training was as effective as exposure and cognitive treatment, and all were more effective than weekly individual therapy sessions[6].

Relaxation has also been used to manage anxiety associated with medical conditions. In patients with newly diagnosed cancer, relaxation improved anxiety as well as other aspects of mood[7]. In similar patients, there was a reduction in state anxiety after relaxation compared with untreated controls, but there was no significant effect on trait anxiety[8].

In addition, relaxation reduces anxiety and dyspnea in patients with chronic obstructive pulmonary disease (COPD). When patients with COPD were randomized to receive relaxation training or standard management alone[9], dyspnea, anxiety and airway obstruction were reduced in the relaxation group, while the condition in the control group remained the same or became worse.

Relaxation training has also been used to reduce anxiety associated with a variety of medical and surgical procedures and to improve some aspects of healing[10]. For minor surgery there is considerable evidence of patient benefit, and one study found relaxation to be superior to attention control in facilitating the ease of general anesthesia in day-case surgery[11]. Audiotapes with relaxation instructions were superior to music tapes or blank tapes at reducing both anxiety and pain during femoral angiography[12]. A relaxation procedure before a magnetic resonance imaging (MRI) scan reduced the anxiety associated with the scan more than no intervention, in a randomized controlled trial[13]. In addition, in a controlled trial of 53 women undergoing radiation therapy for early-stage breast cancer, relaxation with guided imagery was an effective intervention for reducing anxiety and enhancing comfort, compared to no intervention[14].

Exercise

In a controlled trial, where 85 volunteers were randomized to aerobic exercise, relaxation or no treatment, the exercise and relaxation groups decreased anxiety more than the control group[15]. In addition, in another controlled trial with panic disorder and agoraphobia, 10 weeks of walking was less effective than clomipramine, but superior to placebo[16].

Herbal medications

Kava extract

A meta-analysis of three trials showed that kava extract was superior to placebo as a symptomatic treatment for anxiety. There was a significant difference in the reduction of the total score on the Hamilton rating scale for anxiety in favor of kava extract[17]. The use of kavalactones is approved in Germany for 'states of nervous anxiety, tension, and agitation' in doses of 60–120 mg for up to 3 months[18,19]. In spite of safety concerns in recent reports of liver toxicity related to use of kava products in humans[20,21], the US Food and Drug Administration (FDA) has not taken any action against kava products.

Other herbs

Herbs such as German chamomile, lemon balm, passion flower and valerian may be effective in the treatment of anxiety[22], but more studies are required to prove their efficacy.

Massage

Massage therapy given to depressed pregnant adolescents twice a week for 5 weeks was shown to be more effective than relaxation therapy in a clinical trial. Both groups scored lower in anxiety, but the effect in the massage group was accompanied by improvements in mood, sleep and back pain and confirmed by objective measurement of behavior and urinary steroid concentrations[23]. In another controlled trial of elderly institutionalized patients, massage was shown to reduce anxiety to a greater extent than no intervention[24].

Aromatherapy

Aromatherapy is widely used for the treatment of stress. However, a systematic review concluded that, although there are clearly significant effects, modest and short-term effects are unlikely to be clinically relevant[25].

Meditation

There is evidence that meditation can reduce anxiety levels and neuroendocrine responses to stress more effectively than situation control in volunteers placed in stressful conditions[26], and uncontrolled studies have suggested benefits in patients with anxiety. In one randomized controlled trial, 28 individuals were randomized to receive an 8-week stress-reduction program based on mindfulness meditation. Compared with the non-intervention control group, the investigators observed greater reductions in overall psychological symptoms, improvements in sense of control and measure of spiritual experiences[27].

A systematic review, which included observational studies as well as controlled trials on relaxation techniques for trait anxiety, found the effect for meditation to score 0.70 compared with progressive muscle relaxation (0.38). However, there are very few good-quality randomized controlled trials to make a convincing case for the effectiveness of meditation for clinical practice.

Spiritual healing

In a controlled trial, therapeutic touch in the treatment of anxiety has been compared with no treatment in 40 healthy professional care-givers/students. The reduction of anxiety in the high-anxiety group was greater for those who had received therapeutic touch than for those who had not[28]. In addition, effectiveness of therapeutic touch in reducing anxiety was observed in 20 HIV-infected children[29] and 99 hospitalized burn patients[30] in controlled trials.

Biofeedback

In a controlled trial, eight sessions of electromyogram (EMG) and electroencephalogram (EEG) biofeedback were both superior to meditation control at reducing trait anxiety in individuals with generalized anxiety disorder. Improvements persisted for 6 weeks[31]. In another controlled trial, combined alpha wave EEG and EMG biofeedback training improved test anxiety in students with examination phobia, compared with no training[32]. Regular EEG biofeedback sessions have also been proved superior to standard medication treatment in post-traumatic stress disorder[32].

References

1. Kessler RC, McGonagle KA, Zhao S, *et al*. Lifetime and 12-month prevalence of DSM-III-R psychiatric disorders in the United States. *Arch Gen Psychiatry* 1994;51:8–19

2. Gorman JM, Papp LA. Chronic anxiety: deciding the length of treatment. *J Clin Psychiatry* 1990;51(Suppl):11–15

3. Hunt C, Singh M. Generalized anxiety disorder. *Int Rev Psychiatry* 1991;3:215–29

4. Eisenberg DM, Davis R, Ettner SL, *et al*. Trends in alternative medicine use in the United States, 1990-1997. *J Am Med Assoc* 1998;280:1569–75

5. Beck JG, Stanley MA, Baldwin LE, Deagle EA 3rd, Averill PM. Comparison of cognitive therapy and relaxation training for panic disorder. *J Consult Clin Psychol* 1994;62:818–26

6. Ost LG, Westling BE, Hellstrom K. Applied relaxation, exposure *in vivo* and cognitive methods in the treatment of panic disorder with agoraphobia. *Behav Res Ther* 1993;31:383–94

7. Bindemann S, Soukop M, Kaye SB. Randomised controlled study of relaxation training. *Eur J Cancer* 1991;27:170–4

8. Bridge LR, Benson P, Pietroni PC, Priest RG. Relaxation and imagery in the treatment of breast cancer. *Br Med J* 1988;297:1169–72

9. Gift AG, Moore T, Soeken K. Relaxation to reduce dyspnea and anxiety in COPD patients. *Nurs Res* 1992;41:242–6

10. Holden-Lund C. Effects of relaxation with guided imagery on surgical stress and wound healing. *Res Nurs Health* 1988;11:235–44

11. Markland D, Hardy L. Anxiety, relaxation and anaesthesia for day-case surgery. *Br J Clin Psychol* 1993;32:493–504

12. Mandle CL, Domar AD, Harrington DP, *et al*. Relaxation response in femoral angiography. *Radiology* 1990;174:737–9

13. Lukins R, Davan IG, Drummond PD. A cognitive behavioural approach to preventing anxiety during magnetic resonance imaging. *J Behav Ther Exp Psychiatr* 1997;28:97–104

14. Kolcaba K, Fox C. The effects of guided imagery on comfort of women with early stage breast cancer undergoing radiation therapy. *Oncol Nurs Forum* 1999;26:67–72

15. Crocker PR, Grozelle C. Reducing induced state anxiety: effects of acute aerobic exercise and autogenic relaxation. *J Sports Med Phys Fitness* 1991;31:277–82

16. Broocks A, Bandelow B, Pekrun G, *et al*. Comparison of aerobic exercise, clomipramine and placebo in the treatment of panic disorder. *Am J Psychiatr* 1998;155:603–9

17. Pittler M, Ernst E. Efficacy of kava extract for treating anxiety: systematic review and meta-analysis. *J Clin Psychopharmacol* 2000;20:84–9

18. Schulz V, Hansel R, Tyler VE. *Rational Phytotherapy: a Physician's Guide to Herbal Medicine*, 3rd edn. Berlin: Springer-Verlag, 1998

19. Cass H, McNally T. *Kava: Nature's Answer to Stress, Anxiety, and Insomnia*. Rocklin, CA: Prima Health, 1998

20. Russmann S, Lauterburg BH, Helbling A. Kava hepatotoxicity. *Ann Intern Med* 2001;35:68–9

21. Escher M, Desmeules J, Giostra E, Mentha G. Hepatitis associated with kava, a herbal remedy for anxiety. *Br Med J* 2001;322:139

22. Wong AHC, Smith M, Boon HS. Herbal remedies in psychiatric practice. *Arch Gen Psychiatry* 1998;55:1033–44

23. Field T, Grizzle N, Scafidi F, Schanberg S. Massage and relaxation therapies' effects on depressed adolescent mothers. *Adolescence* 1996;31:903–11

24. Fraser J, Kerr JR. Psychophysiological effects of back massage on elderly institutionalized patients. *J Adv Nurs* 1993;18:238–45

25. Cooke B, Ernst E. Aromatherapy: a systematic review. *Br J Gen Pract* 2000;50:493–6

26. MacLean CRK, Walton KG, Wenneberg SR, *et al*. Altered response of cortisol, GH, TSH and testosterone to acute stress after four months' practice of transcendental meditation. *Ann NY Acad Sci* 1994;746:381–4

27. Astin JA. Stress reduction through mindfulness meditation. Effects on psychological symptomatology, sense of control and spiritual experiences. *Psychother Psychosom* 1997;66:97–106

28. Olson M, Sneed N. Anxiety and therapeutic touch. *Issues Mental Health Nurs* 1995;16:97–108

29. Ireland M. Therapeutic touch with HIV-infected children: a pilot study. *J Assoc Nurs AIDS Care* 1998;9:68–77

30. Turner JG, Clark AJ, Gauthier DK, Williams M. The effect of therapeutic touch on pain and anxiety in burn patients. *J Adv Nurs* 1998;28:10–20

31. Rice KM, Blanchard EB, Purcell M. Biofeedback treatments of generalized anxiety disorder: preliminary results. *Biofeedback Self Reg* 1993;18:93–105

32. Moore NC. A review of EEG biofeedback treatment of anxiety disorders. *Clin Electroencephalogr* 2000;31:1–6

DEPRESSION

Depression is a common disorder with an estimated 17% lifetime prevalence for the US population[1]. There are varying degrees of depression. Normal depression occurs when one finds disappointment in not reaching one's personal goals or encountering setbacks in one's life. Pathological depression, however, disrupts normal activities of daily living. Pathological depression may be caused by lack of important neurohormones, such as norepinephrine (noradrenaline), serotonin and dopamine, which most antidepressant medications target. However, many individuals suffering from depression are turning to CAM therapies to treat their illness. Among these are included St John's wort herbal medicine, transcranial magnetic stimulation and religious/spiritual stimulation. Other treatments not discussed at length are massage, relaxation, music, acupuncture and yoga.

Hypericum perforatum (St John's wort) is believed to be an effective antidepressant therapy with fewer side-effects than standard antidepressants[2]. It works by increasing serotonin receptors, weakly inhibiting monoamine oxidases, and decreasing serotonin and norepinephrine uptake. It is also postulated that hyperfornin has a novel, and as yet unknown, action[3]. With pooled data, there was a 60–70% response rate for mild and moderate depression. Great tolerability, low side-effects and high compliance make this a useful medication, especially for the elderly[4]. One multi-center observational study showed St John's wort efficacy and low side-effects with both 600 mg and 1200 mg taken daily for mild and moderate depression[5]. Another controlled trial demonstrated that St John's wort, at a dose of 1050 mg/day, was effective at reducing depression compared to placebo and was just as effective as the tricyclic antidepressant imipramine (100 mg/day) in patients with moderate depression[6].

Reported side-effects include gastrointestinal upset and dizziness. However, in a randomized, double-blind study of patients with major depression, 1200 mg of St John's wort taken daily did not show marked improvement over placebo. Therefore, St John's wort was not considered to be an effective treatment for major depression[7]. It is important to note that St John's wort can have important contra-indications if used concomitantly with antidepressants, such as selective serotonin reuptake inhibitors (SSRIs), leading to serotonin excess called 'serotonin syndrome', which can cause a fast heart rate, mental status changes, restlessness, sweating and rigidity.

Another alternative therapy for treating depression is repetitive transcranial magnetic stimulation (rTMS). An electric coil generates magnetic fields that stimulate the cerebral cortex, a procedure well tolerated by individuals. In one controlled study, medication-resistant patients with major depression underwent either rTMS or sham rTMS. Results indicated that there was no significant difference between the treatment and control groups[8]. However, in another similar study in which the patients suffering from major depression were not medication-resistant, the treatment group receiving rTMS in ten daily sessions for 2 weeks showed a significant improvement in their depression scores over the control group[9]. Therefore, rTMS may have short-term therapeutic effects in depressed patients who are not medication-resistant.

Religion and spirituality has been found to reduce depressive symptoms, and lead to a more rapid remission. In one observational study conducted in the Netherlands, being religious was highly correlated with improvement of depression, especially in those with poor physical health[10]. In another study, patients over the age of 60 with major depression were followed for almost a year. The study showed that intrinsic religiosity was an independent prognostic factor of recovery, and demonstrated a shorter time to remission. Church attendance and private services did not show any correlation[11]. Even cognitive behavioral therapy with religious content or pastoral counselling was shown in another study to lower post-treatment depression significantly more than the standard protocol[12].

Other less studied approaches to treating depression include massage, relaxation, music therapy, acupuncture and yoga. These methods stimulate blood and lymph flow in the body and relieve tension in muscles[13]. These therapies also promote self-worth and a feeling of control over one's mood and performance. They may work physiologically by relieving stress through the release of natural endorphins in the body. In a meta-analysis reporting on four studies comparing cognitive behavioral therapy to standard

antidepressant medication in severely depressed outpatients, cognitive behavioral therapies were shown to be as effective as antidepressant medication in the treatment of acute severe depression. Consequently, prescribed medication should not necessarily be considered a superior treatment to other therapies[14].

Depression is a common mood disorder that can disable individuals and prevent them from continuing with their normal activities of daily living. Depression has been treated extensively with prescribed antidepressant medications that seem to work well. However, there is no compelling evidence to suggest that CAM therapies will not provide the same benefit. Many people may choose to treat their depression with herbal medications, lifestyle modifications, or even rTMS to find relief from their disorder and gain a sense of control over their emotional and psychological problems.

References

1. Kessler RC, McGonagle KA, Zhao S, *et al.* Lifetime and 12-month prevalence of DSM-III-R psychiatric disorders in the United States. Results from the National Comorbidity Survey. *Arch Gen Psychiatry* 1994;51:8–19.
2. Linde K, Ramirez G, Mulrow CD, Pauls A, Weidenhammer W, Melchart D. St John's wort for depression – an overview and meta-analysis of randomised clinical trials. *Br Med J* 1996;313:253–8
3. Kasper S, Schulz V. St John's wort extract as plant antidepressant. [In German.] *Schweiz Rundsch Med Prax* 2000;89:2169–77
4. Hippius H. St John's wort (*Hypericum perforatum*) – a herbal antidepressant. *Curr Med Res Opin* 1998;14:171–84
5. Rychlik R, Siedentop H, von den Driesch V, Kasper S. [St. John's wort extract WS 5572 in minor to moderately severe depression. Effectiveness and tolerance of 600 and 1200 mg active ingredient daily.] *Fortschr Med Orig* 2001;119:119–28
6. Philipp M, Kohnen R, Hiller KO. Hypericum extract versus imipramine or placebo in patients with moderate depression: randomised multicentre study of treatment for eight weeks. *Br Med J* 1999;319:1534–8
7. Shelton RC, Keller MB, Gelenberg A, *et al.* Effectiveness of St John's wort in major depression: a randomized controlled trial. *J Am Med Assoc* 2001;285:1978–86
8. Loo C, Mitchell P, Sachdev P, McDarmont B, Parker G, Gandevia S. Double-blind controlled investigation of transcranial magnetic

stimulation for the treatment of resistant major depression. *Am J Psychiatry* 1999;156:946–8
9. Klein E, Kreinin I, Chistyakov A, *et al.* Therapeutic efficacy of right prefrontal slow repetitive transcranial magnetic stimulation in major depression: a double-blind controlled study. *Arch Gen Psychiatry* 1999;56:315–20
10. Braam AW, Beekman AT, Deeg DJ, Smit JH, van Tilburg W. Religiosity as a protective or prognostic factor of depression in later life; results from a community survey in The Netherlands. *Acta Psychiatr Scand* 1997;96:199–205
11. Koenig HG, George LK, Peterson BL. Religiosity and remission of depression in medically ill older patients. *Am J Psychiatry* 1998;155:536–42
12. Propst LR, Ostrom R, Watkins P, Dean T, Mashburn D. Comparative efficacy of religious and nonreligious cognitive–behavioral therapy for the treatment of clinical depression in religious individuals. *J Consult Clin Psychol* 1992;60:94–103
13. Field TM. Massage therapy effects. *Am Psychol* 1998;53:1270–81
14. DeRubeis RJ, Gelfand LA, Tang TZ, Simons AD. Medications versus cognitive behavior therapy for severely depressed outpatients: mega-analysis of four randomized comparisons. *Am J Psychiatry* 1999;156:1007–13

HEADACHE

Thirty-two per cent of Americans with headache have used CAM in the previous 12 months[1]. Relaxation and chiropractic are the most frequently used CAM therapies. Other therapies, such as herbal medicines, homeopathy and acupuncture, are also employed.

Relaxation

A systematic review of relaxation and biofeedback concluded that relaxation was effective, with a mean effect size of 36%. In children and adolescents, several randomized controlled trials have indicated that relaxation has a positive effect on tension headache. Relaxation can be taught efficiently by school nurses; more than two-thirds of the children in one study recorded at least 50% improvement at follow-up after 6 months, compared with only a quarter of controls[2]. Follow-up over an average of 4 years found that continuing to practice relaxation maintained the improvements in days free of headache and headache severity, compared with an untreated control group[3].

Spinal manipulation

A systematic review suggested that spinal manipulation has a useful effect on tension, cervicogenic and post-traumatic headaches. In the two studies of patients with tension headache, manipulation had marginally better outcomes than amitriptyline in one study and was no better than placebo laser in the other. No clear conclusion can be drawn from the latter study, since the placebo effect of sham laser is unknown, and both groups also received soft tissue massage, the effectiveness of which is also unknown[4].

Herbal medicines

Peppermint oil

In a randomized controlled trial involving 41 adults with a history of tension headache, 164 acute headache attacks were treated with either peppermint oil or placebo oil locally and either acetaminophen or placebo tablet orally[5]. Peppermint oil was superior to placebo and not significantly different from the analgesic drug in reducing headache parameters.

Tiger balm

The use of tiger balm was supported in one multicenter randomized controlled trial in which 57 patients were given either tiger balm to apply locally, placebo balm or standard analgesic medication[6]. There was a statistically significant difference in headache relief between tiger balm and placebo. The difference between tiger balm and medication was not significant. However, subjective blinding was questionable, since tiger balm produces local warmth.

Homeopathy

One controlled trial was conducted to determine the efficacy of classical homeopathic therapy in patients with chronic headaches. The 98 subjects included patients with tension headache as well as those with migraine, and the study found no benefit from individualized homeopathy compared with placebo[7]. There was no significant difference in any parameter between homeopathy and placebo.

Acupuncture

In a meta-analysis, evidence suggested that acupuncture has a role in the treatment of recurrent headaches. However, the quality and amount of evidence was not fully convincing. There is an urgent need for well-planned, large-scale studies to assess the effectiveness of acupuncture[8].

References

1. Eisenberg DM, Davis R, Ettner SL, Appel S, Wilkey S, Rompay MV. Trends in alternative medicine use in the United States, 1990–1997. *J Am Med Assoc* 1998;280:1569–75
2. Larsson B, Melin L. Chronic headaches in adolescents: treatment in a school setting with relaxation training as compared with information-contact and self-registration. *Pain* 1986;25:325–36
3. Engel JM, Rapoff MA, Pressman AR. Long-term follow-up of relaxation training for pediatric headache disorders. *Headache* 1992;32:152–6
4. Vernon H, McDermaid CS, Hagino C. Systematic review of randomized clinical trials of complementary/alternative therapies in the treatment of tension-type and cervicogenic headache. *Complement Ther Med* 1999;7:142–55
5. Gobel H, Fresenius J, Heinze A, Dworschak M, Soyka D. Effectiveness of oleum menthae piperitae and paracetamol in therapy of headache of the tension type. *Nervenarzt* 1996;67:672–81
6. Schattner P, Randerson D. Tiger balm as a treatment of tension headache. A clinical trial in general practice. *Aust Fam Physician* 1996;25:216–20
7. Walach H, Haeusler W, Lower T, *et al*. Classical homeopathic treatment of chronic headaches. *Cephalalgia* 1997;17:119–26
8. Melchart D, Linde K, Fischer P, *et al*. Acupuncture for recurrent headaches: a systematic review of randomized controlled trials. *Cephalalgia* 1999;19:779–86

FIBROMYALGIA

Fibromyalgia is a syndrome of unknown etiology characterized by chronic, diffuse musculoskeletal pain. Other common symptoms include fatigue, sleeping problems, mood disorders and headaches[1]. Fibromyalgia is more common in women and tends to increase with age[2]. This syndrome affects both muscles and soft tissues, but no inflammation is present. Therefore, non-steroidal anti-inflammatory drugs (NSAIDs) are of no use in controlling the pain, and individuals suffering from fibromyalgia have looked to alternative therapies to find a relief from their symptoms[3].

It has been reported that 91% of people are using CAM therapies for fibromyalgia compared to other rheumatological disorders[4]. CAM therapies commonly used for fibromyalgia are acupuncture, EMG biofeedback, S-adenosyl methionine dietary supplement, capsicum pain plaster, manipulation and various mind–body therapies including relaxation, meditation, hypnosis, imagery and cognitive behavioral therapy[5]. At this time, there are mostly small, poorly designed studies investigating the use of CAM therapies in fibromyalgia.

Seven clinical trials have shown that electro-acupuncture, which stimulates blood flow and relieves muscle spasm, is effective in treating the chronic musculoskeletal pain associated with fibromyalgia. Of these, a well-designed controlled study investigating the use of acupuncture randomly assigned fibromyalgia patients to receive either electroacupuncture of tai chi meridians or sham acupuncture in six sessions over a 3-week period. Seven of eight parameters improved in the treatment group. No parameters showed improvement in the sham group. Pain threshold, the main parameter, was shown to improve by 70% in the treatment group as compared to 4% in the sham group. Usually acupuncture is used for acute pain, but strong evidence shows that electroacupuncture is an effective treatment for the chronic pain associated with fibromyalgia. The only negative finding was that acupuncture exacerbated the pain to the point that approximately 20% of participants dropped out of the study[6].

Another effective alternative treatment is EMG biofeedback. Patients receive auditory feedback, which is a pulse of sounds, of their chronic muscle tension transmitted by electrodes. In this manner, individuals hear what their muscle activity sounds like while experiencing the muscle tension. This type of neuromuscular rehabilitation gives patients a type of mind–body control over their internal muscle tension, and thus promotes muscle relaxation. In one study comparing EMG biofeedback and sham biofeedback given in 20-min sessions twice a week for a total of 15 sessions, persistent long-term benefit was seen in 56% of the treatment group, confirmed in a control study.

The only pertinent negative finding was that there was a poor response in patients with psychopathological disturbances. Therefore, EMG biofeedback is not recommended for depressed patients[7].

A dietary supplement, called *S*-adenosyl methionine, has been found to help those suffering from fibromyalgia. This compound, composed of the amino acid methionine and the energy molecule ATP, is an anti-inflammatory drug with both analgesic and antidepressant effects. In a small but well-designed study, 800 mg of *S*-adenosyl methionine taken daily showed improvement in clinical disease activity, pain, fatigue, morning stiffness and mood[8]. The setback is that *S*-adenosyl methionine is expensive, and interactions with other drugs such as antidepressants have been documented[9]. Also, *S*-adenosyl methionine should not be used in patients with bipolar disorder, because manic episodes may be precipitated.

Capsaicin, a topically applied alternative medicine, is an active derivative of cayenne, better known as the chili pepper. It has been discovered through a double-blind, randomized clinical trial that application of capsicum plaster for diffuse back pain is quite effective compared to placebo. There was a 61% response to capsicum compared to 42% with placebo, and better tolerance of the plaster. Capsaicin works by releasing substance P, a neurotransmitter from special nerve pain fibers, thus depleting this painful effector. This results in desensitization to pain and increases the pain threshold[10]. This therapy can be effectively utilized for the non-specific chronic pain in joints and muscles of fibromyalgia. Capsaicin cream did have irritant skin effects or burning sensations in some patients, but these wore off in time.

Manipulation of either the chiropractic or massage technique may improve pain control and use of muscles. Manipulation relies on the belief that, by correcting the misalignment of bones and joints or by manipulating soft tissues, optimal function of those body parts can be returned. More satisfaction has been documented with light massage. In a small study of chiropractic manipulation with rheumatology patients, treatment consisted of spinal manipulation, soft tissue therapy and passive stretching for 1 month. Patients' cervical and lumbar ranges of motion, straight leg raising and reported pain levels improved, and it is believed that these results can be generalized to fibromyalgia patients, but more research is needed[11].

The other alternative therapies such as spa treatments and mind–body therapies including relaxation, hypnosis, imagery, cognitive behavioral therapy and meditation have not been well studied, but are inexpensive and may offer relief to some from both the musculoskeletal pain and the mood disorders present in fibromyalgia patients. Since not much is known about this debilitating syndrome and traditional pain medications do not seem to offer much relief, CAM therapies may provide individuals with fibromyalgia a safe and inexpensive alternative to deal with both the physical and the psychological symptoms.

References

1. Goldenberg DL. Clinical manifestations and diagnosis of fibromyalgia, 2001. http://uptodateonline.com
2. Wolfe F, Ross K, Anderson J, Russell IJ, Hebert L. The prevalence and characteristics of fibromyalgia in the general population. *Arthritis Rheum* 1995;38:19–28
3. Goldenberg DL. Pathogenesis and treatment of fibromyalgia, 2001. http://uptodateonline.com
4. Pioro-Boisset M, Esdaile JM, Fitzcharles M-A. Alternative medicine use in fibromyalgia syndrome. *Arthritis Care Res* 1996;9:13–17
5. Berman BM, Swyers JP. Complementary medicine treatments for fibromyalgia syndrome. *Baillière's Best Pract Res Clin Rheumatol* 1999;13:487–92
6. Deluze C, Bosia L, Zirbs A, Chantraine A, Vischer TL. Electroacupuncture in fibromyalgia: results of a controlled trial. *Br Med J* 1992;305:1249–52
7. Ferraccioli G, Bhirelli L, Scita F, *et al*. EMG-biofeedback in fibromyalgia syndrome. *J Rheumatol* 1989;16:1013–14
8. Jacobsen S, Danneskiold-Samsoe B, Andersen RB. Oral *S*-adenosylmethionine in primary fibromyalgia. Double-blind clinical evaluation. *Scand J Rheumatol* 1991;20:294–302
9. Beck E. How effective are complementary/alternative medicine (CAM) therapies for fibromyalgia? *J Fam Pract* 2001;50:400–1

10. Keitel W, Frerick H, Kuhn U, Schmidt U, Kuhlmann M, Bredehorst A. Capsicum pain plaster in chronic non-specific low back pain. *Arzneimittelforschung* 2001;51:896–903

11. Blunt KL, Rajwani MH, Guerriero RC. The effectiveness of chiropractic management of fibromyalgia patients: a pilot study. *J Manipulative Physiol Ther* 1997;20:389–99

CHRONIC FATIGUE SYNDROME

Chronic fatigue syndrome (CFS) is a condition of unknown etiology characterized by disabling fatigue of at least 6 months' duration, and other symptoms such as muscle pain, pharyngitis and changes in mood, sleep and neurocognition[1]. In clinical settings, CFS is most commonly diagnosed in relatively young, educated and previously healthy women[2]. There are no consistent laboratory findings or diagnostic tests for CFS[2,3].

As defined by the Centers for Disease Control and Prevention (CDC), CFS is a diagnosis of exclusion[1]. The treatment of CFS has focused on symptoms[4]. While these treatments may work for some patients and some symptoms, there are no specific and definitive treatments for CFS. In addition, family, friends and physicians often dismiss CFS patients' complaints as psychosomatic and therefore 'not real'[5].

Individuals with CFS also report the use of CAM. For example, between 19% and 35% of 208 patients with CFS from a clinic sample visited an acupuncturist, chiropractor or naturopath[6]. A small study showed that all CFS patients had seen an acupuncturist, massage therapist, or other allied health professional in the previous year[7]. Individuals with CFS have indicated that the failure of conventional medicine in treating their illness and the lack of satisfaction with the support received from medical professionals are the primary reasons for seeking alternative care[8]. Treatment by CAM practitioners, however, has not been predictive of improvement in CFS symptoms[9].

Exercise

Three randomized controlled trials evaluating graded exercise therapy (GET) found an overall beneficial effect of the intervention in the treated group compared with the control group. One of these studies also looked at the combined effects of GET and fluoxetine, but found no additional benefits[10]. The studies did not report any adverse effects of GET, although two studies did report study withdrawals that may have been related to the intervention[10,11].

Cognitive behavioral therapy

Three of the four controlled trials[12–16] comparing cognitive behavioral therapy to control conditions found a positive overall effect of the intervention, and these studies also scored highly on validity assessment. One of these studies also included a support group as an additional control and found that cognitive behavioral therapy was significantly more effective than either of the control conditions, but that there was no difference between the two control groups[14].

Another randomized controlled trial, which also included immunological therapy[16], and one controlled trial[17] did not find overall beneficial effects of cognitive behavioral therapy. However, the study that included immunological therapy found no effect of either dialyzable leukocyte extract or cognitive behavioral therapy when used alone, but did find a beneficial effect on one of the outcomes investigated in the group receiving both interventions. The duration of the intervention in both of these studies was much shorter than in the three randomized controlled trials that did report overall benefits (9 and 16 weeks vs. 26, 52 and 35 weeks, respectively). The cognitive behavioral therapy used in the controlled trial differed from that used in the four randomized controlled trials, focusing more on limiting activities rather than trying to increase activity, and so it is questionable as to whether it should be classified as cognitive behavioral therapy. This study was methodologically poor, scoring only one out of a possible 20 on the validity assessment.

A controlled trial compared cognitive behavioral theapy with counselling and found that both interventions had a similar effect for patients with CFS[18]. This study included participants from general practice, of whom a small subset had CFS. Only the results for the CFS patients are included in the review. The studies evaluating cognitive behavioral theapy did not report any adverse effects of the intervention, although in one controlled trial two participants dropped out of the study group because they felt that a deterioration in their symptoms was due to the intervention[12]. A second randomized controlled trial showed very high drop-out rates in all three intervention groups; the rates were highest in the cognitive behavioral theapy group, but reasons for drop-outs were not reported[14].

Herbal medicines and other dietary supplements

Herbs and other antioxidants

The botanical antioxidants such as oligomeric proanthocyanidins (OPCs) from grape seed extract and *Ginkgo biloba* should also be considered. Bagchi and colleagues found that OPCs are highly bioavailable, and provide significantly greater protection against free radical damage than β-carotene and vitamins C and E[19]. These authors also reported the ability of OPCs to provide protection from radical-induced lipid peroxidation and DNA damage, which is of particular importance to CFS patients.

Ginkgo biloba is another antioxidant demonstrating strong neuroprotective properties in animals[20]. It has been shown to reduce mitochondrial reactive oxygen species, in particular peroxynitrite[21]. The capacity of ginkgo to increase cerebral blood flow[22] and improve memory and cognition associated with cerebral insufficiency[23] suggests that it may be useful for CFS symptoms related to hypoperfusion.

Plant-based antioxidant support should be maximized through dietary intake. Cao and associates found that a diet high in fruits and vegetables can increase plasma antioxidant capacity in humans, as measured by the oxygen radical absorbance capacity (ORAC) assay[24]. Blueberries had the highest ORAC scores among 30 fruits and vegetables tested[25,26], and

may be of significant benefit, owing to their high potential antioxidant activity[27], neuroprotective properties[28] and specific ability to protect red blood cells from *in vivo* oxidative damage[29]. Of the blueberry species, *Vaccinium myrtillus* has the highest combined anthocyanidin, phenol and ORAC scores[27].

In a double-blind, placebo-controlled, cross-over study, administration of pure anthocyanidins (80 mg daily) showed a small but statistically significant benefit in a group of patients with the related disorder of fibromyalgia[30]. The trial was 3 months in duration for active treatment and involved an anthocyanidin combination derived from grape seed, bilberry and cranberry. Improvements were observed in sleep quality and fatigue. Based on these findings a similar trial is warranted in CFS patients.

In summary, despite extensive international research, both the etiology and the pathogenesis of CFS are far from clear. A number of recent studies demonstrated that oxidative stress is a component of the illness, although further research is needed to elucidate whether the oxidative damage is the cause or an effect. Since it is apparent from the research presented that some degree of oxidative stress is present in CFS patients, various antioxidants show promise as part of a CFS protocol. The antioxidants glutathione, *N*-acetylcysteine, α-lipoic acid, OPCs, *Ginkgo biloba* and *Vaccinium myrtillus* very possibly hold promise, although controlled clinical studies are necessary to demonstrate their efficacy among CFS patients. Other supplements should be considered for potential therapeutic intervention, including selenium, necessary to support glutathione peroxidase activity[31].

Glutathione, N-acetylcysteine, α-lipoic acid and coenzyme Q_{10}

Although there is conflicting evidence, a number of studies have shown that oral administration of glutathione can directly increase plasma and tissue glutathione concentration[32–34]. Alternatively, *N*-acetylcysteine and α-lipoic acid can increase the glutathione concentration indirectly[35,36]. *N*-acetylcysteine provides cysteine for glutathione synthesis, and α-lipoic acid is believed to increase intracellular glutathione levels by reducing extracellular cystine to cysteine, bypassing the cystine transporter[37]. Glutathione is neuroprotective and may play a role in preventing additional central nervous system (CNS) lesions[38]. α-Lipoic acid is also neuroprotective, scavenging nitric oxide and peroxynitrite, and may be especially promising as an antioxidant against mitochondrial dysfunction[37]. The supplement coenzyme Q_{10} has similar neuroprotective qualities, and has the ability to improve mitochondrial function[39].

Essential fatty acids

Two randomized controlled trials of essential fatty acids reported some beneficial effects of the intervention[40,41] and one also found an overall beneficial effect[40].

Magnesium

Magnesium supplements were found to have an overall beneficial effect in a controlled trial[42]. In studies that evaluated general supplements, one study found a positive effect[43] and a controlled trial reported no effect[44]. One study reported that two participants left the intervention group after experiencing a generalized rash[42]; the other studies did not report adverse effects.

Homeopathic remedies

Alternative therapies were evaluated in several controlled trials[45–47]. In one study, participants given homeopathic remedies reported some beneficial effects of the intervention, but the results were not analyzed statistically[46].

Massage therapy

An overall beneficial effect of massage therapy was found in one small randomized controlled trial[45]. More research is required to confirm the efficacy of massage therapy.

Osteopathy

A controlled trial of osteopathy[47] found overall beneficial effects. There were no reports of adverse effects from the interventions in any of these studies.

In summary, the interventions described above demonstrated overall mixed results in terms of effectiveness. All conclusions about effectiveness should be considered together with the methodology used for the studies.

References

1. Fukuda K, Straus SE, Hickie I, Sharpe MC, Dobbins JG, Komaroff A. The chronic fatigue syndrome: a comprehensive approach to its definition and study. International Chronic Fatigue Syndrome Case Definition Study Group. *Ann Intern Med* 1994;121:953–9
2. Komaroff AL, Buchwald D. Symptoms and signs in chronic fatigue syndrome. *Rev Infect Dis* 1991;13:S8–11
3. Buchwald D, Komaroff AL. Laboratory findings in chronic fatigue syndrome. *Rev Infect Dis* 1991;13:S12–18
4. Komaroff AL, Buchwald D. Chronic fatigue syndrome: an update. *Annu Rev Med* 1998;49:1–13
5. Ware NC. Suffering and the social construction of illness: the delegitimation of illness experience in chronic fatigue syndrome. *Med Anthropol Q* 1992;6:347–61
6. Bombardier CH, Buchwald D. Chronic fatigue, chronic fatigue syndrome, and fibromyalgia: disability and health-care use. *Med Care* 1996;34:924–30
7. Buchwald D, Garrity D. Comparison of patients with chronic fatigue syndrome, fibromyalgia, and multiple chemical sensitivities. *Arch Intern Med* 1994;154:2049–53
8. Ax S, Gregg VH, Jones D. Chronic fatigue syndrome: sufferers' evaluation of medical support. *J R Soc Med* 1997;90:250–4
9. Vercoulen JH, Swanink CM, Fennis JF, Galama JM, van der Meer JW, Bleijenberg G. Prognosis in chronic fatigue syndrome: a prospective study on the natural course. *J Neurol Neurosurg Psych* 1996;60:489–94

10. Wearden AJ, Morriss RK, Mullis R, *et al.* Randomised, double-blind, placebo-controlled treatment trial of fluoxetine and graded exercise for chronic fatigue syndrome. *Br J Psychiatry* 1998;172:485–92

11. Fulcher KY, White PD. Randomised controlled trial of graded exercise in patients with the chronic fatigue syndrome. *Br Med J* 1997;314:1647–52

12. Sharpe M, Hawton K, Simkin S, *et al.* Cognitive behaviour therapy for the chronic fatigue syndrome: a randomised controlled trial. *Br Med J* 1996;312:22–6

13. Deale A, Chalder T, Marks I, Wessely S. Cognitive behavior therapy for chronic fatigue syndrome: a randomized controlled trial. *Am J Psychiatry* 1997;154:408–14

14. Prins J, Bleijenberg G, Bazelmans E, *et al.* Cognitive behavior therapy for chronic fatigue syndrome: a multicentre randomised controlled trial. *Lancet* 2001;357:841–7

15. Deale A, Hussain K, Chalder T, Wessely S. Long-term outcome of cognitive behaviour therapy versus relaxation for chronic fatigue syndrome: a 5-year follow-up study. *Am J Psychiatry* 2001;158:2038–42

16. Lloyd AR, Hickie I, Brockman A, *et al.* Immunologic and psychologic therapy for patients with chronic fatigue syndrome: a double-blind, placebo-controlled trial. *Am J Med* 1993;94:197–203

17. Friedberg F, Krupp LB. A comparison of cognitive behavioral treatment for chronic fatigue syndrome and primary depression. *Clin Infect Dis* 1994;18(Suppl 1):S105–10

18. Risdale L, Godfrey E, Chalder T, *et al.* Chronic fatigue in general practice: is counselling as good as cognitive behaviour therapy? A UK randomised trial. *Br J Gen Pract* 2001;51:19–24

19. Bagchi D, Bagchi M, Stohs SJ, *et al.* Free radicals and grape seed proanthocyanidin extract: importance in human health and disease prevention. *Toxicology* 2000;148:187–97

20. Diamond BJ, Shiflett SC, Feiwel N, *et al.* Ginkgo biloba extract: mechanisms and clinical indications. *Arch Phys Med Rehabil* 2000;81:668–78

21. Bastianetto S, Ramassamy C, Dore S, *et al.* The Ginkgo biloba extract (EGb 761) protects hippocampal neurons against cell death induced by beta-amyloid. *Eur J Neurosci* 2000;12:1882–90

22. Krieglstein J, Beck T, Seibert A. Influence of an extract of Ginkgo biloba on cerebral blood flow and metabolism. *Life Sci* 1986;39:2327–34

23. Rai GS, Shovlin C, Wesnes KA. A double-blind, placebo controlled study of Ginkgo biloba extract ('tanakan') in elderly outpatients with mild to moderate memory impairment. *Curr Med Res Opin* 1991;12:350–5

24. Cao G, Booth SL, Sadowski JA, Prior RL. Increases in human plasma antioxidant capacity after consumption of controlled diets high in fruit and vegetables. *Am J Clin Nutr* 1998;68:1081–7

25. Cao G, Sofic E, Prior RL. Antioxidant capacity of tea and common vegetables. *J Agric Food Chem* 1996;44:3426–31

26. Wang H, Cao G, Prior RL. Total antioxidant capacity of fruits. *J Agric Food Chem* 1996;44:701–5

27. Prior RL, Cao G, Martin A, *et al.* Antioxidant capacity as influenced by total phenolic and anthocyanin content, maturity, and variety of *Vaccinium* species. *J Agric Food Chem* 1998;46:2686–93

28. Joseph JA, Shukitt-Hale B, Denisora NA, *et al.* Reversals of age-related declines in neuronal signal transduction, cognitive, and motor behavioral deficits with blueberry, spinach, or strawberry dietary supplementation. *J Neurosci* 1999;19:8114–21

29. Youdim KA, Shukitt-Hale B, MacKinnon S, *et al.* Polyphenolics enhance red blood cell resistance to oxidative stress: *in vitro* and *in vivo*. *Biochim Biophys Acta* 2000;1523:117–22

30. Edwards AM, Blackburn L, Christie S, *et al.* Food supplements in the treatment of fibromyalgia: a double-blind, crossover trial of anthocyanidins and placebo. *J Nutr Environ Med* 2000;10:189–99

31. Arthur JR. The glutathione peroxidases. *Cell Mol Life Sci* 2000;57:1825–35

32. Aw TY, Wierzbicka G, Jones DP. Oral glutathione increases tissue glutathione *in vivo*. *Chem Biol Interact* 1991;80:89–97

33. Jones DP, Hagen TM, Weber R. Oral administration of glutathione (GSH) increases plasma GSH concentration in humans. *FASEB J* 1989;3:A1250 (abstr)

34. Favilli F, Marraccini P, Iantomasi T, Vincenzini MT. Effect of orally administered glutathione on glutathione levels in some organs of rats: role of specific transporters. *Br J Nutr* 1997;78:293–300

35. Kelly GS. Clinical applications of N-acetylcysteine. *Altern Med Rev* 1998;3:114–27

36. Han D, Tritschler HJ, Packer L. Alpha-lipoic acid increases intracellular glutathione in a human T-lymphocyte Jurkat cell line. *Biochem Biophys Res Commun* 1995;207:258–64

37. Packer L, Tritschler HJ, Wessel K. Neuroprotection by the metabolic antioxidant alpha-lipoic acid. *Free Radic Biol Med* 1997;22:359–78

38. Bridges RJ, Koh JY, Hatalski CG, Cotman CW. Increased excito-toxic vulnerability of cortical cultures with reduced levels of glutathione. *Eur J Pharmacol* 1991;192:199–200

39. Matthews RT, Yang L, Browne S, *et al.* Coenzyme Q10 administration increases brain mitochondrial concentrations and exerts neuro-protective effects. *Proc Natl Acad Sci USA* 1998;95:8892–7

40. Behan PO, Behan WM, Horrobin D. Effect of high doses of essential fatty acids on the postviral fatigue syndrome. *Acta Neurol Scand* 1990;82:209–16

41. Warren G, McKendrick M, Peet M. The role of essential fatty acids in chronic fatigue syndrome: a case-controlled study of red-cell membrane essential fatty acids (EFA) and a placebo-controlled treatment study with high dose of EFA. *Acta Neurol Scand* 1999;99:112–16

42. Cox IM, Campbell MJ, Dowson D. Red blood cell magnesium and chronic fatigue syndrome. *Lancet* 1991;337:757–60

43. Stewart W, Rowse C. Supplements help ME says Kiwi study. *J Altern Complement Med* 1987;5:19–22

44. Martin RWY, Ogston SA, Evans JR. Effects of vitamin and mineral supplementation on symptoms associated with chronic fatigue syndrome with Coxsackie B antibodies. *J Nutr Med* 1994;4:11–23

45. Field TM, Sunshine W, Hernandez-Reif M, *et al.* Massage therapy effects on depression and somatic symptoms in chronic fatigue syndrome. *J Chronic Fatigue Syndrome* 1997;3:43–51

46. Awdry R. Homeopathy may help ME. *Int J Altern Complement Med* 1996;14:12–16

47. Perrin RN, Edwards J, Hartley P. An evaluation of the effectiveness of osteopathic treatment on symptoms associated with myalgic encephalomyelitis: a preliminary report. *J Med Eng Technol* 1998;22:1–13

COMMON COLD

The common cold (acute viral respiratory tract infection) is one of the most frequent acute illnesses, with major economic impact. *Echinaceae purpureae* and vitamin C supplement are widely used by people for treatment of the common cold.

Echinaceae purpureae

Considered to have immunostimulating activity, extracts of the plant *Echinacea* (family Compositae) are widely used in some European countries and the USA as a phytomedicinal treatment of the common cold and upper respiratory tract infections (URTIs)[1].

Literature review of 12 clinical studies published from 1961 to 1997 concluded that echinacea was efficacious for treating the common cold, but the results are unclear, owing to inherent flaws in the study design. Five trials have been published since 1997; two showed that echinacea lacked efficacy for treating and preventing URTI symptoms, and three concluded that it was effective in reducing the frequency, duration and severity of common cold symptoms. Again, these results are unclear because of methodologic uncertainties, such as small populations and use of dosage forms that were not commercially available and not standardized. Although evidence for echinacea's efficacy is inconclusive, it appears to be safe. Patients without contraindications to it may not be dissuaded from using an appropriate preparation to treat the common cold[2].

The majority of the available studies which evaluate the effects of preparations containing extracts of echinacea in the prevention and treatment of the common cold reported positive results. However, one article indicated that there was not enough evidence to recommend a specific echinacea product, or echinacea preparations for the treatment or prevention of common colds[1]. Recently, in a randomized, double-blind, placebo-controlled clinical trial, *Echinaceae purpureae* herba (Echinacin, EC31J0), compared to placebo, has shown promising results in the relief of common cold symptoms and the time taken to improvement[3].

Other herbs

A clinical trial of a commercially available fixed combination herbal remedy (radix echinaceae, radix baptisiae, herba thujae) reported that the herbal remedy was effective and safe. The therapeutic benefit consists of a rapid onset of improvement of cold symptoms. If patients with colds are able to start the application of the herbal remedy as soon as practical after the occurrence of the initial symptoms, the benefit is expected to increase[4].

Megavitamin C

Effects of megavitamin C on the common cold are controversial. In a double-blind, randomized clinical trial, doses of vitamin C in excess of 1 g daily taken shortly after onset of a cold did not reduce the duration or severity of cold symptoms in healthy adult volunteers when compared with a vitamin C dose less than the minimum recommended daily intake[5].

References

1. Melchart D, Linde K, Fischer P, Kaesmayr J. Echinacea for preventing and treating the common cold. *Cochrane Database Syst Rev* 2000;2:CD000530
2. Giles JT, Palat CT 3rd, Chien SH, Chang ZG, Kennedy DT. Evaluation of echinacea for treatment of the common cold. *Pharmacotherapy* 2000;20:690–7
3. Schulten B, Bulitta M, Ballering-Bruhl B, Koster U, Schafer M. Efficacy of *Echinacea purpurea* in patients with a common cold. A placebo-controlled, randomised, double-blind clinical trial. *Arzneimittelforschung* 2001;51:563–8
4. Henneicke-von Zepelin H, Hentschel C, Schnitker J, Kohnen R, Kohler G, Wustenberg P. Efficacy and safety of a fixed combination

phytomedicine in the treatment of the common cold (acute viral respiratory tract infection): results of a randomized, double blind, placebo controlled, multicenter study. *Curr Med Res Opin* 1999;15:214–27

5. Audera C, Patulny RV, Sander BH, Douglas RM. Mega-dose vitamin C in treatment of the common cold: a randomised controlled trial. *Med J Aust* 2001;175:359–62

ASTHMA

Asthma is a condition of the lungs in which there is generalized reversible narrowing of airways due to mucosal edema, spasm of smooth muscle and mucus in bronchi and bronchioles, leading to dyspnea, cough, chest tightness and wheezing. In the UK, patients with asthma have reported CAM usage in up to 70% of adults[1] and 55% of children[2–4]. Breathing techniques, relaxation, herbal medicine, homeopathy, yoga and hypnotherapy are commonly used CAM therapies.

Breathing techniques

Breathing techniques have been systematically reviewed[1]. Although yoga and physiotherapy exercises are promising, there is insufficient evidence to conclude that these are effective.

The Buteyko Breathing Technique (BBT) is based on the concept that people with asthma are under stress, and therefore breathe too rapidly and too deeply. The training involves learning to make breathing shallow and slow. In a randomized controlled trial with asthmatic patients, those trained in BBT showed greater reduction in asthma medication use and improvement in quality of life than controls who received asthma education alone[5]. However, there were no significant differences in objective changes in measures of airway caliber between the groups. Further rigorous trials are needed.

Relaxation

Emotional stress can either precipitate or exacerbate both acute and chronic asthma. There is a large body of literature available on the use of relaxation techniques for the treatment of asthma symptoms[6–8]. In a systematic review[9] of randomized controlled trials, 15 trials were identified, of which nine compared the treatment group with the control group appropriately. Five trials tested progressive muscle relaxation or mental and muscular relaxation, two showing significant effects of therapy. There is a lack of evidence for the efficacy of relaxation therapies in the management of asthma. This deficiency is due to the poor methodology of the studies as well as the inherent problems of conducting such trials. There is some evidence that muscular relaxation improves lung function of patients with asthma, but no evidence exists for any other relaxation technique. More well-designed trials are required.

Herbal medicines

A survey by the National Asthma Campaign found that 60% of people with moderate asthma and 70% with severe asthma have used complementary and alternative medicines to treat their condition. Herbal medicine is the third most popular choice of both adults (11%) and children (6%) suffering from asthma[2,3].

Many randomized clinical trials on the use of herbal medicinal products in the treatment of asthma have been found in the literature. However, a number of the studies had significant methodological flaws, and the majority were not conducted with products of standardized quality.

Trials with ginkgo liquor[10], IKPA tablets[11], WTM[12], and dried ivy extract[13] reported clinically relevant improvements in lung function, significantly better than placebo or control treatment. Trials with *Tylophora indica*[14–16] and the TJ-96 study[17] resulted in a significant improvement in asthma symptoms. One trial with *Tylophora indica*[18] and marijuana[19] did not produce any clinically relevant or statistically significant improvement in lung function or asthma symptoms compared with the control. Two trials, one with *Tylophora indica*[20] and the other with *Boswellia serrata*[18], reported a clinically significant improvement in FEV_1, but the data were presented in such a way that the percentage change could not be calculated. *Ligusticum wallichii* mixture[21], SBR and RKISP decoctions[22,23], *Picrorrhiza kurroa*[24], *Solanum xanthocarpum* and *Solanum trilobatum*[25] were also used in other studies.

A systematic review[26] found some promising evidence in single studies with *Picrorrizia kurroa*, *Solanum* spp., *Boswellia serrata*, Saibuko-to, marijuana and dried ivy extract, but insufficient data exist to make firm judgements.

Homeopathy

Homeopathic immunotherapy was superior to placebo in improving symptom in patients with allergic asthma, although the study was short in duration and had a small sample size; only a small effect on lung function was demonstrated[27]. In a systematic review, the reviewers concluded that there was not enough evidence for a reliable assessment of the possible role of homeopathy in asthma. There is a need for observational data to document the different methods of prescribing homeopathic remedies and how patients respond[28].

Yoga

In a controlled trial, patients who continued to practice yoga regularly during a follow-up period of 4.5 years showed a significant reduction in asthma medication use and number of asthma attacks, and an increase in peak flow rate, compared with the matched controls[29]. However, two randomized controlled trials failed to find any effect on lung function, although mental improvements were noted[30,31].

Hypnotherapy

Certain patients with bronchial asthma can benefit, often greatly, from hypnotherapy. In a retrospective analysis of 121 asthmatic patients who were treated by hypnotherapy, 21% had an excellent response to treatment, becoming completely free from asthma and requiring no drug therapy. Another 33% had a good response, with a decrease in the frequency and severity of the attacks of asthma, or a decrease in drug requirements. Approximately half of the 46%, who had a poor response, had a marked subjective improvement in general well-being. Statistical evaluation of the six variables (age, sex, result, trance depth, psychological factors and severity of the asthma) confirmed that hypnotherapy may be effective, especially if there are significant etiological psychological factors present and the asthma is not severe[32]. More well-designed controlled studies are required to test the efficacy of hypnotherapy.

References

1. Ernst E. Breathing techniques – adjunctive treatment modalities for asthma? A systematic review. *Eur Respir J* 2000;15:969–72
2. Ernst E. Complementary therapies for asthma: what patients use. *J Asthma* 1998;35:667–71
3. Ernst E. Use of complementary therapies in childhood asthma. *Pediatr Asthma Allergy Immunol* 1998;21:29–32
4. Andrews L, Lokuge S, Sawyer M, Lillywhite L, Kennedy D, Martin J. The use of alternative therapies by children with asthma: a brief report. *J Paediatr Child Health* 1998;34:131–4
5. Bowler SD, Green A, Mitchell CA. Buteyko breathing techniques in asthma: a blinded randomised controlled trial. *Med J Aust* 1998;169:575–8
6. Alexander AB, Miklich DR, Hershkoff H. The immediate effects of systematic relaxation training on peak expiratory flow rates in asthmatic children. *Psychosom Med* 1972;34:388–94
7. Erskine J, Schonell M. Relaxation therapy in bronchial asthma. *J Psychosom Res* 1979;23:131–9
8. Hock RA, Bramble J, Kennard DW. A comparison between relaxation and assertive training with asthmatic male children. *Biol Psych* 1977;12:593–6

9. Huntley A, White AR, Ernst E. Relaxation therapies for asthma: a systematic review. *Thorax* 2002;57:127–31

10. Li M, Zhang H, Yang B. Effects of ginkgo leaf concentrated oral liquor in treating asthma. *Chung Kuo Ching Hsi I Chieh Ho Tsa Chih* 1997;17:216–18

11. Xu D, Shen Z, Wang W, *et al*. Study on effect of reinforcing kidney and invigorating spleen principle on severe asthma. *Chung Kuo Ching Hsi I Chieh Ho Tsa Chih* 1997;17:584–6

12. Zou JP, Gu FQ, Liao WJ. Clinical study on treating asthma of cold type with Wenyang Tonglulo mixture. *Chung Kuo Ching Hsi I Chieh Ho Tsa Chih* 1996;16:529–32

13. Mansfeld HJ, Hohre H, Repges R, *et al*. Therapy of bronchial asthma with dried ivy leaf. *Münch Med Wochenschr* 1998;140:26–30

14. Shivpuri DN, Menon MPS, Parkash D. Preliminary studies in *Tylophora indica* in the treatment of asthma and allergic rhinitis. *J Assoc Physicians* 1968;16:9–15

15. Shivpuri DN, Singal SC, Parkash D. Treatment of asthma with an alcoholic extract of *Tylophora indica*: a cross-over, double blind study. *Ann Allergy* 1972;30:407–12

16. Thiruvengadam KV, Haranath K, Sudarsan S, *et al*. *Tylophora indica* in bronchial asthma. *J Indian Med Assoc* 1978;71:172–7

17. Egashira Y, Nagano H. A muticenter clinical trial of TJ-96 in patients with steroid-dependent bronchial asthma. *Ann NY Acad Sci* 1993;685:580–3

18. Gupta S, George P, Gupta V, *et al*. *Tylophora indica* in bronchial asthma: a double-blind study. *Indian J Med Res* 1979;69:981–9

19. Tashkin DP, Shapiro BJ, Frank IM. Acute effects of marihuana on airway dynamics in spontaneous and experimentally induced bronchial asthma. In Braude MC, Szara S, eds. *The Pharmacology of Marihuana*. New York, NY: Raven Press, 1976:785–801

20. Mathew KK, Shivpuri DN. Treatment of asthma with alkaloids of *Tylophora indica*: a double-blind study. *Aspects Allergy Appl Immunol* 1974;7:166–79

21. Shao C, Chen F, Tang Y, *et al*. Clinical and experimental study on *Ligusticum wallichii* mixture in preventing and treating bronchial asthma. *Chung Kuo Ching Hsi I Chieh Ho Tsa Chih* 1994;14:465–8

22. Xu DS, Shen ZY, Wang WJ, *et al*. Study on effect of strengthing body resistance method on asthmatic attack. *Chung Kuo Ching Hsi I Chieh Ho Tsa Chih* 1996;16:198–200

23. Xu D, Xu RH. Prevention and treatment of seasonal asthmatic patients by combined invigorating kidney for preventing asthma tablets and beclomethasone dipropionate. *Chung Kuo Ching Hsi I Chieh Ho Tsa Chih* 1997;17:721–3

24. Doshi VB, Shetye M, Mahashur AA, *et al*. *Picrorrhiza kurroa* in bronchial asthma. *J Postgrad Med* 1983;29:89–95

25. Govindan S, Viswanathan S, Vijayasekaran V, *et al*. A pilot study on the clinical efficacy of *Solanum xanthocarpum* and *Solanum trilobatum* in bronchial asthma. *J Ethnopharmacol* 1999;66:205–10

26. Huntley A, Ernst E. Herbal medicines for asthma: a systematic review. *Thorax* 2000;55:925–9

27. Reilly D, Taylor M, Beattie NGM *et al*. Is evidence for homoeopathy reproducible? *Lancet* 1994;344:1601–6

28. Linde K, Jobst KA. Homeopathy for chronic asthma. *Cochrane Database Syst Rev* 2000;2:CD000353

29. Nagarathna R, Nagendra HR. Yoga for bronchial asthma: a controlled study. *Br Med J* 1985;291:1077–9

30. Fluge T, Richter J, Fabel H, Zysno E, Weller E, Wagner TO. Long-term effects of breathing exercises and yoga in patients with bronchial asthma. *Pneumologie* 1994;48:484–90

31. Vedanthan PK, Kesavalu LN, Murthy KC, *et al*. Clinical study of yoga techniques in university students with asthma: a controlled study. *Allergy Asthma Proc* 1998;19:3–9

32. Collison DR. Which asthmatic patients should be treated by hypnotherapy? *Med J Aust* 1975;1:776–81

IRRITABLE BOWEL SYNDROME

Irritable bowel syndrome (IBS) is a functional disorder of the lower gastrointestinal tract that affects between 11 and 22% of American adults between the ages of 30 and 64[1,2]. It is usually characterized by abdominal pain and altered bowel habits, such as diarrhea and constipation. Because there are no known physiological, biochemical or structural abnormalities that characterize the disorder, IBS is ordinarily a diagnosis of exclusion[3]. Current treatment options include high-fiber diets, bulking agents, muscle relaxants, psychotherapy and even antidepressants, but none of these is fully satisfactory[4,5]. Among CAM therapies, herbal medicine, relaxation therapy and hypnotherapy may be effective.

Herbal medicines

Peppermint and caraway oil

Peppermint oil is obtained by steam distillation of arial parts of flowering *Mentha × piperita* L. The active principle of peppermint oil is menthol, a cyclic monoterpene with a Ca^{2+}-channel blocking activity and a pharmacological profile similar to that of dihydropyridine calcium antagonists[6,7].

A meta-analysis assessed the available evidence for peppermint oil[8]. Of eight randomized controlled trials of peppermint oil monopreparations, seven trials included patients who were not diagnosed according to accepted criteria. A double-blind randomized controlled trial, which became available after the meta-analysis, reported beneficial effects for abdominal pain, distension and stool frequency, but also failed to diagnose patients according to the accepted Rome or Manning criteria[9].

A double-blind randomized controlled trial compared two different preparations of a fixed combination of peppermint and caraway oil[10]. A total of 223 patients with non-ulcer dyspepsia in combination with IBS received either enteric-coated capsules containing 90 mg peppermint oil and 50 mg caraway oil or an enteric-soluble formulation containing 36 mg peppermint oil and 20 mg caraway oil. Compared with baseline, the results indicated a reduction in pain intensity with equivalent effectiveness of the preparations. In another controlled trial, 42 children with IBS were given pH-dependent, enteric-coated peppermint oil capsules or placebo. After 2 weeks, 75% of those receiving peppermint oil had reduced severity of pain associated with IBS. Therefore, peppermint oil may be useful as a therapeutic agent during the symptomatic phase of IBS[11].

Appital

A combination preparation (Appital) containing various herbal extracts, e.g. caraway oil, was tested in a double-blind randomized controlled trial, which included 59 patients who were diagnosed according to the Manning criteria[12]. At the end of an 8-week treatment period, there were no differences in symptom scores in the treatment group compared with placebo.

Asafetida

A double-blind placebo-controlled trial assessed the effects of asafetida and asafetida in a combination preparation also containing nux vomica[13]. The results indicated some beneficial effect in the global improvement of symptoms in the active groups, but this did not reach significance when compared with placebo.

Iberogast

Another controlled trial tested a combination of extracts from bitter candytuft, matricaria flower, peppermint leaves, caraway fruit, licorice root and melissa balm (Iberogast) in 103 patients[14]. After 4 weeks of treatment the authors report a significant improvement in the global IBS symptom score compared with placebo.

Chinese herbal medicines

A controlled trial compared individualized standard Chinese herbal formulations and placebo in 103 patients, who were diagnosed according to accepted criteria[15]. After 16 weeks, global improvements in symptoms were reported in both treatment groups compared with placebo. Individualized treatment was no better than with the standard Chinese herbal formulation.

Ayurvedic herbs

In a double-blind randomized placebo-controlled trial, 169 patients were treated for 6 weeks with either standard therapy consisting of clidinium bromide, chlordiazepoxide and isphagula or an Ayurvedic preparation containing *Aegle marmelos correa* and *Bacopa monniere*[16]. Results showed that neither form of therapy was better than placebo.

Relaxation

There have been few studies that have tested relaxation training alone as a treatment for IBS. One study demonstrated that a progressive muscle relaxation program in itself was a clinically significant treatment, especially for the relief of abdominal pain and, to a lesser extent, constipation[17]. In that study, patients attended ten sessions over an 8-week period, and were taught progressive muscle relaxation. Those patients who received the relaxation training had a higher composite primary symptom reduction score than those undergoing symptom monitoring only.

Benson's Relaxation Response Meditation appears to be moderately effective for treating patients with IBS. Patients underwent 6 weeks of treatment, where they received training in the technique and assistance in solving problems that they may have had in implementing regular practice of the technique.

Hypnotherapy

Hypnotherapy may be an effective treatment for IBS. It may be less useful in males with diarrhea-predominant bowel habit, a finding that may have pathophysiological implications[18]. More research is required to assess its efficacy.

References

1. Dancey CP, Whitehouse A, Painter J, Backhouse S. The relationship between hassles, uplifts and irritable bowel syndrome: a preliminary study. *J Psychosom Res* 1995;39:827–32

2. Dancey CP, Taghavi M, Fox RJ. The relationship between daily stress and symptoms of irritable bowel syndrome: a time-series approach. *J Psychosom Res* 1998;44:537–45

3. Thompson WG, Creed F, Drossman DA, Heaton KW, Mazzacca G. Functional bowel disease and functional abdominal pain. *Gastroenterology* 1992;5:75–91

4. Shaw G, Srivastava ED, Sadlier M, *et al.* Stress management for irritable bowel syndrome: a controlled trial. *Digestion* 1991;50:36–42

5. Krag E. Irritable bowel syndrome: current concepts and future trends. *Scand J Gastroenterol* 1985;20(Suppl 109):107–15

6. Taylor BA, Duthie HL, Luscombe DK. Calcium antagonist activity of menthol on gastrointestinal smooth muscle. *Br J Clin Pharm* 1985;20:293–4

7. Hills JM, Aaronson PI. The mechanism of action of peppermint oil on gastrointestinal smooth muscle. *Gastroenterology* 1991;101:55–65

8. Pittler MH, Ernst E. Peppermint oil for irritable bowel syndrome: a critical review and metaanalysis. *Am J Gastroenterol* 1998;93:1131–5

9. Liu J-H, Chen G-H, Yeh H-Z, Huang C-K, Poon S-K. Enteric-coated peppermint-oil capsules in the treatment of irritable bowel syndrome: a prospective, randomized trial. *J Gastroenterol* 1997;32:765–8

10. Freise J, Köhler S. Pfefferminzöl/Kümmelöl-Fixkombination bei nicht-säurebedingter Dyspepsie – Vergleich der Wirksamkeit und Verträglichkeit zweier galenischer Zubereitungen. *Pharmazie* 1999;54:210–15

11. Kline RM, Kline JJ, Di Palma J, Barbero GJ. Enteric-coated, pH-dependent peppermint oil capsules for the treatment of irritable bowel syndrome in children. *J Pediatr* 2001;138:125–8

12. Pedersen BS, Helø OH, Jørgensen FB, Kromann-Andersen H. Behandling af colon irritabile med kosttilskuddet Appital. *Ugeskr Læger* 1998;160:7259–62

13. Rahlfs VW, Mössinger P. Zur Behandlung des Colon irritabile. *Arzneim-Forsch Drug Res* 1976;26:2230–4

14. Madisch A, Plein K, Mayr G, Buchert D, Hotz J. Benefit of a herbal preparation in patients with irritable bowel syndrome: results of a double-blind, randomized placebo-controlled, multicenter trial. *Dig Dis Week* 2002; in press

15. Bensousson A, Talley NJ, Hing M, Menzies R, Guo A, Ngu M. Treatment of irritable bowel syndrome with Chinese herbal medicine. A randomized controlled trial. *J Am Med Assoc* 1998;280:1585–9

16. Yadav SK, Jain AK, Tripathi SN, Gupta JP. Irritable bowel syndrome: therapeutic evaluation of indigenous drugs. *Indian J Med Res* 1989;90:496–503

17. Blanchard EB, Greene B, Scharff L, Schwarz-McMorris SP. Relaxation training as a treatment for irritable bowel syndrome. *Biofeedback Self Regul* 1993;18:125–32

18. Gonsalkorale WM, Houghton LA, Whorwell PJ. Hypnotherapy in irritable bowel syndrome: a large-scale audit of a clinical service with examination of factors influencing responsiveness. *Am J Gastroenterol* 2002;97:954–61

A pediatric perspective on alternative medicines

32

N. A. Lass

INTRODUCTION

Use of alternative medicines (in this chapter, denoting herbal and/or natural compounds) is widespread in the pediatric population. Few scientific data exist about many of these agents, and even less information is available for use in children.

Within the past 20 years, significant advances have been made in the area of developmental pharmacology. Application of this research has resulted in many changes to pediatric therapeutics and safer use. Drug dosing in children continues to be modified, as knowledge accumulates regarding drug distribution, metabolism and elimination. The importance of these scientific advances is reflected in recent US legislation (www.fda.gov/cder/pediatric), including the 1994 Pediatric Labeling Rule, Section 111 (pediatric) of the 1997 Food and Drug Administration (FDA) Modernization Act (FDAMA), the 1998 Pediatric Rule and the 2002 FDAMA Reauthorization (Best Pharmaceuticals for Children Act; Public Law 107-109), which mandate pediatric clinical trials as part of new pharmaceutical drug development. Similar changes have not occurred for alternative medicines, mainly because the clinical pharmacology of these agents is not well understood, making it difficult to apply principles of developmental pharmacology to their use, and because they are not regulated under the Food, Drug, and Cosmetic Act.

Little information is available regarding the trends in alternative medicine use in children. Many studies are relatively old and do not reflect the recent increase in use or the use in a small sample of a subpopulation. Sawyer and colleagues reported that 46% of Australian children with cancer (aged 4–16 years) used

alternative medicines, mainly to reduce the side-effects from their disease or chemotherapy[1]. Mottonen and Uhari reported that 40% of nine Finnish children with leukemia used alternative medicines[2]. It is widely recognized that many patients disclose alternative medicine use only when asked specifically, making it difficult to estimate the frequency of their use.

Specific pediatric issues regarding alternative medicine use, including an overview of developmental pharmacology and the prevention of adverse reactions, are illustrated through the application of a pediatric oncology case study.

CASE STUDY

Your 6-year-old patient, Scott, has recently relapsed leukemia and has restarted chemotherapy. His mother is very concerned about the relapse and asks numerous questions.

When Scott is admitted for his second cycle, you notice his gentle demeanor has been replaced by irritability and restlessness. He complains of a headache and his mother says he is not sleeping well. The nurse tells you he bled 'a long time' after having his blood drawn for tests. He is also vomiting before receiving any medications.

You visit Scott later that evening, after his chemotherapy has begun. He is actively vomiting and very irritable. His mother is encouraging him to drink a cup of tea from a thermos she brought. As you chat with them, the mother explains that she is determined that Scott will not 'get sick' from his chemotherapy or have another relapse. She is surprised the ginger root she gave him did not prevent his vomiting. She mentions that the cup is filled with green tea, which she has been giving Scott for its cancer-prevention properties. She had given him 2 quarts (1.8 l) of green tea today before he was admitted. Upon further questioning, you learn that Scott's mother is also giving him *Ginkgo biloba*, echinacea, lemon balm and valerian to help him through his relapse.

PEDIATRIC PHARMACOLOGY: IMPACT OF DEVELOPMENTAL CHANGES ON THERAPEUTICS

Until recently, pediatric drug dosing and administration was based on adult data. During the early 1980s, researchers began to focus on pediatric aspects of clinical pharmacology. Gentamicin and theophylline, both commonly used drugs in the pediatric population and easily accessible through widely available assays, were among the first to be studied in detail and today are among the best understood. Previously, dosing for gentamicin and theophylline was based on adult recommendations, and varied little by age. Today, developmental changes in fluid compartments, metabolism and renal function form the basis for different dosing recommendations for different ages.

Pharmacodynamics

Drugs are often developed and used for a medical condition based on their specific mechanism of action. As noted above, until recently the FDA did not require pediatric clinical trials for new drug approval. Dosing information carried precautionary statements such as 'the safety and efficacy in pediatric patients below the age of 18 years have not been evaluated' and 'long-term effects in children have not been well established'. Pediatricians treated their patients with the best knowledge of the day, often using drugs for indications not present in adults or for what appeared to be paradoxical reasons. Methylphenidate, theophylline and indomethacin, for example, are used for therapeutic effects and conditions unique to the pediatric age group. Methylphenidate (marketed as Ritalin®, Concerta®, Metadate® and Methylin®), a

central nervous system stimulant, is used in pediatrics for attention deficit hyperactivity disorder (ADHD), although its mechanism of action in children is not completely understood. This appears to be a paradoxical effect, allowing children to become less hyperactive and have more focused attention. Methylphenidate may or may not have the same effect in adults. Theophylline, once a first-line agent in the treatment of pediatric reactive airway disease for its bronchodilating effects, is also used in newborns as a central nervous system stimulant to treat apnea of prematurity. Indomethacin, a non-steroidal anti-inflammatory drug (NSAID) used in adults for the treatment of arthritis symptoms, is also used in an intravenous formulation for the treatment of patent ductus arteriosus in the newborn.

Dose–response relationships may be different in children. Theophylline, when used for bronchodilatation in adolescents and adults, generally requires a serum concentration of 10–20 μg/ml to be effective. Toxicity is often seen when concentrations exceed 20–30 μg/ml. When used in newborns for apnea of prematurity, effects are seen with much lower serum concentrations (< 10 μg/ml). Recommendations for effective serum concentrations have varied from 5–12 μg/ml[3] to as low as 2–3 μg/ml[4–6]. Toxicity, including tachycardia, arrhythmias and symptomatic gastroesophageal reflux, can be seen in children at lower concentrations, suggesting that the therapeutic index is different in this population.

Pharmacokinetics

Pharmacokinetic changes are seen throughout childhood. Absorption can be affected by changes in gastric pH in the first months of life[7]. Concentrations of β-glucuronidase in the first months of life may increase seven-fold over adult levels, leading to reabsorption of substances that may be excreted as glucuronide conjugates[8]. As a result of these and other changes, many drugs may not be well absorbed in the first year of life; an example is diphenylhydantoin (Dilantin®)[9].

Changes in distribution may be due to a variety of factors. Protein binding may differ between children and adults. Protein binding of theophylline in the adult is 52–60%[10], but it is only 30–40% in the first months of life[11]. Developmental changes in protein binding occur in many drugs, reaching adult levels at different ages. Drugs whose effect is directly related to percentage of free drug in the serum may need to have dose adjustments for pediatric patients. Many drugs compete with endogenous substances for protein binding sites. For example, numerous drugs displace bilirubin from albumin. This may have negative effects in the immediate newborn period when bilirubin may be elevated, resulting in seriously elevated serum levels of unconjugated bilirubin and increasing the risk for kernicterus. The presence of maternal hormones, such as estrogen, or the concentration of free fatty acids may also alter distribution. The volume of distribution for digoxin is greater in full-term newborns (approximately 12–16 l/kg) than adults (5 l/kg), and has been shown to be related to greater myocardial binding[12]. The volume of distribution remains at intermediate levels from 9 months through adolescence[13].

The developmental changes in ratios among total body water, intracellular and extracellular fluid also affect distribution. At 12 weeks' gestation, total body water comprises 92% of the fetus' total body weight. At 32 weeks' gestation, total body water is about 80% of the total body weight. By birth at 40 weeks' gestation (full term), approximately 70–75% of the newborn's body weight is total body water. During the first year, total body water gradually stabilizes, and it remains fairly constant during childhood. During adolescence, a further decrease is seen, ultimately resulting in adult levels. Changes occur in the intra- and extracellular fluid compartments as well. Prior to birth, extracellular fluid volume is greater than intracellular fluid volume. Extracellular fluid volume gradually decreases throughout gestation, while intracellular fluid volume increases. Immediately following birth, extracellular fluid volume continues to decrease while intracellular fluid volume increases, reversing the pattern by approximately 3 months of life. Intracellular fluid rises during early childhood, then remains constant until adolescence, when both compartments' volume decreases. These changes, together with others, such as renal function (see below), play an important role in the comprehensive

dosing recommendations (e.g. for gentamicin) in the newborn for different gestational ages (e.g. 26 weeks versus 40 weeks) as well as for different postnatal ages (e.g. <7 days versus >7 days).

Similar changes are seen in the total body lipid content. At 29 weeks' gestation, total body lipid content is 1% of the fetus' total body weight. By birth at 40 weeks, this has increased to 10–15%[14]. Further changes are seen in the first years of life, stabilizing in childhood and then assuming adult levels in adolescence. Drugs such as phenobarbital, which have a significant distribution to the lipid compartment, may be affected by these changes.

Developmental changes also occur in metabolism or biotransformation. As in adults, the main site for drug metabolism is the liver, but the lung and gastrointestinal tract also play a role. The placenta plays a major role in drug metabolism for the fetus. It is well known that maturation of liver enzymes occurs postnatally and variations are seen between species. Dehydrogenation, demethylation, oxidation, reduction and hydrolysis pathways are known to undergo developmental maturation at different rates. Development of hepatic cytoplasmic proteins also occurs postnatally. Phase II reactions such as glucuronidation, sulfation, acetylation and glutathione conjugation also undergo developmental maturation. Developmental expression of genetic polymorphisms for cytochrome P450 (CYP) enzymes such as CYP 2D6 may also play a role.

The developmental pathway of theophylline metabolism has been well studied. In the first year of life, theophylline is metabolized by methylation to form caffeine. This pathway is most active during the first year of life, and is not utilized in the adult. During middle childhood, the predominant pathway is through C8 oxidation, forming 1,3-dimethyl uric acid. During this period, the clearance of theophylline may increase to twice the rate seen in adults. Widely published age-specific dosing guidelines reflect these changes in clearance. During adolescence, the adult pathway takes precedence, demethylating theophylline to methylxanthine and 3-methylxanthine.

Finally, elimination also undergoes developmental changes. In the fetus, the glomerular filtration rate (GFR) gradually rises as gestation progresses.

Immediately following birth at full term, the GFR rapidly rises in the first few days. For those infants born prematurely prior to 34 weeks' gestation, however, this rapid increase does not occur, but rather, the GFR gradually increases, reaching levels of the term infant by approximately 40 weeks' postconceptional age[15–18]. For infants born at term, the GFR does not reach adult levels until approximately 4–6 months of life. For renally excreted drugs such as gentamicin, rapid changes in GFR as well as changes in fluid compartments contribute to the need for changing dosing recommendations based on both gestational as well as postnatal age. Nephron elongation may continue for the first 10 years of life, impacting filtration, reabsorption and secretion of drugs.

Additional factors to consider

Pediatric patients often require different formulations of medications from adults. Small children may be unable to swallow tablets or capsules whole. Liquid formulations, such as elixirs or syrups, can be used if the drug is soluble and bioavailable in the new medium. Pleasant-tasting medications are important for compliance. Dosing is usually by weight (mg/kg) to accommodate for growth. If no pediatric clinical trials have been conducted to determine appropriate dosing, formulas based on proportionality rules may be used to suggest a dose[19]. Commonly used formulas are as follows.

Young's Rule (based on age):

$$\text{Child's dose} = \text{adult dose} \times \frac{\text{age (years)}}{\text{age} + 12}$$

Clarke's Rule (based on weight):

$$\text{Child's dose} = \text{adult dose} \times \frac{\text{weight (kg)}}{70}$$

$$\text{Child's dose} = \text{adult dose} \times \frac{\text{weight (lb)}}{150}$$

A drug's effect on growth and development is an important consideration in pediatrics. Physical growth and development can be adversely affected by medications. Chronic steroid use, for example, can result in growth retardation and short stature[20–22]. Chemotherapy may affect fertility[23–25]. Effects on memory and learning must also be considered. Children who are on chronic medications may not do as well in the classroom if a drug makes them lethargic or hyperactive, or affects memory. This is especially important for children in early childhood and primary grades, when brain development is considered most formative.

Parents play an important role in a child's treatment. It is important to include parents as members of the health-care team and to understand their views. Parents may have a different understanding of their child's medical condition and treatment, leading them to become less compliant with the treatment prescribed. Parents may choose alternative forms of treatment in hopes of providing better care for their child without understanding the impact on the medical condition, concurrent medications and overall treatment plan. A parent's good intentions may not always have the desired effect, making communication and education critical adjuncts to treatment.

SPECIFIC CONSIDERATIONS FOR PEDIATRICS

Should alternative medicines be used?

The clinical pharmacology principles briefly outlined above demonstrate that development does impact therapeutics. Most information regarding drugs and developmental pharmacology is based on studies and case reports using drugs approved by the FDA for pharmaceutical use. While these drugs have demonstrated efficacy and safety in clinical trials for adults when approved, the potential always exists for adverse effects and drug interactions, particularly for pediatric patients. Likewise, alternative medicines such as herbal or natural compounds have active chemical ingredients (not unlike their FDA-approved counterparts), which also exert effects on the body and can produce adverse events and drug–herb interactions. Greater caution must be used with herbal or natural compounds, because they are not subjected to the rigorous scientific trials that pharmaceutical agents are and, therefore, less reliable data exist, particularly for pediatric use[26,27].

Should alternative medicines be used, then, in children? If a potential benefit for the child exists, alternative medicines can be considered as well as standard pharmaceutical agents. Each alternative medicine, like pharmaceutical agents, should be considered individually. What are the benefits of using this alternative medicine? What is known about its effects? Will it provide therapeutic benefit for this medical condition? Are any scientific data available? Risks should also be considered. What adverse events are known to occur with this alternative medicine? Does it have any known interactions with drugs or with other alternative medicines? Will its benefits or risks interfere negatively with the medical condition or current treatment plan?

Once benefits and risks are assessed from the available reliable data, a responsible decision can be made. The treating physician should discuss alternative medicines with the patient and patient's family whenever possible, to provide maximum benefit for treatment. Proactive discussions about alternative medicines can prevent self-prescribing and reduce unnecessary risks for the patient. Alternative medicines can be considered and used safely in children, when thoughtful and responsible decisions are based on consideration of available data and development pharmacology.

Available scientific data

Locating available pediatric scientific data for pharmaceutical agents and alternative medicines can be difficult. FDA-approved pharmaceutical agents require rigorous scientific testing and adult clinical trials prior to approval, but, until very recently, the FDA did not require submission of pediatric data. The FDA now mandates testing in children for new drug approvals and provides procedures for pediatric testing in off-patent drugs. Scientific testing of alternative medicines in adults or children is not required under the Dietary Supplement Health and Education Act (DSHEA), making it more difficult to assess these agents. Information on pediatric effectiveness

and adverse events is dependent on case reports and academic clinical trials from the scientific literature. Additional information may be obtained from spontaneous reports submitted to the FDA on marketed products (MedWatch program). Spontaneous reports are often anecdotal and may provide little detail. Unfortunately, few scientific data have been published regarding the safety and efficacy of alternative medicine use in pediatrics.

A common way to apply scientific data to the pediatric population is by extrapolating results from adult clinical trials and animal studies. For FDA-approved drugs, preclinical (animal) and toxicology data are required for new drug applications. While these data are generally from adult animals, often different ages may be studied. For specific species (e.g. dog, sheep) and organ systems (e.g. cardiovascular, renal), extrapolation of newborn and young animal data may be possible to pediatrics. Data regarding CYP enzyme metabolism are more difficult to extrapolate, as considerable species variation exists (not all species use the same CYP enzymes to metabolize a given compound) and developmental pathways within species are not completely understood. Human clinical trial data will also be available in normal volunteers as well as individuals with the indicated disease state.

Historically, data extrapolation has been widely used, but this has limitations. Gentamicin use in a premature newborn using adult data extrapolations could lead to supratherapeutic serum concentrations, given our recent understanding of fluid compartments, volume of distribution changes and renal maturation. Likewise, theophylline use in middle childhood using adult data could lead to subtherapeutic serum concentrations, given the accelerated clearance now known to exist for that age group. Indomethacin given in a suspension by nasogastric tube to a ventilated premature newborn with a patent ductus arteriosus may be erratically absorbed and not attain therapeutic serum concentrations. While important information can be derived from adult data, this is not always an accurate predictor for safe and effective pediatric use.

Alternative medicines provide few adult scientific data from which to extrapolate. As mentioned earlier, the DSHEA does not require scientific testing for adults or children. More recently, many academic centers have begun to study these agents in controlled clinical trials. These studies are primarily in adults, and, while they provide important information, they do not give specific data for pediatric patients. Manufacturers' labels must be interpreted cautiously. The DSHEA provides few regulations regarding product labels, unlike the FDA regulations for pharmaceutical agents. A 'claim' made on the product label should not be assumed to be based on scientific clinical trials.

Prevention of adverse events

Using available scientific data on pediatric clinical pharmacology parameters, limited pediatric data on FDA-approved drugs and scarce data on alternative medicine use in pediatrics, how can alternative medicines be prescribed safely for pediatric patients? As with adults, safety should focus on the prevention of adverse events and drug–drug or drug–herb interactions.

It is often assumed that the average physician knows and prescribes about 50 drugs well. Among these should be the most common alternative medicines (and their active substances) used by patients in their practice. The physician should also have a general understanding of developmental pharmacology principles if caring for pediatric patients. Most importantly, the physician should stay current with the literature and, if in doubt, take time to look up information.

It is also important for the physician to know their patients and families. What does the patient and their parent(s) understand about the medical condition? What do they understand about the treatment regimen and how it works for that disease? What is the patient's and their parents' view about alternative medicine use? What agents have they used? Do they understand what the active substance is, and how it works? What is the risk of adverse events and drug interactions? Where do they obtain their information?

Finally, it is crucial that the physician be able to discuss both pharmaceutical agents as well as alternative medicines openly with their patients. Patients may be reluctant to volunteer information about their use, particularly if they feel that the physician may not be

open-minded or well-informed. Given the scarcity of pediatric data for alternative medicines, one way to prevent adverse events is to know all medications a patient is taking, both pharmaceutical (prescription and over-the-counter) and alternative, and be able to keep the lines of communication open between physician and patient.

As noted above, improper pediatric dosing regimens can result in adverse events, such as supratherapeutic serum gentamicin concentrations and resultant renal dysfunction. How should a child's dose be selected if none is given? Generally, for FDA-approved drugs, a dose is provided or the product information states that the drug is not approved for use in children. Pediatricians have long used these medications by adjusting the dose according to the adult data or using proportionality rules as discussed above. Similar dosing adjustments may be difficult with alternative medicines. How much of the active ingredient is in the formulation? Can a mg/kg dose be calculated for an adult? Can this be extrapolated for children? Caution should be used when applying proportionality rules to calculate pediatric dosages. As already discussed, volume of distribution, metabolism, clearance and elimination may change throughout childhood. Dosages that may be well tolerated in adults may not be easily tolerated in children. The therapeutic index in children may also be narrower than in adults. Without knowing the clinical pharmacology of an alternative medicine, these dose calculations are 'guesstimates' at best and may lead to adverse events or toxicity. The physician should be ever vigilant for adverse events and signs of toxicity, lowering doses or discontinuing medications as needed. It is always prudent and safer to begin with the lowest possible dose and gradually increase as needed when little or no dosage guidelines are available.

If an alternative preparation (e.g. elixir, syrup) is desired to facilitate administration, careful attention should be directed to the vehicle used. Does the medication crush into a powder? Does it dissolve? Is the medication combined with a chemical moiety that may negatively interact (e.g. chelate) with other substances in the gut and decrease bioavailability or cause gastric irritation? These principles also apply to alternative medicines that may be prepared as 'home remedies'. The child's parent or guardian may administer a home remedy without adequate knowledge about the ingredients. Preparation of a given remedy may vary – quantities of active ingredients may differ, different combinations of ingredients may be used and the preparation itself may alter (e.g. longer boiling time making the active substance in the remedy more concentrated). It is important to understand the parent or guardian's knowledge of these remedies, what effect they are believed to have on the child's care as well as how the home remedy was prepared. Again, caution should be exercised to prevent adverse events and toxicity.

Preventing adverse events and drug–herb interactions

The potential for drug–herb and herb–herb interactions exists for alternative medicines as it does for FDA-approved drugs. Alternative medicines may be natural, but they contain chemically active substances and can interact with each other as well as FDA-approved drugs. It is equally important that, with less scientific data available, many adverse events or interactions may not be known, may not be recognized as adverse events or may not yet have been reported in the literature. This makes preventing adverse events and drug–herb and herb–herb interactions much more difficult.

It is always prudent to be cautious and vigilant when prescribing or recommending medications, including alternative agents. The physician should understand the pharmacodynamics and pharmacokinetics of medicines commonly prescribed as well as basic principles of developmental pharmacology if caring for young patients. This includes the mechanism(s) of action and metabolic (CYP family) enzyme pathways, if known. For example, St John's wort is now known to induce the CYP 3A4 pathway, both in the liver and intestine and the intestinal P-glycoprotein transporter[28–34]. By inducing the CYP 3A4 pathway, it accelerates or induces the metabolism of any medication, herbal or otherwise, utilizing this pathway and may render it less efficacious. Transplant patients taking cyclosporin for immunosuppression

may have subtherapeutic drug levels and risk organ rejection[35]. Simvastatin serum concentrations may also be reduced when combined with St John's wort[36]. This interaction is very important, since CYP 3A4 is the most common pathway used for drug metabolism. Many drugs are substrates for CYP 3A4 (such as clarithromycin, diltiazem, ethinyl estradiol, felodipine, nifedipine, progesterone, tamoxifen, warfarin and verapamil) and may be subject to serum concentration changes if concurrent medications or herbals induce (St John's wort) or inhibit this pathway.

Open communication between the physician, patient and parents is critical for understanding the views of patient and parents, providing good care and preventing adverse events. Most older pediatric patients and their parents are interested in participating in their health-care treatment plans and decisions. By establishing conversation that is both frank and non-judgemental, the physician encourages discussion. Patients and their parents are more likely to mention that they are considering alternative medicines as well as those they may already be using. Discussion provides the physician the opportunity to teach responsibility. Patient and parent education is critical for their understanding, not only of the benefits of alternative medicine use, but also of the risks, including negative effects on their medical condition (e.g. accelerating tumor growth), scarcity of safety data and the dangers of self-prescribing and drug–herb interactions.

ALTERNATIVE MEDICINES USED IN PEDIATRICS

Common conditions for which alternative medicines are used

Use of alternative medicines in pediatrics is thought to be widespread[37], although few data are available. Common conditions for which pediatric patients may take alternative medicines include, but are not limited to, general health, preventive medicine (e.g. influenza, colds), general symptoms (e.g. vomiting, diarrhea, constipation), asthma, insomnia and sleep disturbances, ADHD and childhood cancer. Gardiner and Kemper provide a brief overview of common herbs used in pediatrics[38].

Managing alternative medicines in pediatric practice

Pediatric patients use many of the same alternative medicines as adults. How is the management of pediatric patients different? Developmental pharmacology and pediatric medicine both play important roles. Lack of scientific data and dosing recommendations as well as the risk for adverse events and drug–herb interactions can complicate care. These principles are now applied to the patient care setting using the initial case study.

> Your 6-year-old patient, Scott, has recently relapsed leukemia and has restarted chemotherapy. His mother is very concerned about the relapse and asks numerous questions.

Scott's mother cares for her son and is understandably upset by the recurrence of his illness and the anticipated chemotherapy side-effects. She may also be afraid that his leukemia will not go into remission or that he will die. She wants to be an active participant and do everything possible for Scott. Her viewpoint is critical in understanding her motivation for using specific alternative medicines.

> When Scott is admitted for his second cycle, you notice his gentle demeanor has been replaced by irritability and restlessness. He complains of a headache and his mother says he is not sleeping well. The nurse tells you he bled 'a long time' after having is blood drawn for tests. He is also vomiting before receiving any medications.

Scott's irritability and restlessness may be the result of anxiety. He undoubtedly remembers his last course of chemotherapy. You are concerned about his change in demeanor and interval history of headaches and sleeping disturbances. The nurse has listed only

prescription medications on the admission sheet. You notice Scott is vomiting prior to receiving any medications and decide to return later in the day to take a more detailed history and talk further with his mother.

> You visit Scott later that evening, after his chemotherapy has begun. He is actively vomiting and very irritable. His mother is encouraging him to drink a cup of tea from a thermos she brought. As you chat with them, the mother explains that she is determined that Scott will not 'get sick' from his chemotherapy or have another relapse. She is surprised the ginger root she gave him did not prevent his vomiting. She mentions that the cup is filled with green tea, which she has been giving Scott for its cancer-prevention properties. She had given him 2 quarts (1.8 l) of green tea today before he was admitted. Upon further questioning, you learn that Scott's mother is also giving him *Ginkgo biloba*, echinacea, lemon balm and valerian to help him through his relapse.

It is clear that Scott's mother has made a careful assessment of her son's condition and the effects of chemotherapy. She has designed a medication regimen hoping to prevent adverse events from chemotherapy as well as a future relapse. She has Scott's best interests at heart and assumes that the medicines she has chosen are both safe and effective. A closer look reveals their interaction with Scott's disease and treatment.

Scott's mother chose ginger root *(Zingiber officinale)* to prevent the anticipated chemotherapy-induced nausea. Ginger root is used to relieve nausea and vomiting and for the prevention of nausea due to pregnancy and motion sickness. It has also been used as a preoperative medication. There is clinical evidence to support its use as an anti-emetic[39–41]. Ginger root, however, is also known to potentiate effects of anticoagulants such as warfarin[42,43]. In this case, ginger root was not effective as an anti-emetic, owing to toxicity from another herbal remedy.

Chemoprevention is very important to Scott's mother, motivating her to add green tea to Scott's diet. Green tea has been used for chemoprevention, atherosclerosis prevention and the treatment of vomiting and diarrhea. Clinical research suggests that green tea may be effective in preventing caries[44], providing photoprotection[45,46] and prevention of oral and colon cancer[47–49]. Scott's mother understood green tea to be a general chemopreventive agent and was aware of preliminary reports suggesting benefit in the treatment of leukemia[50–52].

Tea is a common beverage rarely associated with severe adverse effects. Scott's mother assumed that green tea, as an herbal tea, was 'safe'. Green tea's adverse effects are mainly related to caffeine content. Restlessness, tremor and hyper-reflexia may be seen with ingestion of more than 300 mg of caffeine. Irritability, insomnia, palpitations, vertigo, vomiting, diarrhea, anorexia and headache can all be seen with chronic ingestion of more than 1 g of caffeine per day. It is not clear how long prior to admission Scott's mother had been giving him green tea. She states that he drank 2 quarts on the day of admission. While amounts vary, Scott may have ingested approximately 480 mg of caffeine on the day of admission (assuming one cup contains 60 mg of caffeine). Since Scott's mother was using this as a chemopreventive agent, one might suspect chronic use. Scott's change in demeanor, irritability, restlessness, headache, sleep disturbance and vomiting are probably related to excessive green tea consumption. Caffeine is metabolized to theophylline, which has an accelerated clearance in children Scott's age as discussed above. As a result, Scott may be able to tolerate higher doses of caffeine before reaching toxic levels. It is important to discuss green tea's effects with Scott's mother. She has inadvertently caused Scott to become ill during chemotherapy (making the ginger root appear ineffective), while intending to prevent a relapse.

Scott also received *Ginkgo biloba*. This agent is used primarily for the improvement of circulation to the brain and periphery, but has also been used in the treatment of Alzheimer's disease, arthritis, bronchial congestion and ADHD in pediatrics. Clinical research supports improvement in cerebral blood flow and memory[53–55] as well as benefit in ADHD[56]. *Ginkgo biloba* is known to potentiate anticoagulants such as aspirin, NSAIDs, warfarin and heparin by inhibiting platelet-activating factors[57]. Daily ginger root and

Ginkgo biloba may have contributed to Scott's prolonged bleeding time. Furthermore, his chemotherapy will lead to bone marrow depression and low platelet counts. Impaired platelet activation with a low platelet count will further increase his risk for bleeding. Scott's mother was less sure why this herb would be beneficial to Scott's care, citing friends who had suggested it. It is important to discuss with her the risk for adverse events and drug interactions whether or not an alternative medicine is beneficial. If there is no benefit, it should not be given. Again, Scott's mother was concerned about her son's welfare and was not aware that alternative medicines might interact with his chemotherapy.

Echinacea (*Echinacea angustifolia, Echinacea pallida, Echinacea purpurea*) is an herb commonly used as an immune stimulant for general health and to prevent infections such as influenza and upper respiratory infections. It has also been used to treat colon cancer and arthritis. Clinical research supports its use as an immune stimulant[58–60]. Scott's mother's intention was to prevent the febrile neutropenia syndrome often seen following chemotherapy. There are no data to suggest that the incidence of febrile neutropenia is decreased with echinacea use. Recent data suggest, however, that *Echinacea purpurea* may have therapeutic value in the treatment of leukemia by increasing the number of natural killer cells[61].

Scott's mother understood the value of sleep and added lemon balm (*Melissa officinalis*) and valerian (*Valeriana officinalis*) to her son's regimen. Both of these herbs are used for insomnia as well as ADHD in children. Clinical research has shown that valerian improves sleep quality[62], and may enhance lemon balm's effects when used together.

Advising patients and parents

This case illustrates a caring mother's attempt to do everything possible to help her son cope with the treatment of a chronic disease. It also demonstrates how good intentions can have negative effects. Scott's adverse events from the green tea, ginger root and *Ginkgo biloba* may have been averted if his mother had better understood these medicines in the context of the leukemia chemotherapy, and if the physician had been aware that she was administering them.

Physicians must take the lead with their patients and parents to discuss alternative medicine use. When asked 'What medications are you taking?' patients often assume that this means prescription drugs and occasionally over-the-counter drugs. Rarely do they include alternative medicines. It is important that the physician specifically ask about alternative medications in a non-judgemental way. Furthermore, when taking a history, it is important to understand the patient and parent's reasons for using herbal medications. In this case, Scott's mother had chosen alternative medicines very specifically for what she thought were benefits. It is also important to ask why a specific agent is used as well as the patient and parent's understanding of how it works, and the adverse effects and drug interactions it may have. Patient education regarding the medical condition, standard therapy and how alternative medications might have benefit or risk is critical for optimum care and compliance. It may be helpful to develop materials for the office staff to distribute to patients and parents discussing common issues and alternative medicines.

The patient's complaints should be listened to carefully. Adverse event profiles are sketchy to incomplete for many alternative medicines. An effort should be made to differentiate signs and symptoms that might be related to alternative medicines as opposed to a medical condition or standard therapy. If new adverse events are seen, it is prudent to report these directly to the FDA (1-800-FDA-1088 or online at www.fda.gov/medwatch) and the manufacturer, as well as in case reports in the scientific literature. The more reports are published, the easier it will be to prescribe and recommend alternative medicines safely.

CONCLUSIONS

With increasing use of alternative medicines in pediatrics, it is important for the patient, parents and physician to be responsible about treatment. Physicians should consider a 'holistic' approach to their patients. Time should be taken to learn which alternative medicines patients are using and why. Patients should be encouraged to discuss their concerns. Education enables them to be more responsible and to be more likely to understand the dangers of self-prescribing.

Physicians should also know the clinical pharmacology of the drugs they most commonly prescribe, including alternative medicines. By understanding pathways of metabolism, for example, many drug interactions can be avoided. Those physicians caring for children also need to be aware of how a child's development impacts the pharmacodynamics and pharmacokinetics of a drug. Staying current with the literature and understanding general principles of clinical pharmacology are critical.

Given the paucity of scientific data available for alternative medicines, particularly for pediatrics, it is important to be vigilant for possible adverse events and report them. Communication with other physicians and health-care providers through the FDA and scientific literature is important. The area of alternative medicine use in pediatrics is fertile for basic and clinical research.

Physicians approach patient care with the concept 'first do no harm'. To provide the best treatment for pediatric patients, this must extend to the use of alternative medicines. Responsible use allows their benefits to be utilized and their adverse effects to be avoided.

References

1. Sawyer MG, Gannoni AF, Toogood IR, Antoniou G, Rice M. The use of alternative therapies by children with cancer. *Med J Aust* 1994;160:320–2

2. Mottonen M, Uhari M. Use of micronutrients and alternative drugs by children with acute lymphoblastic leukemia. *Med Pediatr Oncol* 1997;28:205–8

3. Jones RA, Baillie E. Dosage schedule for intravenous aminophylline in apnoea of prematurity, based on pharmacokinetic studies. *Arch Dis Child* 1979;54:190–3

4. Dietrich J, Krauss AN, Reidenberg M, Drayer DE, Auld PA. Alterations in state in apneic pre-term infants receiving theophylline. *Clin Pharmacol Ther* 1978;24:474–8

5. Milsap RL, Krauss AN, Auld PA. Oxygen consumption in apneic premature infants after low-dose theophylline. *Clin Pharmacol Ther* 1980;28:536–40

6. Myers TF, Milsap RL, Krauss AN, Auld PA, Reidenberg MM. Low-dose theophylline therapy in idiopathic apnea of prematurity. *J Pediatr* 1980;96:99–103

7. Agunod M, Yamaguchi N, Lopez R, Luhby AL, Glass GB. Correlative study of hydrochloric acid, pepsin, and intrinsic factor secretion in newborns and infants. *Am J Dig Dis* 1969;14:400–14

8. Roberts RJ. *Drug Therapy in Infants: Pharmacologic Principles and Clinical Experience.* Philadelphia, PA: WB Saunders, 1984

9. Painter MJ, Pippenger C, MacDonald H, Pitlick W. Phenobarbital and diphenylhydantoin levels in neonates with seizures. *J Pediatr* 1978;92:315–19

10. Taburet AM, Schmit B. Pharmacokinetic optimisation of asthma treatment. *Clin Pharmacokinet* 1994;26:396–418

11. Aranda JV, Sitar DS, Parsons WD, Loughnan PM, Neims AH. Pharmacokinetic aspects of theophylline in premature newborns. *N Engl J Med* 1976;295:413–16

12. Park MK, Ludden T, Arom KV, Rogers J, Oswalt JD. Myocardial vs. serum digoxin concentrations in infants and adults. *Am J Dis Child* 1982;136:418–20

13. Wagner JG, Dick M 2nd, Behrendt DM, Lockwood GF, Sakmar E, Hees P. Determination of myocardial and serum digoxin concentrations in children by specific and nonspecific assay methods. *Clin Pharmacol Ther* 1983;33:577–84

14. Poissonnet CM, Burdi AR, Garn SM. The chronology of adipose tissue appearance and distribution in the human fetus. *Early Hum Dev* 1984;10:1–11

15. Arant BS Jr. Developmental patterns of renal functional maturation compared in the human neonate. *J Pediatr* 1978;92:705–12

16. Coulthard MG. Maturation of glomerular filtration in preterm and mature babies. *Early Hum Dev* 1985;11:281–92

17. Aperia A, Broberger O, Elinder G, Herin P, Zetterstrom R. Postnatal development of renal function in pre-term and full-term infants. *Acta Paediatr Scand* 1981;70:183–7

18. Strauss J, Daniel SS, James LS. Postnatal adjustment in renal function. *Pediatrics* 1981;68:802–8

19. Koren G. Special aspects of perinatal and pediatric pharmacology. In Katzung BG, ed. *Basic and Clinical Pharmacology*, 7th edn. Stamford, CT: Appleton and Lange, 1998:988

20. Simon D, Touati G, Prieur AM, Ruiz JC, Czernichow P. Growth hormone treatment of short stature and metabolic dysfunction in juvenile chronic arthritis. *Acta Paediatr Suppl* 1999;88:100–5

21. Allen DB, Julius JR, Breen TJ, Attie KM. Treatment of glucocorticoid-induced growth suppression with growth hormone. National Cooperative Growth Study. *J Clin Endocrinol Metab* 1998; 83:2824–9

22. Hokken-Koelega AC, van Zaal MA, van Bergen W, *et al.* Final height and its predictive factors after renal transplantation in childhood. *Pediatr Res* 1994;36:323–8

23. Thomson AB, Wallace WH. Treatment of paediatric Hodgkin's disease. A balance of risks. *Eur J Cancer* 2002;38:468–77

24. Gleeson HK, Shalet SM. Endocrine complications of neoplastic diseases in children and adolescents. *Curr Opin Pediatr* 2001;13:346–51

25. Leung W, Hudson MM, Strickland DK, *et al.* Late effects of treatment in survivors of childhood acute myeloid leukemia. *J Clin Oncol* 2000;18:3273–9

26. Angell M, Kassirer JP. Alternative medicine – the risks of untested and unregulated remedies. *N Engl J Med* 1998;339:839–41

27. Ernst E. Harmless herbs? A review of the recent literature. *Am J Med* 1998;104:170–8

28. Obach RS. Inhibition of human cytochrome P450 enzymes by constituents of St. John's Wort, an herbal preparation used in the treatment of depression. *J Pharmacol Exp Ther* 2000; 294:88–95

29. Wentworth JM, Agostini M, Love J, Schwabe JW, Chatterjee VK. St. John's wort, a herbal antidepressant, activates the steroid X receptor. *J Endocrinol* 2000;166:R11–16

30. Moore LB, Goodwin B, Jones SA, *et al.* St John's wort induces hepatic drug metabolism through activation of the pregnane X receptor. *Proc Natl Acad Sci USA* 2000;97:7500–2

31. Wang Z, Gorski JC, Hamman MA, Huang SM, Lesko LJ, Hall SD. The effects of St. John's wort (*Hypericum perforatum*) on human cytochrome P450 activity. *Clin Pharmacol Ther* 2001;70:317–26

32. Roby CA, Anderson GD, Kantor E, Dryer DA, Burstein AH. St. John's wort: effect on CYP3A4 activity. *Clin Pharmacol Ther* 2000;67:451–7

33. Durr D, Stieger B, Kullak-Ublick GA, *et al.* St. John's Wort induces intestinal P-glycoprotein/MDR1 and intestinal and hepatic CYP3A4. *Clin Pharmacol Ther* 2000;68:598–604

34. Johne A, Brockmoller J, Bauer S, Maurer A, Langheinrich M, Roots I. Pharmacokinetic interaction of digoxin with an herbal extract from St. John's wort (*Hypericum perforatum*). *Clin Pharmacol Ther* 1999;66:338–45

35. Ernst E. St. John's wort supplements endanger the success of organ transplantation. *Arch Surg* 2002;137:316–19

36. Sugimoto K, Ohmori M, Tsuruoka S, *et al.* Different effects of St. John's wort on the pharmacokinetics of simvastatin and pravastatin. *Clin Pharmacol Ther* 2001;70:518–24

37. Ottolini MC, Hamburger EK, Loprieato JO, *et al.* Complementary and alternative medicine use among children in the Washington, DC area. *Ambul Pediatr* 2001;1:122–5

38. Gardiner P, Kemper KJ. Herbs in pediatric and adolescent medicine. *Pediatr Rev* 2000;21:44–57

39. Bone ME, Wilkinson DJ, Young JR, McNeil J, Charlton S. Ginger root – a new antiemetic. The effect of ginger root on postoperative nausea and vomiting after major gynaecological surgery. *Anaesthesia* 1990;45:669–71

40. Holtmann S, Clarke AH, Scherer H, Hohn M. The anti-motion sickness mechanism of ginger. A comparative study with placebo and dimenhydrinate. *Acta Otolaryngol* 1989;108:168–74

41. Phillips S, Ruggier R, Hutchinson SE. *Zingiber officinale* (ginger) – an antiemetic for day case surgery. *Anaesthesia* 1993;48:715–17

42. Heck AM, DeWitt BA, Lukes AL. Potential interactions between alternative therapies and warfarin. *Am J Health Syst Pharm* 2000;57:1221–7

43. Miller LG. Herbal medicinals: selected clinical considerations focusing on known or potential drug–herb interactions. *Arch Intern Med* 1998;158:2200–11

44. Hamilton-Miller JM. Anti-cariogenic properties of tea (*Camellia sinensis*). *J Med Microbiol* 2001;50:299–302

45. Elmets CA, Singh D, Tubesing K, Matsui M, Katiyar S, Mukhtar H. Cutaneous photoprotection from ultraviolet injury by green tea polyphenols. *J Am Acad Dermatol* 2001; 44:425–32

46. Katiyar SK, Elmets CA. Green tea polyphenolic antioxidants and skin photoprotection. *Int J Oncol* 2001;18:1307–13

47. Hsu SD, Singh BB, Lewis JB, *et al.* Chemoprevention of oral cancer by green tea. *Gen Dent* 2002;50:140–6

48. Masuda M, Suzui M, Weinstein IB. Effects of epigallocatechin-3-gallate on growth, epidermal growth factor receptor signaling path-

ways, gene expression, and chemosensitivity in human head and neck squamous cell carcinoma cell lines. *Clin Cancer Res* 2001;7:4220–9

49. Suganuma M, Ohkura Y, Okabe S, Fujiki H. Combination cancer chemoprevention with green tea extract and sulindac shown in intestinal tumor formation in Min mice. *J Cancer Res Clin Oncol* 2001;127:69–72

50. Li HC, Yashiki S, Sonoda J *et al*. Green tea polyphenols induce apoptosis *in vitro* in peripheral blood T lymphocytes of adult T-cell leukemia patients. *Jpn J Cancer Res* 2000;91:34–40

51. Otsuka T, Ogo T, Eto T, Asano Y, Suganuma M, Niho Y. Growth inhibition of leukemic cells by (−)-epigallocatechin gallate, the main constituent of green tea. *Life Sci* 1998;63:1397–403

52. Asano Y, Okamura S, Ogo T, Eto T, Otsuka T, Niho Y. Effect of (−)-epigallocatechin gallate on leukemic blast cells from patients with acute myeloblastic leukemia. *Life Sci* 1997; 60:135–42

53. Kleijnen J, Knipschild P. *Ginkgo biloba* for cerebral insufficiency. *Br J Clin Pharmacol* 1992;34:352–8

54. Curtis-Prior P, Vere D, Fray P. Therapeutic value of *Ginkgo biloba* in reducing symptoms of decline in mental function. *J Pharm Pharmacol* 1999;51:535–41

55. Wesnes KA, Ward T, McGinty A, Petrini O. The memory enhancing effects of a *Ginkgo biloba/Panax ginseng* combination in healthy middle-aged volunteers. *Psychopharmacology (Berl)* 2000; 152:353–61

56. Lyon MR, Cline JC, Totosy de Zepetnek J, Shan JJ, Pang P, Benishin C. Effect of the herbal extract combination *Panax quinquefolium* and *Ginkgo biloba* on attention–deficit hyperactivity disorder: a pilot study. *J Psychiatry Neurosci* 2001;26:221–8

57. Lamant V, Mauco G, Braquet P, Chap H, Douste-Blazy L. Inhibition of the metabolism of platelet activating factor (PAF-acether) by three specific antagonists from *Ginkgo biloba*. *Biochem Pharmacol* 1987;36:2749–52

58. Percival SS. Use of echinacea in medicine. *Biochem Pharmacol* 2000;60:155–8

59. Rehman J, Dillow JM, Carter SM, Chou J, Le B, Maisel AS. Increased production of antigen-specific immunoglobulins G and M following *in vivo* treatment with the medicinal plants *Echinacea angustifolia* and *Hydrastis canadensis*. *Immunol Lett* 1999;68:391–5

60. See DM, Broumand N, Sahl L, Tilles JG. *In vitro* effects of echinacea and ginseng on natural killer and antibody-dependent cell cytotoxicity in healthy subjects and chronic fatigue syndrome or acquired immunodeficiency syndrome patients. *Immunopharmacology* 1997;35:229–35

61. Currier NL, Miller SC. *Echinacea purpurea* and melatonin augment natural-killer cells in leukemic mice and prolong life span. *J Altern Complement Med* 2001;7:241–51

62. Leathwood PD, Chauffard F, Heck E, Munoz-Box R. Aqueous extract of valerian root (*Valeriana officinalis* L.) improves sleep quality in man. *Pharmacol Biochem Behav* 1982;17:65–71

Further reading

Avery GB, Fletcher MA, MacDonald MG, eds. *Neonatology: Pathophysiology and Management of the Newborn*, 4th edn. Philadelphia, PA: JB Lippincott, 1994

Behrman RE, Kliegman RM, Arvin AM, eds. *Nelson Textbook of Pediatrics*, 15th edn. Philadelphia, PA: WB Saunders, 1996

Carruthers SG, Hoffman BB, Melmon KL, Nierenberg DW, eds. *Melmon and Morrelli's Clinical Pharmacology*, 4th edn. New York, NY: McGraw-Hill, 2000

Ernst E, ed. *The Desktop Guide to Complementary and Alternative Medicine: An Evidence-Based Approach*. St Louis, MO: Mosby, 2001

Pizzorno JE Jr, Murray MT, eds. *Textbook of Natural Medicine*, 2nd edn. New York, NY: Churchill Livingstone, 1999

Radde IC, MacLeod SM, eds. *Pediatric Pharmacology and Therapeutics*, 2nd edn. St Louis, MO: Mosby, 1993

Skidmore-Roth L. *Mosby's Handbook of Herbs and Natural Supplements*. St Louis, MO: Mosby, 2001

Yaffe SJ, Aranda JV, eds. *Pediatric Pharmacology: Therapeutic Principles in Practice*, 2nd edn. Philadelphia, PA: WB Saunders, 1992

What you and your patients should know before surgery

33

M. K. Ang-Lee, J. Moss and C.-S. Yuan

INTRODUCTION

There is enormous public enthusiasm for herbal medications. Two recent surveys have found widespread use among the presurgical population[1,2]. Morbidity and mortality associated with herbal medications may be more likely in the perioperative period because of the polypharmacy and physiological alterations that occur[3]. Such complications include myocardial infarction, stroke, bleeding, inadequate oral anticoagulation, prolonged or inadequate anesthesia, organ transplant rejection and interference with medications indispensable for patient care.

Of the herbal medications that clinicians are likely to encounter, we have identified the eight herbs that potentially pose the greatest impact on the care of patients undergoing surgery. These account for over 50% of all single herb preparations among the 1500–1800 herbal medications sold in the USA[4,5]. Non-herbal dietary supplements such as vitamins, minerals, amino acids and hormones are beyond the scope of this review. Some of the non-herbal dietary supplements that surgical patients are most likely to take, such as glucosamine and chondroitin for osteoarthritis[6,7], appear to be safe. There is limited information, however, on the use of these supplements in the presurgical population.

In this chapter, we consider herbal medicine safety and USA regulatory issues; review the literature on eight commonly used herbal medications as they affect perioperative care; and propose rational strategies for managing the preoperative use of these agents. The prevention, recognition and treatment of complications begin with explicitly eliciting and documenting a history of herbal medicine use. Familiarity with the scientific literature on herbal medications is necessary because the current regulatory mechanism for commercial herbal preparations sold in the USA does not necessarily protect against unpredictable or undesirable effects. Our goal is to provide a framework for physicians practicing in the contemporary environment of widespread herbal medicine use.

PREOPERATIVE USE OF HERBAL MEDICATIONS

The most extensive surveys on the use of complementary and alternative medicines in the USA revealed that approximately 12% of the population used herbal medications in 1997[8,9]. This figure represented a 380% increase from 1990. Patients undergoing surgery appear to use herbal medications significantly more frequently than the general population. Tsen and co-workers[1] reported that 22% of patients who underwent evaluation in their preoperative clinic took herbal medications. Kaye and colleagues[2] found that 32% of patients admitted to their use in an ambulatory surgery setting.

Over 70% of these patients fail to disclose their herbal medicine use during routine preoperative assessment[2]. Explanations for this phenomenon include patient-held beliefs that physicians are unknowledgeable about herbal medications or prejudiced against their use[10]. Some patients may fear admitting reliance on unconventional therapies to their physicians[11]. Others may neglect to mention herbal medications when using them for reasons perceived as unrelated to their medical care[12]. Still others would not consider these substances to be medications and may neglect to report them during routine questioning. For these reasons, it is necessary for physicians specifically to seek out a history of herbal medicine use in pre-surgical patients.

REGULATION AND SAFETY OF HERBAL MEDICATIONS

Herbal medications were classified as dietary supplements in the Dietary Supplement Health and Education Act (DSHEA) of 1994[13]. This exempts them from the proof of safety and efficacy required of prescription and over-the-counter drugs. The burden is shifted to the Food and Drug Administration (FDA) to prove a product unsafe before it can be removed from the market[14]. Manufacturers are not required to conduct preclinical animal studies, premarketing controlled clinical trials, or postmarketing surveillance and the inability to patent herbal medications discourages them from performing this costly research[15].

The current regulatory mechanism provides little assurance that commercial preparations have predictable pharmacological effects and that product labels are accurate. The potency of herbal medications can vary from manufacturer to manufacturer and from lot to lot[16–18]. Plants may be misidentified or deliberately replaced with cheaper or more readily available alternatives[19–22]. Moreover, herbal medications, especially those of Eastern origin, can be adulterated with heavy metals, pesticides and even conventional drugs[23–25]. Some herbal manufacturers have tried to standardize products to fixed concentrations of selected chemical constituents[26]. The benefit of this effort is uncertain, however, because many products achieve their effects through the combined or synergistic actions of different compounds[27]. Even when they are advertised and labelled as standardized, potency can still vary considerably[28].

Because there is no mechanism for postmarketing surveillance, the incidence and exact nature of adverse events is unknown. Empirical evidence gained from a long history of use supports the notion that most herbal medications are safe[29]. Nevertheless, some have been associated with serious harm[30,31]. Over 5000 suspected herb-related adverse reactions were reported to the World Health Organization before 1996[32]. Between January 1993 and October 1998, 2621 adverse events, including 101 deaths, associated with dietary supplements were reported to the FDA[33]. Adverse events are underreported, however, because there is no central mechanism for mandatory reporting as there is for conventional medications. Other factors that contribute to underreporting are that physicians do not recognize adverse events[34] and that patients are reluctant to report and seek treatment for adverse reactions associated with herbal medications[35]. This reluctance has been attributed to the belief that physicians cannot be consulted in the use of unconventional therapies and to patients' unwillingness to admit use of these remedies to physicians. The deficiencies in monitoring adverse events mean that safety profiles are usually limited to animal studies, case reports, or predictions derived from known pharmacology.

COMMONLY USED HERBAL MEDICATIONS

Despite many uncertainties in commercial preparations, herbal medications adhere to the principles of modern pharmacology. A single herbal medication may adversely impact the perioperative period through a number of different mechanisms. These are direct effects (intrinsic pharmacological effects), pharmacodynamic interactions (alteration of the action of conventional drugs at effector sites) and pharmacokinetic interactions (alteration of the absorption, distribution, metabolism and elimination of conventional drugs).

Echinacea

Three species of echinacea, a member of the daisy family, are used for the prophylaxis and treatment of viral, bacterial and fungal infections, particularly those of upper respiratory origin[36]. Pharmacological activity cannot be attributed to a single compound, although the lipophilic fraction, which contains the alkylamides, polyacetylenes and essential oils, appears to be more active than the hydrophilic fraction.

Echinacea had a number of immunostimulatory effects in preclinical studies[37–39]. While there are no studies specifically addressing interactions between echinacea and immunosuppressive drugs, expert opinion generally warns against the concomitant use of echinacea and these drugs, owing to the probability of diminished effectiveness[37,40,41]. Therefore, patients who may require perioperative immunosuppression, such as those awaiting organ transplants, should be counselled to avoid echinacea. In contrast to the immunostimulatory effects with short-term use, long-term use of more than 8 weeks is accompanied by the potential for immunosuppression[41] and a theoretically increased risk of certain post-surgical complications such as poor wound healing and opportunistic infections.

Echinacea has also been associated with allergic reactions, including one reported case of anaphylaxis[42]. Therefore, echinacea should be used with caution in patients with asthma, atopy, or allergic rhinitis. Concerns of potential hepatoxicity have also been raised, although documented cases are lacking[17]. In the absence of definitive information, patients with pre-existing liver dysfunction should be cautious using echinacea. Furthermore, since the pharmacokinetics of echinacea have not been studied, it may be prudent to discontinue this herb as far in advance of surgery as possible when compromises in hepatic function or blood flow are anticipated. These situations often occur secondary to concomitant anesthetic drug administration or as an effect of surgical manipulation.

Ephedra

Ephedra, known as ma huang in Chinese medicine, is a shrub native to central Asia. It is used to promote weight loss, increase energy and treat respiratory conditions, such as asthma and bronchitis. Ephedra contains alkaloids including ephedrine, pseudoephedrine, norephedrine, methylephedrine and norpseudoephedrine[43]. Commercial preparations may be standardized to a fixed ephedrine content.

Ephedra causes dose-dependent increases in blood pressure and heart rate. Ephedrine, the predominant active compound, is a non-catecholamine sympathomimetic that exhibits α_1, β_1 and β_2 activity by acting directly at adrenergic receptors and indirectly by releasing endogenous norepinephrine (noradrenaline). These sympathomimetic effects have been associated with more than 1070 reported adverse events, including fatal cardiac and central nervous system complications[44].

Although ephedrine is widely used as first-line therapy for intraoperative hypotension and bradycardia, the unsupervised preoperative use of ephedra raises certain concerns. Vasoconstriction and, in some cases, vasospasm of coronary and cerebral arteries may cause myocardial infarction and thrombotic stroke[45]. Patients who have consumed ephedra and are later anesthetized with halothane may be at risk of developing intraoperative ventricular arrhythmias, because halothane sensitizes the myocardium to ventricular arrhythmias caused by exogenous catecholamines[46]. Ephedra may also affect cardiovascular function by causing hypersensitivity myocarditis, characterized by cardiomyopathy with myocardial lymphocyte and eosinophil infiltration[47]. Long-term use results in tachyphylaxis from depletion of endogenous catecholamine stores and may contribute to perioperative hemodynamic instability. In these situations, direct-acting sympathomimetics may be preferred as first-line therapy for intraoperative hypotension and bradycardia. Concomitant use of ephedra and monoamine oxidase inhibitors can result in life-threatening hyperpyrexia, hypertension and coma. Finally, heavy ephedra use has been documented as a very rare cause of radiolucent kidney stones[48,49].

The pharmacokinetics of ephedrine have been studied in humans[50,51]. Ephedrine has an elimination half-life of 5.2 h with 70–80% of the compound excreted unchanged in the urine. Based upon the pharmacokinetic data and the known cardiovascular risks of ephedra, including myocardial infarction, stroke and cardiovascular collapse from catecholamine depletion, this herb should be discontinued at least 24 h prior to surgery.

Garlic

Garlic is one of the most extensively researched medicinal plants. It has the potential to modify the risk of developing atherosclerosis by reducing blood pressure, thrombus formation and serum lipid and cholesterol levels[52]. These effects are primarily attributed to the sulfur-containing compounds, particularly allicin and its transformation products. Commercial garlic preparations may be standardized to a fixed alliin and allicin content.

Garlic inhibits platelet aggregation *in vivo* in a dose-dependent fashion. The effect of one of its constituents, ajoene, appears to be irreversible and may potentiate the effect of other platelet inhibitors such as prostacyclin, forskolin, indomethacin and dipyridamole[53,54]. Although these effects have not been consistently demonstrated in volunteers, there is one case in the literature of an octogenarian who developed a spontaneous epidural hematoma that was attributed to heavy garlic use[55]. In addition to bleeding concerns, garlic has the potential to lower blood pressure. Allicin decreased systemic and pulmonary vascular resistance[56] and lowered blood pressure in laboratory animals[57]. In humans, however, the antihypertensive effect of garlic is marginal[58].

Although there are insufficient pharmacokinetic data on garlic's constituents, the potential for irreversible inhibition of platelet function may warrant the discontinuation of garlic at least 7 days prior to surgery, especially if postoperative bleeding is a particular concern or other platelet inhibitors are given.

Ginkgo

Ginkgo is derived from the leaf of *Ginkgo biloba*. It has been used for cognitive disorders, peripheral vascular disease, age-related macular degeneration, vertigo, tinnitus, erectile dysfunction and altitude sickness. Studies have suggested that ginkgo may stabilize or improve cognitive performance in patients with Alzheimer's disease and multi-infarct dementia[59,60]. The compounds believed to be responsible for its pharmacological effects are the terpenoids and flavonoids. The two ginkgo extracts used in clinical trials are standardized to ginkgo-flavone glycosides and terpenoids.

Ginkgo appears to alter vasoregulation[61], act as an antioxidant[62], modulate neurotransmitter and receptor activity[63] and inhibit platelet-activating factor (PAF)[64]. Of these effects, the inhibition of PAF raises the greatest concern for the perioperative period, since platelet function may be altered. Clinical trials in a small number of patients have not demonstrated bleeding complications, but four reported cases of spontaneous intracranial bleeding[65–68], one case of spontaneous hyphema[69] and one case of postoperative bleeding following laparoscopic cholecystectomy[70] have been associated with ginkgo use.

Terpenoids are highly bioavailable when administered orally. Glucuronidation appears to be part of the metabolism of the flavonoids[71]. The elimination half-lives of the terpenoids after oral administration are between 3 and 10 h[72]. Based upon the pharmacokinetic data and the risk of bleeding, particularly in the surgical population, ginkgo should be discontinued at least 36 h prior to surgery.

Ginseng

Among the several species used for their pharmacological effects, Asian ginseng and American ginseng are the most commonly described. Ginseng has been labelled an 'adaptogen' since it reputedly protects the body against stress and restores homeostasis[73]. Most pharmacological actions are attributed to the ginsenosides that belong to a group of compounds known as steroidal saponins. Commercially available ginseng preparations may be standardized to ginsenoside content.

Ginseng has a broad but incompletely understood pharmacological profile because of the many heterogeneous and sometimes opposing effects of different ginsenosides[74]. The underlying mechanism appears to be similar to that classically described for steroid hormones. A potential therapeutic use for this herb has to do with its ability to lower postprandial blood glucose in both type 2 diabetics and non-diabetics[75], but this effect may create unintended hypoglycemia, particularly in patients who have fasted before surgery.

There is a concern about ginseng's effect on coagulation pathways. Ginsenosides inhibit platelet aggregation *in vitro*[76,77] and prolong both thrombin time and activated partial thromboplastin time in rats[78]. One early study suggested that the antiplatelet activity of panaxynol, a constituent of ginseng, may be irreversible in humans[79]. These findings await further confirmation. Although ginseng may inhibit the coagulation cascade, ginseng use was associated with a significant decrease in warfarin anticoagulation in one reported case[80].

The pharmacokinetics of ginsenosides Rg_1, Re and Rb_2 have been investigated in rabbits, with elimination halflives between 0.8 and 7.4 h[81]. These data suggest that ginseng should be discontinued at least 24 h prior to surgery. However, because ginseng platelet inhibition may be irreversible, it is probably prudent to discontinue ginseng use at least 7 days prior to surgery.

Kava

Kava is derived from the dried root of the pepper plant *Piper methysticum*. Kava has gained widespread popularity as an anxiolytic and sedative. Clinical trials suggest therapeutic potential in the symptomatic treatment of anxiety[82]. The kavalactones appear to be the source of kava's pharmacological activity[83].

Because of its psychomotor effects, kava was one of the first herbal medications expected to interact with anesthetics. The kavalactones have dose-dependent effects on the central nervous system including antiepileptic[84], neuroprotective[85] and local anesthetic properties[84]. Kava may act as a sedative/hypnotic by potentiating inhibitory neurotransmission of γ-aminobutyric acid (GABA). The kavalactones increase barbiturate sleep time in laboratory animals[86]. This effect may explain the mechanism underlying the report of a coma attributed to an alprazolam–kava interaction[87]. Although kava has abuse potential, whether long-term use can result in addiction, tolerance and acute withdrawal after abstinence has not been satisfactorily investigated. With heavy use, kava produces 'kava dermopathy', characterized by reversible scaly cutaneous eruptions[88].

Peak plasma levels occur 1.8 h after an oral dose and the elimination halflife of kavalactones is 9 h[83]. Unchanged kavalactones and their metabolites undergo renal and fecal elimination[89]. The pharmacokinetic data and possibility for the potentiation of the sedative effects of anesthetics suggest that this herbal medication should be discontinued at least 24 h prior to surgery.

St John's wort

St John's wort is the common name for *Hypericum perforatum*. A number of clinical trials have reported efficacy in the short-term treatment of mild-to-moderate depression[90]. However, a multicenter clinical trial recently concluded that St John's wort is not effective in the treatment of major depression[91]. The compounds believed to be responsible for pharmacological activity are hypericin and hyperforin[92]. Commercial preparations are often standardized to a fixed hypericin content of 0.3%.

St John's wort exerts its effects by inhibiting serotonin, norepinephrine and dopamine reuptake[93,94]. Concomitant use of this herb with or without serotonin reuptake inhibitors may create a syndrome of central serotonin excess[95,96]. Although early *in vitro* data implicated monoamine oxidase inhibition as a possible mechanism of action[97], a number of later investigations have demonstrated that monoamine oxidase inhibition is insignificant *in vivo*[98,99].

The use of St John's wort can significantly increase the metabolism of many concomitantly administered drugs, some of which are vital to the perioperative care of certain patients. There is induction of the cytochrome P450 3A4 isoform, approximately doubling its metabolic activity[100,101]. Interactions with substrates of the 3A4 isoform including indinavir sulfate[102], ethinylestradiol[103] and cyclosporin have been documented. In one series of 45 organ transplant patients, St John's wort was associated with an average decrease of 49% in blood cyclosporin levels[104]. Another group reported two cases of acute heart transplant rejection associated with this particular pharmacokinetic interaction[105]. Other P450 3A4 substrates commonly used in the perioperative period include alfentanyl, midazolam, lidocaine, calcium channel blockers and 5-hydroxytryptamine (HT)$_3$ receptor antagonists. In addition to the 3A4 isoform, the cytochrome P450 2C9 isoform may also be induced. The anticoagulant effect of warfarin, a substrate of the 2C9 isoform, was reduced in seven reported cases[103]. Other 2C9 substrates include the non-steroidal anti-inflammatory drugs. Furthermore, the enzyme induction caused by St John's wort may be more pronounced when other enzyme inducers, which could include other herbal medications, are taken concomitantly. St John's wort also affects digoxin pharmacokinetics[106].

The single-dose and steady-state pharmacokinetics of hypericin, pseudohypericin and hyperforin have been determined in humans[107,108]. After oral administration, peak plasma levels of hypericin and hyperforin are obtained in 6.0 and 3.5 h, and their median elimination halflives are 43.1 and 9.0 h, respectively. The long halflife and alterations in the metabolism of many drugs make concomitant use of St John's wort a particular risk in the perioperative setting. The pharmacokinetic data suggest that this herbal medication should be discontinued at least 5 days prior to surgery. This is especially important in patients waiting for organ transplantation or in those who may require oral anticoagulation postoperatively. Moreover, these patients should be counselled to avoid taking St John's wort postoperatively.

Valerian

Valerian is an herb native to the temperate areas of the Americas, Europe and Asia. It is used as a sedative, particularly in the treatment of insomnia and virtually all herbal sleep-aids contain valerian[109]. Valerian contains many compounds acting synergistically, but the sesquiterpenes are the primary source of valerian's pharmacological effects. Commercially available preparations may be standardized to valerenic acid.

Valerian produces dose-dependent sedation and hypnosis[110]. These effects appear to be mediated through modulation of GABA neurotransmission and receptor function[111,112]. Valerian increases barbiturate sleep time in experimental animals[113]. In one case, valerian withdrawal appeared to mimic an acute benzodiazepine withdrawal syndrome after the patient presented with delirium and cardiac complications following surgery and his symptoms were attenuated by benzodiazepine administration[114]. Based upon these findings, valerian should be expected to potentiate the sedative effects of anesthetics and adjuvants, such as midazolam, that act at the GABA receptor.

The pharmacokinetics of valerian's constituents have not been studied, although their effects are thought to be short-lived. Caution should be used with abrupt discontinuation in patients who may be physically dependent upon valerian, owing to the risk of benzodiazepine-like withdrawal. In these individuals, it may be prudent to taper this herbal medication with close medical supervision over the course of several weeks before surgery. If this is not feasible, physicians can advise patients to continue taking valerian up until the day of surgery. Based upon the mechanism of action and a reported case of efficacy[114], benzodiazepines can be used to treat withdrawal symptoms should they develop in the postoperative period.

MANAGING PREOPERATIVE USE OF HERBAL MEDICATIONS

Because most patients may not volunteer this information in the preoperative evaluation[2], physicians should specifically elicit and document a history of herbal medication use. Obtaining such a history may be difficult. Written questionnaires for information on herbal medication use have not proved to be beneficial in identifying patients taking these remedies, since half of the patients who use alternative therapies fail to report this information unless questioned in person[115]. An oral history, however, may also be inadequate. Unless this information is directly solicited, patients may not be forthcoming. Even when a positive history of herbal medication use is obtained, one in five patients is unable properly to identify the preparation they are taking[116]. Therefore, patients should be asked to bring their herbal medications and other dietary supplements with them at the time of the preoperative evaluation.

Table 1 Clinically important effects and perioperative concerns of eight herbs and recommendations for discontinuation before surgery

Herb and common name(s)	Important pharmacological effects	Perioperative concerns	Preoperative discontinuation
Echinacea (purple coneflower root)	activation of cell-mediated immunity	allergic reactions decreased effectiveness of immunosuppressants potential for immunosuppression with long-term use	no data
Ephedra (ma huang)	increased heart rate and blood pressure through direct and indirect sympathomimetic effects	risk of myocardial ischemia and stroke from tachycardia and hypertension ventricular arrhythmias with halothane long-term use depletes endogenous catecholamines and may cause intraoperative hemodynamic instability life-threatening interaction with MAO inhibitors	at least 24 h before surgery
Garlic (ajo)	inhibition of platelet aggregation (may be irreversible) increased fibrinolysis equivocal antihypertensive activity	potential to increase risk of bleeding, especially when combined with other medications that inhibit platelet aggregation	at least 7 days before surgery
Ginkgo (duck foot tree, maidenhair tree, silver apricot)	inhibition of platelet-activating factor	potential to increase risk of bleeding, especially when combined with other medications that inhibit platelet aggregation	at least 36 hours before surgery
Ginseng (American ginseng, Asian ginseng, Chinese ginseng, Korean ginseng)	lowers blood glucose inhibition of platelet aggregation (may be irreversible) increased PT/PTT in animals many other diverse effects	hypoglycemia potential to increase risk of bleeding potential to decrease anticoagulant effect of warfarin	at least 7 days before surgery
Kava (awa, intoxicating pepper, kawa)	sedation anxiolysis	potential to increase sedative effect of anesthetics ability to increase anesthetic requirements with long-term use unstudied	at least 24 h before surgery
St John's wort (amber, goat weed, hardhay, hypericum, klamathweed)	inhibition of neurotransmitter reuptake MAO inhibition is unlikely	induction of cytochrome P450 enzymes, affecting cyclosporin, warfarin, steroids, protease inhibitors and possibly benzodiazepines, calcium channel blockers and many other drugs decreased serum digoxin levels	at least 5 days before surgery
Valerian (all heal, garden heliotrope, vandal root)	sedation	potential to increase sedative effect of anesthetics benzodiazepine-like acute withdrawal potential to increase anesthetic requirements with long-term use	no data

PT, prothrombin time; PTT, partial thromboplastin time; MAO, monoamine oxidase

Patients who use herbal medications may be more likely than those who do not to avoid conventional diagnosis and therapy[117]. Hence, a history of herbal medicine use should prompt physicians to suspect the presence of undiagnosed disorders causing symptoms that may lead to self-medication. These recommendations also apply to pediatric patients, because caretakers may treat children with herbal medications without medical supervision[118]. One in six parents reported giving dietary supplements to their children[10].

Although the American Society of Anesthesiologists has no official standards or guidelines on the preoperative use of herbal medications, public and professional educational information released by this organization suggest that they be discontinued at least 2–3 weeks before surgery[119,120]. Our review of the literature favors a more targeted approach. Pharmacokinetic data on selected active constituents indicate that some herbal medications are eliminated quickly and may be discontinued closer to the time of surgery. This may be necessary, since evaluating patients 2–3 weeks before elective surgery may be impossible in

practice. Moreover, some patients require non-elective surgery or are non-compliant with instructions to discontinue herbal medications preoperatively. These factors and the high frequency of herbal medicine use may mean that many patients will take herbal medications until the time of surgery. Therefore, clinicians should be familiar with commonly used herbal medications in order to recognize and treat complications that may arise. Table 1 summarizes the clinically important effects, perioperative concerns and recommendations for discontinuation before surgery of the eight herbal medications discussed in this chapter.

Clinicians should also recognize that presurgical discontinuation of all herbal medications may not free a patient from risk. Withdrawal of regular medications is associated with increased morbidity and mortality after surgery[121]. In alcoholics, preoperative abstinence may result in poorer postoperative outcome than continued preoperative drinking[122]. The danger of abstinence after long-term use may be similar with herbal medications, such as valerian, which have the

Table 2 Herbal medicine and other dietary supplement-related sites on the World Wide Web

Center for Food Safety and Applied Nutrition, Food and Drug Administration
http://vm.cfsan.fda.gov/~dms/supplmnt.html
Clinicians should use this site to report adverse events associated with herbal medicines and other dietary supplements. Sections also contain safety, industry and regulatory information.

National Center for Complementary and Alternative Medicine, National Institutes of Health
http://nccam.nih.gov
This site contains fact sheets about alternative therapies, consensus reports and databases.

Agricultural Research Service, United States Department of Agriculture
www.ars-grin.gov/duke
This site contains an extensive phytochemical database with search capabilities.

Quackwatch
www.quackwatch.com
Although this site addresses all aspects of health care, there is a considerable amount of information covering complementary and herbal therapies.

National Council Against Health Fraud
www.ncahf.org
This site focuses on health fraud with a position paper on over-the-counter herbal remedies.

HerbMed
www.herbmed.org
This site contains information on over 120 herbal medications, with evidence for activity, warnings, preparations, mixtures and mechanisms of action. There are short summaries of important research publications with Medline links.

ComsumerLab
www.consumerlab.com
This site is maintained by a corporation that conducts independent laboratory investigations of dietary supplements and other health products.

potential for producing acute withdrawal after long-term use.

Because this field is rapidly evolving, sources for reliable and updated information are important in helping physicians stay abreast of new discoveries about the effects of herbal medications and other dietary supplements. Several resources that are available on the World Wide Web as clinical aides are listed in Table 2.

SUMMARY

The task of caring perioperatively for patients who use herbal medications is an evolving challenge. The limited evidence-based information about the safety and efficacy of herbal medications, the absence of a standard regulatory mechanism for herbal medicine approval and surveillance, and improper patient assumptions about herbal medications represent important medical issues. Although there has been initiation of herbal medicine into medical school curricula at several institutions including ours, many practicing physicians remain unaware of potential perioperative interactions. Physicians should be familiar with all medications, whether conventional or herbal, that their patients are taking. This information is necessary to prevent, recognize and treat potentially serious problems associated with herbal medications, whether these are taken alone or in conjunction with conventional medications.

References

1. Tsen LC, Segal S, Pothier M, Bader AM. Alternative medicine use in presurgical patients. *Anesthesiology* 2000;93:148–51
2. Kaye AD, Clarke RC, Sabar R, *et al.* Herbal medications: current trends in anesthesiology practice – a hospital survey. *J Clin Anesth* 2000;12:468–71
3. Bovill JG. Adverse drug interactions in anesthesia. *J Clin Anesth* 1997;9:3S–13S
4. Anon. NBJ herbal and botanical U.S. consumer sales. *Nutrition Business Journal.* San Diego, CA: Nutrition Business International, 2000
5. Commission on Dietary Supplement Labels. *Report of the Commission on Dietary Supplement Labels, Report to the President, Congress and The Secretary of the Department of Health and Human Services.* Washington, DC: US Government Printing Office, 1997
6. McAlindon TE, La Valley MP, Gulin JP, Felson DT. Glucosamine and chondroitin for treatment of osteoarthritis. *J Am Med Assoc* 2000;283:1469–75
7. Reginster JY, Deroisy R, Rovati LC, *et al.* Long–term effects of glucosamine sulphate on osteoarthritis progression: a randomized, placebo-controlled clinical trial. *Lancet* 2001;357:251–6
8. Eisenberg DM, Davis RB, Ettner SL, *et al.* Trends in alternative medicine use in the United States, 1990–1997: results of a follow-up study. *J Am Med Assoc* 1998;280:1569–75
9. Eisenberg DM, Kessler RC, Foster C, Norlock FE, Calkins DR, Delbanco TL. Unconventional medicine in the United States. Prevalence, costs and patterns of use. *N Engl J Med* 1993;328: 246–52
10. Blendon RJ, DesRoches CM, Benson JM, Brodie M, Altman DE. American's views on the use and regulation of dietary supplements. *Arch Intern Med* 2001;161:805–10
11. Eisenberg DM. Advising patients who seek alternative medical therapies. *Ann Intern Med* 1997;127:61–9
12. Elder NC, Gillcrist A, Minz R. Use of alternative health care by family practice patients. *Arch Fam Med* 1997;6:181–4
13. 103rd Congress. *Dietary Supplement Health and Education Act of 1994.* Pub. Law 103–417. 108 Stat. 4325. 1994
14. Marwick C. Growing use of medicinal botanicals forces assessment by drug regulators. *J Am Med Assoc* 1995;273:607–9
15. Matthews HB, Lucier GW, Fisher KD. Medicinal herbs in the United States: research needs. *Environ Health Perspect* 1999;107:773–8
16. Winslow LC, Kroll DJ. Herbs as medicines. *Arch Intern Med* 1998;158:2192–9
17. Miller LG. Herbal medicinals: selected clinical considerations focusing on known or potential drug–herb interactions. *Arch Intern Med* 1998;158:2200–11
18. Anon. Herbal roulette. *Consumer Reports*, November 1995:698–705
19. Ernst E. Harmless herbs? A review of the recent literature. *Am J Med* 1998;104:170–8
20. Slifman NR, Obermeyer WR, Aloi BK, *et al.* Contamination of botanical dietary supplements by *Digitalis lanata*. *N Engl J Med* 1998;339:806–11
21. Kessler DA. Cancer and herbs. *N Engl J Med* 2000;342:1742–3
22. Nortier JL, Martinez MC, Schmeiser HH, *et al.* Urothelial carcinoma associated with the use of a Chinese herb (*Aristolochia fangchi*). *N Engl J Med* 2000;342:1686–92
23. Ko RJ. Adulterants in Asian patent medicines. *N Engl J Med* 1998;339:847
24. Vander Stricht BI, Parvais OE, Vanhaelen-Fastre RJ, Vanhaelen MH, Quertinier D. Safer use of traditional remedies. Remedies may contain cocktail of active drugs. *Br Med J* 1994;308:1162
25. Espinoza EO, Bleasdell B. Arsenic and mercury in traditional Chinese herbal balls. *N Engl J Med* 1995;333:803–4
26. Thompson CA. Herbal quality seems to be growing. *Am J Health Syst Pharm* 1998;55:2341–2

27. Wagner H. Phytomedicine research in Germany. *Enivron Health Perspect* 1999;107:779–81

28. Monmaney T. Label's potency claims often inaccurate, analysis finds. *Los Angeles Times*, August 31, 1998:A10

29. Abbot NC, White AR, Ernst E. Complementary medicine. *Nature (London)* 1996;381:361

30. Windrum P, Hull DR, Morris TCM. Herb–drug interactions. *Lancet* 2000;355:1019–20

31. Fugh-Berman A. Herb–drug interactions. *Lancet* 2000;355:134–8

32. Edwards R. Monitoring the safety of herbal medicine. WHO project is under way. *Br Med J* 1995;311:1569–70

33. Anon. Herbal Rx – the promises and pitfalls. *Consumer Reports*, March 1999:44–8

34. Perharic L, Shaw D, Murray V. Toxic effects of herbal medications and food supplements. *Lancet* 1993;342:180–1

35. Barnes J, Mills SY, Abbot NC, Willoughby M, Ernst E. Different standards for reporting ADRs to herbal remedies and conventional OTC medicines: face-to-face interviews with 515 users of herbal remedies. *Br J Clin Pharmacol* 1998;45:496–500

36. Melchart D, Linde K, Fischer P, Kaesmayr J. Echinacea for preventing and treating the common cold. *Cochrane Database Syst Rev* 2000;2:CD000530

37. Pepping J. Echinacea. *Am J Health Syst Pharm* 1999;56:121–2

38. See DM, Broumand N, Sahl L, Tilles JG. *In vitro* effects of echinacea and ginseng on natural killer and antibody-dependent cell cytotoxicity in healthy subjects and chronic fatigue syndrome or acquired immunodeficiency syndrome patients. *Immunopharmacology* 1997;35:229–35

39. Rehman J, Dillow JM, Carter SM, Chou J, Le B, Maisel AS. Increased production of antigen-specific immunoglobulins G and M following *in vivo* treatment with the medicinal plants *Echinacea angustifolia* and *Hydrastis canadensis*. *Immunol Lett* 1999;68:391–5

40. Anon. Echinacea. In Gruenwald J, Brendler T, Jaenicke C, eds. *PDR for Herbal Medicines*, 2nd edn. Montvale, NJ: Medical Economics Company, 2000:261–6

41. Boullata JI, Nace AM. Safety issues with herbal medicine. *Pharmacotherapy* 2000;20:257–69

42. Mullins RJ. Echinacea-associated anaphylaxis. *Med J Aust* 1998;168:170–1

43. Gurley BJ, Gardner SF, Hubbard MA. Content versus label claims in ephedra-containing dietary supplements. *Am J Health Syst Pharm* 2000;57:963–9

44. Nightingale SL. From the Food and Drug Administration. *J Am Med Assoc* 1997;278:15

45. Haller CA, Benowitz NL. Adverse cardiovascular and central nervous system events associated with dietary supplements containing ephedra alkaloids. *N Engl J Med* 2000;343:1833–8

46. Roizen MF. Anesthetic implications of concurrent diseases. In Miller RD, ed. *Anesthesia*, 4th edn. New York, NY: Churchill Livingstone. 1994:903–1014

47. Zaacks SM, Klein L, Tan CD, Rodriguez ER, Leikin JB. Hypersensitivity myocarditis associated with ephedra use. *J Toxicol Clin Toxicol* 1999;37:485–9

48. Blau JJ. Ephedrine nephrolithiasis associated with chronic ephedrine abuse. *J Urol* 1998;160:825

49. Powell T, Hsu FF, Turk J, Hruska K. Ma-huang strikes again: ephedrine nephrolithiasis. *Am J Kidney Dis* 1998;32:153–9

50. White LM, Gardner SF, Gurley BJ, Marx MA, Wang PL, Estes M. Pharmacokinetics and cardiovascular effects of ma-huang (*Ephedra sinica*) in normotensive adults. *J Clin Pharmacol* 1997;37:116–22

51. Gurley BJ, Gardner SF, White LM, Wang PL. Ephedrine pharmacokinetics after the ingestion of nutritional supplements containing *Ephedra sinica* (ma huang). *Ther Drug Monit* 1998;20:439–45

52. Stevinson C, Pittler MH, Ernst E. Garlic for treating hypercholesterolemia: a meta-analysis of randomized clinical trials. *Ann Intern Med* 2000;133:420–9

53. Srivastava KC. Evidence for the mechanism by which garlic inhibits platelet aggregation. *Prostaglandins Leukot Med* 1986;22:313–21

54. Apitz-Castro R, Escalante J, Vargas R, Jain MK. Ajoene, the antiplatelet principle of garlic, synergistically potentiates the antiaggregatory action of prostacyclin, forskolin, indomethacin and dipyridamole on human platelets. *Thromb Res* 1986;42:303–11

55. Rose KD, Croissant PD, Parliament CF, Levin MB. Spontaneous spinal epidural hematoma with associated platelet dysfunction from excessive garlic ingestion: a case report. *Neurosurgery* 1990;26:880–2

56. Kaye AD, De Witt BJ, Anwar M, et al. Analysis of responses of garlic derivatives in the pulmonary valscular bed of the rat. *J Appl Physiol* 2000;89:353–8

57. Ali M, Al-Qattan KK, Al-Enezi F, Khanafer RM, Mustafa T. Effect of allicin from garlic powder on serum lipids and blood pressure in rats fed with a high cholesterol diet. *Prostaglandins Leukot Essent Fatty Acids* 2000;62:253–9

58. Silagy CA, Neil HA. A meta-analysis of the effect of garlic on blood pressure. *J Hypertens* 1994;12:463–8

59. Le Bars PL, Katz MM, Berman N, Itil TM, Freedman AM, Schatzberg AF. A placebo-controlled, double-blind, randomized trial of an extract of *Ginkgo biloba* for dementia. North American Egb Study Group. *J Am Med Assoc* 1997;278:1327–32

60. Oken BS, Storzbach DM, Kaye JA. The efficacy of *Ginkgo biloba* on cognitive function in Alzheimer disease. *Arch Neurol* 1998;55:1409–15

61. Jung F, Mrowietz C, Kiesewetter H, Wenzel E. Effect of *Ginkgo biloba* on fluidity of blood and peripheral microcirculation in volunteers. *Arzneimittelforschung* 1990;40:589–93

62. Maitra I, Marcocci L, Droy-Lefaix MT, Packer L. Peroxyl radical scavenging activity of *Ginkgo biloba* extract EGb 761. *Biochem Pharmacol* 1995;49:1649–55

63. Hoyer S, Lannert H, Noldner M, Chatterjee SS. Damaged neuronal energy metabolism and behavior are improved by *Ginkgo biloba* extract (EGb 761). *J Neural Transm* 1999;106:1171–88

64. Chung KF, Dent G, McCusker M, Guinot P, Page CP, Barnes PJ. Effect of a ginkgolide mixture (BN 52063) in antagonizing skin and platelet responses to platelet activating factor in man. *Lancet* 1987;1:248–51

65. Rowin J, Lewis SL. Spontaneous bilateral subdural hematomas associated with chronic *Ginkgo biloba* ingestion. *Neurology* 1996;46:1775–6

66. Vale S. Subarachnoid haemorrhage associated with *Ginkgo biloba*. *Lancet* 1998;352:36

67. Gilbert GJ. *Ginkgo biloba*. *Neurology* 1997;48:1137

68. Matthews MK Jr. Association of *Ginkgo biloba* with intracerebral hemorrhage. *Neurology* 1998;50:1933–4

69. Rosenblatt M, Mindel J. Spontaneous hyphema associated with ingestion of *Ginkgo biloba* extract. *N Engl J Med* 1997;336:1108

70. Fessenden JM, Wittenborn W, Clarke L. *Gingko biloba*: a case report of herbal medicine and bleeding postoperatively from a laparoscopic cholecystectomy. *Am Surg* 2001;67:33–5

71. Watson DG, Oliveira EJ. Solid-phase extraction and gas chromatography–mass spectrometry determination of kaempferol and

quercetin in human urine after consumption of *Ginkgo biloba* tablets. *J Chromatogr B Biomed Sci Appl* 1999;723:203–10

72. Anon. Ginkgo. In Mills S, Bone K, eds. *Principles and Practice of Phytotherapy*. New York, NY: Churchill Livingstone, 2000:404–17

73. Brekham II, Dardymov IV. New substances of plant origin which increase nonspecific resistance. *Annu Rev Pharmacol* 1969;9:419–30

74. Attele AS, Wu JA, Yuan CS. Ginseng pharmacology: multiple constituents and multiple actions. *Biochem Pharmacol* 1999;58:1685–93

75. Vuksan V, Sievenpiper JL, Koo VY, *et al.* American ginseng (*Panax quinquefolius* L) reduces postprandial glycemia in nondiabetic subjects and subjects with type 2 diabetes mellitus. *Arch Intern Med* 2000;160:1009–13

76. Kimura Y, Okuda H, Arichi S. Effects of various ginseng saponins on 5-hydroxytryptamine release and aggregation in human platelets. *J Pharm Pharmacol* 1988;40:838–43

77. Kuo SC, Teng CM, Lee JC, Ko FN, Chen SC, Wu TS. Antiplatelet components in *Panax ginseng*. *Planta Med* 1990;56:164–7

78. Park HJ, Lee JH, Song YB, Park KH. Effects of dietary supplementation of lipophilic fraction from *Panax ginseng* on cGMP and cAMP in rat platelets and on blood coagulation. *Biol Pharm Bull* 1996;19:1434–9

79. Teng CM, Kuo SC, Ko FN, *et al.* Antiplatelet actions of panaxynol and ginsenosides isolated from ginseng. *Biochim Biophys Acta* 1989;990:315–20

80. Janetzky K, Morreale AP. Probable interaction between warfarin and ginseng. *Am J Health Syst Pharm* 1997;54:692–3

81. Chen SE, Sawchuk RJ, Staba EJ. American ginseng. III. Pharmacokinetics of ginsenosides in the rabbit. *Eur J Drug Metab Pharmacokinet* 1980;5:161–8

82. Pittler MH, Ernst E. Efficacy of kava extract for treating anxiety: systematic review and meta-analysis. *J Clin Psychopharmacol* 2000;20:84–9

83. Pepping J. Kava: *Piper methysticum*. *Am J Health Syst Pharm* 1999;56:957–60

84. Meyer HJ. Pharmacology of kava – 1. *Psychopharmacol Bull* 1967;4:10–11

85. Backhauss C, Krieglstein J. Extract of kava (*Piper methysticum*) and its methysticin constituents protect brain tissue against ischemic damage in rodents. *Eur J Pharmacol* 1992;215:265–9

86. Jamieson DD, Duffield PH, Cheng D, Duffield AM. Comparison of the central nervous system activity of the aqueous and lipid extract of kava (*Piper methysticum*). *Arch Int Pharmacodyn Ther* 1989;301:66–80

87. Almeida JC, Grimsley EW. Coma from the health food store: interaction between kava and alprazolam. *Ann Intern Med* 1996;125:940–1

88. Norton SA, Ruze P. Kava dermopathy. *J Am Acad Dermatol* 1994;31:89–97

89. Rasmussen AK, Scheline RR, Solheim E, Hansel R. Metabolism of some kava pyrones in the rat. *Xenobiotica* 1979;9:1–16

90. Gaster B, Holroyd J. St. John's wort for depression: a systematic review. *Arch Intern Med* 2000;160:152–6

91. Shelton RC, Keller MB, Gelenberg A, *et al.* Effectiveness of St. John's wort in major depression. *J Am Med Assoc* 2001;285:1978–86

92. Muller WE, Singer A, Wonnemann M, Hafner U, Rolli M, Schafer C. Hyperforin represents the neurotransmitter reuptake inhibiting constituent of hypericum extract. *Pharmacopsychiatry* 1998;31 (Suppl 1):16–21

93. Neary JT, Bu Y. Hypericum LI 160 inhibits uptake of serotonin and norepinephrine in astrocytes. *Brain Res* 1999;816:358–63

94. Franklin M, Chi J, McGavin C, *et al.* Neuroendocrine evidence for dopaminergic actions of hypericum extract (LI 160) in healthy volunteers. *Biol Psychiatry* 1999;46:581–4

95. Lantz MS, Buchalter E, Giambanco V. St. John's wort and antidepressant drug interactions in the elderly. *J Geriatr Psychiatry Neurol* 1999;12:7–10

96. Brown TM. Acute St. John's wort toxicity. *Am J Emerg Med* 2000;18:231–2

97. Suzuki O, Katsumata Y, Oya M, Bladt S, Wagner H. Inhibition of monoamine oxidase by hypericin. *Planta Med* 1984;50:272–4

98. Yu PH. Effect of the *Hypericum perforatum* extract on serotonin turnover in the mouse brain. *Pharmacopsychiatry* 2000;33:60–5

99. Muller WE, Rolli M, Schafer C, Hafner U. Effects of hypericum extract (LI 160) in biochemical models of antidepressant activity. *Pharmacopsychiatry* 1997;30(Suppl 2):102–7

100. Obach RS. Inhibition of human cytochrome P450 enzymes by constituents of St. John's wort, an herbal preparation used in the treatment of depression. *J Pharmacol Exp Ther* 2000;294:88–95

101. Ernst E. Second thoughts about safety of St. John's wort. *Lancet* 1999;354:2014–16

102. Piscitelli SC, Burstein AH, Chaitt D, Alfaro RM, Falloon J. Indinavir concentrations and St. John's wort. *Lancet* 2000;355: 547–8

103. Yue QY, Bergquist C, Gerden B. Safety of St. John's wort. *Lancet* 2000;355:576–7

104. Breidenbach T, Hoffmann MW, Becker T, Schlitt H, Klempnauer J. Drug interaction of St. John's wort with cyclosporin. *Lancet* 2000;355:1912

105. Ruschitzka F, Meier PJ, Turina M, Luscher TF, Noll G. Acute heart transplant rejection due to Saint John's wort. *Lancet* 2000;355:548–9

106. Johne A, Brockmoller J, Bauer S, Maurer A, Langheinrich M, Roots I. Pharmacokinetic interaction of digoxin with an herbal extract from St. John's wort (*Hypericum perforatum*). *Clin Pharmacol Ther* 1999;66:338–45

107. Kerb R, Brockmoller J, Staffeldt B, Ploch M, Roots I. Single-dose and steady-state pharmacokinetics of hypericin and pseudohypericin. *Antimicrob Agents Chemother* 1996;40:2087–93

108. Biber A, Fischer H, Romer A, Chatterjee SS. Oral bioavailability of hyperforin from hypericum extracts in rats and human volunteers. *Pharmacopsychiatry* 1998;31(Suppl 1):36–43

109. Houghton PJ. The scientific basis for the reputed activity of valerian. *J Pharm Pharmacol* 1999;51:505–12

110. Hendriks H, Bos R, Allersma DP, Malingre TM, Koster AS. Pharmacological screening of valerenal and some other components of essential oil of *Valeriana officinalis*. *Planta Med* 1981;42:62–8

111. Ortiz JG, Nieves-Natal J, Chavez P. Effects of *Valeriana officinalis* extracts on [3H]flunitrazepam binding, synaptosomal [3H]GABA uptake and hippocampal [3H]GABA release. *Neurochem Res* 1999;24:1373–8

112. Santos MS, Ferreira F, Cunha AP, Carvalho AP, Ribeiro CF, Macedo T. Synaptosomal GABA release as influenced by valerian root extract – involvement of the GABA carrier. *Arch Int Pharmacodyn Ther* 1994;327:220–31

113. Leuschner J, Muller J, Rudmann M. Characterization of the central nervous depressant activity of a commercially available valerian root extract. *Arzneimittelforschung* 1993;43:638–41

114. Garges HP, Varia I, Doraiswamy PM. Cardiac complications and delirium associated with valerian root withdrawal. *J Am Med Assoc* 1998;280:1566–7

115. Hensrud DD, Engle DD, Scheitel SM. Underreporting the use of dietary supplements and nonprescription medications among patients undergoing a periodic health examination. *Mayo Clin Proc* 1999;74:443–7

116. Kassler WJ, Blanc P, Greenblatt R. The use of medicinal herbs by human immunodeficiency virus-infected patients. *Arch Intern Med* 1991;151:2281–8

117. Cirigliano M, Sun A. Advising patients about herbal therapies. *J Am Med Assoc* 1998;280:1565–6

118. Coppes MJ, Anderson RA, Egeler RM, Wolff JEA. Alternative therapies for the treatment of childhood cancer. *N Engl J Med* 1998;339:846–7

119. Leak JA. Herbal medicines: what do we need to know? *ASA Newslett* 2000;64:6–7

120. Anesthesiologists warn: if you're taking herbal products, tell your doctor before surgery. Available at: http://www.asahq.org/PublicEduction/herbal.html. (Accessed 10 May 2001)

121. Kennedy JM, van Rij AM, Spears GF, Pettigrew RA, Tucker IG. Polypharmacy in a general surgical unit and consequences of drug withdrawal. *Br J Clin Pharmacol* 2000;49:353–62

122. Tonnesen H, Rosenberg J, Nielsen HJ, *et al*. Effect of preoperative abstinence on poor postoperative outcome in alcohol misusers: randomized controlled trial. *Br Med J* 1999;318:1311–16

Index